Recent Results in Cancer Research 64

Fortschritte der Krebsforschung
Progrès dans les recherches sur le cancer

Lymphoid Neoplasias I

Classification Categorization Natural History

Edited by
G. Mathé M. Seligmann M. Tubiana

With 167 Figures and 88 Tables

Springer-Verlag
Berlin Heidelberg New York 1978

CNRS International Colloquium.
Held in Paris on June 22–24, 1977

Professor GEORGES MATHÉ
Institut de Cancérologie et d'Immunogénétique
Hôpital Paul-Brousse, 14–16, Avenue Paul-Vaillant-Couturier
F-94800 Villejuif

Professor MAXIME SELIGMANN
Laboratory of Immunochemistry and Immunopathology
INSERM (U 108), and Laboratory of Cytology
Research Institute on Blood Diseases, Hôpital Saint-Louis
2, Place du Docteur-A. Fournier, F-75010 Paris

Dr. MAURICE TUBIANA
Department of Radiations, Institut Gustave-Roussy
16bis, Avenue Paul-Vaillant-Couturier, F-94800 Villejuif

Sponsored by the Swiss League against Cancer

ISBN-13: 978-3-642-81248-4 e-ISBN-13: 978-3-642-81246-0
DOI: 10.1007/ 978-3-642-81246-0

Library of Congress Cataloging in Publication Data. Main entry under title: Lymphoid neoplasias. (Recent results in cancer research; 64–65) Papers presented at a CNRS international colloquium, held in Paris, June 22–24, 1977, sponsored by the Swiss League against Cancer. Bibliography: p. Includes index. CONTENTS: 1. Classification, categorization, natural history.—2. Clinical and therapeutic aspects. 1. Lymphoma—Congresses. I. Mathé, Georges, 1922– II. Seligmann, Maxime, 1927– III. Tubiana, Maurice, 1920– IV. France. Centre national de la recherche scientifique. V. Schweizerische Nationalliga für Krebsbekämpfung und Krebsforschung. VI. Series. RC261.R35 vol. 64–65, etc. [RC280.L9] 616.9′94′008s [616.9′94′46] 78–19077

Softcover reprint of the hardcover 1st edition 1978

Typeset by CCC at William Clowes & Sons Limited, London and Beccles

87 Würzburg, Germany
2125/3140-543210

Contents

Part I: Current Morphologic Categorizations

Part II: Membrane Markers and Immunologic Categorization

Part III: Natural History of Lymphoid Neoplasias: Human and Experimental Models

List of Contributors

V. A. Bedoya, Labor für Immunopathologie, Pathologisches Institut der Universität Köln, Lindenburg, D-5000 Köln 41 (visiting Humboldt Foundation Professor from the University of Antioquia Medical School, Medellin, DC/USA)

D. Belpomme, Institut de Cancérologie et d'Immunogénétique, Hôpital Paul-Brousse, and Institut Gustave-Roussy, 14–16, Avenue Paul-Vaillant-Couturier, F-94800 Villejuif

M. H. Bennett, Department of Histiopathology, Mount Vernon Hospital, Northwood, Middlesex/U.K.

C. W. Berard, Hematopathology Section, Laboratory of Pathology, National Cancer Institute, National Institutes of Health, Bethesda, MD 20014/USA

I. Botto, Institut de Cancérologie et d'Immunogénétique, Hôpital Paul-Brousse, 14–16, Avenue Paul-Vaillant-Couturier, F-94800 Villejuif

H. Bouman, Institut für Biochemie der Universität Kiel, Olshausenstraße, D-2300 Kiel

R. C. Braylan, Department of Pathology, University of Florida College of Medicine P.O. Box 7275 JHMHG, Gainesville, FL 32610/USA

J. Breton-Gorius, Unité de Recherches sur les Anémies, INSERM (U 91), Hôpital Henri-Mondor, F-94010 Créteil

J. C. Brouet, Laboratory of Immunochemistry and Immunopathology, INSERM (U 108), Research Institute on Blood Diseases, Hôpital Saint-Louis, 2, Place du Docteur-A. Fournier, F-75010 Paris

B. Caillou, Institut Gustave-Roussy, 16bis, Avenue Paul-Vaillant-Couturier, F-94800 Villejuif

D. Catovsky, M. R. C. Leukaemia Unit, Royal Postgraduate Medical School, Du Cane Road, London W12 0HS/U.K.

M. Cherchi, M. R. C. Leukaemia Unit, Royal Postgraduate Medical School, Du Cane Road, London W12 0HS/U.K.

J. A. Child, Department of Haematology, The General Infirmary, Leeds LS1 3EX, Yorkshire/U.K.

M. Cibull, Department of Pathology, Stanford University Medical Center, Stanford, CA 94305/USA

E. H. COOPER, Department of Experimental Pathology and Cancer Research, University of Leeds, Leeds, Yorkshire/U.K.

F. DANON, Laboratory of Immunochemistry and Immunopathology, INSERM (U 108), Hôpital Saint-Louis, 2, Place du Docteur-A. Fournier, F-75010 Paris

D. DANTCHEV, Institut de Cancérologie et d'Immunogénétique, Hôpital Paul-Brousse, 14–16, Avenue Paul-Vaillant-Couturier, F-94800 Villejuif

A. J. S. DAVIES, Institute of Cancer Research, Chester Beatty Research Institute, London SW3 6JB/U.K.

L. DENARD, Address not communicated

J. DIEBOLD, Service Central "Jacques-Delarue" d'Anatomie et de Cytologie Pathologiques Hôpital Hôtel-Dieu, 1, Place du Parvis Notre-Dame, F-75181 Paris Cédex 4

R. F. DORFMAN, Department of Pathology, Stanford University Medical Center, Stanford, CA 94305/USA

B. DREYFUS, Unité de Recherches sur les Anémies, INSERM (U 91), Hôpital Henri-Mondor, F-94010 Créteil

A. L. EPSTEIN, Cancer Biology Research Laboratory, Department of Radiology, Stanford University School of Medicine, Stanford, CA 94305/USA

J. P. FARCET, Unité de Recherches sur les Anémies, INSERM (U 91), Hôpital Henri-Mondor, F-94010 Créteil

G. FARRER-BROWN, Fitzroy Nuffield Hospital, 10–12 Bryanston Square, London, W1H 8BB/U.K.

H. FELIX, Abteilung für Krebsforschung, Institut für Pathologie, Universität Zürich, Birchstraße 95, CH-8050 Zürich

G. FLANDRIN, Laboratoire de Cytologie, Institut de Recherches sur les Leucémies et les maladies du Sang, Hôpital Saint-Louis, 2, Place du Docteur-A. Fournier, F-75475 Paris Cédex 10

J. FUCHS, Abteilung für Allgemeine Pathologie und Pathologische Anatomie der Universität Kiel, Hospitalstraße 42, D-2300 Kiel

A. GALIAN, Department of Pathology, Hôpital Lariboisière, 2, Rue Ambroise Paré, F-75010 Paris

R. GERARD-MARCHANT, Institut Gustave-Roussy, 16bis, Avenue Paul-Vaillant-Couturier, F-94800 Villejuif

E. GLEICHMANN, Department of Immunohistopathology, Central Laboratory of the Netherlands Red Cross Blood Transfusion Service, and Laboratory of Experimental and Clinical Immunology, University of Amsterdam, P.O. Box 9190, Amsterdam, The Netherlands

H. GLEICHMANN, Institut für Pathologie der Medizinischen Hochschule Hannover, D-3000 Hannover 61

M. F. GOURDIN, Unité de Recherches sur les Anémies, INSERM (U 91), Hôpital Henri-Mondor, F-94010 Créteil

M. HADAM, Institut für Immunologie der Universität München, Schillerstraße 42, D-8000 München 2

G. HAEMMERLI, Abteilung für Krebsforschung, Institut für Pathologie, Universität Zürich, Birchstraße 95, CH-8050 Zürich

K. HENRY, Department of Histopathology, Westminster Medical School, London SW1P 2PP/U.K.

H. W. v. HEYDEN, Abteilung Innere Medizin II, Medizinische Universitätsklinik, D-7400 Tübingen

S. ILLINGWORTH, Department of Experimental Pathology and Cancer Research, University of Leeds, Leeds, Yorkshire/U.K.

E. S. JAFFE, Hematopathology Section, Laboratory of Pathology, National Cancer Institute, National Institutes of Health, Bethesda, MD 20014/USA

F. JAUBERT, Groupe de Pathologie Pédiatrique, INSERM (U 77), 149, Rue de Sévres, F-75730 Paris Cédex 15

H. S. KAPLAN, Cancer Biology Research Laboratory, Department of Radiology, Stanford University School of Medicine, Stanford, MD 94305/USA

H. KIM, City of Hope National Medical Center, 1500 East Duarte Road, Duarte, California 91010/USA

G. R. F. KRUEGER, Labor für Immunopathologie, Pathologisches Institut der Universität Köln, Lindenburg, D-5000 Köln 41

N. LELARGE, Institut de Cancérologie et d'Immunogénétique, Hôpital Paul-Brousse, 14–16, Avenue Paul-Vaillant-Couturier, F-94800 Villejuif

K. LENNERT, Abteilung für Allgemeine Pathologie und Pathologische Anatomie der Universität Kiel, Hospitalstraße 42, D-2300 Kiel

R. P. LINKE, Institut für Immunologie der Universität München, Schillerstraße 42, D-8000 München 2

R. J. LUKES, Department of Pathology, University of Southern California, School of Medicine, 2025 Zonal Avenue, Los Angeles, CA 90033/USA

R. M. MANN, Department of Surgical Pathology, Johns Hopkins Hospital, Baltimore, MD 21205/USA

G. MATHÉ, Institut de Cancérologie et d'Immunogénétique, Hôpital Paul-Brousse, 14–16, Avenue Paul-Vaillant-Couturier, F-94800 Villejuif

C. MATUCHANSKY, Gastroenterology Unit and Research Unit on Pathophysiology of Digestion, INSERM (U 54), Hôpital Saint-Lazare, 107, Rue du Faubourg Saint-Denis, F-75010 Paris

C. J. MELIEF, Department of Tumor Immunology, Central Laboratory of the Netherlands Red Cross Blood Transfusion Service and Laboratory of Experimental and Clinical Immunology, University of Amsterdam, P.O. Box 9190, Amsterdam, The Netherlands

C. MICHAEU, Institut Gustave-Roussy, 16bis, Avenue Paul-Vaillant-Couturier, F-94800 Villejuif

E. M. MORAN, University of California Irvine and the Veterans Administration Hospital, Long Beach, CA/USA

K. NANBA, Department of Pathology, Kure Mutual Hospital, Niskí-Chuoh, Kure, 737, Japan

B. N. NATHWANI, City of Hope National Medical Center, 1500 East Duarte Road, Duarte, CA 91010/USA

C. NEZELOF, Groupe de Pathologie Pédiatrique, INSERM (U 77), 149, Rue de Sèvres, F-75730 Paris Cédex

M. O'BRIEN, M. R. C. Leukemia Unit, Royal Postgraduate Medical School, Du Cane Road, London W12 0HS/U.K.

G. T. O'CONOR, Department of Health, Education and Welfare, National Cancer Institute, National Institute of Health, Bethesda, MD 20014/USA

G. A. PANGALIS, Univerisity of Athens, School of Medicine, 1st Department of Internal Medicine, Hospital Visselevs Pavlos, Athens, Greece

C. S. PAPADIMITRIOU, Abteilung für Allgemeine Pathologie und Pathologische Anatomie der Universität Kiel, Hospitalstraße 42, D-2300 Kiel

A. POLLIACK, Department of Hematology, Hadassah University Hospital, Hadassah Medical School, Jerusalem, Israel

J.-L. PREUD'HOMME, Laboratory of Immunochemistry and Immunopathology, INSERM (U 108), Research Institute on Blood Diseases, Hôpital Saint-Louis, 2, Place du Docteur-A. Fournier, F-75010 Paris

E. PUJADE LAURAINE, Address not communicated

J. C. RAMBAUD, Gastroenterology Unit and Research Unit on Pathophysiology of Digestion, INSERM (U 54), Hôpital Saint-Lazare, 107, Rue du Faubourg Saint-Denis, F-75010 Paris

H. RAPPAPORT, City of Hope National Medical Center, 1500 East Duarte Road, Duarte, California 91010/USA, and Institut de Cancérologie et d'Immunogénétique, Hôpital Paul-Brousse, 14–16, Avenue Paul-Vaillant-Couturier, F-94800 Villejuif

A. RAUSING, University Institute of Pathology, General Hospital, S-214 01 Malmö

F. REYES, Unité de Recherches sur les Anémies, INSERM (U 91), Hôpital Henri-Mondor, F-94010 Créteil

E. P. RIEBER, Institut für Immunologie der Universität München, Schillerstraße 42, D-8000 München 2

G. A. RIETHMÜLLER, Abteilung für Experimentelle Chirurgie und Immunologie, Chirurgische Universitätsklinik, D-7400 Tübingen

J. G. SAAL, Robert-Bosch-Krankenhaus, D-7000 Stuttgart

S. E. SALMON, Section of Hematology and Oncology, and The University of Arizona Cancer Center, Health Sciences Center, Tucson, AZ 85724/USA

M. SELIGMANN, Laboratory of Immunochemistry and Immunopathology, INSERM (U 108), Research Institute on Blood Diseases, Hôpital Saint-Louis, 2, Place du Docteur-A. Fournier, F-75010 Paris

L. H. SOBIN, Cancer Unit, World Health Organization, CH-1211 Geneva 27

P. SPERANDIO, M. R. C. Leukaemia Unit, Royal Postgraduate Medical School, Du Cane Road, London W12 0HS/U.K.

H. STEIN, Abteilung für Allgemeine Pathologie und Pathologische Anatomie der Universität Kiel, Hospitalstraße 42, D-2300 Kiel

P. STRÄULI, Abteilung für Krebsforschung, Institut für Pathologie, Universität Zürich, Birchstraße 95, CH-8050 Zürich

N. TALAL, Clinical Immunology, Veterans Administration Hospital, University of California, San Francisco, CA 94121/USA

C. R. TAYLOR, Los Angeles County and University of Southern California Medical Center, Department of Immunopathology, 2025 Zonal Avenue, Los Angeles, CA 90033/USA

B. H. TINDLE, Department of Pathology, University of Southern California School of Medicine, 2025 Zonal Avenue, Los Angeles, CA 90033/USA

H. D. WALLER, Abteilung Innere Medizin II, Medizinische Universitätsklinik, D-7400 Tübingen

N. L. WARNER, Departments of Pathology and Medicine, University of New Mexico, School of Medicine, Albuquerque, NM/USA

T. S. WORTHY, The Regional Radiotherapy Centre, Cookridge Hospital, Leeds, Yorkshire/U.K.

Part I

Current Morphologic Categorizations

Lymphomas We Must Classify

L. H. Sobin

Lymphomas we must classify
 By rubrics with codes and in lists.
The reason I'm sure you know why
 Clear thinking it seems to assist.

It helps when assessing the rates,
 Causes, effects, and raw data,
Comparing prognosis and fates,
 And whether the treatment does matter.

But when I relate to my friends,
 In a language I learned in my youth,
We find ourselves at our wit's ends
 Cause we cannot arrive at the truth.

For what I once thought lymphocytic,
 A form of malignant lymphoma,
I find someone calls centrocytic,
 Another hematosarcoma.

Lymphomas of histiocytes,
 I am sure we have all used the name,
Today several say is not right,
 But the tumor must still be the same.

Separating on differentiation
 Was once well-accepted by all,
But now cellular transformation
 Makes one group use large mixed and small.

There are those who eye nuclear form,
 Cleaved, convoluted, and round.
Follicular structure's the norm
 Perhaps here the basis is sound.

Some fear old terms dear and quite classic
 Imply they're no longer of use,
Prefer words like germinoblastic
 Follicular tumor diffuse.

It's a problem for all labs and nations
 To seek now a language that's one,
Agree on a classification,
 Until that our work is not done.

Integration of Modern Data in WHO Categorization of Lymphosarcomas. Its Value for Prognosis Prediction and Therapeutic Adaptation to Prognosis

G. MATHÉ

There is no real simplicity
There are only simplifications
L. P. FARGUE

Many classifications of hematosarcomas or malignant non-Hodgkin's lymphosarcomas have been proposed [3, 9, 16, 17, 23, 20, 29]. Some are still used, mainly that of Rappaport [29], which were conceived before the establishment of the concept of lymphocyte transformation by antigen(s) into large pyroninophilic cells (Fig. 1), which were confused with "histiocytes" before this concept and have been called immunoblasts by DAMESHEK [7]. The recent availability of immune and/or cytochemical markers (Fig 2) able to recognize T- and B- and so-called null lymphocytes (Table 1) [6,13, 31, 36, 38] have not only subtracted from the so-called

Table 1. T- and B- immune markers

Markers	T	B
Immune	Sheep red blood cell rosette forming assay + [13.38]	Ig secretion demonstrated by immunofluorescence assays [see 31], by immunoperoxidase [36] ?
Cytochemical	Acid phosphatase activity + [6]	

histiocytic tumors, the immunoblastic lymphosarcoma [22], but also mycosis fungoides which have been shown to be a T-lymphosarcoma [18]. Hence, the field of histiocytic sarcomas has been restricted and may be still further restricted if not suppressed in the future when we are able to identify the tumors composed of reticulum and/or dentritic cells, such as the cells recently studied by STEINMAN et. al. [33,34,35]. For this reason, the WHO Reference Center for the Classification of Neoplasias of Hematopoietic and Lymphoid tissues [23] has decided to use the term reticulosarcoma to designate the sarcomas of so-called mononuclear phagocytes, according to a WHO monograph [37] because it is historical [26] and because there is no proof that the cells which constitute this tumor in a strict sense are not reticulum cells and/or dentritic cells. Simultaneously, the fields of lymphosarcomas in a broad sense have been extended not only by the inclusion of the above-mentioned immunoblastic lymphosarcomas [22] and mycosis fungoides [18], but also by that of plasmocytic and lymphoplasmocytic lymphosarcomas [16, 17] (Table 2). However, if the old term lymphosarcoma is now justified by the immune categorization, we cannot pretend to use it always in a strict sense, as there are tumors composed of cells which do not carry the markers of differentiated T or B cells which are called null (Table 2) and the prognosis of which is better than that of T- or B-lymphosarcomas [1]. A cytochemical marker of certain populations of prothymocytes (the terminal deoxynucleotidyl transferase) [28] and immune markers of pre-B-lymphocytes [4, 14, 30] will show us soon if all such null cell tumors (Table 2) are composed of precursors of lymphocytes, hence are really lymphosarcomas, or if there are sarcomas of undifferentiated stem cells.

The purpose of this paper is to discuss the three most *common types* of lymphosarcomas as far as their nomenclature and subtyping, especially with immune markers, are concerned. They are called in WHO nomenclature [23]: 1) prolymphocytic (centrofollicular), nodular, or diffuse, 2) lymphoblastic, and 3) immunoblastic. The correlation between this adapted WHO categorization and prognosis, and hence its value for therapeutic indications, will be shown. This nomenclature is based on the simplistic concept shown on Table 3 which has not been disproved by recent data. It does recognize several steps of differentiation: 1) one comprising cells, deriving from undifferentiated stem cells and engaged in lymphoid differentiation, which

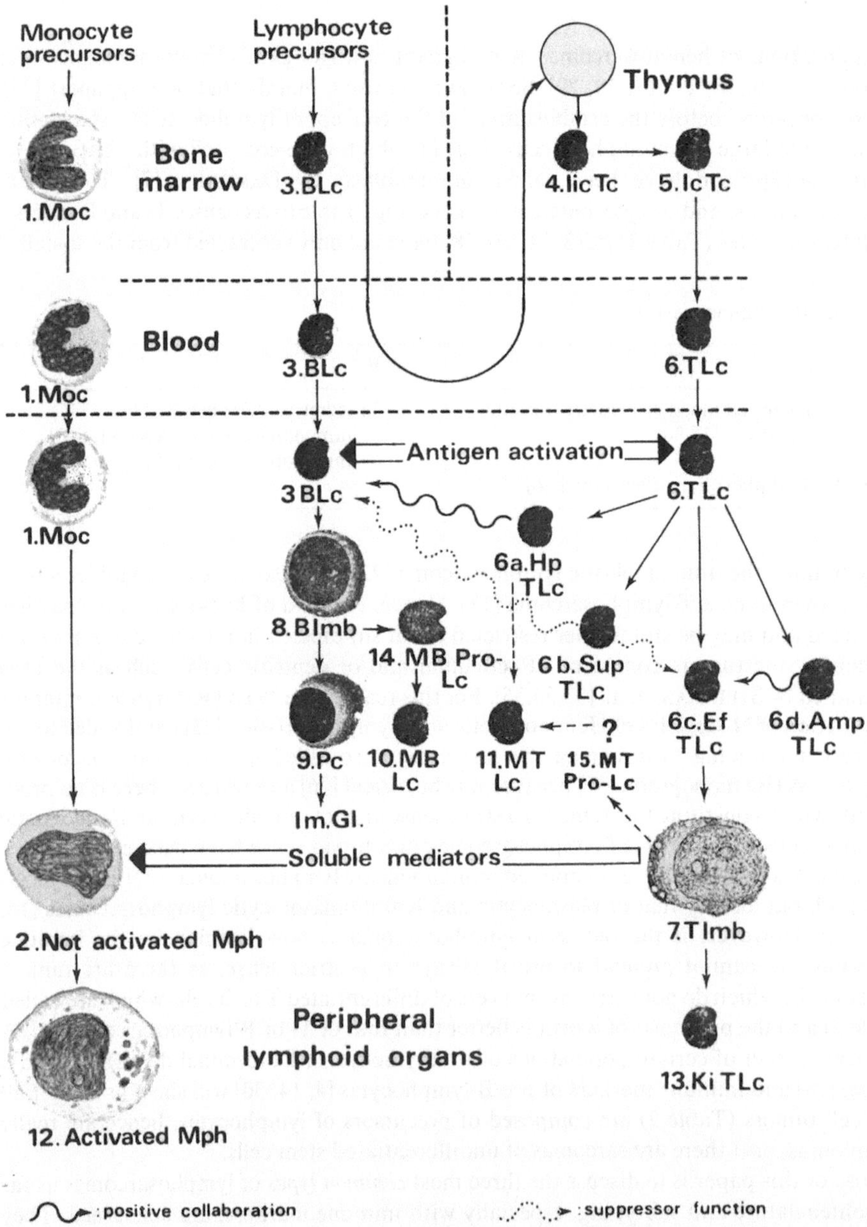

Fig. 1. Known morphologic correspondences to some functional steps of mononuclear cells. Not activated and activated macrophages are also called histiocytes. They should not be confused with reticulum cells and/or dendritic cells which may not be macrophages [33, 34, 35]

can be called lymphoblasts, 2) one comprising the cells presenting an intermediate aspect between lymphoblasts and lymphocytes which are called prolymphocytes, 3) one comprising nonprimed lymphocytes, 4) one comprising the immunoblasts or large pyroninophilic blast cells resulting from lymphocyte transformation by the antigen(s), 5) one comprising promemory lymphocytes, 6) one comprising memory lymphocytes, and 7) one which finally accepts that B-immunoblasts generate plasma cells via a proplasma cell step. We know that nonprimed lymphocytes, memory lymphocytes, and plasma cells do not divide; they result from the division of blasts and of intermediate cells (prolymphocytes). We do not know how many divisions are necessary at each blastic or prolymphocytic or proplasmocytic step to produce the resting lymphocytes or plasma cells. Do these physiologically conceived cells of the various steps of lymphoid differentiation correspond to cells given the above names on morphologic criteria? The answer is different for the three morphologic types of cells which compose the three most common lymphosarcomas, so-called, in WHO nomenclature, "immunoblastic," "prolymphocytic (centrofollicular)," and "lymphoblastic."

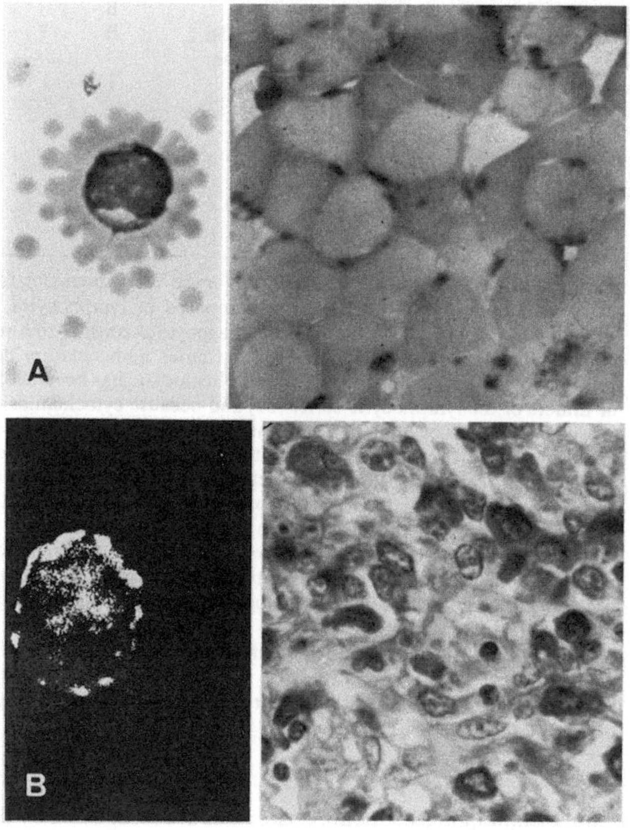

Fig. 2. (A) Markers of T-lymphocytes.
Left: the sheep red blood cell marker as a cell surface immune marker [13, 38];
Right: acid phosphatase activity [6].
(B) Markers of B-lymphocytes.
Left: immunoglobulin shown by the classic cytologic immunofluorescence method [see 31] as a cell surface immune marker;
Right: immunoglobulin shown by the immunoperoxidase method adapted to histologic section [36]

Immunoblastic Lymphosarcoma

The T- and B-immunoblasts result from blastic transformation by an antigen of T- and B-lymphocytes, respectively (Fig. 1). T-Immunoblasts have been described in graft-versus-host reaction [5] as large blasts with pyroninophilic cytoplasm, which corresponds with its high content of ribosomes and polyribosomes seen under the electron microscope (Fig. 3). B-Immunoblasts may be induced by the transformation of B-lymphocytes by B-antigens. They may differ from T-immunoblasts by a tendency to form an ergastoplasm and to evolute toward plasma cells.

Table 2. Modern frame of lymphosarcoma (LS) in a broad sense[a]

Microscopic types		*Markers*
Plasmocytic		B
Lymphoplasmocytic		B
Lymphocytic		B
Prolymphocytic (centrofollicular) LS[b c]	nodular / diffuse	B
Mycosis fungoides		T
Lymphoblastic LS[c]	convoluted	T
	nonconvoluted	T / Null / B
Burkitt's LS		B
Immunoblastic LS[c]		B / T

[a] The term reticulosarcoma has been chosen for the WHO nomenclature to design those hematosarcomas which are not composed of lymphocytes but of cells belonging to the so-called mononuclear phagocyte according to a recent WHO nomenclature [37]. The WHO Reference Center nomenclature does not call them histiocytic sarcoma because the term histiocytic has been used in the past for tumors of the lymphocytic series [29] and because cytochemical studies [39] as well as studies of functions in immunity [33, 34, 35] have shown that histiocytes, which are highly differentiated tissue monocytes, do not share cytochemical features or immune functions with fixed cells such as dendritic cells [33, 34, 35], which exercise none of the functions of the so-called macrophages (spleen and peritoneum histiocytes) in immunity. Until our knowledge is increased, the WHO Reference Center has retained the term reticulosarcoma for tumors of the conventional mononuclear phagocytes. In fact, the cells do not resemble immunologists' histiocytes on smears [23] or under scanning electron microscopy [8].

[b] The term centrofollicular is added when the centrofollicular nature of the cells can be proved.

[c] The common lymphosarcomas which are the object of this study are in italics.

T- and B-immunoblastic lymphosarcomas are recognized by LUKES and COLLINS [17], LENNERT et al. [16], MATHÉ et al. [22], and included in WHO nomenclature [7]. Their cells are large, have regular shape, with blastic nuclei (regular chromatin) containing usually several nucleoli. Their cytoplasms are red in sections stained with pyronin and dark blue in sections or smears stained with Giemsa. They usually contain vacuoles and always many ribosomes and polyribosomes visible under the electron microscope (Fig. 3). One can microscopically distinguish B-immunoblastic lymphosarcomas (Fig. 4) from the T-immunoblastic types (Fig. 5) owing to the frequent plasmocytoid features seen under the light microscope and to the ergastoplasmic

Table 3. Concept of lymphoid cell differentiation

			Stem cells	→	Lymphoblasts
→	Immunoblasts	→	Prolymphocytes[a] Memory prolymphocytes	→	Lymphocytes Memory lymphocytes
	(B) ↓				
	Proplasma cells				
	↓				
	Plasma cells				

[a] Divisions

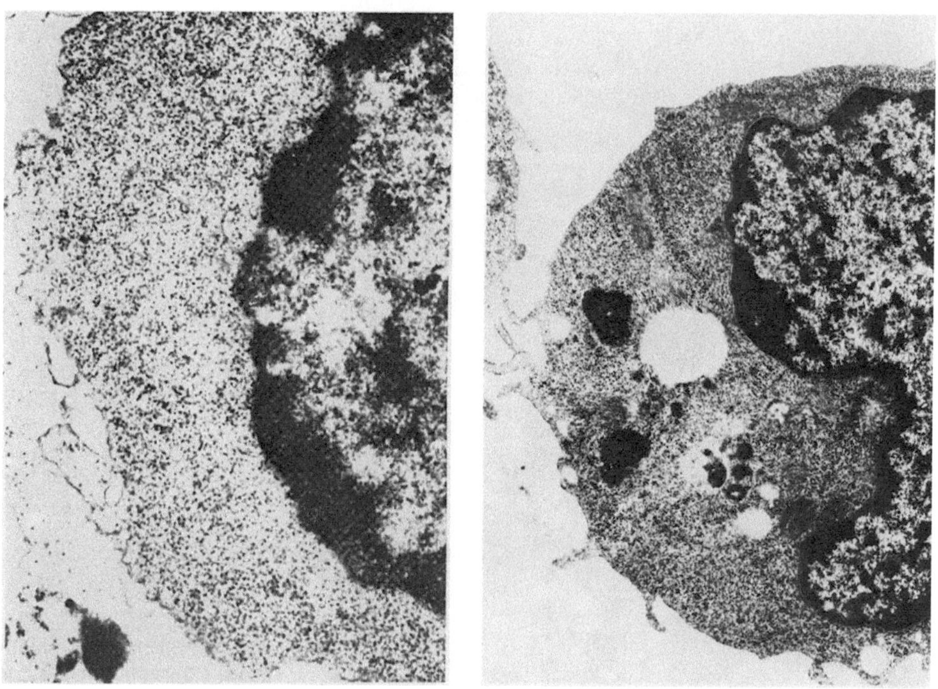

Fig. 3. Left: a graft-versus-host reaction (T) immunoblast under electron microscopy [5];
Right: an immunoblast of a T-immunoblastic lymphosarcoma [22]. Note the abundance of ribosomes and of polyribosomes in both cells

formation tendency of the B-type under the electron microscope. The immunoperoxidase test may be an easy method of confirming the B-nature of the cells.

There are some pathologists who do not use the term "immunoblast," either because they prefer a descriptive term such as "large lymphoid pyroninophilic cell" [9] which is homonymous

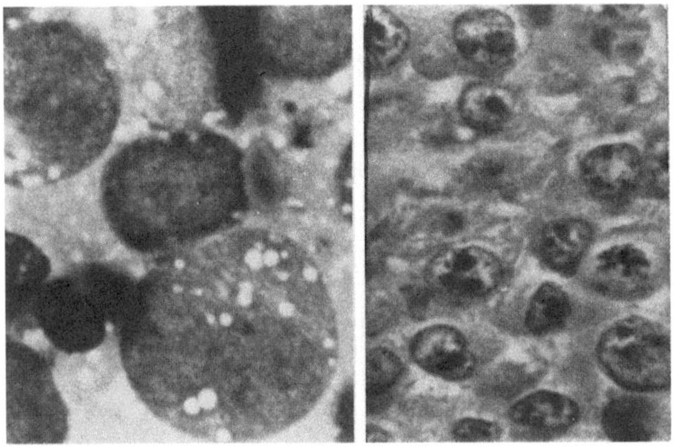

Fig. 4. A B-immunoblastic lymphosarcoma: cytologic appearance on a smear (left) and histologic appearance of a section (right)

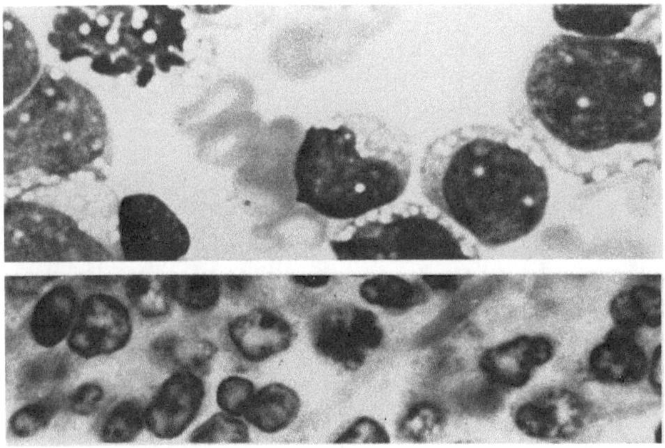

Fig. 5. A T-immunoblastic lymphosarcoma: cytologic appearance (above) on a smear and histologic appearance of a section (below)

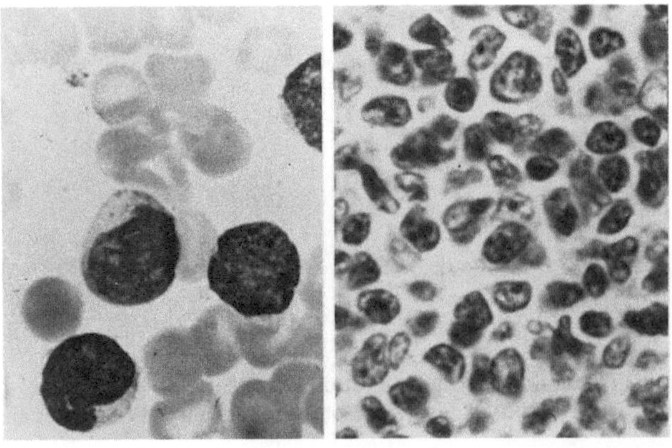

Fig. 6 Prolymphocyte centrofollicular lymphosarcoma, large cleaved nucleus cell type.
Left: cytologic appearance on a smear;
Right: histologic appearance of a section

and hence does not induce confusion, or because they do not accept the concept. This is the case of BENNETT et al. [3]; if they describe, as is probably the case, immunoblastic lymphosarcomas under the name of "undifferentiated large cells," they use an incorrect term, as immunoblasts are differentiated cells and carry T- or B- differentiation markers.

Prolymphocytic (Centrofollicular) Lymphosarcomas

If all prolymphocytes, in the morphologic sense of the term, are not centrofollicular cells [we have described a T- or null prolymphocytic acute lymphoid leukemia [2, 21]], most centrofollicular cells may be considered to be B-memory prolymphocytes. As a matter of fact, secondary follicules, those which have germinal centers, only appear after antigenic stimulation. Thus, they contain daughter cells of B-immunoblasts. As their appearance is intermediate between that of blasts and that of lymphocytes, the term "prolymphocytes" describes them best. Hence, the WHO categorization of lymphosarcomas calls the tumors composed of those cells B-prolymphocytic (centrofollicular) lymphosarcomas. We prefer this term to that of "centrocytic" or "centrocytocentroblastic lymphoma" proposed by LENNERT et al. [16] and to that of "follicle cell lymphoma" proposed by BENNETT et al. [3], as they use a parameter which is not the morphologic differentiation parameter used for the types of lymphosarcomas. Moreover, if it is accepted that the nodular form of prolymphocytic lymphosarcoma is composed of follicular center cells, it is less easy, and it is imprudent to affirm that a given diffuse form of lymphosarcoma is composed of follicular center cells, except perhaps if one has proof that the cells are B, which is far from always being the case in routine practice. The description of several types of those cells by LUKES and COLLINS [17], according to the appearances of the nuclei (cleaved or not cleaved) and to the size (small, large, or mixed) Figs. 6 and 7), is sufficient to underline the difficulty and the risk of concluding a centrofollicular nature of a diffuse lymphosarcoma. As a result, the choice for the WHO categorization of lymphosarcomas is the term "prolymphocytic," which is based on the same differentiation criteria as the terms used for other types, and which is completed by the term "centrofollicular" only when the pathologist has the certitude that the cells are follicular center cells (nodular form; cleaved nuclei and/or B-markers for the diffuse form).

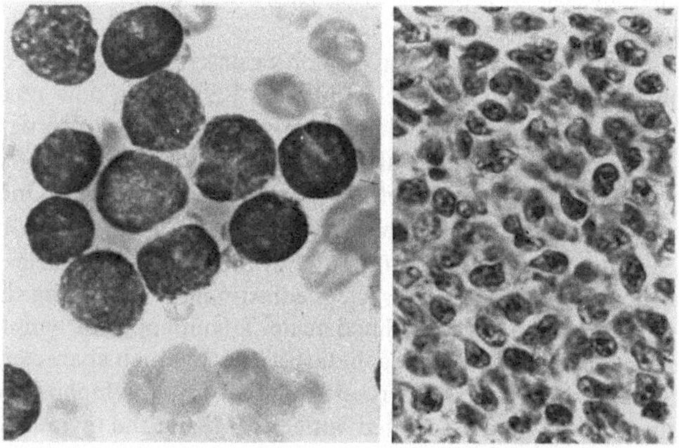

Fig. 7. Prolymphocyte centrofollicular lymphosarcoma, small cell type with some cleaved nucleus cells.
Left: cytologic appearance on a smear;
Right: histologic appearance of a section

Lymphoblastic Lymphosarcomas

The cytologists call lymphoblasts the cells of certain types of so-called acute lymphoid leukemia (Fig. 8) [22, 21]. They are blast cells with regular chromatin, of median or small size, having usually no more than one nucleolus in their nuclei. The classic morphologists considered these

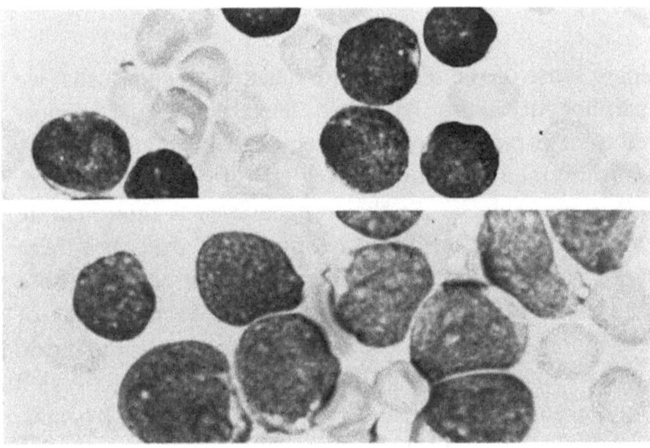

Fig. 8 Two types of so-called acute lymphoid leukemia cells called lymphoblasts.
Above: microlymphoblasts;
Below: macrolymphoblasts [21, 23]

cells to be progenitors of nonprimed lymphocytes. This concept cannot currently be disproved, but our present knowledge indicates that there are several types of lymphoblasts as far as differentiation is concerned: 1) some are thymic or postthymic cells as they form SRBC rosettes [2] and may be acid phosphatase positive [6], 2) some null lymphoblasts may be prethymic cells as they have a terminal deoxynucleotidyl transferase activity which is a possible marker of certain population(s) of prothymocytes [28], 3) some other null lymphoblasts may be pre-B-secreting lymphocytes, as they carry the B-antigens described by Billing [4], Kadin [14] and Schlossmann [30]. We cannot eliminate the possibility according to which some so-called morphologic lymphoblasts could be undifferentiated stem cells as suggested by Greaves' [10] study on lymphoblast-like cell chronic myeloid leukemia blastic crisis; the cells carry the Phl chromosome and have terminal deoxynucleotidyl transferase activity [12]. However, as long as we call the typical blasts of so-called acute lymphoid leukemia, lymphoblastic (Fig. 8) we cannot use another term for the morphologically and immunologically similar cells which characterize a form of lymphosarcoma called lymphoblastic lymphosarcoma in WHO nomenclature (Fig. 9).

The form of lymphosarcoma which we described in our first classification [20] was not identified in Rappaport's classic classification [29] but is now recognized by this author [25]. It is included in most other classifications [3, 16] but not recognized by Lukes and Collins [17]. Recognizing a lymphosarcoma as lymphoblastic is not enough, especially for prognosis prediction [24], and therefore, therapeutic indications. One must distinguish between the T- and the null types [1]. The T-types may be microscopically recognized when the cells have convoluted nuclei (Fig. 10) [16], but the convoluted nuclei T-lymphoblastic lymphosarcoma, which frequently involves the mediastinum by enlarging the thymus, does not include the T-type. There is a nonconvoluted nuclei T-lymphoblastic lymphosarcoma, hence the great interest in the search for acid phosphatase activity, which characterizes these T-cell forms and, if cells are available, the SRBC rosette assay. Most T-lymphosarcomas might also carry the human thymus leukemia-associated antigens [15] and the thymus leukemia antigen described by Sen

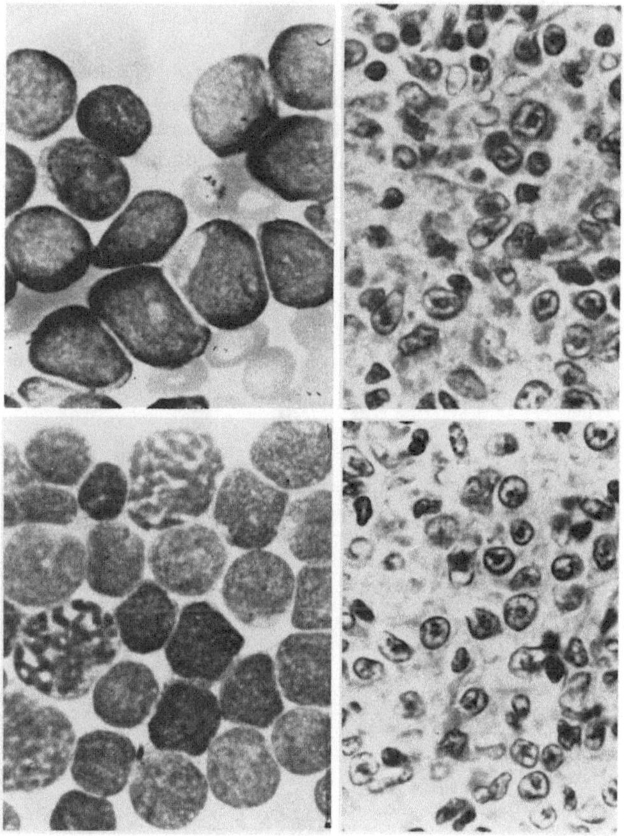

Fig. 9. Two lymphoblastic lymphosarcomas. The cells of the lower case are larger than those of the upper case.
Above: cytologic appearance of a smear;
Below: histologic appearance of a section

and BORELLA [32]. A microscopically typical lymphoblastic lymphosarcoma may be negative in the T-cell bioassays, including the SRBC rosette test, and also may be negative in the B-cell assays (Ig production). It is typed as null cell lymphoblastic lymphosarcoma [1], and the future will tell if the cells are prothymocytes [28], pro-B-secreting cells (new B-antigens) [4, 14, 30], or less differentiated stem cells.

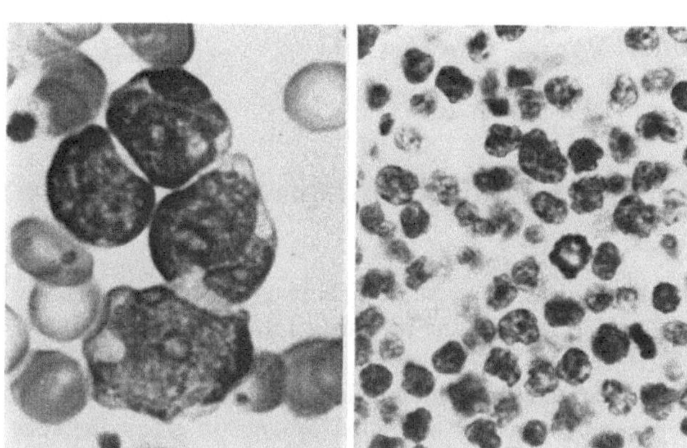

Fig. 10. Lymphoblastic lymphosarcoma with convoluted nucleus cells.
Left: cytologic appearance of a smear;
Right: histologic appearance of a section

Age Distribution

Figure 11 shows that the age distribution is different for the three types. The immunoblastic type occurs in all ages with a slight increase in incidence after 30 years of age. The prolymphocytic type does not occur in childhood and is distributed between the ages of 20 and 60 years, with a peak incidence at 45 years. The lymphoblastic type predominates in children and young adults with two peaks, at 5 and 25 years of age.

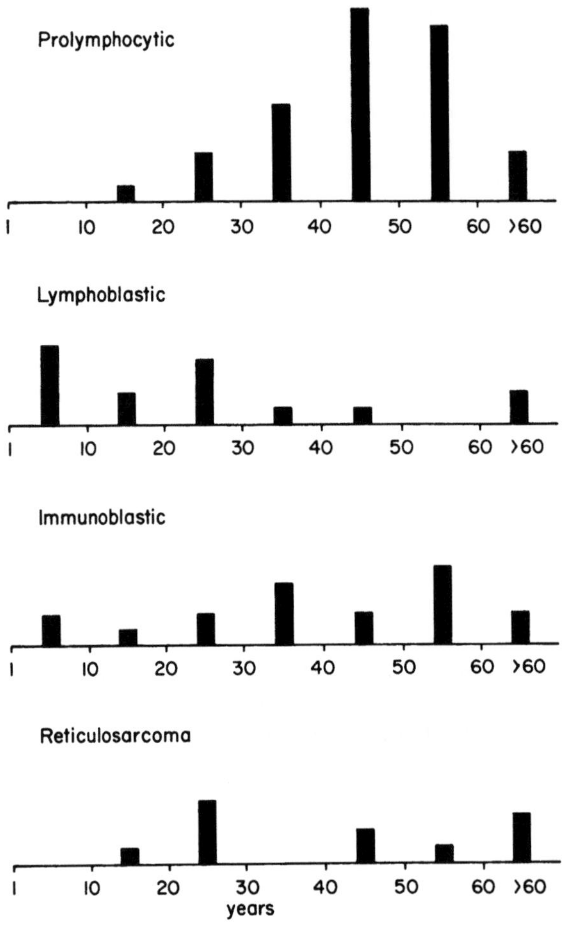

Fig. 11. Age distribution of the main types of lymphosarcomas compared with that of reticulosarcomas

Prognostic Value of Adapted WHO Categorization

For the present, differentiating between a null lymphoblastic lymphosarcoma and a T-subtype is essential, because the prognosis for these two subtypes is very different, as seen in Fig. 12, which also shows the great value of WHO nomenclature for the other main types of lymphosarcomas and their different subtypes. It allows us to distinguish two groups according to present prognosis: the good prognostic group includes the prolymphocytic and the null lymphoblastic lymphosarcoma, and the poor prognosis group the T-lymphoblastic and both T-

and B-immunoblastic lymphosarcomas. The treatment which we have applied until now [24] gives remarkable results for the first group, while its results are no better than those of the past for the second group, which needs intensive research on new drugs, new combinations, and new protocols.

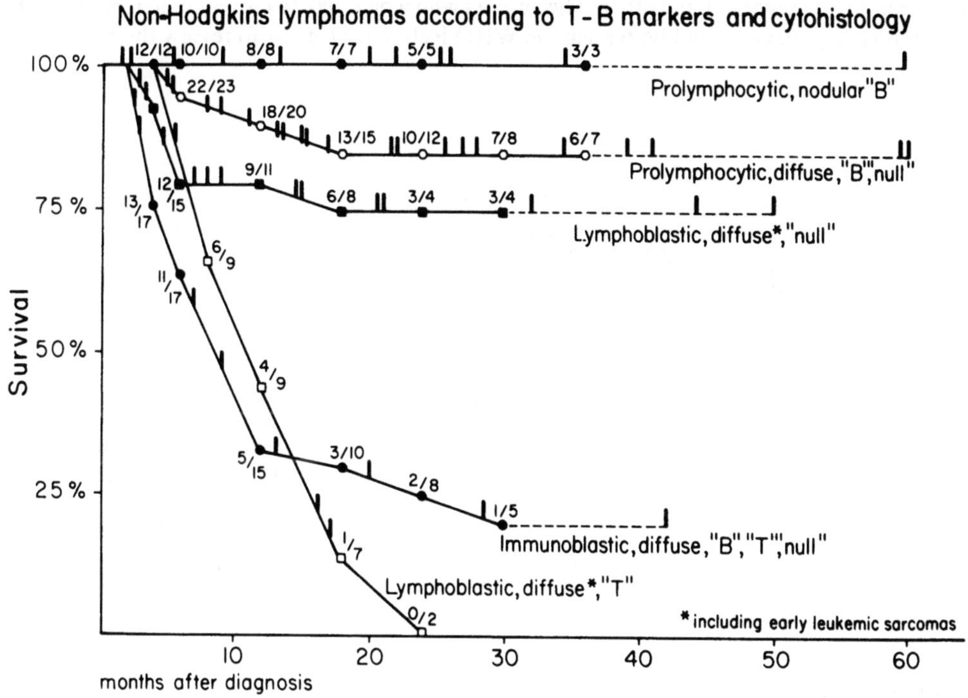

Fig. 12. Prognosis of lymphosarcomas according to the double histocytologic and immune categorization. See the value of the histolocytologic classification in MISSET et al. [24] and that of the immune classification in BELPOMME et al. [1]

Table 4. Comparison of WHO and RAPPAPORT's non-Hodgkin's common hematosarcoma classification

WHO	RAPPAPORT
	Nodular diffuse
	(i) Undifferentiated
Lymphoplasmocytic (B) LS Lymphocytic (B) LS	(ii) Lymphocytic, well-differentiated
Nodular or diffuse prolymphocytic centrofollicular (B) LS	(iii) Lymphocytic, poorly differentiated
Lymphoblastic Convoluted n (T) LS Common (T) LS Common (null) LS	(iv) Mixed (Lymphocytic and histiocytic)
Immunoblastic TS Immunoblastic BS Reticulosarcoma	(v) Histiocytic

Correlations Between WHO Nomenclature and the Rappaport Classification

Table 4 gives the correspondence of the terms of the WHO categorization and the RAPPAPORT classification. As seen in this Table, the translation is not simple, one term in one classification corresponding to several in the other. The authors who would like to correlate their results with the WHO categorization had better ask the WHO Reference Center to review their sections.

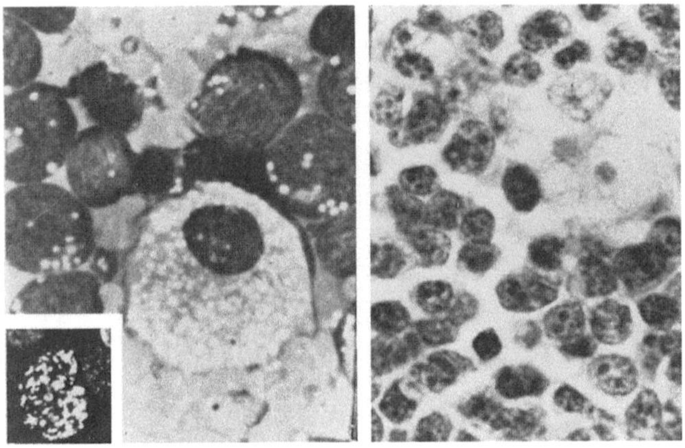

Fig. 13. Burkitt's tumor: Burkitt's cells infiltrated with nonneoplastic macrophages. Left: cytologic appearance of a smear;
Right: histologic appearance of a section. Lower left corner: the EBNA test

Burkitt's Tumor

If the simplistic concept given in Table 3 greatly helps in finding a practically useful classification for common lymphosarcomas, it does not help one to know the differentiation stage of the B-lymphoid cells involved in Burkitt's lymphosarcoma [27]. The true African Burkitt's tumor is composed of blast cells which resemble immunoblasts by their cytoplasm (basophilia, pyroninophilia, vacuoles) but which are of a smaller size than the cells of the common B-cell immunoblastic lymphosarcoma (Fig. 13). Their size is that of lymphoblasts. If we do not know the differentiation stage of those cells, there is no difficulty in identifying the African tumor which is usually EBNA positive [11].

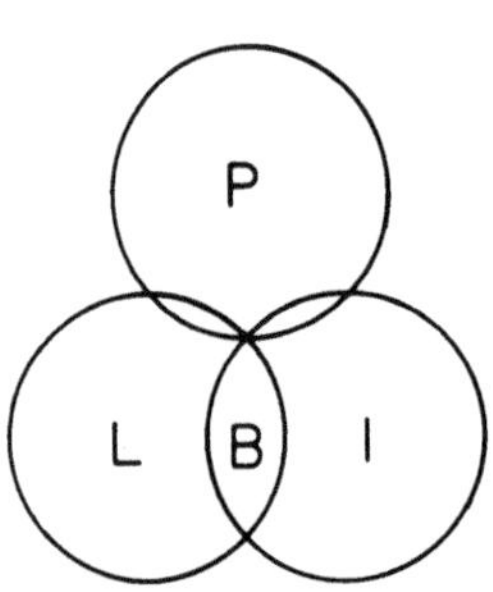

Fig. 14. Burkitt's tumor (B) is at the intersection of the three main types of lymphosarcomas. As its neoplastic cells arise in the germinal centers, it is related to the prolymphocytic centrofollicular types (P); the cells resemble immunoblasts (I) but are the size of lymphoblasts (L)

The problem is much more complex with so-called non-African Burkitt's tumor, which is most often EBNA negative [11]. It has recently been shown that the prognosis of non-African Burkitt's tumor is similar to that of the African type [40]. As this does not prove that it is the same disease, it provides a strong argument in favor of the maintenance of this entity. The neoplastic cells have been shown by MANN et al. [19] to arise in the germinal centers. Thus, Burkitt's tumor is at the intersection of the three main types of lymphosarcomas (Fig. 14).

Summary

The categorization of lymphosarcomas with immune markers has enriched the prognosis value of the WHO classification. The prolymphocytic (centrofollicular) B-type and the null lymphoblastic subtype have a good prognosis, while the (T- or B-) immunoblastic type and the T-lymphoblastic subtype have a poor prognosis.

References

1. BELPOMME, D., LELARGE, N., MATHÉ G., DAVIES, A. J. S.: Etiological, clinical and prognostic significance of the T-B immunological classification of primary acute lymphoid leukaemias and non-Hodgkin's lymphomas. In: Immunological Diagnosis of Leukemias and Lymphomas. THIERFELDER, S., ROFT, H., THIEL, E. (eds) Heidelberg-New York: Springer-Verlag 1977a, p. 33.
2. BELPOMME, D., MATHÉ, G., DAVIES, A. J. S.: Clinical significance and prognostic value of the T-B immunological classification of human primary acute lymphoid leukaemias. Lancet 1977b I, 555.
3. BENNETT, M. H., FARRER-BROWN, G., HENRY, K., JELIFFE, A. M.: Classification of non-Hodgkin's lymphomas. Lancet 1974 I, 1295.
4. BILLING, R., RAFIZADEH, B., DREW, I., HARTMAN, G., GALE, R., TERASAKI, P.: Human B-lymphocyte antigen expressed by lymphocytic and myelocytic leukaemia cells. J. Exp. Med. *144*, 167 (1976).
5. BINET, J. L., MATHÉ, G.: Optical and electron microscopy studies of the immunological competent cells during the reaction of the graft versus host. Ann. NY. Acad. Sci. *99*, 426 (1962).
6. CATOWSKY, D., GALETTO, J., OKOS, A., MILIANI, E., GALTON, D. A. G.: Cytochemical profile of B and T leukaemic lymphocytes with special reference to acute lymphoblastic leukaemia. J. Clin. Pathol. *27*, 767 (1974).
7. DAMESHEK, W.: "Immunoblasts" and "Immunocytes"; an attempt at a functional nomenclature. Blood *21*, 243 (1963).
8. DANTCHEV, D., BELPOMME, D.: Critical study of the mononuclear leukocyte morphology based on scanning electron microscopy in normal subjects and in patients with lymphoid or monocytoid proliferative disorders. Comparison with the T, B or null cell membrane phenotypes. Biomedicine *26*, 202 (1976).
9. DORFMAN; R. F.: the non-Hodgkin's lymphomas. In: The Reticulo Endothelial System. REBUCK, J. W., BERARD, C. W., ABELL, M. R. (eds) Baltimore: Williams and Wilkins 1975, p. 262.
10. GREAVES, M. F., BROWN, G., RAPSON, N., LISTER, T. A. Antisera to acute lymphoblastic leukaemia cells. Clin. Immunol. Immunopathol. *4*, 67 (1975).
11. HAUSEN, H. zur: Oncogenic herpes virus. Biochim. Biophys. Acta. *417*, 25 (1975).
12. JANOSSY, G., ROBERTS, M., GREAVES, M. F.: Target cell in chronic myeloid leukemia and its relationship to acute lymphoid leukemia. Lancet 1976 I, 1058.
13. JONDAL, M., HOLM, G., WIGZELL, H.: A large population of lymphocytes forming non-immune rosettes with sheep red blood cells. J. Exp. Med. *136*, 207 (1972).
14. KADIN, M. E., GARRATTY, E., SCALAPINO, J.: Detection of a new B-membrane antigen in Hodgkin's disease and non-Hodgkin's lymphomas. Proc. Assoc. Cancer Res. *18*, 29 (abstr. 113) (1977).
15. KERSEY, J., SABAD, A., GAJL-PECZALSKA, K., HALLGREN, H., YUNIS, E., NESBIT, M.: Acute lymphoblastic leukemia cells with markers of T (thymus derived) lymphocytes. Science *182*, 1355 (1973).
16. LENNERT, K., MOHRI, N., STEIN, H., KAISERLING, E. The histopathology of malignant lymphoma. Br. J. Haematol. *31* (suppl.), 193 (1975).

17. LUCKES, R. J., COLLINS, R. D.: A functional classification of malignant lymphomas. In: The Reticulo-Endothelial System. REBUCK, J. W., BERARD, C. W., ABELL, M. R. (eds) Baltimore: Williams and Wilkins 1975, p. 213.
18. LUTZNER, M., EDELSON, R., SCHEIN, P., GREEN, I., KIRKPATRICK, C., AHMED, A.: Cutaneous T-cell lymphomas: the Sezary syndrome, mycosis fungoides and related disorders. Ann. Intern. Med. *83*, 534 (1975).
19. MANN, R. B., JAFFE, E. S., BRAYLAN, R. C., NANBA, K., FRANK, M. M., ZIEGLER, J. L., BERARD, C. W.: Non-endemic Burkitt's lymphoma. A B-cell tumor related to germinal centers. N. Engl. J. Med. *295*, 685 (1976).
20. MATHÉ, G., SEMAN, G.: Aspects Histologiques et Cytologiques des Leucémies et Hématosarcomes. Maloine: Paris 1963.
21. MATHÉ, G., POUILLART, P., STERESCU, M., AMIEL, J. L., SCHWARZENBERG, L., SCHNEIDER, M., HAYAT, M., DE VASSAL, F., JASMIN, C., LAFLEUR, M.: Subdivision of clinical varieties of acute leukemia. Correlation with prognosis and cure expectancy. Eur. J. Clin. Biol. Res. *16*, 554 (1971).
22. MATHÉ, G., BELPOMME, D., DANTCHEV, D., KHALIL, A. M., AFIFI, A. M., TALEB, N., POUILLART, P., SCHWARZENBERG, L., HAYAT, M., DE VASSAL, F., JASMIN, C., MISSET, J. L., MUSSET, M.: Immunoblastic lymphosarcoma. A cytological and clinical entity? Biomedicine *22*, 473 (1975).
23. MATHÉ, G., RAPPAPORT, H., O'CONOR, G. T., TORLONI, H.: Histological and Cytological Typing of Neoplastic Diseases of Haematopoietic and Lymphoid Tissues. World Health Organization: Geneva 1976.
24. MISSET, J. L., MATHÉ, G., TUBIANA, M., CAILLOU, B., POUILLART, P., GIL, M., TENTAS, C., DELGADO, M.: Preliminary results of chemoradiotherapy followed or not by active immunotherapy of stage III and IV lymphosarcoma and reticulosarcoma. Correlation of the results with WHO categorisation. In: Lymphoid Neoplasias. MATHÉ, G., SELIGMANN, M., TUBIANA, M. (eds) Heidelberg-New York: Springer-Verlag, 1978 (in press).
25. NATHWANI, B. N., KIM, H., RAPPAPORT, H.: Malignant lymphoma, lymphoblastic. Cancer *38*, 964 (1976).
26. OBERLING, G.: Les réticulosarcomes et les réticulo-endothélio-sarcomes de la moelle osseuse (sarcome d'Ewing). Bull. Cancer (Paris) *17*, 259 (1928).
27. O'CONOR, G. T. Histopathological classification of Burkitt's tumour. Bull. W.H.O. *40*, 601 (1969).
28. PAZMINO, N. H., MACEWAN, R. N., IHLE, J. N.: Terminal transferases: enzyme marker for a specific prothymocyte cell populations. Proc. Am. Assoc. Cancer Res. *18*, 81 (abstr. 332) (1977).
29. RAPPAPORT, H.: Tumors of the Hematopoietic Systems. In Atlas of Tumor Pathology. Section 3, Fasc. 8. Armed Forces Institute Pathology: Washington 1966.
30. SCHLOSSMANN, S. S.: personal communication.
31. SELIGMANN, M., PREUD'HOMME J. L., BROUET, J. C.: B and T cell markers in human proliferative blood diseases and primary immuno-deficiencies with special references to membrane bound immunoglobulins. Transplant. Rev. *16*, 85 (1973).
32. SEN, L., BORELLA, L.: Clinical importance of lymphoblasts with T markers in childhood acute leukaemia, N. Engl. J. Med. *292*, 828 (1975).
33. STEINMAN, R. M., COHN, Z. A.: Identification of a novel cell type in peripheral lymphoid organs of mice. I Morphology, quantitation, tissue distribution. J. Exp. Med. *137*, 1142 (1973).
34. STEINMAN, R. M., LUSTIG, D. S., COHN, Z. A.: Identification of a novel cell type in peripheral lymphoid organs of mice. II. Functional properties in vivo. L. Exp. Med. *139*, 1431 (1974).
35. STEINMAN, R. M., ADAMS, J. C., COHN, Z. A.: Identification of a novel cell type in peripheral lymphoid organs of mice. III. Identification and distribution in mouse spleen. J. Exp. Med. *141*, 804 (1975).
36. TAYLOR, C, R., BURNS, J.: The demonstration of plasma cells and other immunoglobulin-containing cells in formalin-fixed, paraffin-embedded tissues using peroxidase-labelled antibody. J. Clin. Pathol. *27*, 14 (1974).
37. VAN FURTH, R., COHN, Z. A., HIRSCH, J. G., HUMPHREY, J. H., SPECTOR, W., LANGEVOORT, H. L.: The mononuclear phagocyte system: a new classification of macrophages, monocytes and their precursor cells. Bull. W.H.O. *46*, 845 (1972).
38. WYBRAN, J., CAN, M. C., FUDENBERG. H. H.: The human rosette forming cells as a marker of a population of thymus derived cells. J. Clin. Invest. *51*, 2537 (1972).
39. YAM, L. T., TAVASSOLI, M., JACOBS, P.: Differential characterization of the "reticulum cell" in lymphoreticular neoplasms. Am. J. Clin. Pathol. *64*, 171 (1975).
40. ZIEGLER, J. L.: Treatment result of 54 American patients with Burkitt's lymphoma are similar to the African experience. N. Engl. J. Med. *297*, 75 (1977).

Functional Classification of Malignant Lymphoma of Lukes and Collins

R. J. LUKES

Introduction

Malignant lymphomas in our functional approach are regarded as neoplasms of the immune system. They involve the T- and B-cell systems, commonly develop from alterations in lymphocyte transformation, and often develop in abnormal immune disorders [24, 25, 26, 27]. The lymphoma cells in this concept are defective immune cells that resemble to varying degrees their normal counterparts in their site of origin, migration, and function. We have proposed that the nodular lymphomas of RAPPAPORT [36] are lymphomatous follicles composed of follicular center cell (FCC) types and each type represents a stage in FCC transformation [24, 25, 26, 27]. It was also proposed that histiocytic lymphomas or reticulum cell sarcomas of the past, for the most part, involve lymphomas of transformed lymphocytes or T- or B-cell types. The results of our recent multiparameter investigation, including immunologic surface marker studies on 384 cases of non-Hodgkin's lymphomas and related disorders [28], as well as those of others [1, 4, 5, 6, 7, 9, 12, 15, 17, 20, 29], provide support for our above proposals.
The terminology and classifications of the past, including that of RAPPAPORT [36], were proposed long before the recent dramatic advances in immunology. It is evident that the cytologic types of previous classifications, particularly the diffuse types of RAPPAPORT [36], are all heterogeneous which probably accounts for their variability in clinical expression and the differences in therapeutic responsiveness. The new homogeneous cytologic types of our classification, such as the convoluted T cell, the four FCC types, and immunoblastic sarcoma of T- and B-cell types are emerging as distinctive clinical-morphologic-immunologic entities. In this presentation, I will briefly review 1) the morphologic and conceptual basis of our functional approach to the malignant lymphomas, 2) the functional classification, 3) the significance of the results of the multiparameter studies, and 4) the implications of the heterogeneity of the cytologic types of the past and the homogeneous cytologic types of our functional classification.

Immunologic and Morphologic Bases of Functional Approach

The basis of our approach has previously been presented in detail [24, 25, 26, 27] and therefore will only be outlined briefly here. The new approach is based upon three principles that are interrelated with our morphologic observations. Beginning in 1971 and in a series of papers [24, 25, 26, 27], we presented the new approach on the basis of the following proposals: 1) malignant lymphomas involve the T- and B-lymphocytic systems and rarely the histiocyte-monocyte group, 2) lymphomas commonly involve alterations in lymphocyte transformation, either as a block or as a "switch on" (derepression) and result in lymphomas developing at various positions in the T- and B-cell transformation sequence, 3) the follicular center is a B-cell area, and the interfollicular or paracortical area of lymph nodes is a T-cell zone. The techniques developed in the experimental animal systems for defining T and B cells could be applied to human lymphoma cells as part of a multiparameter study for the redefinition of the malignant lymphomas according to modern immunology. The multiparameter approach included special morphology, cytochemistry, ultrastructural studies, immunologic surface marker techniques, and immunoperoxidase stains for cytoplasmic immunoglobulin and muramidase.

An appreciation of the morphologic expressions of in vitro lymphocyte transformation in both smears and histologic sections is essential for the understanding of malignant lymphomas. There is a remarkable change in vitro of the lymphocytes exposed to mitogens from the small lymphocyte to the large metabolically active dividing form known as the hyperbasophilic blast cell. We suggested that small lymphocytes represented the dormant form and the hyperbasophilic blast cell the dividing expression of lymphocytes. Because of the bidirectional character of in vitro lymphocyte transformation, it seems most appropriate to regard the in vivo lymphocyte transformation phenomenon as modulation rather than lymphocyte differentiation. On this basis it is considered inappropriate to use the term "lymphoblast", since the small lymphocyte usually regarded as a mature lymphocyte appears to be the dormant form of the primitive appearing dividing lymphocyte. Thus, there seem to be three basic forms of lymphocytes in each system: 1) the dormant small lymphocytes, 2) the large transformed dividing form, and 3) the functional expressions such as the plasma cell. In our experience, human lymphomas often seem to develop from either a block in this transformation mechanism with accumulation of small dormant lymphocytes or from a switch on (derepression) to the large transformed lymphocyte, the dividing active form in which high turnover rate proliferations are found. In the latter, there seems to be an inability to revert to the dormant form or switch off lymphocyte transformation. Intermediate expressions have also been identified. Finally, lymphomas of the small lymphocytes in both T- and B-cell systems have varying tendencies in the course of the disease to change into lymphomas of the large transformed lymphocytes in the same system. This change in morphology is accompanied by a dramatic alteration in the aggressiveness of the process, from the low turnover rate small lymphocytes to the high turnover rate transformed lymphocytes.

From my experience with the appearance of in vitro transformed lymphocytes in histologic sections, there was a striking similarity between their features and the large pyroninophilic cytoplasmic cells in normal reactive follicular centers. This similarity suggested that the follicular center as a B-cell region might be the site of B-cell transformation and the large pyroninophilic cytoplasmic cell the transformed B cell. Camera lucida studies of normal FCC revealed four cell types: 1) cleaved cells, 2) noncleaved cells, 3) phagocytic starry-sky histiocytes, and 4) dendritic reticulum cells. There was a wide range in the size of both the cleaved and noncleaved FCC. The follicular center was proposed as the site of B-cell transformation, with the cellular sequence illustrated schematically in Figure 1. We proposed

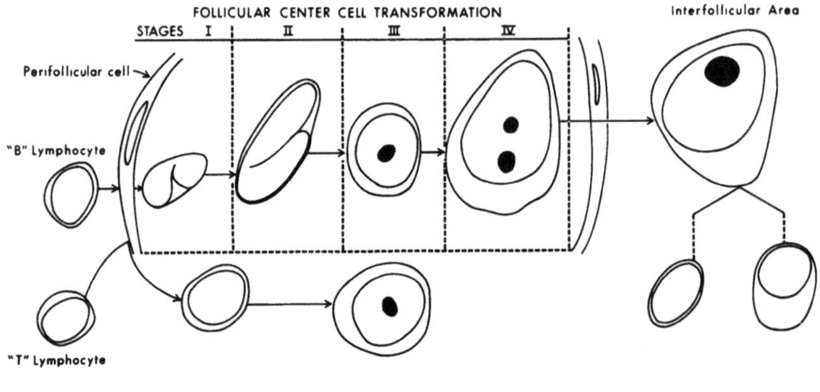

Fig. 1. Schematic representation of malignant lymphomas of follicular center cells

that in this transformation the small B-lymphocyte from the follicular lymphocytic mantle is induced to undergo transformation under the influence of antigen on the surface of the dendritic reticulum cell to form the large noncleaved FCC type, with intermediate stages. In the initial stage, the small lymphocyte develops nuclear cleavage as the small cleaved FCC. It gradually enlarges to the large cleaved cell as it acquires pyroninophilic cytoplasm. In the next sequence, the nucleus becomes round and the cell adds more pyroninophilic cytoplasm as it becomes a small noncleaved FCC. By further enlargement of the nucleus and acquisition of more cytoplasm, a large noncleaved or fully transformed FCC is formed. The small and large cleaved cells are believed to be essentially nondividing cells, while the small and large noncleaved FCC are regarded as the dividing cells of the follicular center. In light microscopy sections, the large noncleaved cell seems at times to be moving out of the follicular center into the interfollicular tissue where it is designated the B-immunoblast. This observation is supported by the recent ultrastructural studies of KOJIMA & TSUNODA [19] in which immunoperoxidase demonstration of cytoplasmic immunoglobulin labels the large noncleaved cells. These cells, in the view of KOJIMA & TSUNODA [19], seem to be passing through channels in the lymphocytic mantle into the interfollicular tissue. The B-immunoblast of the interfollicular tissue is a dividing cell and the immediate precursor of the plasma cell. It may continue to divide and form daughter cells and ultimately more plasma cells as required or revert to the small lymphocyte capable of prompt reactivation to form the immunoblast on subsequent exposure to this antigen. The sequence of transformation in the FCC concept is acknowledged to be in conflict with the generally held view of germinal cell development. Our view is based upon the acknowledged in vitro change from the small lymphocyte to the large transformed lymphocyte. This is supported by the immunoperoxidase studies of TAYLOR [40] in which a gradual increase in cytoplasmic immunoglobulin was demonstrated in normal FCC from the large cleaved FCC stage through the noncleaved FCC to the interfollicular immunoblast and plasma cell.

Transformation in the T-cell system seems to occur in a parallel fashion in the interfollicular tissue without the formation of plasma cells. Camera lucida studies of the cells of nodular lymphomas demonstrated that they were composed of cleaved and noncleaved FCC of varying size and closely resemble cleaved and noncleaved FCC of the normal follicular center. Support for this observation was provided by the ultrastructural stůdy of GLICK et al. [14] and LEVINE & DORFMAN [23].

The cytologic types of malignant lymphoma can all be related to positions in T- or B-cell transformation with the exception of three T-cell types: the convoluted lymphocyte which is proposed as a pre-T cell [39], the cerebriform cell of Sezary's syndrome and mycosis fungoides, and the new T cell found in association with epithelioid clusters of histiocytes [21, 27].

Functional Classification

The functional classification listed in Table 1 originally included five major groups: 1) U cells (undefined), 2) T cells, 3) B cells, 4) histiocytes, and 5) unclassifiable. A sixth group, cells of uncertain origin, which includes Hodgkin's disease, has been added. Previously, Hodgkin's disease was listed in a questionable position in the T-cell group. There is growing evidence that the T cells in Hodgkin's disease may be fundamentally abnormal [11, 18]. We have proposed that the Reed-Sternberg cell is possibly a polyploid transformed lymphocyte [32, 41] as TAYLOR has presented elsewhere in this symposium, but the precise nature of the Reed-Sternberg cells remains debatable [18].

Two new cytologic types of lymphoma have been added since our initial presentation of this classification [25, 26, 27], the small lymphocyte of T cells that now appears to be established as a separate lymphoma and a distinctive type of T-cell lymphoma that has emerged from the

Table 1. Functional classification

U Cell (undefined)
T Cell
Small lymphocyte
Convoluted lymphocyte
Sézary—mycosis fungöides
Immunoblastic sarcoma of T cells
B Cell Lymphoepithelioid cell
Small lymphocyte
Plasmacytoid lymphocyte
Follicular center cell (FCC)
Follicular, diffuse, follicular and diffuse, and with or without sclerosis
Small cleaved
Large cleaved
Small noncleaved (transformed)
Large noncleaved (transformed)
Immunoblastic sarcoma of B cells
Hairy cell leukemia
Histiocytic
Cell of uncertain origin
Hodgkin's disease—origin of neoplastic cell uncertain
Unclassifiable

heterogeneous group of disorders described by LENNERT under the term epithelioid type of lymphogranulomatosis [21]. LENNERT has also observed this distinctive lymphoma and proposed the term lymphoepithelioid-cell lymphoma [22].

The U cell (undefined) was created as a theoretic group for those primitive cellular proliferations without distinctive morphologic features in which the existing techniques were unable to characterize the cells specifically. The so-called null cell type of acute lymphocytic leukemia (ALL) of childhood that lacks surface markers falls within the U-cell group. Using highly specific B-cell antiserum, SCHLOSSMAN et al. [37] and WINCHESTER et al. [43] have recently presented evidence that this process involves a special B-lymphocyte. The small proportion of cases previously included in the histiocytic group that morphologically resemble transformed lymphocytes but fail to mark specifically are classified according to their morphologic features, rather than in the U-cell group.

The T- and B-cell groups each contain a small lymphocytic type and a large, fully transformed lymphocyte, immunoblastic sarcoma (IBS). The T-cell group includes lymphocytes of peculiar configuration: the primitive convoluted T cell [25, 26, 27] that is commonly observed as a lymphoma-leukemia process in the second decade of life and interrelates with T-cell ALL, the cerebriform cell of Sézary's syndrome and mycosis fungoides [33], and the peculiar lymphocytic lymphoma associated with epithelioid clusters of histiocytes and formerly included in LENNERT'S lesion [21]. The B-cell group, in addition to the small B-lymphocyte and IBS, contains the plasmacytoid lymphocyte and the FCC variants which are plasma cell precursors. Each of the FCC types may occur in follicular, follicular and diffuse, or diffuse histologic patterns, and with or without sclerosis [3].

The most appropriate placement of the neoplasms of true histiocytic type is uncertain. The diagnosis at the present time in our view requires a specific histiocyte marker, either the α-naphthyl butyrate on tissue imprints or frozen fresh tissue [44], or the immunoperoxidase stain for cytoplasmic muramidase (lysozyme). In the future, it seems likely that this neoplasm, which involves the macrophage-monocyte system and even fibroblasts, will most appropriately be included in the mesenchymal, stromal, and malignant histiocytoma proliferations, all of which have numerous designations, rather than in the malignant lymphomas. The term malignant lymphoma should possibly be reserved for malignancies with the varied expressions of lymphocytes.

The unclassifiable group permits categorization of those processes that are technically unsatisfactory for specific cytologic classification but of sufficient quality to permit recognition of the process as a malignant lymphoma. Hodgkin's disease listed in the group, cells of uncertain origin, is subclassified according to the Rye modification of the LUKES-BUTLER classification [30, 31] and includes the four well-known types: lymphocyte predominance, nodular sclerosis, mixed cellularity, and lymphocyte depletion.

It is uncertain whether any new cytologic types will be added in the immediate future. The principal work in progress at present concerns the characterization of the function of the cytologic types. A detailed morphologic description of the individual cytologic types has already been presented [24, 25, 26, 27].

Significance of Results of Multiparameter Studies

For the redefinitional studies of malignant lymphomas, a panel of techniques have been employed by both Dr. Robert COLLINS' group at Vanderbilt University and by my group at the University of Southern California. These include special morphology, cytochemistry, electron microscopy, and immunologic surface marker studies. Frequently, immunoperoxidase stains have been used on paraffin sections for cytoplasmic immunoglobulin and muramidase, and at times, in vitro lymphocyte transformation studies. More recently, cell kinetic studies have been added to characterize their proliferative features. At the recent National Cancer Institute Symposium on Malignant Lymphomas, the results of parallel studies carried out at both institutions on 384 cases of non-Hodgkin's lymphomas and related leukemias were presented [28]. To date, my group at the University of Southern California alone has completed studies on over 350 cases of these disorders, and the results are essentially similar to those of the above report.

The results indicate that malignant lymphomas mark as T- or B-cell types with the exception of the rare histiocytic type and the unmarked portion of ALL. Of the 384 cases, 67% were included in the B-cell group, 15% in the T-cell, 17% in the U-cell, and 1% in the histiocytic group. The large number of cases of Hodgkin's disease investigated were not included in this report. The majority of all cytologic types included in the B-cell group marked in a monoclonal fashion with surface immunoglobulin and presented conclusive evidence of their B-cell nature. In each of the cytologic types, several cases exhibited only a small percentage of cells with surface immunoglobulin and a few had a polyclonal type of surface immunoglobulin, even though the morphologic features in each situation were identical. Of the 17 cases diagnosed as hairy cell leukemia, eight marked with the monoclonal surface immunoglobulin, and three of these cases resynthesized the immunoglobulin after stripping with trypsin. The monoclonal nature of the surface immunoglobulin on the B-cytologic types provides strong support for the B-cell nature of these cytologic types, but immunoglobulin synthesis by the lymphoma cells is acknowledged to provide the most ideal evidence.

Confirmation of the T-cell nature of lymphomas in this study was based on the morphologic demonstration of E-rosette formation about the lymphoma cells in cytocentrifuge preparations along with the lack of monoclonal surface immunoglobulin and the absence of cytochemical evidence of histiocytes. The frequency of E-rosettes is not considered a reliable determinant of a T-cell lymphoma because of the frequent admixture of nonlymphomatous T cells. Only the identification of morphologically demonstrated lymphoma cells forming valid E-rosettes is regarded as essential proof. The convoluted T-cell lymphoma (26 cases) was the most common type in the T-cell group. It exhibited a wide range in the frequency of E-rosettes, from 5%–90%, with 61% of the cases having E-rosettes in excess of 20%. The three cases exhibiting features of the new T-cell lymphoma that is associated with clusters of epithelioid histiocytes all demonstrated a high frequency of E-rosette formation. Of the 21 cases interpreted as IBS of T cells, all had sufficient cells for study. The range of E-rosettes was from 27%–84% with a median of 55%, and all were shown to form E-rosettes morphologically. The histiocyte group contained only four cases (1%), and the lymphoma cells of these cases marked with the histiocyte enzyme, α-naphthyl butyrate, and lacked monoclonal surface immunoglobulins. They were variable in morphologic expression and at times exhibited both histiocytic and monocytoid features. Several cases eventually presented with diffuse leukemic-type marrow involvement during relapse.

Our multiparameter prospective study of 49 cases of lymphomas and leukemias of childhood and the morphologic retrospective evaluation of 114 cases of childhood lymphomas indicate that the B- and T-cell type neoplasms in this age group are basically lymphoma-leukemic processes [38, 42]. The convoluted T-cell process often presents outside the marrow in peripheral lymph nodes with or without mediastinal masses, while the small noncleaved FCC Burkitt-like B-cell type primarily presents in the abdomen and less frequently in the nasopharynx, paranasal sinuses, or orbital tissues [38]. Both processes in our experience frequently develop a diffuse leukemic marrow involvement in the course of the process and commonly relapse in the central nervous system. Classification of these processes in the past as a leukemia or a lymphoma has been dependent upon whether the initial prominent manifestation was in the marrow or in the extramarrow sites. Commonly, leukemic manifestations of convoluted lymphocytes in the peripheral blood were the initially recognized findings and only several days later was a mediastinal mass incidentally discovered in a routine x-ray examination of the chest. Such patients in the past have been included in ALL and not regarded as lymphomas. In our experience, the convoluted T cell is a process with features of both lymphoma and leukemia that may be observed essentially in four forms: 1) lymphadenopathy only, 2) lymphadenopathy and a mediastinal mass, 3) lymphadenopathy, mediastinal mass, and marrow involvement, at times with a leukemic peripheral blood, and 4) bone marrow involvement, usually with leukemic peripheral blood involvement and lymphadenopathy. The convoluted T-cell process presents distinctive morphologic features and consists of noncohesive primitive-appearing cells with primitive, finely dispersed nuclear chromatin, distinctive nuclear convolutions, numerous mitoses, and scanty cytoplasm. The distinctiveness of the morphologic features is most discernible in histologic sections since the nuclear convolutions are obscured considerably in the technique of preparing smears or tissue imprints. The convoluted T cell has a number of other distinctive markers forming E-rosettes, often EAC-rosettes as an expression of a C_3 receptor and also a single positive acid phosphatase area in the region of the Golgi apparatus [39]. Similar findings have been reported by CATOVSKY et al. [8] in T-cell ALL.

It is obvious that the distinctiveness of the morphologic features of the convoluted lymphocyte we described is not based solely on nuclear convolutions as the critical report of NATHWANI et al. [35] suggests. Furthermore, we did not indicate that mediastinal masses were found only with the convoluted lymphocytic type. In addition, the report of NATHWANI et al. [35] lacks immunologic surface marker studies. It also fails to emphasize the importance of pyroninophilic cytoplasm that is essentially lacking in the convoluted lymphocyte and prominent in the small noncleaved FCC type, the two histologic types in this age group that may not be distinguished readily by inexperienced observers. Our retrospective and prospective studies have also provided confirmatory evidence of the distinctiveness of the morphologic features and the associated clinical entity. Finally, the convoluted lymphocyte appears to be a counterpart of the pre-T cell on the basis of its membrane C_3 receptor, according to STEIN et al. [39], rather than a lymphoblast or prolymphocyte.

The findings in the above studies are sufficient to indicate that the lymphomas can be classified principally as subtypes of the T- and B-cell systems, and that the terminology of the past is incorrect. The diffuse histologic cytologic types, such as the histiocytic and poorly differentiated lymphocytic types of RAPPAPORT [36], are heterogeneous and include both T- and B-cell types.

The morphologic features of the lymphomas for the most part are predictive of their T- and B-cell nature, if the histologic material is optimal and the observer is experienced.

The results also indicate that the lymphomas can now be approached as neoplasms of the immune system in a manner similar to the investigation of immune defects. This observation is of particular importance in immunoblastic sarcoma, the disorder we described developing in a variety of abnormal immune states, such as Sjögren's disease, immunoblastic lymphadenopathy [29], the immune suppressed graft rejection patient, systemic lupus erythematous, α-chain disease, and the senescent state [25, 26, 27]. It appears that these abnormal immune disorders are predisposed to the development of lymphomas and provide a basis for investigating the abnormality of the control mechanism of the switch on (derepression) of the lymphocyte transformation mechanism that allows the development of this lymphoma. The process described by MATHÉ et al. [34] under the term immunoblastic lymphosarcoma [34] is in our view not immunoblastic sarcoma. Morphologically, it appears to relate to the small noncleaved FCC type. It is a smaller cell and approaches the Burkitt cell in morphologic appearance. It often develops leukemic manifestations, a feature essentially lacking in immunoblastic sarcoma in our experience.

The major goal of our multiparameter studies, the redefinition of the malignant lymphomas as neoplasms of the immune system that involve the T- and B-cell systems, has been fulfilled. Only the characterization of the function and cell kinetics of the T- and B-cell subtypes remain to be determined. The realization of the major goal and the associated demonstration of the heterogeneity of the cytologic types of the past clearly indicate that the time has come to change to a modern functional and immunologic classification of the malignant lymphomas.

Heterogeneity of the Cytologic Types of the Past and Homogeneity of the Immunologic Cytologic Types of the Future

It is now readily apparent from a comparison of our classification with those of the past that all of the previous diffuse cytologic types whether of small, intermediate, or large cell types are heterogeneous. The recently proposed classifications [3, 10, 13], with the exception of the Kiel classification [13], are modifications of the RAPPAPORT classification [36]. The diffuse types are to varying extents heterogeneous. The cytologic types of the Kiel classification have been developed on a conceptual basis similar to our own but lack the recognition of T- and B-cell types. Until a comparative study is accomplished using both classifications on a similar population, it is uncertain whether the cytologic types of the Kiel classification and our own are identical. Immunoblastic sarcoma, as used in the Kiel classification, appears to include almost all of the large cell types, judging from its high frequency in the recent case series of LENNERT et al. [22], and it therefore does not appear to be equivalent to our definition of immunoblastic sarcoma. The data presented by LENNERT elsewhere at this meeting has attempted to correct the difference.

Table 2. Heterogeneity of histiocytic lymphoma of RAPPAPORT [36]. Comparison of histologic types

	LUKES and COLLINS
Histiocytic RAPPAPORT [36]	Large cleaved FCC
	Large noncleaved FCC
	IBS—B cell
	IBS—T cell
	Histiocytic

FCC = follicular center cell
IBS = immunoblastic sarcoma

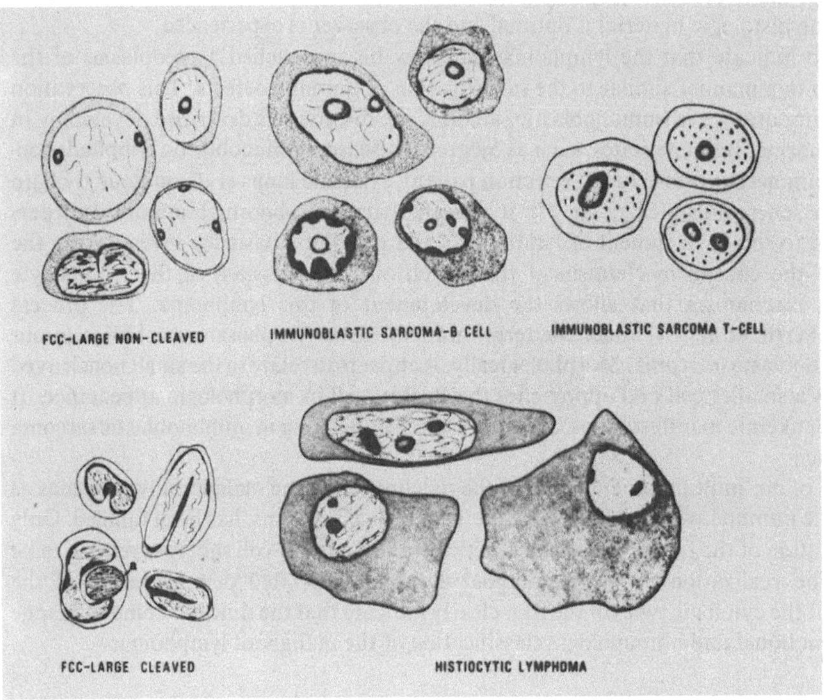

Fig. 2. Heterogeneity of histiocytic lymphoma (RAPPAPORT)

The diffuse histiocytic type of RAPPAPORT [36] exemplifies the heterogeneity of all the cytologic types of lymphoma of the past. Identification of the histiocytic type has been based essentially on cell size and therefore includes all of our large cell types. When compared with our cytologic types as shown in Table 2, it includes the large cleaved, the large noncleaved FCC types, along with IBS-B cell, IBS-T cell, and the rare true histiocytic type. The morphologic features of these cytologic types are shown in Figure 2, using camera lucida studies of photomicrographs of cases characterized by our multiparameter studies. The similar size range is readily apparent in all types, although the large cleaved cell type is the smallest. It frequently exhibits, however, a wide range in cell size and an extreme irregularity in nuclear configuration, and as a result is usually included in the histiocytic type of RAPPAPORT [36]. The diversity of cell types included in the histiocytic type of RAPPAPORT [36] may account for the variability in therapeutic responsiveness. It also seems likely that the clinical expressions of these disorders may vary widely. At present, we are attempting to collect clinical information and survival data on the individual cytologic types previously included in the histiocytic types of RAPPAPORT [36] in an attempt to answer these important questions regarding clinical expression and therapeutic responsiveness. Our preliminary studies on cell kinetics also suggest that there may be considerable differences in their proliferative characteristics.

Childhood ALL has also been acknowledged to be heterogeneous [16] and has included the T- and B-cell types as well as the so-called null cell or unmarked cell. Nevertheless, this heterogeneous disorder has been used as a demonstration of the remarkable improvement in effectiveness of chemotherapy. Lost within the ALL group, however, are the T- and B-cell types that respond poorly to ALL therapy and usually relapse within six months with few individuals surviving, in our experience, beyond 1 year [38]. It is estimated that approximately

20%–25% of ALL are of T-cell type and less than 5% are of B-cell type. Since these two groups represent a small component, the ineffective therapy for the T- and B-cell types has been obscured in the heterogeneous ALL group. It seems likely that the therapeutic regimen for ALL may be excessive for good responders, the U-cell group, and inappropriate for the T- and B-cell types. The lack of appreciation of the lymphoma-leukemia nature of the T- and B-cell types has also distorted the composition of case series of ALL, since the T- and B-cell types are included in ALL if the marrow is involved at initial presentation and excluded if uninvolved. Because of the lymphoma-leukemic character of the convoluted T cell and the small noncleaved FCC (B cell), they have been included in an inconsistent fashion in ALL, and in my view they must be separated consistently from ALL. From therapeutic and clinical considerations, it appears that the term acute lymphocytic leukemia should be restricted to the U-cell type that according to SCHLOSSMAN et al. [37] and WINCHESTER et al. [43] may prove to be a special B-cell type. The term ALL as used in the past is an excellent example of the problem of the heterogeneous types. It demonstrates the importance of distinguishing homogeneous cytologic types with uniform morphologic, cytochemical, and immunologic characteristics. Only when homogeneous cytologic types are identified will the effective definition of their clinical expressions and therapeutic responsiveness of the disease be achieved. The use of a new functional classification and cytologic types seems initially difficult, but it permits the identification of homogeneous cytologic types with uniform clinical features. In addition, the future will unquestionably bring more helpful techniques, such as highly specific antisera that will ultimately permit the achievement of both precision and reproducibility in the widespread application of the immunologic approach.

Conclusions

1. The malignant lymphomas of the past were all proposed long before modern developments in immunology and do not bear any relationship to our modern understanding of immunology.

2. Our recently proposed functional approach to the malignant lymphomas as neoplasms of the immune system relates these disorders to the T- and B-cell systems and alterations in lymphocyte transformation. The cytologic types of our new classification attempt to identify specific functional subtypes of the T- and B-cell systems as defective expressions of their normal counterparts.

3. Our multiparameter studies on over 384 cases of non-Hodgkin's lymphomas using special morphology, cytochemistry, immunologic surface markers, electron microscopy, and immunoperoxidase studies of cytoplasmic immunoglobulin and muramidase, and those of others have demonstrated that the malignant lymphomas for the most part mark as T- or B-cell types with the exception of a rare lymphoma of true histiocytic type and the unmarked portion of acute lymphocytic leukemia of childhood.

4. The results of the multiparameter studies confirm our original prediction that the cytologic types of the past were heterogeneous. The other recently proposed classifications, with the exception of the Kiel classification, are modifications of the RAPPAPORT classification and consist of heterogeneous cytologic types. The basic concept of the Kiel classification is similar to our approach, but the degree of identity of its cytologic types with our types is uncertain.

5. Each of the diffuse histologic types of RAPPAPORT appears to be heterogeneous and includes a number of T- and B-cytologic subtypes. The diffuse histiocytic type encompasses the five large cytologic types of our classification, the immunoblastic sarcomas of both T- and B-cell types, the large cleaved and large noncleaved FCC types, and the rare true histiocytic

lymphoma. The poorly differentiated lymphocytic type similarly includes four medium size types of T- and B-cell types, and even the diffuse well-differentiated lymphocytic type includes three cytologic types. The undifferentiated and mixed types are applied in a variable fashion, and it is difficult to forecast the cytologic types included.

6. The heterogeneity of the cytologic types of the past unquestionably account for much of the variability of their clinical expressions and therapeutic responsiveness. Childhood ALL is a dramatic example of the heterogeneity of the past. It includes the convoluted T cell, the diffuse small noncleaved FCC type, a B cell, and the U cell, which includes the so-called null cell type. This heterogeneity obscures the recognition of poorly responding T- and B-cell types and interferes with the effective design and evaluation of therapeutic regimens. It is proposed that these disorders be designated separately as the above types.

7. The cytologic types of our functional approach recognized by morphologic features and confirmed by multiparameter studies permit the identification of homogeneous cytologic proliferations and assure a greater uniformity of biologic behavior, clinical expression, and prediction of therapeutic responsiveness. As a result, a number of distinctive clinical, morphologic, and immunologic entities are merging, including the convoluted T cell, the immunoblastic sarcoma of T- and B-cell type, and the FCC types.

8. The effective identification of the cytologic types of malignant lymphoma according to the T- and B-cell systems will in the future necessitate greater care in the collection of and processing of biopsy material for more ideal diagnostic histologic material and considerable experience in the interpretation of their complex morphologic expressions. A limited number of special techniques will be required for proper evaluation and diagnosis, such as the E-rosettes for ALL and immunoblastic sarcoma of T cells. The immunoperoxidase studies for cytoplasmic immunoglobulin on paraffin sections will be invaluable in the evaluation of the diffuse types, including those presently in the histiocytic type of Rappaport. The cytochemical procedure, α-naphthyl butyrate for the histiocyte or the immunoperoxidase stain for muramidase, will be required for the identification of the true histiocytic lymphoma.

9. The future development of greater precision in cytologic identification and the resultant characterization of the functional expressions of the subtypes of the T- and B-cell systems will ultimately lead to improvement in the understanding of their basic biology and permit the redesign of the biologic approaches to therapy.

Acknowledgements

This investigation has been supported in part by National Institutes of Health training grant No. CA 19449-02 and the Beaumont Foundation.

References

1. Aisenberg, A. C., Long, J. C.: Lymphocyte surface characteristics in malignant lymphoma. Am. J. Med. *58*, 300–306 (1975).
2. Barcos, M. P., Lukes, R. J.: Malignant lymphoma of convoluted lymphocytes: A new entity of possible T-cell type. In: Conflicts in Childhood Cancer. Sinks, L. F, Godden, J. E. (eds.) New York: Alan R. Liss 1975, p. 147.
3. Bennett, M. H., Farrer-Brown, G., Henry, K., Jelliffe, A. M.: Classification of non-Hodgkin's lymphomas. Lancet *1974 II*, 405 (Letters).

4. BERARD, C. W., GALLO, R. C., JAFFE, E., GREEN, I., DEVITA, V. T.: Current concepts of leukemia and lymphoma: Etiology, pathogenesis and therapy. Ann. Intern. Med. *85*, 351–366 (1976).
5. BRAYLAN, R. C., JAFFE, E. S., BERARD, C. W.: Malignant lymphomas: current classification and new observations. In: Hematologic and Lymphoid Pathology Decennial 1966–1975. SOMMERS, S. C. (ed.) New York: Appleton-Century-Crofts 1975.
6. BROUET, J., FLANDRIN, G., SELIGMANN, M.: Thymus-derived nature of the proliferating cells in Sézary's syndrome. N. Engl. J. Med. *289*, 341–344 (1973).
7. BROUET, J., LABAUME, S., SELIGMANN, M.: Evaluation of T and B lymphocyte membrane markers in human non-Hodgkin's malignant lymphomas. Br. J. Cancer *31*, suppl. II, 121–127 (1975).
8. CATOVSKY, D., GALETTO, J., OKOS, A., MILLIANI, E., GALTON, D. A. G.: Cytochemical profile of B and T leukaemic lymphocytes with special reference to acute lymphoblastic leukaemia. J. Clin. Pathol. *27*, 767–771 (1974).
9. DAVEY, F. R., GOLDBERG, J., STOCKMAN, J., GOTTLIEB, A. J.: Immunologic and cytochemical cell markers in non-Hodgkin's lymphomas. Lab. Invest. *35*, 430–438 (1976).
10. DORFMAN, R. F.: Classification of non-Hodgkin's lymphomas. Lancet *1974 I*, 1295 (Letters).
11. FUKS, Z., STROBER, S., KAPLAN, H. S.: Interaction between serum factors and T lymphocytes in Hodgkin's disease. Use as a diagnostic test. N. Engl. J. Med. *295*, 1273–1278 (1976).
12. GAHL-PECZALSKA, K. J., BLOOMFIELD, C. D., COCCIA, P. F., SOSIN, H., BRUNNING, R. D., KERSEY, J. H.: B and T cell lymphomas. Am. J. Med. *59*, 674–685 (1975).
13. GERHARD-MARCHANT, R., HAMLIN, I., LENNERT, K., RILKE, F., STANSFIELD, A. G., VAN UNNIK, J. A. M.: Classification of non-Hodgkin's lymphomas. Lancet *1974 II*, 405 (Letters).
14. GLICK, A. D., LEECH, J. H., WALDRON, J. A., FLEXNDER, J. M., HORN, R. G., COLLINS, R. D.: Malignant lymphomas of follicular center cell origin in man. II. Ultrastructural and cytochemical studies. J. Natl. Cancer Inst. *54*, 23–36 (1975).
15. GREEN, I., JAFFE, E., SHEVACH, E. M., EDELSON, R. L., FRANK, M. M., BERARD, C. W.: Determination of the origin of malignant reticular cells by the use of surface membrane markers. In: The Reticuloendothelial System, International Academy of Pathology Monograph No. 16. REBECK, BERARD, ABELL (eds.). Baltimore: Williams & Wilkins 1975, p. 282.
16. HAEGERT, D. G., STUART, J., SMITH, J. L.: Acute lymphoblastic leukaemia: A heterogeneous disease. Br. Med. J. *1975/II*, 312–314.
17. JAFFE, E. S., SHEVACH, E. M., FRANK, M. M., BERARD, C. W., GREEN, I.: Nodular lymphoma—evidence for origin from follicular B lymphocytes. N. Engl. J. Med. *290*, 813–819 (1974).
18. KAPLAN, H. S.: Immunological abnormalities of Hodgkin's disease. Am. J. Pathol. (in press).
19. KOJIMA, M., TSUNODA, R.: Localization of immunoglobulins in germinal centers of human tonsils. In: The Reticuloendothelial System in Health and Disease: Immunologic and Pathologic Aspects. FRIEDMAN, H. et al. (eds.) New York: Plenum 1976, p. 77.
20. LEECH, J., GLICK, A., HORN, R., COLLINS, R.: Immunologic, histochemical and ultrastructural studies of malignant lymphomas presumed to be of follicular center cell origin. J. Natl. Cancer Inst. *54*, 11–21 (1975).
21. LENNERT, K., MESTDAGH, J.: Lymphogranulomatosen mit konstant hohem epitheloidzellgehalt. Virchows Arch. [Pathol. Anat.] *344*, 1–20 (1968).
22. LENNERT, K., MOHRI, N., STEIN, H., KAISERLING, E.: Histopathology of malignant lymphomas. Br. J. Haematol. *31*, 193–203 (1975).
23. LEVINE, G. D., DORFMAN, R. F.: Nodular lymphoma: An ultrastructural study of its relationship to germinal centers and a correlation of light and electron microscopic findings. Cancer *35*, 148–164 (1975).
24. LUKES, R. J., COLLINS, R. D.: New observations on follicular lymphoma. In: GANN Monograph on Cancer Research 15, Malignant Diseases of the Hematopoietic System. AKAZAKI, K. et al. (eds.) Baltimore-London-Tokyo: University Park Press 1973, p. 209.
25. LUKES, R. J., COLLINS, R. D.: Immunologic characterization of human malignant lymphomas. Cancer *34*, 1488–1503 (1974a).
26. LUKES, R. J., COLLINS, R. D.: A functional approach to the classification of malignant lymphoma. Recent Results Cancer Res. *46*, 18–30 (1974b).
27. LUKES, R. J., COLLINS, R. D.: New approaches to the classification of the lymphomata. Br. J. Cancer *31*, suppl. II, 1–28 (1975).
28. LUKES, R. J., COLLINS, R. D.: The Lukes-Collins classification and its significance. Conference on The Non-Hodgkin's Lymphomas, San Francisco, September 30–October 2, 1976. In: Cancer Treatment Reports *61*, 971–979, 1977.
29. LUKES, R. J., TINDLE, B. H.: Immunoblastic lymphadenopathy. A hyperimmune entity resembling Hodgkin's disease. N. Engl. J. Med. *292*, 1–8 (1975).
30. LUKES, R. J., BUTLER, J. J., HICKS, E. B.: Natural history of Hodgkin's disease as related to its pathologic picture. Cancer *19*, 317–344 (1966a).

31. Lukes, R. J., Craver, L. L., Hall, T. C., Rappaport, H., Ruben, P.: Hodgkin's disease, report of Nomenclature Committee. Cancer Res. *26*, 1311 (1966b).
32. Lukes, R. J., Tindle, B. H., Parker, J. W.: Reed-Sternberg-like cells in infectious mononucleosis. Lancet *1969 II*, 1003–1004.
33. Lutzner, M., Edelson, R., Schein, P., Green, I., Kirkpatrick, C., Ahmed, A.: Cutaneous T cell lymphoma: The Sézary syndrome, mycosis fungoides and related disorders. Ann. Intern. Med. *85*, 534–552 (1975).
34. Mathé, G., Belpomme, D., Dantchev, D., Khalil, A., Afifi, A. M., Taleb, N., Pouillart, P., Schwarzenberg, L., Hayat, M., De Vassal, F., Jasmin, C., Misset, J. L., Musset, M.: Immunoblastic lymphosarcoma, a cytological and clinical entity? Biomedicine *22*, 473–488 (1975).
35. Nathwani, B. N., Kim, H., Rappaport, H.: Malignant lymphoma, lymphoblastic. Cancer *38*, 964–983 (1976).
36. Rappaport, H.: Tumors of hematopoietic system. In: Atlas of Tumor Pathology, sect. III, fasc. 8. Washington, D.C.: Armed Forces Institute of Pathology 1966.
37. Schlossman, S. F., Chess, L., Humphreys, R. E., Strominger, J. L.: Distribution of Ia-like molecules on the surface of normal and leukemic human cells. Proc. Natl. Acad. Sci. U.S.A. *73*, 1288–1292 (1976).
38. Schneider, B. K., Higgins, G. R., Swanson, V., Isaacs, H., Tindle, B. H., Lukes, R. J.: Malignant lymphomas of childhood. Submitted for publication.
39. Stein, H., Peterson, N., Gaedicke, G., Lennert, K., Landberg, C.: Lymphoblastic lymphoma of convoluted or acid phosphatase type—A tumor of T precursor cells. Int. J. Cancer *17*, 292–295 (1976).
40. Taylor, C. R.: An immunohistological study of follicular lymphoma, reticulum cell sarcoma and Hodgkin's disease. Eur. J. Cancer *12*, 61–75 (1976).
41. Tindle, B. H., Parker, J. W., Lukes, R. J.: "Reed-Sternberg Cells" in infectious mononucleosis? Am. J. Clin. Pathol. *58*, 607–617 (1972).
42. Williams, A. H., Taylor, C. R., Higgins, G. R., Quinn, J. J., Schneider, B. K., Swanson, V., Parker, J. W., Pattengale, P. K., Chandor, S. B., Powars, D., Lincoln, T. L., Tindle, B. H., Lukes, R. J.: Childhood leukemia and lymphoma. I. Correlation of morphology and functional studies. Submitted for publication.
43. Winchester, R. J., Fu, S. M., Wernet, P., Kunkel, H. G., Dupont, B., Jersild, C.: Recognition by pregnancy serums of non-HL-A alloantigens selectively expressed on B lymphocytes. J. Exp. Med. *141*, 924–929 (1975).
44. Yam, L. T., Li, C. Y., Crosby, W. H.: Cytochemical identification of monocytes and granulocytes. Am. J. Clin. Pathol. *55*, 283–290 (1971).

Personal Points of View on the Kiel Classification[1]

K. LENNERT and H. STEIN

In recent years, numerous research groups in all parts of the world have been working on the immunologic definition of lymphomas, e.g., the groups led by AISENBERG in Boston, BERARD in Bethesda, LUKES and COLLINS in Los Angeles and Nashville, and SELIGMANN in Paris, to mention only a few. They have obtained remarkably similar results that also agree with our findings, at least by extrapolation, if not directly. It is not possible to give a detailed report on the results of these immunologic studies here. We shall confine this presentation to the *morphologic* entities and specify the lymphomas that can now be grouped into the B- or T-cell system by means of subtle morphologic analysis *alone*, i.e., the lymphomas that proved, *without exception*, to be B- or T-cell lymphomas in immunologic studies.

At this point, we should define the expression "subtle morphologic analysis." What we mean is the histologic study of biopsies that have been well fixed, embedded carefully in paraffin, and stained by hematologic techniques—we recommend a high-quality Giemsa stain. In some cases, the additional study of imprints with appropriate hematologic stains (Pappenheim or Giemsa) and with a few cytochemical reactions, especially acid phosphatase and nonspecific esterase, is indispensable.

The results of our subtle morphologic analyses of the immunologically defined types of lymphomas are given in Tables 1 and 2. The data apply to our second series of non-Hodgkin's lymphomas, which we collected between October 1973 and December 1976 and studied on the basis of our previous immunologic experience. If we compare these data with those of our earlier series [7], we find a remarkable similarity: in the first series the low-grade malignant lymphomas made up 70%, in the second series 72%; correspondingly, 30% and 28%, respectively, were high-grade malignant lymphomas. The data on the various types of low-grade malignant lymphomas also coincide. We think this is an indication of the reproducibility of our classification. In contrast, a few shifts are evident in the group of high-grade malignant lymphomas. First, a considerable number (about 4%) of cases have been taken out of the group of immunoblastic lymphomas and put into the group of centroblastic lymphomas. Our immunologic studies showed that cells from some tumors that were originally classified as immunoblastic lymphomas formed rosettes with EAC (complexes composed of sheep erythrocytes coated with antierythrocyte antibody of the IgM-type and with mouse complement). These complement receptor-positive lymphomas also contained centroblasts and anaplastic centrocytes as well as immunoblasts. Therefore, we now interpret such tumors as (polymorphic) centroblastic lymphomas. A second significant shift is the decrease in the number of unclassified lymphoblastic lymphomas in favor of the convoluted cell type and, to a lesser extent, the Burkitt type. We found about 3.8% definite and 2.0% probable cases of the convoluted cell type. This increase was due particularly to the routine use of the acid phosphatase reaction in imprints or blood smears. In the 2.0% probable cases it was not possible to perform the acid phosphatase reaction.

---

1 This work was supported by the Deutsche Forschungsgemeinschaft, SFB 111/C7.

Table 1. Incidence of different types of non-Hodgkin's lymphoma in two series. The cases in the first series were collected between July 1965 and September 1973, and those in the second series between October 1973 and December 1976, at the Lymph Node Registry in Kiel

	July '65–Sept. '73 n=841[a] (%)			Oct. '73–Dec. '76 n=1997[a] (%)		
M.L. lymphocytic	22.7			20.7		
B-CLL		20.9			17.3	
T-CLL		—			0.25	
Prolymphocytic leukemia		—			0.05	
Hairy cell leukemia		0.4			1.0	
Mycosis fungoides and Sézary's syndrome		1.4	~70		0.8	~72
T-zone lymphoma		—			1.3	
M.L. lymphoplasmacytic/-cytoid (LP immunocytoma)	16.2			17.8		
M.L. plasmacytic	0.8			0.8		
M.L. centrocytic	8.6			10.0		
M.L. centroblastic/centrocytic	21.6			22.8		
M.L. centroblastic	>1.2			5.5		
M.L. lymphoblastic	12.7			12.1		
Burkitt type		0.7			2.1	
Convoluted cell type			~30			~28
(acid phosphatase type)		0.8			3.8+2.0	
Unclassified		11.2			4.2	
M.L. immunoblastic	<15.9			10.3		
Unclassifiable[a]	(9.9)			(9.8)		

[a] n = classified cases = 100%. The percentage of unclassifiable cases is based on the total number of classified and unclassified cases.

It was astonishing, but at the same time instructive, that the proportion of unclassifiable non-Hodgkin's lymphomas was practically the same, namely, about 10%, in both series. Cases were unclassifiable for several reasons: 1) the slides were of poor technical quality, 2) there were no slides that could be evaluated with cytologic and cytochemical methods, and 3) our knowledge was insufficient. We estimate that our unclassifiable cases are divided about equally among these three categories. Our classification provides a possibility, however, for making the problem tolerable to the clinician; as a rule, it is possible to say whether a given malignant lymphoma is of low- or high-grade malignancy. This is in most cases sufficient for choosing the right therapy.

Let us turn to the 1997 classified lymphomas of the second series and ask how many of them can be regarded as B- or T-cell lymphomas (Table 2). The first notable fact is that virtually all low-grade malignant lymphomas can be identified as B- or T-cell neoplasms by morphologic methods alone. We would like to demonstrate this with a few examples. Chronic lymphocytic leukemia of the B-type (B-CLL) is easy to recognize histologically, especially because of the pseudofollicular proliferation centers, which are never seen in T-CLL. T-CLL can be diagnosed by the following histologic, cytologic, and cytochemical criteria. Histologically, the most prominent feature is the great increase in typical or atypical epithelioid venules, which should immediately lead one to suspect T-CLL when seen with a monotonous lymphocytic infiltration. This suspicion is strengthened by the demonstration of medium-sized convoluted lymphocytes. Because these cells occur in small numbers, they must be looked for by oil immersion, but they are easier to demonstrate in blood smears or imprints. In a number of cases, the lymphocytes show azurophil granules [3], which do not occur in B-lymphocytic leukemias. In T-CLL of

Table 2. Identification of non-Hodgkin's lymphomas as B- or T-cell-derived by means of morphologic methods alone (histology, cytology, cytochemistry). Morphologically unclassifiable cases (9.8%) are not included

		%	B	T	?/null[a]
M.L. lymphocytic					
B-CLL		17.3	17.3		
T-CLL		0.25		0.25	
Prolymphocytic leukemia		0.05	0.05		
Hairy cell leukemia		1.0	1.0		
Mycosis fungoides and Sézary's syndrome		0.8		0.8	
T-zone lymphoma	100%	1.3		1.3	
M.L. lymphoplasmactytic/-cytoid (LP immunocytoma)		17.8	17.8		
M.L. plasmacytic		0.8	0.8		
M.L. centrocytic		10.0	10.0		
M.L. centroblastic/centrocytic		22.8	22.8		
Low-grade malignant lymphomas		72.10	69.75	2.35	—
M.L. centroblastic		5.5	5.5		
M.L. lymphoblastic					
Burkitt type		2.1	2.1		
Convoluted cell type (acid phosphatase type)	~50%	3.8+2.0[b]		3.8	2.0[b]
Unclassified		4.2			4.2
M.L. immunoblastic		10.3	~2.0		~8.3
High-grade malignant lymphomas		27.9	9.6	3.8	14.5
			79.35	6.15	
All malignant lymphomas			85.5		14.5

[a] Non-B/non-T and undefinable cases. [b] Probable cases.

nonazurophilic type, most of the leukemic lymphocytes and the convoluted cells contain small clumps of acid phosphatase, acid nonspecific esterase, and β-glucuronidase activity. Another example of a T-cell neoplasm is T-zone lymphoma, in which all structural elements of T-regions are present, namely, T-lymphocytes, epithelioid venules, interdigitating reticulum cells, and reticulin fibers. In T-zone lymphoma, the 5-nucleotidase reaction is negative in the neoplastic T-regions, whereas it is positive in the remaining nonneoplastic B-regions.

We do not need to provide the participants of this conference with proof that lymphomas that contain plasma cells, i.e., lymphoplasmacytic/-cytoid lymphoma (LP immunocytoma) and plasmacytoma, should be regarded as B-cell neoplasms. The same applies to the germinal center cell tumors, which have been clearly identified as B-cell tumors, because the cells formed EAC-rosettes and revealed surface immunoglobulin. This is especially true for diffuse centrocytic lymphoma, as known since the studies of AISENBERG et al. [1, 2] and LEECH et al. [6]. If we classify all low-grade malignant lymphomas according to their derivation from the B- or T-cell series and look at them in relation to all malignant lymphomas, we find that almost 70% should be regarded as B-cell neoplasms, whereas only 2.35% may be classified as T-cell lymphomas. Taking the group of low-grade lymphomas alone, 96.74% are B-cell tumors and 3.26% are T-cell tumors.

The classification of high-grade malignant lymphomas is more difficult (Table 2). We were able to assign only about 50% of our cases to the B- or T-cell series. Centroblastic lymphoma and lymphoblastic lymphoma of the Burkitt type indisputably belong to the B-cell series. About 20% of the immunoblastic lymphomas are recognizable by light microscopy as B-cell derivatives because of signs of plasmablastic or plasmacytic differentiation. Unfortunately, the rest can only be identified as derived from B- or T- (or null) cells by means of immunologic techniques. Lymphoblastic lymphoma of the convoluted cell type has been proved to be a T-cell lymphoma by numerous investigators. We found not only E-rosettes, but often EAC/E- (mixed) rosettes [11]. This lymphoma cannot always be diagnosed on histologic sections with sufficient certainty, since the nuclear convolutions are often scarce and often simulated because of artifactual shrinkage. We therefore need imprints in order to make a definite diagnosis of this type of lymphoblastic lymphoma: a focally positive acid phosphatase reaction confirms the diagnosis. We have mentioned this finding many times since the lymphoma conference in Chicago in 1973. CATOVSKY et al. [4] and others [5] have confirmed it in T-lymphoblastic leukemias. We usually obtained the same or similar results with the acid nonspecific esterase reaction [8]. Occasionally, however, the acid esterase reaction is negative (Table 3), as was recently shown

Table 3. Comparison of acid phosphatase and acid nonspecific esterase reactions in imprints and smears of M.L. lymphoblastic, convoluted cell type (acid phosphatase type)

	Lymph node imprints	Blood smears	Bone marrow smears	Total
Acid phosph. ≈ acid est.	3	2	—	5
Acid phosph. > acid est.	4	3	1	8
Acid phosph. +/− acid est.	2	2	—	4
Acid phosph. < acid est.	3	1	1	5
Acid phosph. −/+ acid est.	—	—	—	—
Total	12	8	2	22

Study performed by SUGIYAMA.

by SUGIYAMA in our laboratory. We have found indications that there are also T-lymphoblastic lymphomas without nuclear convolutions (nonconvoluted lymphoblastic lymphoma of NATHWANI et al. [9]). In one such case, we found a strong, focal acid nonspecific esterase reaction. The histologically unclassified lymphoblastic lymphomas must be characterized by means of immunologic techniques. Even then, however, a large number of tumors do not show any immunologic markers and are therefore called null lymphoblastic lymphomas.

If we consider all the high-grade malignant lymphomas that we have been able to classify so far, we find that there are more T-cell-derived lymphomas, i.e., more than 13.6%, and fewer B-cell-derived lymphomas (34.4%) than in the group of low-grade malignant lymphomas. About 50% of the high-grade malignant lymphomas in our series have not been classified. We assume that it would be possible to characterize a large number of them as B- or T-cell-derived by means of immunologic techniques, although not by morphologic methods. The rest of the cases would not show any immunologic markers (null cell lymphomas).

When we summed up all our morphologically classified cases, 79% were B-cell lymphomas and 6% were T-cell lymphomas, whereas 14% could not be identified as B- or T-cell lymphomas. At least one third of them should be null cell lymphomas. Taking the unclassified lymphomas into consideration, we estimate that *in our material* about 85% of the lymphomas are B-cell-derived and probably not more than 10% are T-cell-derived, whereas less than 5% belong to the null cell category.

For the last year, we have been using the immunoperoxidase technique of TAYLOR [12] for the further identification of lymphomas in paraffin sections. With this technique, it is often possible to clearly identify intracytoplasmic immunoglobulin and to determine mono- or polyclonality. The results of the studies we have performed with FUCHS, U., MÜLLER-

Table 4. Monoclonal increase in immunoglobulin in the three subtypes of LP immunocytoma demonstrated by means of TAYLOR's immunoperoxidase technique

	IgM		IgG		IgA		Light chains		Total	
	κ	λ	κ	λ	κ	λ	κ	λ	κ	λ
Lymphoplasmacytoid	16	4	1	—	1	—	4	—	22	4
Lymphoplasmacytic	4	4	2	1	—	—	—	—	6	5
Polymorphic	6	4	—	1	—	—	—	1	6	6
All subtypes	26	12	3	2	1	—	4	1	34	15
	38		5		1		5		49	

Study performed with FUCHS, U. MÜLLER-HERMELINK, and PAPADIMITRIOU.

HERMELINK, and PAPADIMITRIOU on LP immunocytoma are shown in Table 4. Most immunocytomas show monoclonal IgM synthesis. κ-chains are about twice as common as λ-chains. In a few cases, the identification of heavy chains was not successful, probably for technical reasons. With this method, it is possible to distinguish monoclonally positive immunocytomas from B-CLL. B-CLL is negative or occasionally contains some nonneoplastic plasma cells with polyclonal immunoglobulin.

We are now in the process of analyzing immunoblastic lymphomas by means of the immunoperoxidase technique, but we are not yet able to state the percentages of monoclonally positive cases. We are convinced that the immunoperoxidase technique, in spite of the difficulties in the preparation of the slides and evaluation of the results, is another useful weapon in the arsenal of methods available to us for the analysis of paraffin sections.

Many people say that the Kiel classification is too complicated and more difficult to reproduce than other classifications. This motivated VAN UNNIK to test the reproducibility of the classification of RAPPAPORT, that of LUKES and COLLINS, and the Kiel classification. The participants in this study were Professor Dr. BUYSSENS, Antwerpen, Dr. VAN HEERDE, Amsterdam, and Dr. HEIMAN, Brussels. They reevaluated 50 cases of the European Lymphoma Club series that the members of the Club had already classified by consensus according to the three classifications. The selected cases were of more than average difficulty. Cytologically, six lymphoma groups were distinguished according to the RAPPAPORT classification. There were nine types of lymphoma according to the LUKES and the Kiel classifications. The agreement on diagnosis between the three observers and the European Lymphoma Club is shown in Table 5.

Table 5. Number of cases (out of 50) in which the diagnosis of the three observers was in agreement with that of the members of the European Lymphoma Club

Observer	Classification					
	RAPPAPORT		LUKES		Kiel	
I	32	97	23	87	30	99
II	30		32		36	
III	35		32		33	

Data provided by VAN UNNIK.

The results for the three classifications were quite close. Although the differences were not significant, one can at least say that the results for the Kiel classification were not worse than those for the other two classifications—they were even slightly better, even though the Kiel classification contains nine main types of lymphoma, as does the LUKES classification, whereas the RAPPAPORT classification contains only six entities.

Mr. HART, statistician of the Netherlands Cancer Institute in Amsterdam, computed the "measure of agreement" (K-value; see Table 6) of these data. According to Mr. HART, the Kiel classification did significantly better than the other two classifications. We realize that these results are preliminary and have to be substantiated in a larger series of unselected cases. Nevertheless, they do show that the Kiel classification can be learned and that it is at least not more difficult to reproduce than the classifications of RAPPAPORT and LUKES.

Table 6. Measure of agreement of the three observers' diagnoses with the diagnoses by the European Lymphoma Club of 50 cases of malignant lymphoma according to three classifications

Observer	Classification					
	RAPPAPORT		LUKES		Kiel	
I	0.52		0.37		0.54	
II	0.48	0.53	0.58	0.50	0.67	0.60
III	0.59		0.56		0.59	

Data provided by VAN UNNIK.

Conclusions

We are not here to defend the Kiel classification. If it is scientifically correct, it will find its own way. If it is incorrect, it does not deserve anything more than to be forgotten. Since we are convinced that scientific correctness will sooner or later acquire clinical relevance, we believe that the overestimation of clinical relevance at the cost of scientific correctness is an unjustifiable simplification, which, in the long run, will not serve our patients. It has already been shown, however, that the Kiel classification is of great clinical relevance in a retrospective study by BRITTINGER et al. of cases provided by the Kiel Lymphoma Study Group (see BRITTINGER et al. in this volume).

References

1. AISENBERG, A. C., BLOCH, K. J., LONG, J. C.: Cell-surface immunoglobulins in chronic lymphocytic leukemia and allied disorders. Am. J. Med. *55*, 184–191 (1973).
2. AISENBERG, A. C., LONG, J. C.: Lymphocyte surface characteristics in malignant lymphoma. Am. J. Med. *58*, 300–306 (1975).
3. BROUET, J.-C., FLANDRIN, G., SASPORTES, M., PREUD'HOMME, J.-L., SELIGMANN, M.: Chronic lymphocytic leukaemia of T-cell origin. Immunological and clinical evaluation in eleven patients. Lancet *II*, 890–893, 1975.
4. CATOVSKY, D., GALETTO, J., OKOS, A., MILIANI, E., GALTON, D. A. G.: Cytochemical profile of B and T leukaemic lymphocytes with special reference to acute lymphoblastic leukaemia. J. Clin. Pathol. *27*, 767–771 (1974).
5. LANDBECK, G., GAEDICKE, G., WINKLER, K., STEIN, H.: Besonderheiten der malignen Lymphome im Kindesalter. In: Maligne Lymphome und Monoklonale Gammopathien. Hämatologie und Bluttransfusion. LÖFFLER, H. (ed.). München: J. F. Lehmanns Verlag Vol. XVIII pp. 225–235 (1976).

6. Leech, J. H., Glick, A.D., Waldron, J. A., Flexner, J. M., Horn, R. G., Collins, R. D.: Malignant lymphomas of follicular center cell origin in man. I. Immunologic studies. J. Natl. Cancer Inst. *54*, 11–21 (1975).
7. Lennert, K., Mohri, N., Stein, H., Kaiserling, E.: The histopathology of malignant lymphoma. Br. J. Haematol. *31* (suppl.), 193–203 (1975).
8. Mueller, J., Brun del Re, G., Buerki, H., Keller, H.-U., Hess, M. W., Cottier, H.: Nonspecific esterase activity: A criterion for differentiation of T and B lymphocytes in mouse lymph nodes. Eur. J. Immunol. *5*, 270–274 (1975).
9. Nathwani, B. N., Kim, H., Rappaport, H.: Malignant lymphoma, lymphoblastic. Cancer *38*, 964–983 (1976).
10. Ritter, J., Gaedicke, G., Winkler, K., Beckmann, H., Landbeck, G.: Possible T-cell origin of lymphoblasts in acid-phosphatase-positive acute lymphatic leukaemia. Lancet *II*, 75, 1975.
11. Stein, H., Petersen, N., Gaedicke, G., Lennert, K., Landbeck, G.: Lymphoblastic lymphoma of convoluted or acid phosphatase type—a tumor of T precursor cells. Int. J. Cancer *17*, 292–295 (1976).
12. Taylor, C. R.: The nature of Reed-Sternberg cells and other malignant "reticulum" cells. Lancet *II*, 802–807, 1974.

Morphological Classification of Non-Hodgkin's Lymphomas

Kristin Henry, M. H. Bennett, and G. Farrer-Brown

Lymphomas by definition are those tumors arising from peripheral lymphoreticular tissue and thus exclude the neoplastic proliferations of bone marrow—the leukemias—and the primary tumors of thymus—the thymomas. In practice most lymphomas arise in lymph nodes in the first instance and are thus derived from the lymphoreticular mononuclear phagocytic system of cells (LRMPS). Therefore, before embarking on a description of our classification of non-Hodgkin's lymphomas, a brief account will first be given of some of the normal component cells of the lymph node. As a result of electron microscopic studies of both normal and neoplastic lymphoreticular tissue (Figs 1–4), we recognize five main types of cells indigenous to lymph nodes [12], which are as follows:

1. Lymphoid cell series including plasma cells
2. Mononuclear phagocytic cells (histiocytes and other variants)
3. Dendritic cells
4. Endothelial cells
5. Fiber-forming cells

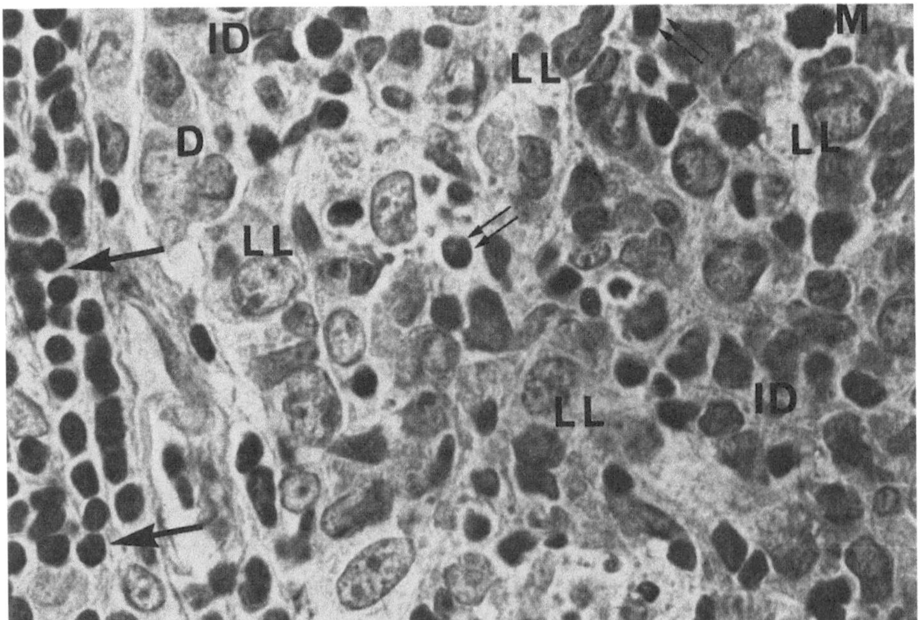

Fig. 1. Part of a germinal center showing a mixture of large lymphoid cells (LL) and dendritic cells (D) with the smaller irregular follicle center (intermediate) lymphocytes (ID). Note in comparison the round regular nuclei of the small lymphocytes in the surrounding lymphoid cuff (arrows) (× 780)

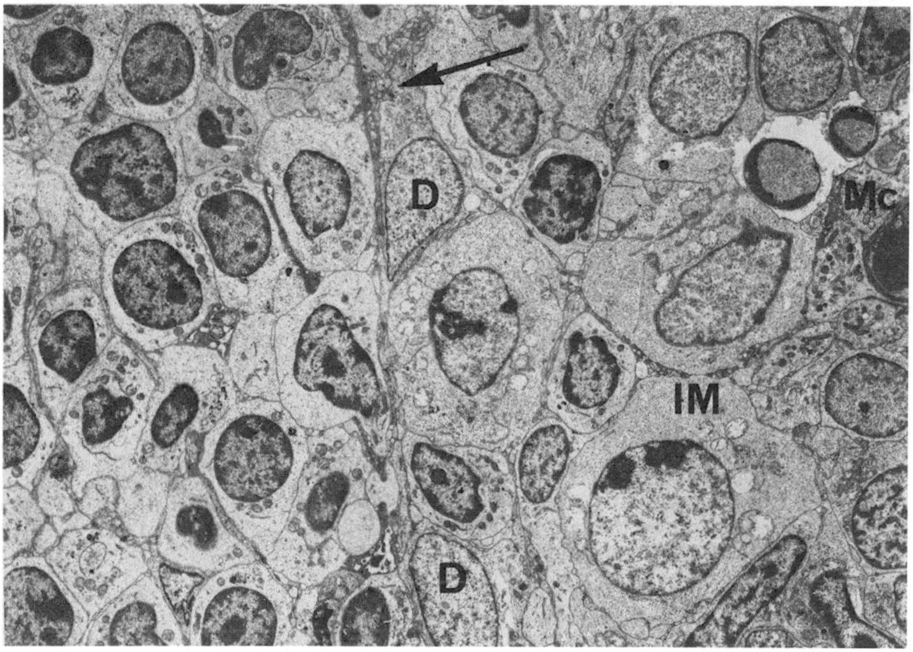

Fig. 2. Electron micrograph of the junctional zone of a germinal center (right) with its lymphoid cuff (left). IM: immunoblast; D: dendritic cell; MC: tingeable body macrophage. Processes of dendritic cells arrowed (×2770)

Our classification is thus based primarily on cell morphology at both light and ultrastructural levels. It is derived from the classical GALL and MALLORY classification [9], but it takes into account recent advances in immunology and redefinition of cell types found in peripheral lymphoreticular tissue as described above. The introduction of new and possibly confusing nomenclature has been avoided, and while we recognize that lymphomas are essentially neoplasms of the immune system there has been no attempt to imply immunological function, the recognition of which requires specialized techniques. Essentially, therefore, it is a classification intended for the surgical histopathologist working at light microscopical level. This working classification on the non-Hodgkin's lymphomas put forward at a workshop on non-Hodgkin's lymphomas held in Chicago in 1973 [3] has now been adopted by the British National Lymphoma Investigation [4]. This classification is now named the National Lymphoma Investigation (NLI) classification and has in its full form (Table 1) proved acceptable to the 38 centers participating in the trial. One of the important aspects for the clinician is the separation of the different groups into grade I (lower) and grade II (higher) malignant categories.

Follicular lymphomas remain a separate entity but have been separated into three groups. The diffuse lymphomas have been broken down into seven main categories based on the degree of "differentiation" and the believed cell of origin. All but one of the seven types of the diffuse tumors are considered to be derived from lymphoid cells and thus include tumors composed of plasma cells (extramedullary plasmacytoma). The remaining seventh type of diffuse lymphoma, the true histiocytic lymphoma, is also included in the classification of non-Hodgkin's lymphomas, as it has been shown that cells of the mononuclear phagocytic system are an integral and functionally essential component of the lymphoreticular system, and because recent ultrastructural studies [12] have confirmed the existence of true histiocytic lymphomas and have shown that they form a not insignificant portion of the large cell group of lymphomas [13]. Tumors derived from dendritic cells and fiber-forming cells (fibroblasts or reticular cells) have been identified (unpublished observations), but since to date they appear to be very uncommon, no provision has yet been made for their separate categorization.

Table 1. National Lymphoma Investigation classification (BENNETT, FARRER-BROWN, and HENRY, 1973)

Follicular lymphoma	
Follicle cells, predominantly small	
Follicle cells, mixed small and large	
Follicle cells, predominantly large	Grade I
Diffuse lymphoma	
Lymphocytic, well-differentiated (small round lymphocyte)	
Lymphocytic, intermediate differentiated (small follicle lymphocyte)	
Lymphocytic, poorly differentiated (lymphoblast)	
1. Non-Burkitt lymphoma	
2. Burkitt's tumor	
3. Convoluted cell mediastinal lymphoma	Grade II
Lymphocytic, mixed small and large cell (mixed follicle cells)	
"Undifferentiated" large cell (large lymphoid cell)	
Histiocytic cell (mononuclear phagocytic cells)	
Plasma cell (extramedullary plasma cell)	Grade I and II
Unclassified	

Plasmacytoid differentiation in lymphocytic tumors, and banded or fine sclerosis recorded.

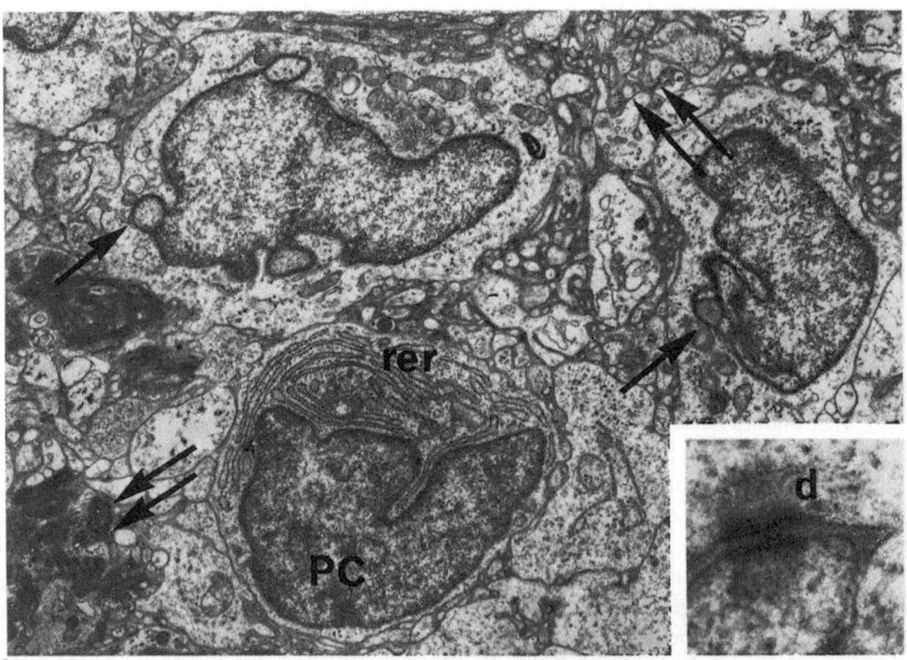

Fig. 3. Electron micrograph of the characteristic irregularly nucleated follicle center lymphocytes. Note the nuclear extrusions or pockets (arrows) in addition to the nuclear indentations and the generally irregular cytoplasmic contour. Electron-dense material is present between the processes of dendritic cells (double arrows) and a desmosomal connection (d) between two such processes is shown in the insert. PC: plasma cell; rer: rough endoplasmic reticulum. ×6250 (Inset: ×60,000)

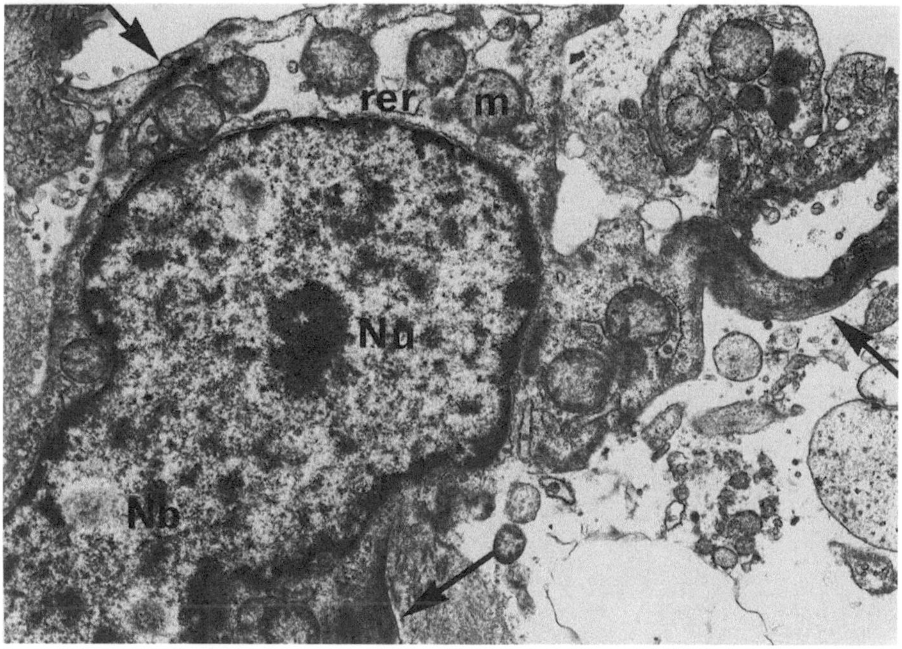

Fig. 4. Part of a fiber-forming reticular cell or myofibroblast. Note the elongated cytoplasmic extensions with characteristic fibrillar material abutting on cytoplasmic margins (arrows) and the dilated rough endoplasmic reticulum (rer). Nb: nuclear bodies; Nu: nucleolus; M: mitochondria (× 10,500)

It must be emphasized, however, that in diagnosing diffuse malignant lymphoma, and especially in the case of plasma cell and histiocytic cell tumors, it is important to establish that the disease is arising in the first instance in peripheral lymphoreticular tissue. Inevitably, there remain a small group of unclassifiable tumors. A detailed account now follows of the histological features of the different types of lymphoma, as shown in Table 1.

Follicular Lymphomas

The neoplastic follicles are composed in varying proportions of small and large lymphoid cells that are considered to derive from their non-neoplastic germinal center counterparts. At light microscopical level (Fig. 5A), the majority of cells are small, but in contrast to the small round nuclei of the resting or interphase "mature" lymphocyte their nuclear irregularity is generally greater than that of the normal counterpart, and at ultrastructural level (Fig. 5B), in addition to the prominent nuclear indentations and convolutions, nuclear blebs, protrusions, and pockets are a prominent feature [12]. For this reason, the term "cleaved cell" introduced by LUKES & COLLINS [19] does not seem quite appropriate, although it is true that in *haematological* preparations the nuclei in addition to an angular appearance may show prominent notching [24]. These were the circulating cells originally described by ROSENTHAL et al.as haematogones in association with follicular lymphomas [23]. The large cell population of the neoplastic follicles is composed of cells either with an ovoid irregular nuclear outline and relatively inconspicuous nucleoli or with a rounded nucleus of smooth outline and prominent nucleoli,

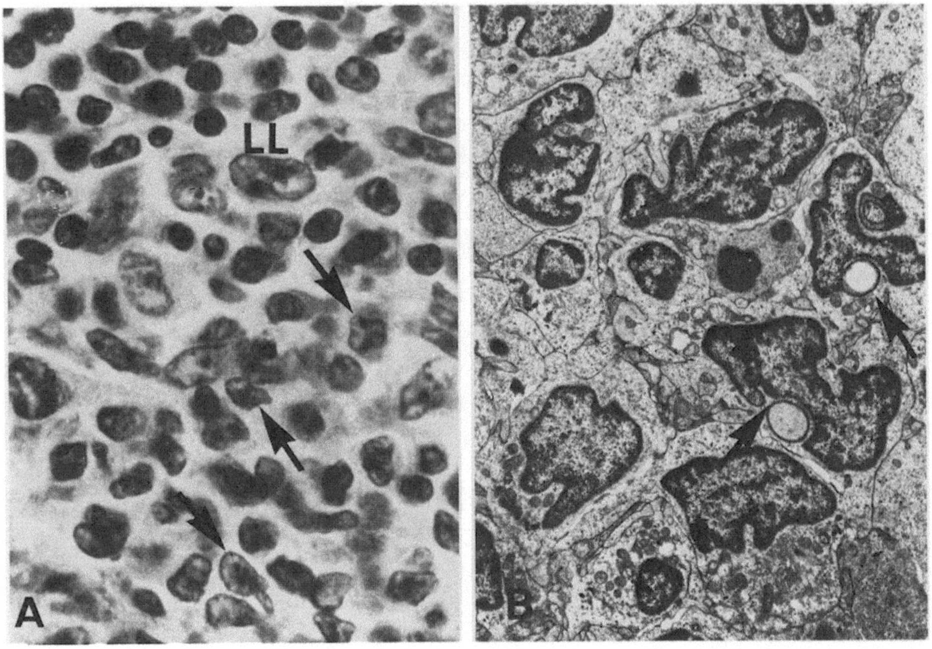

Fig. 5. (A) Follicular lymphoma of predominantly small follicle cell type. There are a few large lymphoid cells (LL), but the majority of cells are the irregular small follicles (intermediate) lymphocytes (arrowed). Note the residual lymphocytic cuff of small well-differentiated lymphocytes above (×750);
(B) Electron micrograph of a follicular lymphoma composed predominantly of small (intermediate) follicle lymphocytes. Note the highly irregular nuclear contour and the presence of nuclear pockets (arrowed) (×3500)

the latter cell type appearing the larger and more prominent of the two. No case has been recorded to date of a follicular lymphoma composed either of malignant histiocytes or of malignant dendritic cells.

Since prognosis has in the past been generally believed to be related to the proportion of large lymphoid cells present, the follicular lymphomas have been subdivided as follows: 1) a predominantly small cell type (less than one-third large cells), 2) a mixed small and large cell type (between one-third and two-thirds large cells), and 3) a predominantly large cell type (more than two-thirds large cells)—the least common type. The small cell population in any of the three subtypes is composed of the small lymphocytes with irregularly contoured, or "groovy" nuclei, while the large cells are usually the large, round, smoothly nucleated follicle "blast" cells (Fig. 5). It is this mixture of cells that is the single most reliable criterion in differentiating malignant from benign reactive follicles. Nodes showing only a partial or minimal neoplastic follicular pattern are still called follicular lymphomas since in recent analyzes the presence of diffuse areas does not appear to indicate a significantly worse prognosis [8]. This finding, as well as the proportion of large cells present, is being evaluated further with actuarial survival curves in prospective trials.

In general, follicular lymphomas appear to have a slow evolution, but it is well-recognized that in a proportion of such tumors a diffuse lymphoma of high-grade malignancy may at any time develop. Sclerosis, either in the form of bands or a fine compartmentalizing fibrosis, is more commonly seen in lymphomas of follicular center origin—even if diffuse—than in other types of lymphoma, and appears to indicate a somewhat better prognosis [2, 5].

There are certain features present in some follicular lymphomas which may result in neoplastic nodes being interpreted as reactive follicular hyperplasia. Briefly, these are as follows: 1) the persistence of the small regular lymphocyte mantle around the neoplastic follicle, 2) marked mitotic activity, 3) the presence of tingeable body macrophages, 4) marked variation in size and shape of the neoplastic follicles—even within the same neoplastic node the shape of the follicles may be very variable and range in size from very small to very large, and 5) the presence of eosinophilic proteinaceous debris between the neoplastic follicular cells [22]. These features, which may be found alone or in combination, have in the past been believed to be those associated with reactive follicles [21] and it is therefore important to realize that they may also be seen in neoplastic follicles [8]. Conversely, findings which *are* helpful when present in supporting the diagnosis of follicular lymphomas are: 1) perinodal extension of follicular structures, 2) a reticulin pattern showing increased and condensed reticulin fibers in the interfollicular area, and 3) the pattern of fibrosis.

Diffuse Lymphomas

Lymphocytic Well-Differentiated Type (Small Round Lymphocyte)

These lymphomas are composed of small lymphocytes with small, round, regular darkly staining nuclei due to abundant clumped chromatin, inconspicuous nucleoli, and minimal

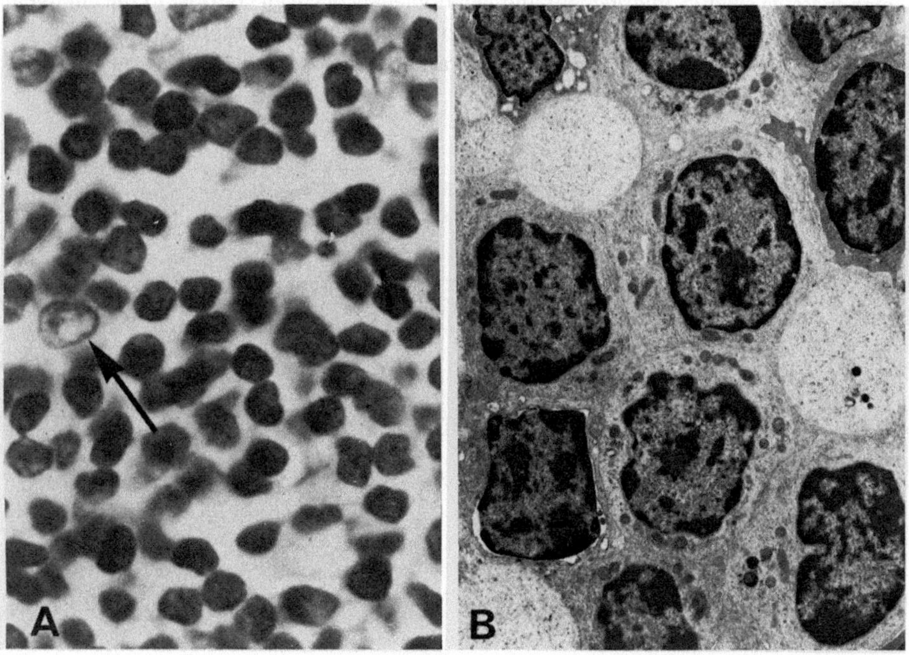

Fig. 6. (A) Diffuse lymphocytic lymphoma of well-differentiated type. The component cells are small, well-differentiated lymphocytes with round, regular nuclei and a compact chromatin arrangement indistinguishable from the lymphocytic cells of chronic lymphocytic leukemia. Occasional larger precursor cells are present (arrow) (×750);
(B) Electron micrograph of infiltrating cells in chronic lymphocytic leukemia. The neoplastic lymphocytes possess generally rounded nuclei with abundant clumped chromatin and an absence of nuclear pockets (×3500)

amounts of cytoplasm (Fig. 6A and B). Mitiotic activity is minimal. In histological sections, they appear similar to the small lymphocyte occurring in the cuff of small lymphocytes surrounding germinal centers. The majority of these "lymphomas" are of B-cell type and are the tissue manifestations of chronic lymphocytic leukemia [1], although many present before the leukemic phase is evident. A feature commonly observed in this type of lymphoma is the presence of small foci of pale staining areas, the so-called proliferation centers (Fig. 7), which are composed of larger lymphoic cells including prolymphocytes and "blasts" [18]. During an accelerated phase of the disease, the proliferating cells may be slightly larger with nuclei showing a less dense chromatin pattern and conspicuous nucleoli approaching the appearance of lymphoblasts.

Some tumors of this group show plasmacytoid differentiation (Fig. 8A) and may or may not be associated with the production of a paraprotein, the most frequent type being the IgM macroglobulin associated with Waldenström's disease. Those lymphomas which show plasmacytoid differentiation have been and are called lymphomas of lymphoplasmacytoid type and placed in a separate category by some workers. In the NLI classification, plasmacytoid differentiation is noted but the lymphomas are not separately categorized unless the *majority* of cells show the morphological features of plasma cells, in which case such lymphomas are placed in the plasmacytoma group. There is, however, some justification for placing tumors with evidence of paraprotein production in the plasmacytoma group right from the start since at ultrastructural level many of the cells, which at light microscopical level appear to be lymphocytes, show the cytoplasmic features of plasma cells with an extensive secretory rough endoplasm reticulum (Fig. 8B).

A rare variant of chronic lymphocytic leukemia (CLL) is prolymphocytic leukemia [10] in which massive splenic enlargement and hepatomegaly occur in contrast to the enlargement of lymph nodes which may be either inconspicuous or absent. The lymphocyte morphology is best appreciated in Romanowsky-stained preparations of blood or bone marrow, or by electron

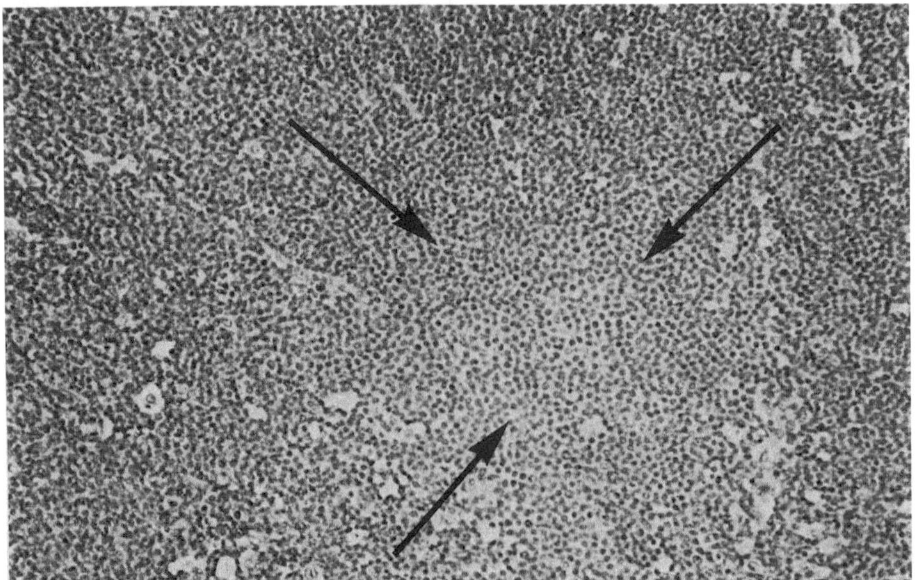

Fig. 7. Low power view of a diffuse, well-differentiated lymphocytic lymphoma showing a paler area (arrowed) composed of larger more immature lymphoid cells—a so-called proliferation center (× 102)

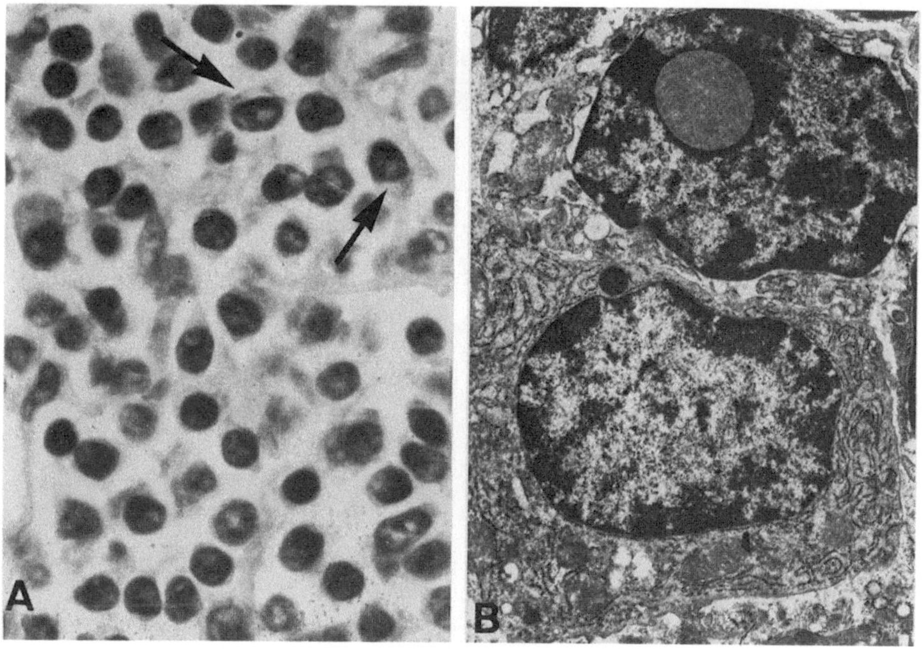

Fig. 8. (A) Diffuse lymphocytic lymphoma composed of small lymphoid cells showing prominent plasmacytoid differentiation. Note the perinuclear haloes or hofs (arrows) (× 750);
(B) Electron micrograph of component cells in a lymph node in macroglobulinaemia. The cytoplasm of both cells contains an abundance of rough endoplasmic reticulum (rer) with secretion product. The nucleus of the upper cell contains a cytoplasmic inclusion or Dutcher body (× 7500)

microscopy, rather than on routinely processed tissue sections. The diagnostic features are the presence of lymphoid cells larger than the small CLL type of lymphocytes which, while retaining the condensed or coarse nuclear chomatin associated with the latter type, also show the presence of a prominent nucleolus. Thus, while the nucleoli are similar to those of lymphoblasts, the cells are neither as large nor do their nuclei show the more open chromatin pattern associated with the lymphoblasts.

Lymphocytic Intermediate Differentiation (Small Follicle Cell)

This tumor is interpreted as the diffuse counterpart of the predominantly small follicle cell type of follicular lymphoma described above and thus by definition represents another type of B-cell lymphoma. A helpful finding in many of these tumors is that in addition to the characteristic irregularly nucleated lymphocytes there are large lymphoid cells scattered singly (Fig. 9), in contrast to the focal aggregates of lymphoid cells comprising the proliferation centers seen in the lymphocytic well-differentiated group (vide supra). Fibrosis both outside and inside the node may be a conspicuous feature of this type of lymphoma [2].

Lymphocytic Poorly Differentiated Type (Lymphoblastic)

This is a heterogeneous group of tumors. It includes: 1) the most common type composed of poorly "differentiated" lymphocytes (or lymphoblasts) which, although resembling Burkitt's

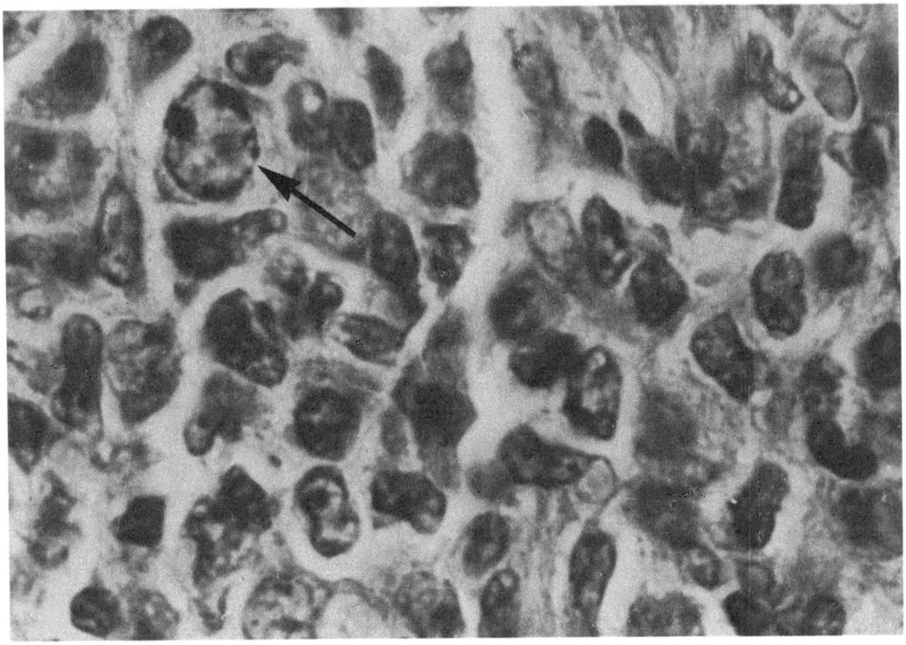

Fig. 9. Diffuse lymphocytic lymphoma of intermediate (small follicle) cell type. The proliferative cells are predominantly small, irregularly nucleated lymphocytes analagous to the irregular follicle centre lymphocyte. Note the occurrence of large immunoblast-like cells (arrow) scattered among the small lymphoid population (× 1150)

tumor, are not—hence the term non-Burkitt type, 2) the Burkitt's tumor proper, and 3) the poorly differentiated convoluted lymphocytic lymphoma or so-called Sternberg sarcoma which usually arises in the mediastinum of young individuals and is often associated with an acute lymphocytic leukemia-like blood picture. The majority of these latter tumors have been identified as of T-cell origin [17] in contrast to the Burkitt and non-Burkitt groups which appear to be of B-cell origin. It is not always easy for the routine diagnostic pathologist to distinguish between these three types of lymphomas. The component cells of both the Burkitt and non-Burkitt types are recognizable as lymphoid cells smaller than immunoblasts. The round nuclei contain chromatin, which is less in amount than that seen in the small mature lymphocytes, and usually a prominent central nucleolus can be identified (Fig. 10A). The cytoplasm is well defined and often strongly pyroninophilic. The accepted histological hallmark of Burkitt's tumor is the presence of numerous scattered tingeable body macrophages seen against a background of neoplastic lymphoblasts, resulting in the so-called "starry sky" appearance. This feature is, however, not pathognomic of the Burkitt lymphoma since it occurs in a significant proportion of the more common "Burkitt-like" poorly differentiated lymphocytic lymphomas (Fig. 10B). Good histological preparations and tumor imprints utilizing special stains enable some pathologists experienced in the field of Burkitt's tumor to separate these two cell types [6]. Both the Burkitt and non-Burkitt lymphoblastic types may show plasmacytoid differentiation.

With regard to the often mediastinal T-cell lymphoma, again, given good histological preparations, it is possible to recognize certain features, the most characteristic of which is the convoluted or cerebroid nucleus containing linear condensations of chromatin—the appearance of which has been likened to the imprint of a chicken's foot [19]—and the rather discrete arrangement of the cells (Fig. 11A). A cell that shares similarities with the mediastinal T cell is the Sézary/Lutzner cell—also demonstrated to be a T cell [26]. Diagnostic difficulties are not likely to occur when interpreting skin biopsies, but lymph nodes involved either in the Sézary syndrome or in mycosis fungoides may present difficulties (Fig. 11B), and it is essential for the certain identification of these cells as convoluted cells that they are either viewed under the oil immersion lens, preferably in plastic embedded sections, or are processed for electron microscopy (Fig. 12).

Lymphocytic Mixed Small and Large Cell Type (Mixed Follicle Cell)

The term "mixed" lymphoma is restricted to tumors composed of a mixture of small and large germinal center-type lymphoid cells thought to be the diffuse counterpart of the mixed type of follicular lymphoma (Fig. 13A) and is not synonymous with the mixed histiocytic-lymphocytic lymphoma of RAPPAPORT [20]. The helpful differential feature which enables this diagnosis to be made is that the smaller lymphocytic cells are analogous to the small follicular center lymphocytes and therefore show the characteristic irregular nuclei. The larger lymphoid cells may be predominantly of the large, regularly nucleated lymphoid cells, the large, irregularly nucleated cell, or both. It is stressed that these "mixed" tumors are uncommon. Most so-called mixed lymphomas are in reality tumors that only present a mixed appearance because, in addition to the neoplastic component, there are other cells present consisting of normal residual cells and/or reactive cells such as small lymphocytes, histiocytes, and plasma cells. With regard

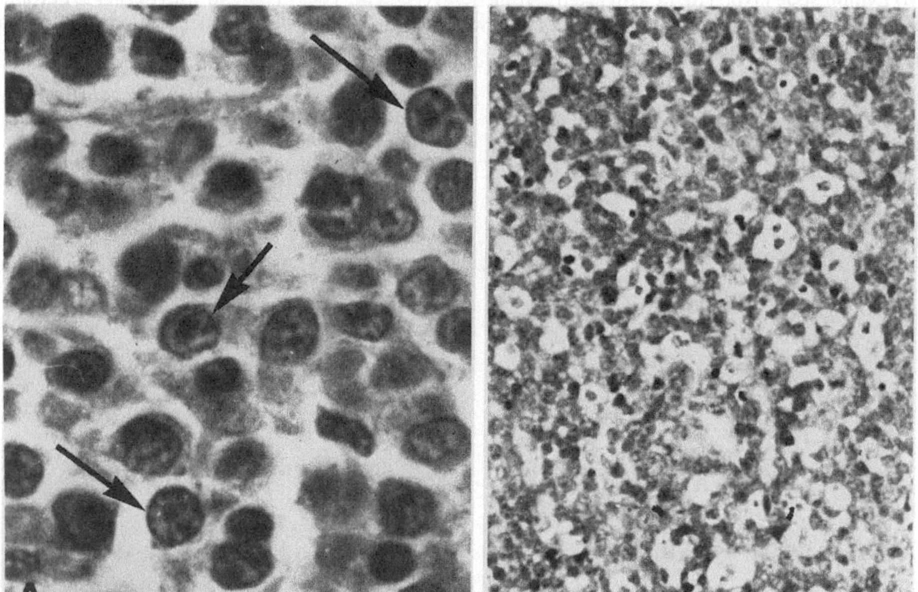

Fig. 10. (A) Diffuse lymphocytic lymphoma of poorly differentiated (lymphoblastic) type. The neoplastic lymphoid cells possess rounded nuclei often with a prominent centrally placed nucleolus (arrows) and a relatively small amount of cytoplasm (× 1010);
(B) Low power view of a non-Burkitt's poorly differentiated lymphocytic lymphoma showing numerous scattered tingeable body macrophages and resulting "starry sky" appearance (× 225)

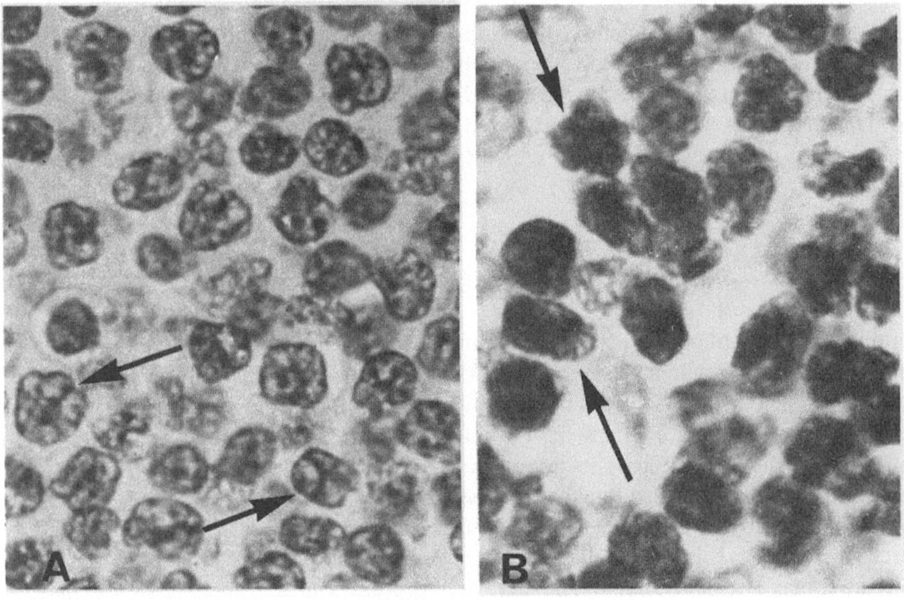

Fig. 11. (A) Diffuse lymphocytic lymphoma of poorly differentiated convoluted cell type. The proliferating cells are rather discretely arranged and the nuclear contour finely irregular. Note the segmented appearance of the nuclei due to the presence of chromatin strands sometimes resulting in a chicken's foot appearance (arrows) (× 1010);
(B) Lymph node involvement with proliferating Sézary/Lutzner cells in patient with Sézary syndrome. The cells are more crowded and possess more darkly staining nuclei, but the crinkled/convoluted nuclear contour (arrows) can be seen (× 1150)

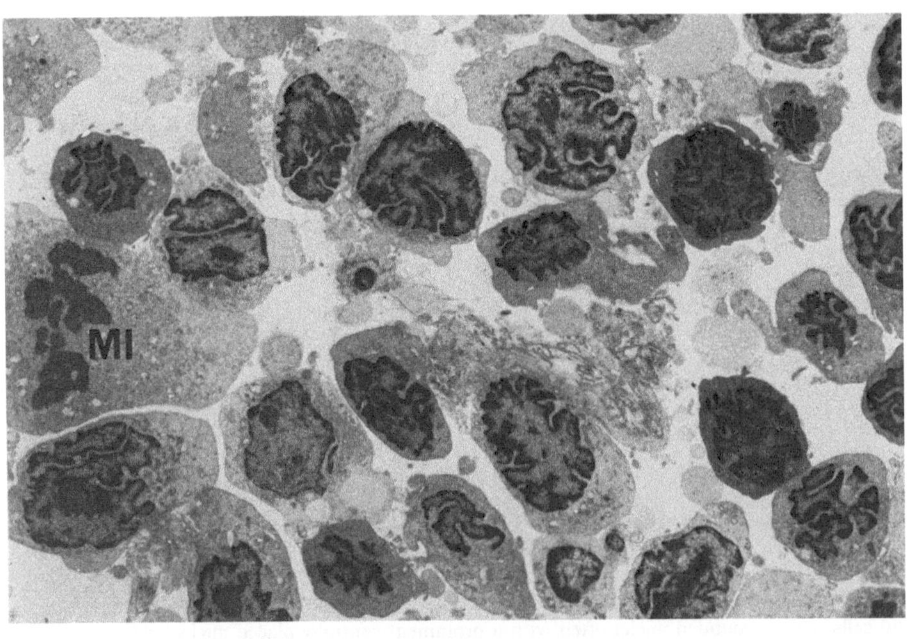

Fig. 12. Low power electron micrograph of the Sézary cell infiltrate shown in Fig. 11B. The very marked crenellated irregularity of the nuclei is now clearly evident (× 2100)

to reactive plasma cells, these must not be confused with neoplastic lymphoid cells showing plasmacytoid differentiation.

Large "Undifferentiated" Cell Type (Large Lymphoid Cell)

This important group consists mainly of tumors composed of large *lymphoid* cells with or without plasmacytoid differentiation. Inevitably, some true histiocytic tumors and possibly other types of large cell lymphomas will be included, since without the benefit of special techniques, such as electron microscopy or immunocytochemistry, it is not always possible to make an accurate histological diagnosis. Immunological techniques for their identification may be the least helpful approach since many of the lymphomas in this group are composed of null cells, i.e., cells without either T- or B-markers, or markers associated with the mononuclearphagocytic series [7]. For this reason, the collective term "undifferentiated"—which is open to criticism—has been retained for this group, since, although one can identify the lymphoid nature of the majority of these large cell tumors, there still remains a small group without any morphologically distinctive features to indicate their cell of origin.

As already stated, the majority of this group are large lymphoid cells (Fig. 14). They possess a large, generally round to ovoid nucleus—larger in volume than that of the tissue histiocyte—with a dispersed nuclear chromatin, and one, two, or more large prominent nucleoli are often present at the nuclear membrane. The pyroninophilic cytoplasm is somewhat variable in

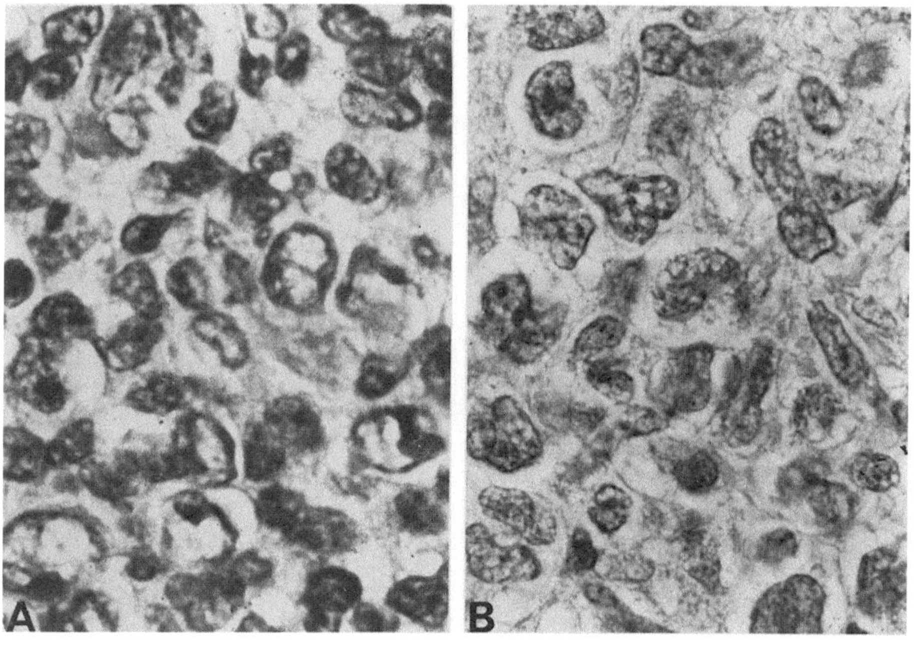

Fig. 13. (A) Diffuse lymphocytic lymphoma of mixed small and large (follicle) cell type. The component cells are a mixture of the intermediate or small, irregularly nucleated follicle lymphocyte and large lymphoid cells with predominantly regular nuclear contours (×820);
(B) Diffuse lymphocytic lymphoma of large cell type in which the neoplastic cells are predominantly large, irregularly nucleated (follicle-type) lymphocytes. Compared to the small (intermediate) follicle lymphocytes (cf. Figs. 1, 3, 5 and 9), the nuclear chromatin is more finely dispersed, and the nuclei much more variable in shape. The cytoplasm is indistinct, and nucleoli are not readily identified (×820)

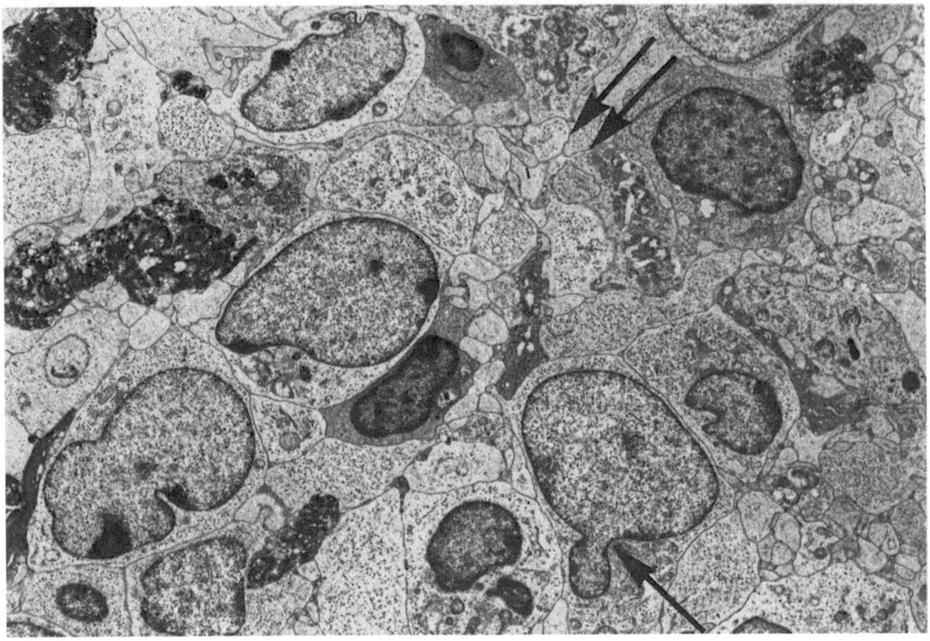

Fig. 14. Electron micrograph of large cell lymphoma composed of large irregular follicle-type lymphocytes. The nuclear irregularity is due to constrictions and protrusions (arrows). Note the presence of nucleoli in relation to the nuclear membrane. Dendritic cell processes (double arrows) (× 3100)

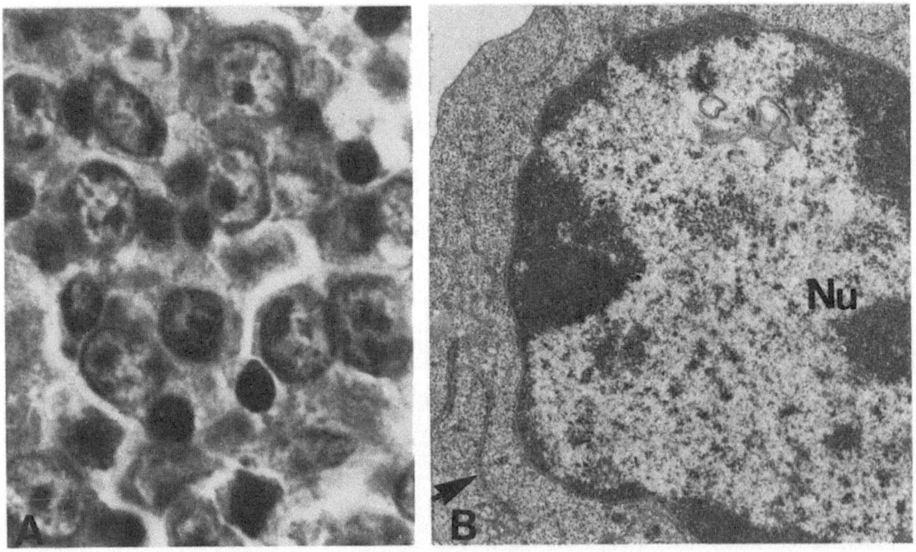

Fig. 15. (A) Diffuse lymphoma of undifferentiated large cell (large lymphoid cell) type. The cells possess large, round nuclei with marginated chromatin and one or more prominent nucleoli often applied to the nuclear membrane. The relatively sparse cytoplasm is intensely pyroninophilic (× 820);
(B) Electron micrograph of a malignant lymphoma of large lymphoid cell (immunoblast) type. The nuclear configuration with its characteristic chromatin arrangement and prominent nucleoli (Nu) are well-shown. The cytoplasm is filled with RNA, and there is only a modicum of rough endoplasmic reticulum (arrow) (× 7600)

amount but never abundant in relation to the nuclear size, and in well-fixed preparations the cytoplasmic boundaries are well-defined. These, essentially, are the features associated with immunoblasts or transformed lymphocytes, and their lymphoid nature has been verified at ultrastructural level (Fig. 15). Reticulin fiber, which is often considerable in amount, is the product of reactive fibroblasts. Occasionally, these large cell tumors are composed of the highly distinctive large irregular follicle center cells (Figs. 13B and 14) or a mixture of these cells and immunoblasts.

Histiocytic Cell Type (Mononuclear Phagocytic Cell)

True histiocytic lymphomas are considered by most contemporary workers to be very uncommon [19] or, if they exist at all, that they should not be included in any classification of malignant lymphomas [11]; and indeed, out of a total of 977 malignant lymphomas entered in the Kiel Lymph Node Registry between the years 1966 and 1973 there is not one reference to a histiocytic lymphoma [18]. We, however, cannot endorse these views. Firstly, tumors showing the features of histiocytic (mononuclear phagocytic) cells—and which on the basis of ultrastructural studies can now be recognized at light microscopical level—form a not insignificant proportion of all large cell lymphomas [13]. Secondly, since the term lymphoma is generally used for tumors of the peripheral lymphoreticular system, and since cells of

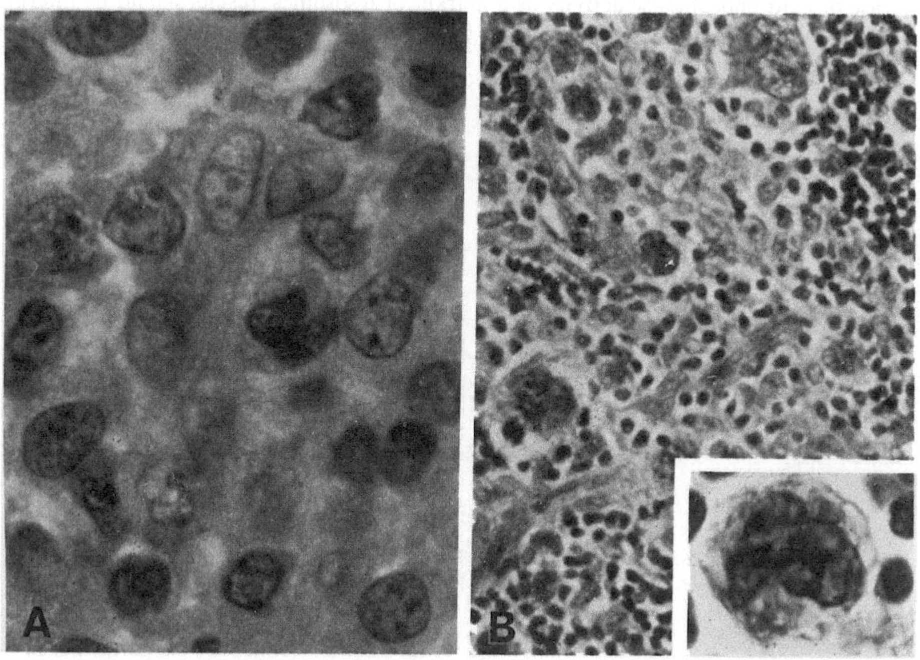

Fig. 16. Diffuse lymphoma of histiocytic cell (mononuclear phagocytic cell) type.
(A) Representative field from a well-differentiated histiocytic tumor. The component cells show round to ovoid nuclei sometimes with a reniform shape—vesiculated chromatin and readily discernible nucleoli. The cytoplasm is abundant with indistinct limits (× 820);
(B) A histiocytic tumor composed of cells showing great variation in size and shape. The nucleoli are lumpy and lobated (see inset) and the cytoplasm foamy or granular. The nuclear features of this giant cell are quite different from those of a typical Reed-Sternberg cell. (The small dark cells are residual small lymphocytes.) (× 250. Inset × 820)

mononuclear phagocytic origin are a major and integral part of this system [25], it seems illogical not to include tumors derived from these cells with the other types of lymphomas. It is of course mandatory that tissue involvement as a manifestation of systemic malignant histiocytosis must be carefully excluded, just as—with the exception of the tissue manifestation of CLL—leukemic infiltrates are excluded.

The neoplastic histiocytes may be divided into three main types. They may be quite well-differentiated (Fig. 16A), approximating closely in appearance to tissue histiocytes; they may be composed of a much more pleomorphic population of large histiocytic cells (Fig. 16B), with lumpy or lobated nuclei occurring frequently in multinucleated form; or they may be composed predominantly of "blast" cells—histioblasts.

In the former types, the cytoplasm tends to be eosinophilic, foamy, or granular, and while often considerable in amount has irregular ill-defined limits. A point worth noting is that the cytoplasm of the less well-differentiated malignant histiocytes and histioblasts is sometimes intensely pyroninophilic due to abundant RNA or to well-developed rough endoplasmic reticulum. Another helpful finding is the apparent fine sclerosis or packeting of cells by reticulin, much of which at electron microscopical level is seen to consist only of proteinaceous electron-dense material. Phagocytosis by the neoplastic histiocytes (Fig. 17), while a helpful feature when present, is not essential for the diagnosis of this group of tumors. It is the pleomorphic type of histiocytic tumor that is most likely to be confused with Hodgkin's disease—usually of reticular type. Not only may the "multinucleate" giant cells be interpreted as Reed-Sternberg cells, but areas of necrosis and the presence of eosinophils and plasma cells are not uncommon. With regard to the use of histochemical techniques such as the non-specific esterase or acid phosphatase activity as a marker of lysosomes, results should be interpreted

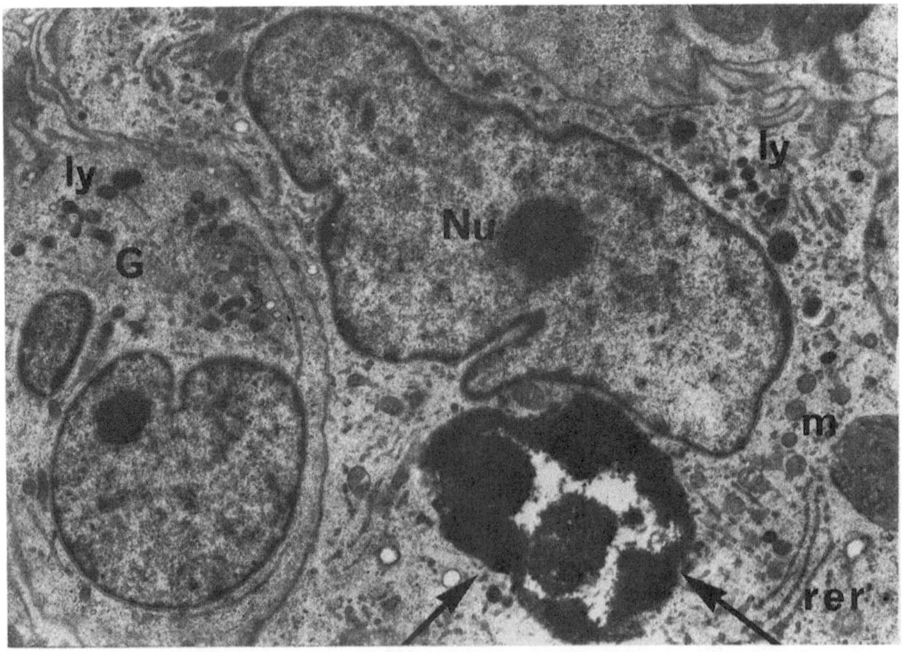

Fig. 17. Electron micrograph of a well-differentiated histiocytic tumor. Note the prominent centrally placed nucleoli (Nu), the voluminous cytoplasm containing lysosomal structures (Ly), short stacks of rough endoplasmic reticulum (rer), prominent Golgi (G), and a phagocytosed lymphocyte (arrows). The mitochondria (m) are small and lozenge-shaped (× 7400)

with extreme caution since, as already mentioned, large numbers of *reactive* histiocytes may be present in many essentially non-histiocytic lymphomas, while in the more malignant or primitive variants of true histiocytic tumors, enzyme activity may be very low or absent. In contrast, ultrastructural studies [14] have provided supportive evidence of the histiocytic nature of these tumors (Figs. 17 and 18). The nuclei and cytoplasm share many features with their non-neoplastic counterparts, such as nuclear pattern, irregular cytoplasmic contour, and an abundance of cytoplasmic organelles including lysosomes.

Plasma Cell Type (Plasma Cell—extramedullary)

Extramedullary plasmacytomas are recognized but are generally regarded as being rare; even when this diagnosis is made, such tumors have not formerly been included in classifications of lymphomas. This seems inconsistent since it is now accepted that the plasma cell is a specialized secretory cell of B-lymphocyte origin. Either the term "plasma cell" should be discarded altogether or, if retained, it is suggested that the term "plasmacytoma" or "lymphoma of plasma cell type" should be applied to those tumors that are essentially composed of plasma cells! Also, with regard to their incidence, they have been found not to be as rare as indicated in the literature; plasma cell tumors form an appreciable component of primary lymphomas of the gastrointestinal tract [16], and they are also seen in other extramedullary sites such as gonads, breast, and salivary glands (unpublished observations). They do, however, appear to be less common in lymph nodes and spleen, although we are now recognizing them with increasing frequency.

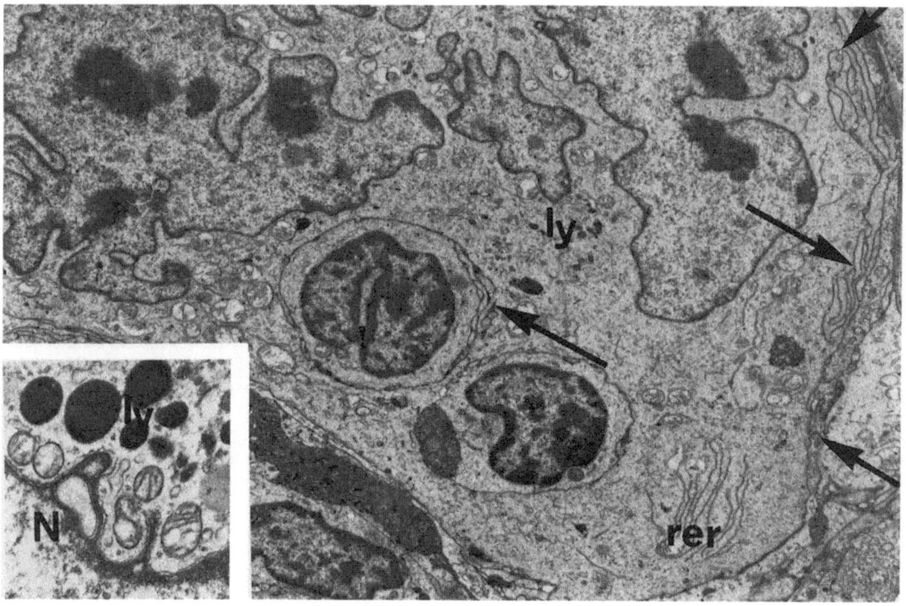

Fig. 18. Electron micrograph of part of a giant cell from the pleomorphic histiocytic tumor shown in Fig. 16B. The lobated nucleus which appears to be several separate nuclei in this thin section preparation is very irregular and clefted with frequent nuclear protrusions. The cytoplasm when it abuts on surrounding cells shows a markedly folded arrangement (arrows). There are short stacks of rough endoplasmic reticulum (rer) and scattered lysosomes (Ly) better seen in the insert (×12,300). The two lymphocytes are not phagocytosed but are invaginating the cytoplasm (N) nucleus (×4000)

In pathology practice, it is surprising to find how tumors composed even of well-differentiated or mature plasma cells have been labelled as lymphosarcoma when occurring in extramedullary sites as, for example, the gastrointestinal tract (Fig. 19A). It is, therefore, less surprising that tumors composed of more immature pleomorphic plasma cell forms (Fig. 19B) still continue to be classified as a variety of lymphomas including reticulum cell sarcoma and Hodgkin's disease. In recognizing these tumors, one of the most helpful features is the perinuclear halo or hof, which may be greatly enhanced by methyl-green pyronin staining. This halo represents the Golgi apparatus of an actively secreting cell and is seen in the mature as well as the immature precursors of the plasma cell. Plasma cells are, of course, pyroninophilic, but this property is seen in other cell types and in itself should not be used to identify plasma cells. The basophilic cytoplasmic borders are well-defined but cell shape may show considerable variation. In the less differentiated plasma cell tumors, multinucleated cells are a common and distinctive finding (Fig. 19B). Their nuclei tend to be of similar rounded shape, to overlap each other, and to show the chomatin arrangement associated with plasma cell nuclei. It is to some members of this group that the term "plasmacytoid reticulum cell sarcoma" was formerly applied. Other workers label this group of tumors as immunoblastic sarcoma, but where the morphological features are identifiable as those of plasma cells (Figs. 19 and 20) as opposed to transformed lymphocytes, and where there is evidence of intracytoplasmic secretory activity, this label seems inappropriate. The term plasmacytoma in our terminology is restricted to tumors in which the majority of cells appear to be plasma cells or their precursors and is not applied to the variety of different lymphomas showing some degree of plasmacytoid differentiation and to which mention has already been made.

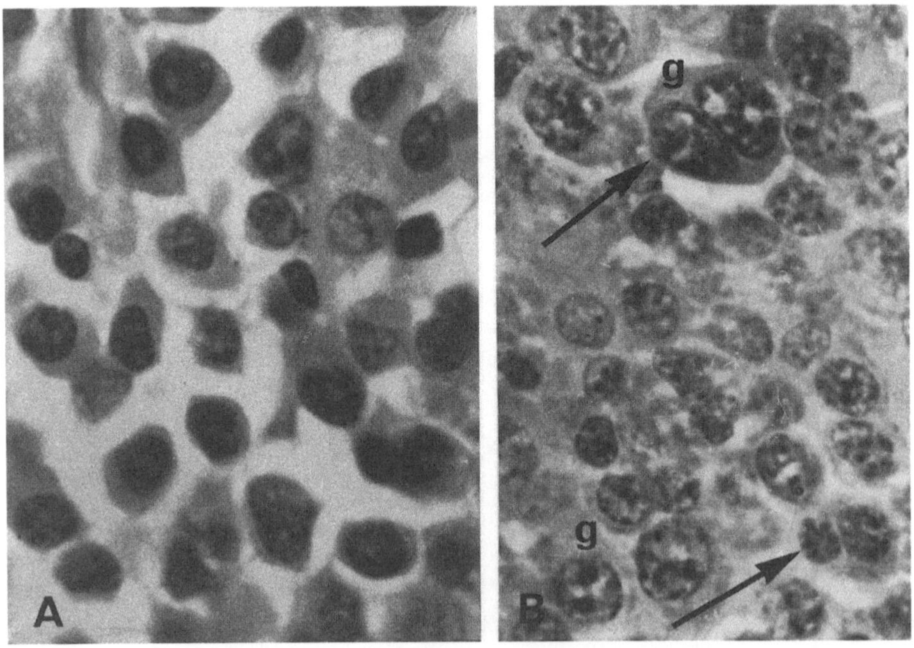

Fig. 19. Diffuse lymphoma of plasma cell type (extramedullary plasmacytoma).
(A) A gastrointestinal plasmacytoma in which the component cells are well-differentiated plasma cells (×820);
(B) Primary nodal plasmacytoma associated with a monoclonal gammopathy. The proliferating cells are much more variable in size, but the nuclei retain the characteristic chromatin arrangement of plasma cells. Perinuclear haloes (g) can often be discerned and there are frequent binucleate forms (arrows) (×820)

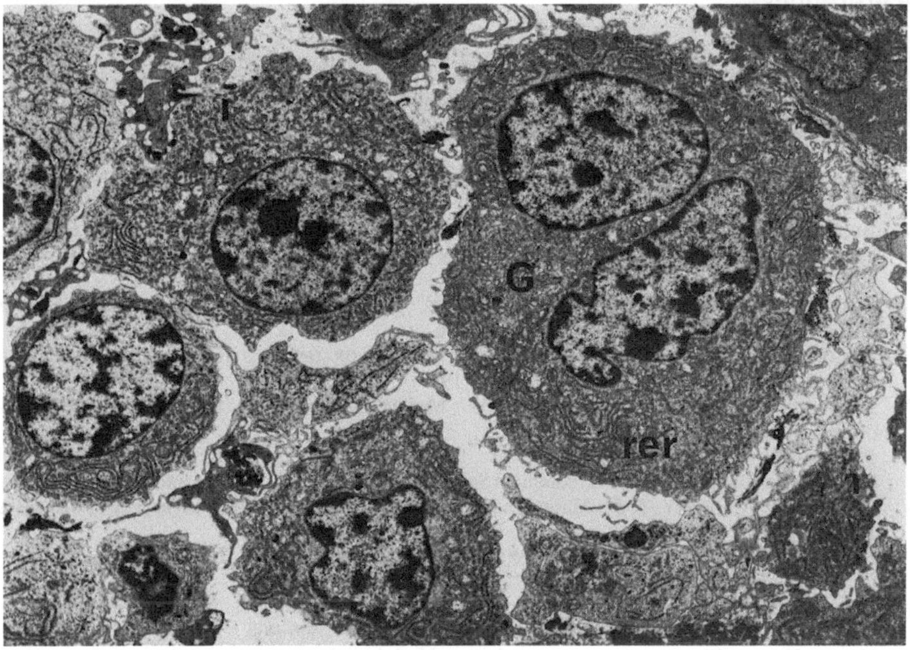

Fig. 20. Electron micrograph of the pleomorphic plasma cell tumor shown in Fig. 19B. Note the abundance of rough endoplasmic reticulum (rer) filling the cytoplasm, the prominent Golgi zone (G), and the binucleate cell at right (×4350)

Unclassified

Only a small proportion of tumors fall into the unclassified group, and these are usually labelled as such on the basis of inadequate or technically unsatisfactory material submitted for diagnosis. Having excluded anaplastic carcinoma—and in difficult cases electron microscopy may be necessary—there are inevitably some tumors which although acceptable as malignant lymphomas should not be forced into an inappropriate category simply because they cannot be accurately identified. What is essential in this small group is to give some indication to the clinician as to the grade of malignancy so that appropriate therapy may be instituted.

In conclusion, we would like to emphasize that whatever classification is ultimately adopted, a good understanding and recognition of the cell types that collectively make up the peripheral LRMPS of cells is absolutely essential [15], since any of them in theory undergo neoplastic transformation.

Acknowledgements

We should like to thank the Editor of the *British Journal of Cancer* for permission to reproduce Figures 2, 3, 8, and 19 and the Editor and Publishers of *Recent Advances in Pathology*, 10th edn., for permission to reproduce the illustrations used. We are grateful to Miss Joan Carter for the preparation of the manuscript. K. Henry is in receipt of a grant from the Cancer Research Campaign.

References

1. AISENBERG, A. C., BLOCH, K. J.: Immunoglobulins on the surface of neoplastic lymphocytes. N. Engl. J. Med. *287*, 272–276 (1972).
2. BENNETT, M. H.: Sclerosis in non-Hodgkin's lymphomata. Br. J. Cancer *31*, suppl. II, 44–52 (1975).
3. BENNETT, M. H., MILLETT, Y.: Nodular sclerotic lymphosarcoma, a possible new clinicopathological entity. Clin. Radiol. *20*, 339–343 (1969).
4. BENNETT, M. H., FARRER-BROWN, G., HENRY, Kristin: A Classification of Non-Hodgkin's Lymphoma Presented at the Workshop on Classification of Non-Hodgkin's Lymphomas. University of Chicago (1973).
5. BENNETT, M. H., FARRER-BROWN, G., HENRY, Kristin, JELLIFFE, A. M.: Classification of non-Hodgkin's lymphomas. Lancet 1974 *II*, 405–406.
6. BERARD, C. W., O'CONNOR, G. T., THOMAS, L. B., TORLONI, H.: Histopathological definition of Burkitt's tumour. Bull. W.H.O. *40*, 601–607 (1969).
7. BRAYLAN, R. C., JAFFE, E. S., BERARD, C. W.: Malignant lymphomas: Current classification and new observations. Pathol. Ann. 213–270 (1975).
8. FARRER-BROWN, G., HOWARTH, Catherine, BENNETT, M. H., HENRY, Kristin: Follicular lymphoma. Communication to the 131st Pathological Society of Great Britain and Ireland 1975.
9. GALL, E. A., MALLORY, T. B.: Malignant lymphoma. A clinico-pathological survey of 618 cases. Am. J. Pathol. *18*, 381–429 (1942).
10. GALTON, D. A. G., GOLDMAN, J. M., WILTSHAW, E., CATOVSKY, D., HENRY, Kristin, GOLDENBERG, G. J.: Prolymphocytic leukaemia. Br. J. Haematol. *27*, 7–23 (1974).
11. GERARD-MARCHANT, R., HAMLIN, I., LENNERT, K., RILKE, F., STANSFELD, A. G., VAN UNNIK, J. A. M.: Classification of non-Hodgkin's lymphoma. Lancet 1974 *II*, 406–408.
12. HENRY, Kristin: Electron microscopy in the non-Hodgkin's lymphomas. Symposium on non-Hodgkin's lymphomata. Br. J. Cancer *31*, suppl. II, 73–93 (1975a).
13. HENRY, Kristin: Malignant lymphomas of Mononuclear Phagocytic (Histiocytic) Type: an Electron Microscopic Study. Communication to the 131st Pathological Society of Great Britain and Ireland 1975.
14. HENRY, Kristin: Tumours of the mononuclear phagocytic system—an ultrastructural study of histiocytic lymphoma. IRCS Med. Sci. *5*, 326–327 (1977).
15. HENRY, Kristin, BENNETT, M. H., FARRER-BROWN, G.: Classification of the non-Hodgkin's lymphomas. In: Recent Advances in Pathology, 10th ed. WOOLF, N., ANTHONY, P. (eds). London: Churchill Livingstone (in press).
16. HENRY, Kristin, FARRER-BROWN, G.: Primary lymphomas of the gastrointestinal tract. I. Plasma cell tumours. Histopathology *1*, 53–76 (1977).
17. KERSEY, J. H., SABAD, A., GAJL-PECZALSKA, K., HALLGREN, H. M., YUNIS, E. J., NESBIT, M. E.: Acute lymphoblastic leukaemia cells with "T" (Thymus-derived) lymphocyte markers. Science *182*, 1355–1356 (1973).
18. LENNERT, K., MOHRI, N., STEIN, H., KAISERLING, E.: The Histopathology of malignant lymphoma. Br. J. Haematol. *31*, suppl., 193–203 (1975).
19. LUKES, R. J., COLLINS, R. D.: New approaches to the classification of the lymphomata. Symposium on non-Hodgkin's lymphomata. Br. J. Cancer *31*, suppl. II, 1–28 (1975).
20. RAPPAPORT, H.: Tumours of the Haematopoietic System. Atlas of Tumour Pathology, sect. 3, fasc. 8. Washington, D.C.: Armed Forces Institute of Pathology 1966.
21. RAPPAPORT, H., WINTERS, W. J., HICKS, E. B.: Follicular lymphoma. A re-evaluation of its position in the scheme of malignant lymphoma based on a survey of 253 cases. Cancer *9*, 792–821 (1956).
22. ROSAS-URIBE, A., VARIAKOJIS, D., RAPPAPORT, H.: Proteinaceous precipitate in nodular (follicular) lymphomas. Cancer *31*, 534–542 (1973).
23. ROSENTHAL, N., DRESKIN, O. H., VARAL, I. K., ZAK, P. G.: The significance of haematogones in blood, bone marrow and lymph node aspiration in giant follicular lymphobastoma. Acta Haematol. (Basel) *8*, 368–377 (1952).
24. SPIRO, S., GALTON, D. A. G., WILTSHAW, E., LOHMANN, R. C.: Follicular lymphoma: a survey of 75 cases with special reference to the syndrome resembling chronic lymphocytic leukaemia. Br. J. Cancer *31*, suppl. II., 60–72 (1975).
25. VAN FURTH, R., COHN, Z. A., HIRSCH, J. G., HUMPHREY, J. H., SPECTOR, W. G., LANGEVOORT, H. L.: The mononuclear phagocytic system: a new classification of macrophages, monocytes and their precursor cells. Bull. W.H.O. *46*, 845–852 (1972).
26. ZUCKER-FRANKLIN, D., MELTON, J. N., QUAGLIATA, F.: Ultrastructural, immunologic and functional studies on Sézary cells: a neoplastic variant of thymus-derived (T) lymphocytes. Proc. Nat. Acad. Sci. U.S.A. *71*, 1877–1881 (1972).

Some Considerations on the Classification of the Lymphoid Neoplasias

J. Diebold

The necessity of a new classification for the lymphoid neoplasias is quite evident to all pathologists. Today, we have too many classifications. More than six were published during the last three years [1, 2, 3, 4, 5, 6, 7, 8, 9, 10]. So many classifications leads to real confusion, particularly for the clinician. My purpose is not to expound upon our own classification used at the Hotel-Dieu of Paris. I want only to emphasize the three following points concerning the general problem of classification:

1. The choice of the criteria
2. The types of neoplasias which are recognized by the greatest number of pathologists
3. The types of lymphoid neoplasias which are discussed by some pathologists

Choice of Criteria

At present, a classification based on etiologic factors is impossible. A clinical one is insufficient; the best classification is a morphologic one. The morphologic criteria are defined by cytologic and histologic studies. But, it is of great importance to emphasize that all these morphologic criteria have to be recognizable by routine techniques. In fact, all pathologists should be able to utilize such a classification.

Undoubtedly, new, more sophisticated techniques are of prime importance for specifying the cellular type of the lymphoma, the exact origin of the proliferating cells. The morphologic and functional characteristics, which enable one to propose a functional classification, can be obtained by transmission and scanning electron microscopy, cyto- and histoenzymology, immunofluorescence, and immunologic studies of the membrane receptors. But we must look at that type of functional classification with a critical eye because the results are often very difficult to interpret and because some of the results can be artifacts. Furthermore, these techniques need expensive material and well-trained technicians; thus, only specialized laboratories can do them and they can only be utilized in a few cases. The results obtained for a few cases can be more or less generalized to apply to all lymphomas possessing the same morphology.

The Different Types of Lymphoid Neoplasias Accepted by all Pathologists

All the classifications agree on the existence of a special kind of B-lymphoid cell which originates from the follicular center. These cells give rise to all the nodular or follicular malignant lymphomas and to some diffuse ones. All the classifications also recognize different sorts of diffuse malignant lymphomas, composed either of:

1. Little round lymphocytes forming a lymphoma indistinguishable from the CLL.
2. Lymphocytes with convoluted nuclei.
3. Cleaved lymphoid cells predominantly infiltrating the skin, forming mycosis fungoides and Sézary's disease.
4. Lymphoblasts with very basophilic cytoplasma, forming Burkitt's disease.

Four Types of Lymphoid Neoplasias Discussed or Not Quite Accepted by All Pathologists

1. The existence of a lymphoplasmocytic sarcoma has been widely demonstrated. Its population is very pleomorphic; besides lymphocytes, we can see plasmocytes, lymphoplasmocytes, and immunoblasts in varying numbers. The reality of an intracellular secretion of a monoclonal immunoglobulin, mainly of IgM-κ, can be easily demonstrated by immunofluorescence on paraffin sections obtained from fixed tissues.

2. Plasmocytic sarcoma is different because its population is only composed of plasmoblasts and plasmocytes secreting mainly monoclonal IgA, IgG, or light chains. This lymphoma corresponds to the late extra osseous myeloma and can be seen during the evolution of α-heavy chain disease.

3. Malignant lymphomas of immunoblastic type are well-known. They were later called reticulosarcomas. The proliferating cells are large cells with clear nuclei, basophilic cytoplasma, and a large number of ribosomes. Many of them are of B-type, one-third showing a differentiation toward a plasmocyte with development of an ergastoplasm, as can be seen at the ultrastructural level and demonstrated by immunofluorescence. Some others are of follicular origin and can be recognized by their two symmetrically disposed nucleoli, as described by Lukes and Lennert [7, 8, 9]. Others are perhaps of T-origin. It is of interest to indicate here that the Reed–Sternberg cells from Hodgkin's disease are probably some kind of B-immunoblasts. Their cytoplasm contains effectively monoclonal immunoglobulin, as demonstrated first by Taylor [10] and as revealed in one of our cases by immunoperoxidase in semithin preparations and during ultrastructural study.

4. The last type of malignant lymphoma I would like to discuss is the reticulo- or histiocytosarcoma. It is the most discussed type. Before considering them, the term reticular cell has to be defined. We have already seen that the immunoblast was described under this name. The other cells are the following:

a) The fibroblast and the endothelial cells, which are sometimes considered to be of reticular origin.

b) The histiocytes and macrophages, which are also sometimes named reticular cells. Their proliferation gives rise to malignant histiocytosis or perhaps histiocytosarcoma, which is probably very rare.

c) The interdigitating cells that lie in the T-dependent lymphoid zones and have distinctive cytoplasmic features. They are probably of histiocytomonocytic origin and do not produce collagen fibers. Rare lymphomas are probably due to the proliferation of this type of cell.

d) The reticulum cells are part of the lymphoid network. They have cytoplasmic extensions surrounding collagen fibers, so-called reticular fibers. Their origin, perhaps fibroblastic, and their capacity to proliferate are unknown.

e) The dendritic cells are specialized cells lying in the follicular center, characterized by their long dendrite-like cytoplasmic arms, attached to one another by desmosomes. At present, it is not certain whether they can give rise to a lymphoma.

So, in my opinion, reticular cell is a term that covered too many types of cells and which must be eliminated because of its imprecision. Reticulosarcoma is a word which has to be avoided as long as knowledge about the so-called reticular cells is insufficient.

References

1. Bennett, M. H., Farrer-Brown, G., Henry, K., Jelliffe, A. M.: Classification of non Hodgkin's lymphomas. Lancet *1974/ii*, 405–406.
2. Diebold, J.: Affections malignes lymphoplasmocytaires et réticulohistiocytaires. Propositions pour une nouvelle classification. Arch. Anat. Pathol. (Paris) *21* (2), 103–111 (1973).
3. Diebold, J.: Classifications morphologiques des hématosarcomes lymphoïdes non hodkiniens. Propositions. Nouv. Press Méd. *3*, 1818 (1974).
4. Diebold, J.: Classifications des sarcomes lymphoïdes non hodkiniens et des proliférations voisines. Arch. Anat. Pathol. (Paris) *23* (2), 97–106 (1975).
5. Dorfman, R. F.: Classification of non-Hodgkin's lymphomas. Lancet *1974/ii*, 1295–1296.
6. Gerard-Marchant, R., Hamlin, I., Lennert, K., Rilke, F., Stansfeld, A. G., Van Unnik, J. A. M.: Letter to the Editor. Lancet *1974/ii*, 406–408.
7. Lennert, K.: Morphology and classification of malignant lymphomas and so-called reticuloses. Acta Neuropathol. (Berl.) *4* (suppl.), 1–16 (1975).
8. Lennert, K., Mohri, N., Stein, H., Kaiserling, E.: The histopathology of malignant lymphoma. Br. J. Haemoatol. *31* (suppl.), 193–203 (1975).
9. Lukes, R. J., Collins, R. D.: Immunologic characterization of human malignant lymphomas. Cancer *34* (4) (suppl.), 1488–1503 (1974).
10. Mathé, G., Rappaport, H., O'Conor, G. T., Portoni, H.: Histological and cytological typing of neoplastic disease of haematopoietic and lymphoid tissues. World Health Organization, Genève 1976 (International Histological Classification of Tumours N° 14).
11. Taylor, C. R.: The nature of Reed Sternberg cells and other malignant reticulum cells. Lancet *1975/ii*, 802–806.

Current Techniques for the Study of Cell Morphology

B. CAILLOU

Today, more and more new techniques are becoming available for studying cell morphology. Besides classic histology and cytology, it is possible to use cytochemistry, immunofluorescence, or immunoperoxidase techniques, semithin sections, transmission, or scanning electron microscopy.

The immunoperoxidase technique applied to tissues embedded in paraffin is a controversial technique. Specificity and interpretation of the results are questionable. Nevertheless, this technique is very interesting because it finely selects some cells from among the others. What does this staining mean? Even if the answer is still unclear, it seems obvious that it will give important information on the physiologic status of the cell. Comparison must be made with electron microscopic results in which the peroxidase staining can be seen inside organelles of the cells. The use of semithin sections is one of the best methods for studying morphology by light microscopy. In the hematopoeitic field, it will become essential, soon probably, for classifying malignant cells.

Transmission and scanning electron microscopy have added a lot of new information on cell structures which is not yet used routinely.

To date, classification of lymphosarcomas was essentially based upon classic histologic and cytologic methods.

What about the other more sophisticated techniques?

As far as nomenclature is concerned, can we really use the same terminology for all of these current techniques, or does each one have to have its own classification?

Classifications of the Malignant Lymphomas: A Survey

R. F. DORFMAN

It is unlikely that a critical review of a controversial topic of this nature can be presented without offending some, if not all, who have proposed new classifications [2, 11, 12, 15, 22, 24] of the so-called non-Hodgkin's lymphomas (a term which, by virtue of its negative implications, is already in some disrepute). Clearly, Rappaport [27, 28, 29] recognizes the need for a change in terminology in keeping with recent observations based on newly devised techniques for cellular indentification [5, 12, 16]. He [28] and I [13] have, nevertheless, challenged some of the recently proposed concepts and nomenclature, based on a so-called functional approach [21, 22].

The new terms *immunocytoma* and *immunoblastic sarcoma* fly in the face of recommendations by COTTIER et al. [10] that *terms should be descriptive* and that they should not be based on "as yet debatable functional interpretations".

My proposed working classification (Table 1) employs descriptive terminology and does not seek to impose contentious and cumbersome designations upon practicing pathologists, hematologists, and oncologists [11, 12, 13].

Table 1. Working classification of non-Hodgkin's lymphomas (DORFMAN—1974, modified 1976)

Follicular lymphomas[a]
(Follicular or follicular and diffuse)
Small lymphoid
Mixed small and large lymphoid
Large lymphoid
Diffuse lymphomas[a]
Small lymphocytic[b]
Atypical small lymphoid
Lymphoblastic
Convoluted
Nonconvoluted
Large lymphoid[b]
Mixed small and large lymphoid
Histiocytic
Burkitt's lymphoma
Mycosis fungoides
Undefined

[a] Composite lymphomas, comprising two well-defined and apparently different types of lymphomas within the same tissue, and lymphomas associated with sclerosis.

[b] Lymphomas showing plasmacytoid differentiation, and those diffuse lymphomas associated with epithelioid cells are suitably designated.

Uncertainty already exists regarding the definition of immunoblastic sarcoma as applied to large cell lymphomas. It would appear that LENNERT et al. [21] apply this term to most large cell lymphomas, whereas LUKES and COLLINS [22] interpret only a minority of these lymphomas as immunoblastic sarcoma. Those lymphomas heretofore termed histiocytic by RAPPAPORT [27] now encompass a variety of tumors defined variably by LUKES and COLLINS as "large cleaved and noncleaved follicular center, B-immunoblastic, T-immunoblastic and histiocytic." Whatever term is applied to the histiocytic or large cell lymphomas, it is clear that they differ considerably from other lymphomas with respect to natural history, organ involvement, and microscopic and gross pathologic manifestations [20]. The large cell lymphomas do not show the homing patterns exhibited by the small lymphocytic lymphomas.

Both LUKES and LENNERT have asserted that the small lymphocytic (well-differentiated lymphocytic) lymphoma (WDLL) is the tissue expression of chronic lymphocytic leukemia (CLL) [21, 22], whether this be of the more common B-cell type or the rare, newly recognized T-cell type [6]. PANGALIS et al. [26] have recently questioned this concept. While WDLL, CLL, and lymphoproliferative disorders with a monoclonal gammopathy are histologically similar, their clinical and hematologic presentations differ sufficiently to justify their separation. They may, nevertheless, represent different expressions of the same basic process, i.e., a proliferation of small lymphocytes usually of the B-cell type.

LUKES and COLLINS have made an important contribution by demonstrating the morphologic identification of the *convoluted lymphocytic lymphoma* and emphasizing its predilection for the mediastinum, its frequency in adolescent boys, and its propensity to involve the bone marrow, peripheral blood, and the central nervous system [1]. On the other hand, NATHWANI et al. [25] have recently reported that mediastinal lymphomas with an identical clinical presentation may be composed of cells with nonconvoluted nuclei and propose the term *malignant lymphoma lymphoblastic convoluted and nonconvoluted* for this form of lymphoma. I have made identical observations and am in full agreement with this concept [13].

Implicit in the LUKES-COLLINS classification is the concept that cellular function can be recognized morphologically and that such functions should constitute the main criteria for nomenclature and classifications. Thus they associate nuclear convolution with T-cell characteristics; however, JAFFE et al. have reported a heterogeneity of immunologic markers and surface morphology in childhood lymphoblastic lymphoma, and similar observations were made by BROUET et al. [7] in their study of acute lymphoblastic leukaemia. Neither of these studies established a correlation of cytologic features with membrane markers.

Techniques for the immunologic characterization of cells have enabled investigators to establish that mycosis fungoides, Sézary's syndrome, a proportion of lymphoblastic lymphomas and leukemias, and rare cases of CLL represent T-cell disorders [7]. Mycosis fungoides is recognized as a malignant lymphoma of T-lymphocytes originating in the skin and subsequently spreading to lymph nodes and other internal organs [28, 29]. This disorder warrants inclusion in all newly devised classifications of the non-Hodgkin's lymphomas.

The cells of *Burkitt's lymphoma*, previously designated as undifferentiated [4], have now been shown to possess B-cell characteristics [18]. LUKES and COLLINS have proposed that Burkitt's lymphoma is of follicular center cell origin, and the recent report by MANN et al. [23] supports the contention that this lymphoma is a B-cell tumor related to germinal centers. In other respects, however, Burkitt's lymphoma, with its distinctive clinicopathologic features and characteristic response to therapy, bears little resemblance to currently recognized follicular (nodular) lymphomas [3, 12]. The latter are *extremely rare* in children and in blacks. Their cellular homing patterns, the topographic distribution of lesions and their relatively benign biologic behavior, stamp the nodular (follicular) lymphomas as a group that must clearly be separated. There is, nonetheless, convincing evidence that the cells of nodular lymphomas derive from follicular B-lymphocytes [12, 16], whether these be small or large and heretofore designated as histiocytic. The importance of identifying a nodular (follicular) pattern, in terms of age, sex, and racial distribution, topographic distribution of lesions, natural history, and response to therapy has clearly been stressed [3, 12, 19, 32]. Moreover, BUTLER et al. [9], utilizing LUKES and COLLINS's classification, indicated that "*as far as survival is concerned the most important histological feature of a lymphoma is its pattern, whether diffuse or follicular.*" Despite these observations, both LENNERT and LUKES contend that follicular center cell lymphomas, which they designate as "centrocytic" and "small cleaved", respectively, all have a favorable prognosis, regardless of the architectural pattern [21].

The WHO classification [24] identifies nodular lymphomas but employs the term "prolymphocytic" for the small cell type. This appears to be in conflict with the entity "prolymphocytic leukemia," described by GALTON et al. [14], which differs cytologically and clinically from the leukemic phase of nodular lymphocytic lymphoma. While it incorporates some of the newly proposed terms such as "immunoblastic" and retains established terms such as "Burkitt's tumor," the WHO classification is retrogressive in its reintroduction of the terms "lymphosarcoma" and "reticulosarcoma."

Yet to be established as a distinct clinicopathologic entity is the lymphoma with a high content of epithelioid cells [8], previously considered to represent a form of Hodgkin's disease, but recently renamed "*lymphoepithelioid cellular lymphoma*" by LENNERT [21]. None of the new classifications pays specific attention to *childhood lymphomas*, virtually all of which have a diffuse pattern (Table 2) [13]. Nodular lymphomas of all types are exceptionally rare in children, and well-differentiated lymphocytic lymphomas have yet to be reported in this age group.

Table 2. Classification of childhood lymphomas[a] (DORFMAN—1976)

Lymphoblastic
Convoluted
Nonconvoluted
Large lymphoid
Histiocytic
Burkitt's lymphoma
Undifferentiated

[a] Virtually all are diffuse.

Many new terms and concepts have been proposed since the introduction of ROBB-SMITH's classification [30] which, on his own admission, was once described "as avoiding the fallacy of over-simplification!" [31]. Pathologists now have the unenviable choice of one of at least five newly proposed classifications [2, 11, 12, 15, 22, 24], as an alternative to that of RAPPAPORT [27]. This state of affairs has dismayed clinicians faced with the choice of therapy and statisticians attempting comparative studies. In an endeavor to resolve this impasse, the United States National Cancer Institute is supporting a large-scale retrospective review of material from 1000 patients with non-Hodgkin's lymphomas. Selected panels of expert hematopathologists will visit four participating institutions in order to subclassify these cases according to one or more of the proffered schemes. It is hoped that this carefully controlled clinicopathologic study will indicate which of the newly proposed classifications is most adaptable to comparative clinical trials and is most easily utilized by practicing pathologists.

References

1. BARCOS, M. P., LUKES, R. J.: Malignant lymphoma of convoluted lymphocytes. A new entity of possible T-cell type. In: Conflicts in Childhood Cancer. New York: Stan R. Liss, Inc. 1975, p. 147–178.

2. Bennett, M. H., Farrer-Brown, G., Henry, K., Jeliffe, A. M.: Classification of non-Hodgkin's lymphomas. Lancet *1974/ii*, 405–405.
3. Berard, C. W., Dorfman, R. F.: Histopathology of malignant lymphomas. In: Clinics in Hematology. Rosenberg, S. A. (ed.). Philadelphia: Saunders 1974, p. 39–76.
4. Berard, C. W., O'Conor, G. T., Thomas, L. B., Torloni, H. (ed.): Histopathological definition of Burkitt's tumor. Bull. W.H.O. *40*, 601–607 (1969).
5. Braylan, R. C., Jaffe, E. S., Berard, C. W.: Malignant lymphomas: Current classification and new observations. Pathol. Annu. *10*, 213–270 (1975).
6. Brouet, J. C., Flandrin, G., Sasportes, M., Preud'Homme, J-L., Seligmann, M.: Chronic lymphocytic leukaemia of T-cell origin. Immunological and clinical evaluation in eleven patients. Lancet *1975/ii*, 890–893.
7. Brouet, J. C., Valensi, R., Daniel, M-T., Flandrin, G., Preud'Homme, J-L., Seligmann, M.: Immunological classification of acute lymphoblastic leukaemias: Evaluation of its clinical significance in a hundred patients. Br. J. Haematol. *33*, 319–328 (1976).
8. Burke, J., Butler, J.: Malignant lymphoma with a high content of epithelioid histiocytes. (Lennert's Lymphoma.) Am. J. Clin. Pathol. *66*, 1–9 (1976).
9. Butler, J. J., Stryker, J. A., Shullenberger, C. C.: A clinico-pathological study of stages 1 & 11 non-Hodgkin's lymphomata using the Lukes–Collins classification. Br. J. Cancer *31* (Suppl. 11), 208–216 (1975).
10. Cottier, H., Turk, J., Sobin, L.: A proposal for a standardized system of reporting human lymph node morphology in relation to immunological function. Bull. W.H.O. *47*, 375–408 (1972).
11. Dorfman, R. F.: Classification of non-Hodgkin's lymphomas. Lancet *1974/i*, 1295.
12. Dorfman, R. F.: The non-Hodgkin's lymphomas. In: The Reticuloendothelial System. IAP Monograph No. 16. Baltimore: Williams and Wilkins 1975, p. 262–281.
13. Dorfman, R. F.: Pathology of the non-Hodgkin's lymphomas: New classifications. Cancer Treat. Rep. *61*, 945–951 (1977).
14. Galton, D. A. G., Goldman, E. W., Catovsky, D., Henry, K., Goldenberg, G. J.: Prolymphocytic leukemia. Br. J. Haematol. *27*, 7–23 (1974).
15. Gerard-Marchant, R., Hamilin, I., Lennert, K., Rilke, F., Stansfeld, A. G., Van Unnik, J. A. M.: Classification of non-Hodgkin's lymphomas. Lancet *1974/ii*, 406–408.
16. Jaffe, E. S., Shevach, E. M., Frank, M. M., Berard, C. W., Green, I.: Nodular lymphoma-evidence for origin from follicular B lymphocytes. N. Engl. J. Med. *290*, 813–819 (1974).
17. Jaffe, E. S., Braylan, R. C., Frank, M. M., Green, I., Berard, C. W.: Heterogeneity of immunologic markers and surface morphology in childhood lymphoblastic lymphoma. Blood *48*, 213–222 (1976).
18. Jondal, M., Klein, G.: Surface markers on human B and T lymphocytes. II. Presence of Epstein–Barr virus receptors on B lymphocytes. J. Exp. Med. *138*, 1365 (1973).
19. Jones, S. E., Fuks, Z., Bull, M., Kadin, M. E., Dorfman, R. F., Kaplan, H. S., Kim, H., Rosenberg, S. A.: Non-Hodgkin's lymphomas. IV. Clinico-pathologic correlation in 405 cases. Cancer *31*, 806–823 (1973).
20. Kim, H., Dorfman, R. F.: Morphological studies of 84 untreated patients subjected to laparotomy for the staging of non-Hodgkin's lymphomas. Cancer *33*, 657–674 (1974).
21. Lennert, K., Mohri, N., Stein, H., Kaiserling, E.: The histopathology of malignant lymphoma. Br. J. Haematol. *31* (suppl.), 193–203 (1975).
22. Lukes, R. J., Collins, R. D.: Immunological characterization of human malignant lymphomas. Cancer *34*, 1488–1503 (1974).
23. Mann, R. B., Jaffe, E. S., Braylan, R. C., Nanba, K., Frank, M. M., Ziegler, J. L., Berard, C. W.: Non-endemic Burkitt's lymphoma. A B-cell tumor related to germinal centers. N. Engl. J. Med. *295*, 685–691 (1976).
24. Mathe, G., Rappaport, H., O'Conor, G. T., Torloni, H.: Histological and Cytological Typing of Neoplastic Diseases of Hematopoietic and Lymphoid Tissues. Geneva. WHO International Histological Classification of Tumors. No. 14 1976.
25. Nathwani, B. N., Kim, H., Rappaport, H.: Malignant lymphoma, lymphoblastic. Cancer *38*, 964–983 (1976).
26. Pangalis, G. A., Nathwani, B. N., Rappaport, H.: Malignant lymphoma well differentiated lymphocytic. Its relationship with chronic lymphocytic leukemia and macroglobulinemia of Waldenstrom. Cancer *39*, 999–1010 (1977).
27. Rappaport, H.: Tumors of the hematopoietic system. In : Atlas of Tumor Pathology. Sect. 3, fasc. 8. Washington, D.C.: Armed Forces Institute of Pathology 1966, pp. 91–204.
28. Rappaport, H.: In: Round Table Discussion of Histopathologic Classification. Proc. Non-Hodgkin's lymphoma Symposium, San Francisco, October 1976. Cancer Treat Rep. *61*, 1037–1042 (1977).

29. RAPPAPORT, H., BRAYLAN, R. C.: Changing concepts in the classification of malignant neoplasms of the hematopoietic system. In: The Reticuloendothelial System. Int. Acad. Pathol. Monogr. *16*, 1–19 (1975).
30. ROBB-SMITH, A. H. T.: Reticulosis and reticulosarcoma. A histological classification. J. Pathol. Bacteriol. *47*, 457–480 (1938).
31. ROBB-SMITH, A. H. T.: Immunotopography of lymphoreticular disorders. Lancet *1974/i*, 513–514.
32. WARNKE, R., KIM, H., FUKS, Z., DORFMAN, R. F.: The coexistence of nodular and diffuse patterns in nodular non-Hodgkin's lymphomas. Significance and clinico-pathologic correlation. Cancer *40*, 1229–1233 (1977).

Surface Morphology of Lymphoreticular Cells: Review of Data Obtained From Scanning Electron Microscopy

A. Polliack

During the past 10 years, scanning electron microscopy (SEM) has been used to study the surface morphology of human leukocytes [2, 9, 17, 18, 33, 39, 44, 47, 50, 51, 59, 62, 68, 69, 70, 73, 74, 75, 76, 78, 88, 105,106]. Initially, it was hoped that this mode of microscopy would have something to contribute to the more accurate definition of different cell types and in particular to cells of the lymphoreticular system and lymphoproliferative disorders. Earlier studies employing air drying techniques in SEM preparation [9, 17, 39, 59] did not provide optimal details of cell surface architecture, and cell shrinkage and collapse of microprojections made it difficult to recognize different cell types with certainty. Nevertheless, it was evident from these earlier studies that lymphocytes and monocytes/macrophages differed in their surface morphology and that transformed lymphocytes had more active surfaces than normal lymphocytes [9, 33, 39]. Much better preservation of cell surface architecture was obtained when freeze and critical point drying techniques [5] were used to prepare cells for SEM [10, 85, 68]. This enabled easier characterization and recognition of different cell types and surface microprojections. Because of the above results [10, 85, 68], air drying has not been recommended for use in the preparation of leukocytes for SEM since 1972.

In our earlier studies using critical point drying and an aspiration-filtration technique [68, 69, 70, 71, 72, 76, 77, 78], it was possible to detect differences in the surface architecture of various leukocytes, based on studies of peripheral circulating cells (derived from normal and leukemic individuals), different cultured cell lines, and tissues obtained from humans and animals. From these and other studies [1, 2, 36, 42, 47, 50, 51, 52, 54, 55, 58, 62, 65, 88, 89, 91, 104], it was clearly evident that monocytes and macrophages could readily be distinguished from lymphocytes under SEM. Lymphocytes have varying numbers of finger-like microvilli and

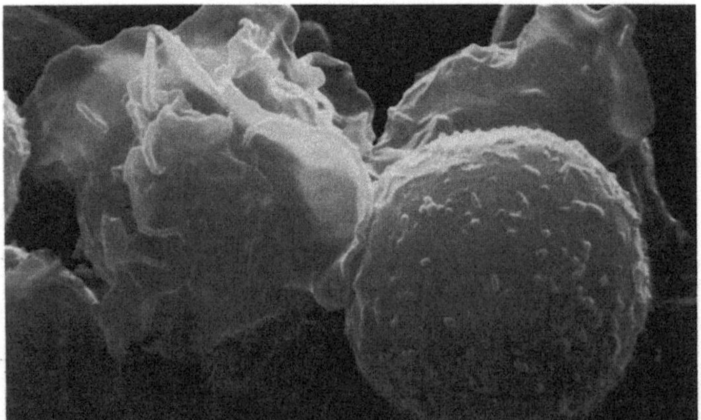

Fig. 1. Ficoll-Hypaque separated mononuclear cells. On the left, a monocyte with well-developed ruffles and on the right, a spherical lymphocyte with small stub-like microvilli (× 8000)

generally lack ridge-like profiles or ruffles, while monocytes and macrophages have characteristic, well-developed ruffles and prominent ridge-like profiles (Figs. 1–3). The latter become even more prominent during activation and phagocytosis [1, 67, 79]. Immunoscanning electron microscopic studies have confirmed these findings conclusively and have shown that lymphocytes rarely have ruffles [37, 54, 55, 60, 61].

Granulocytes have a wider spectrum of surface morphology and are difficult to distinguish from monocytes. Microvilli can be encountered on these cells, particularly basophils and eosinophils [70, 76]. Nevertheless, the most frequent surface features encountered are ridge-like profiles and smaller ruffles, which are sometimes polarized to one end of the cell, particularly during locomotion (Fig. 4). These initial results were encouraging and indicated that SEM may be useful in defining different cell types and justified further research relating to

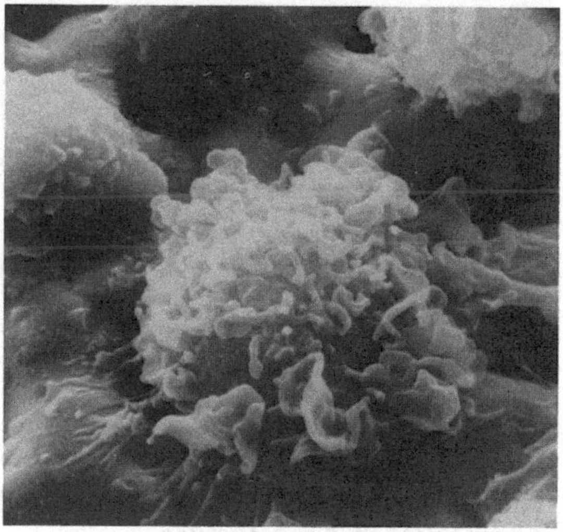

Fig. 2. Typical monocyte/macrophage surface architecture. Ruffles and ridge-like profiles are prominent (× 8200)

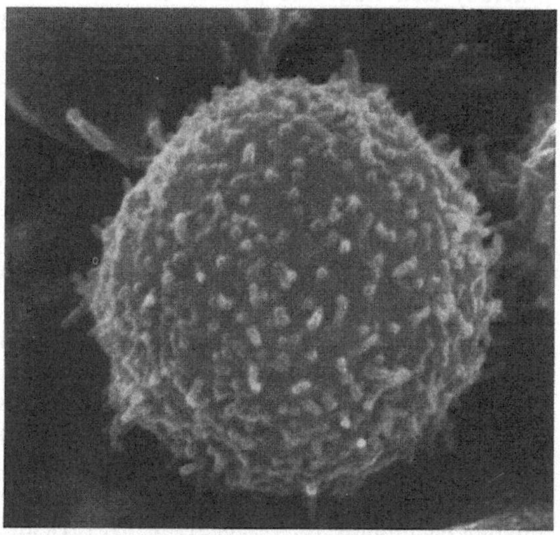

Fig. 3. Typical lymphocyte surface architecture. Microvilli are evident and ruffles seldom seen (× 12,000)

malignant cells in an attempt to establish whether this mode of microscopy could contribute to the diagnosis of malignant lymphoreticular disorders and leukemias.
Before summarizing current knowledge on SEM and malignant disorders, it is appropriate to review the current status of knowledge and available SEM data which relates to normal lymphocytes and thymic cells and the factors which influence and alter their surface architecture.

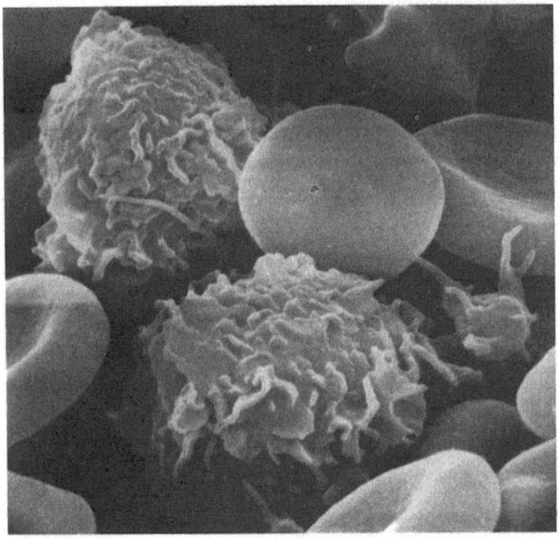

Fig. 4. Ficoll-Hypaque separated granulocytes and erythrocytes. Cells have ridges and ruffles which are frequently polarized to one end of the cell (× 6000)

Normal Lymphocytes and Thymic Cells: Review of Factors Influencing Their Surface Architecture

The above cells can readily be distinguished from monocytes and macrophages under SEM and generally lack ridge-like profiles or ruffles. In 1972, LIN et al. [51] showed that *thymic lymphocytes* differ from circulating lymphocytes and show less microvilli. This finding has been confirmed by others [49, 70, 81, 88, 89] and is consistent and unrelated to the methodologies used for cell preparation. In our studies on thymic cells, we have shown that they show relatively few microvilli irrespective of the manner in which they are fixed or prepared for SEM [81]. Tissue thymic cells studied in vivo show similar features [49], but when these cells are stimulated by mitogens, the number of surface microvilli increases. These "blast" transformed T cells differ from their nonstimulated counterparts (Figs. 5 and 6).
In our earlier studies [68, 69, 70, 71, 72, 78], employing an aspiration filtration technique on cells which were initially *not fixed in cell suspension*, circulating lymphocytes showed varying numbers of microvilli, and it appeared that the majority of cells had relatively few or moderate numbers of microvilli while approximately 25%–30% had more complex villous surfaces. The different proportion of villous and less villous cells correlated well with the proportion of B- and T-derived lymphocytes in the peripheral blood. This impression was confirmed from studies on enriched B- and T-cell populations [70, 72], cultured B- and T-cell lines, and thymic lymphocytes. Accordingly, it was suggested that B cells frequently show more microvilli than their less villous T-derived counterparts. Similar results were obtained by other workers using different techniques [18, 47, 50, 51, 88, 89, 101], and comparison of E-rosetting T-lymphocytes

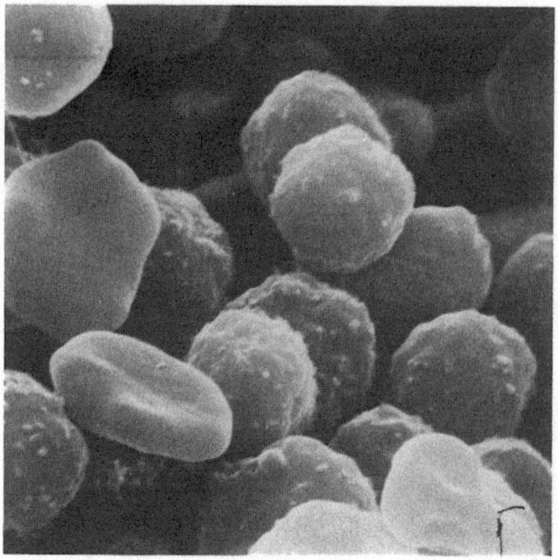

Fig. 5. Thymic lymphocytes (obtained from murine thymus) with only a few surface microvilli. Some discocyte erythrocytes are also seen to the left (×4000). *Cells fixed in suspension prior to collection onto substrate*

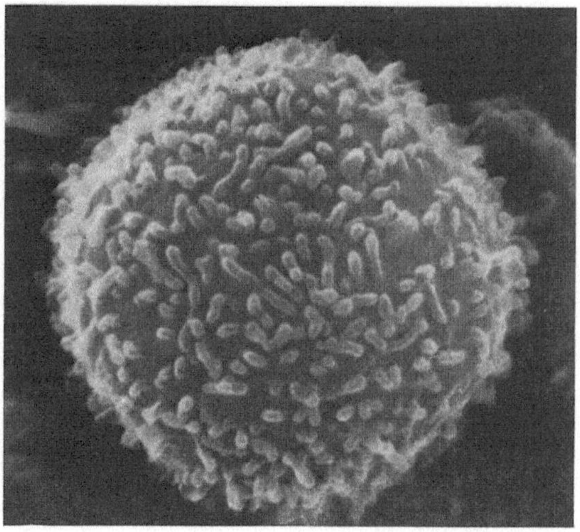

Fig. 6. Typical mitogen transformed thymic lymphocyte which now displays microvilli (×11,000)

and EAC-rosetting B-lymphocytes [42, 50, 71] suggested that this was in fact so. Lymphocytes with intermediate surface features were always encountered in these studies, making classification of subpopulations difficult, and parallel immunologic identification of cells examined under SEM was always recommended (Fig. 7).

In subsequent SEM studies by ALEXANDER and WETZEL and co-authors [2, 3] and other workers [7, 43, 56, 62, 98, 103, 105, 106], differences between B and T cells were not encountered. These authors have demonstrated how variations in the mode of fixation, cell collection and preparation, and other in vitro and microenvironmental factors may alter the number of microvilli seen at a given moment on lymphocytes, and it is clear that these factors play an important role in determining the eventual cell surface architecture as seen by SEM. Different studies during the past 2–3 years have shown that the type and osmolality of the

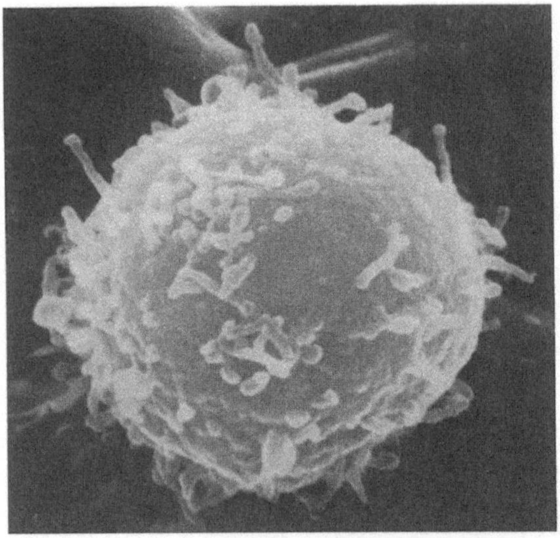

Fig. 7. Peripheral blood lymphocyte with moderate numbers of microvilli (× 15,000)

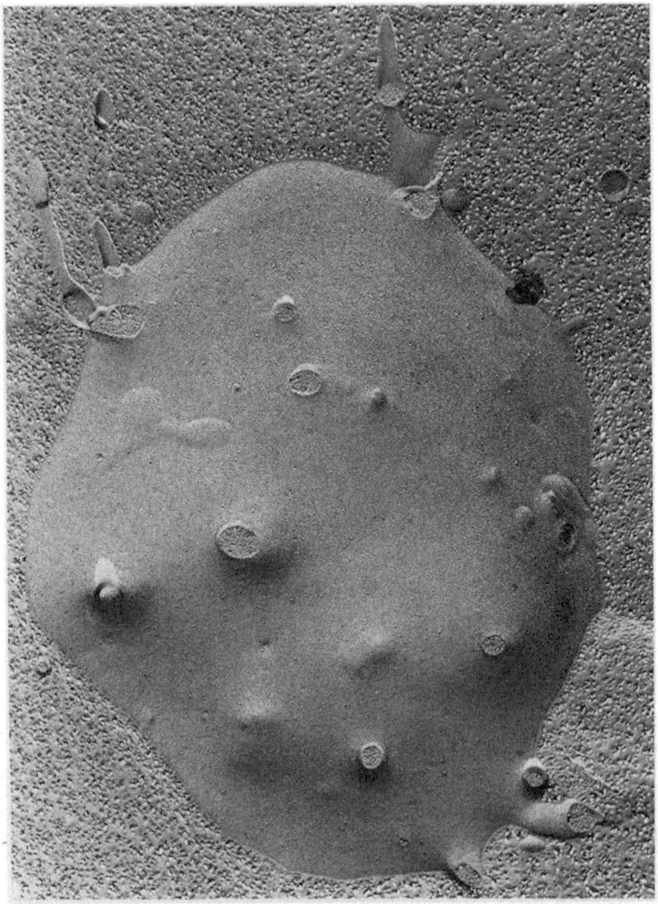

Fig. 8. Cryofractured, freeze-etched human peripheral blood lymphocyte showing few microvilli (× 25,000). Most cells have this surface architecture (Courtesy of Dr. Renau-Piqueras, Valencia, Spain) Human blood lymphocyte (× 25,000). Not published

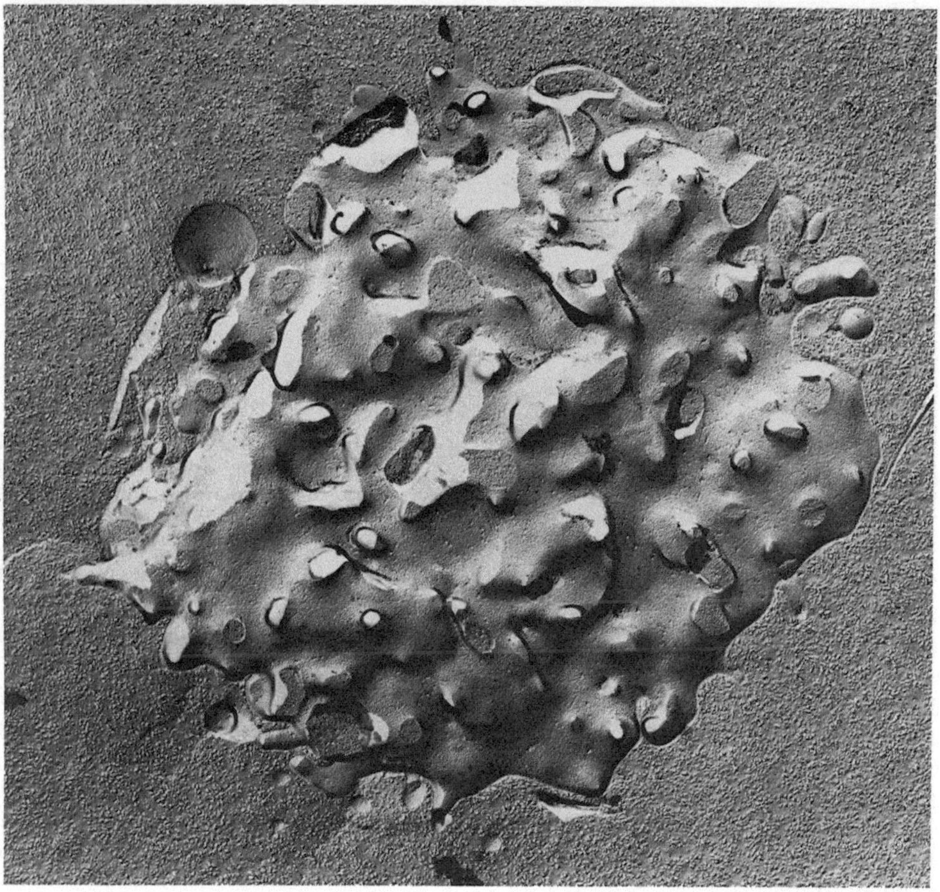

Fig. 9. Cryofractured, freeze-etched human peripheral blood lymphocyte showing multiple microvilli. Only about 25% of circulating cells display this type of surface architecture (×28,000) (Courtesy of Dr. Renau-Piqueras, Valencia, Spain);
Human blood lymphocyte (×28,000). Not published

fixative and buffer used for cell preparation [6], duration of fixation and the interval prior to fixation [106], cell spreading [25], aspiration and filtration of cells [3], intercellular contact and cell density [52, 71, 93], temperature [53], cell cycle [86], contact with viruses [4, 23, 29, 35, 87], chemicals [57], and mitogens [81, 100] are among the factors determining the number and type of microprojections seen on the surface of mammalian cells. In addition, activation, maturation, and the functional state of the lymphocyte may also alter the number of microvilli seen on the surface [7, 44, 56, 103]. Thus, it is apparent that the microvilli, so characteristic of lymphocytes, are labile structures easily modulated by microenvironmental factors in vitro and in vivo, and their presence or absence on lymphocytes does not seem to depend on lymphocyte source. Particularly convincing in this respect are the results of in vivo studies by VAN EWIJK and co-workers [103] on homing and recirculation of lymphocyte populations. These workers showed that B- and T-lymphocytes in lymph nodes and spleens had similar surface topographies under SEM but altered on cell contact with endothelium and during their entry into the circulation. Thus, taking all the above data into consideration, we must conclude that it would be unwise to use the number of microvilli as a consistent and reliable criterion for establishing B- or T-cell origin. Accordingly, we have not attempted in our SEM studies on leukemic and transformed lymphocytes to establish B- or T-cell identity *solely* on the basis of surface architecture.

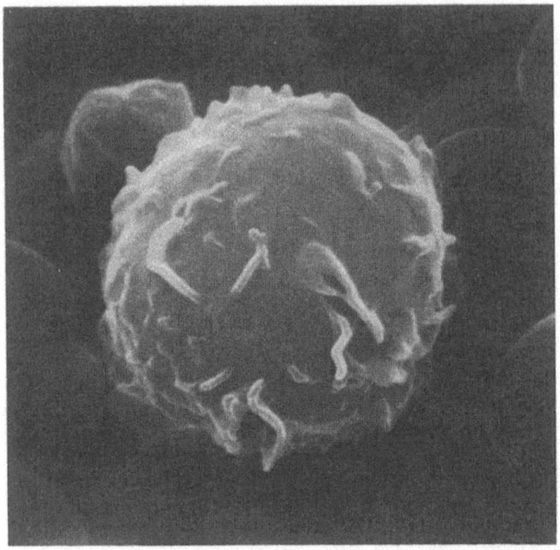

Fig. 10. Circulating leukemic myeloblast from a patient with acute nonlymphoblastic leukemia showing transverse ridges and small ruffles (× 7500)

At this point, however, we must consider the results of other microscopic studies relating to the surface morphology of normal lymphocytes, which have shown major differences between B- and T-lymphocytes. These include studies by phase microscopy, and Nomarski differential interference microscopy [22, 90, 96, 98, 102], Hoffman modulation contrast microscopy [66], fluorescence microscopy [26, 26], transmission and immunoelectron microscopy [34, 36, 91], and freeze-etching with cryofracture [88, 89]. These results, which have frequently been ignored in the discussion of SEM studies on lymphocytes, cannot be reconciled with those of ALEXANDER and WETZEL [2, 3] and raise further questions relating to B- and T-cell identification on the basis of surface morphology. They show that the initial differences described between B and T *cannot all be related* to artifact or other technical factors alone (Figs. 8 and 9).

In summary, from almost all studies performed until now, it is clear that it is possible to distinguish normal lymphocytes from monocytes and macrophages on the basis of their surface architecture. Lymphocytes, which have been positively identified by immuno-SEM techniques [37, 54, 55, 60, 61], have finger-like microvilli and generally lack ruffles, while monocytes and

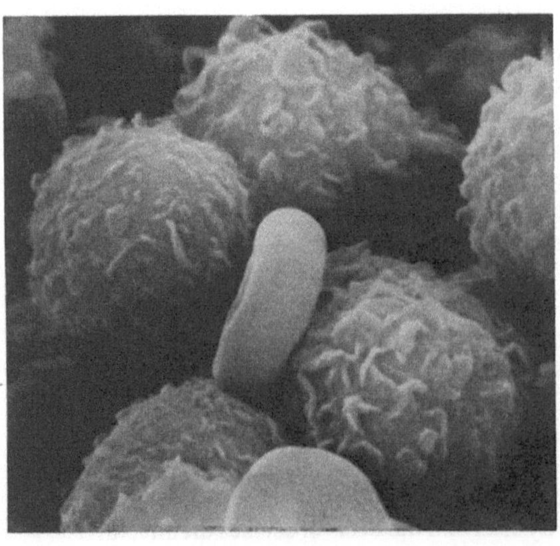

Fig. 11. Circulating leukemic cells from a patient with acute granulocytic leukemia showing transverse ridge-like profiles and small ruffles (× 6200)

macrophages have broad-based ruffles and lack multiple microvilli. In relation to B- and T-lymphocytes—despite differences in surface morphology described in earlier studies and clear-cut differences between these two cell types observed with other modes of microscopy and by cryofracture—*recent data* indicate that it would be *unwise to attempt to distinguish between* them solely on the basis of the number of microvilli seen under SEM. Bearing the above-mentioned factors in mind, let us turn to a review of current knowledge and available data on the surface features of malignant and leukemic cells as seen by SEM.

Leukemias

One of the major problems in the interpretation of SEM photographs in these disorders is related to the spectrum of cell surface topography encountered in some of the cases studied. In

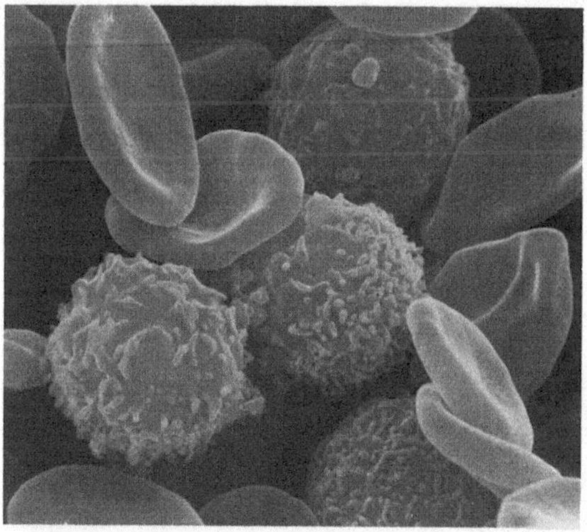

Fig. 12. Circulating leukemic leukocytes and erythrocytes from the buffy coat of a patient with eosinophilic leukemia (× 5900). Cells show mainly ridge-like profiles but can also display microvilli

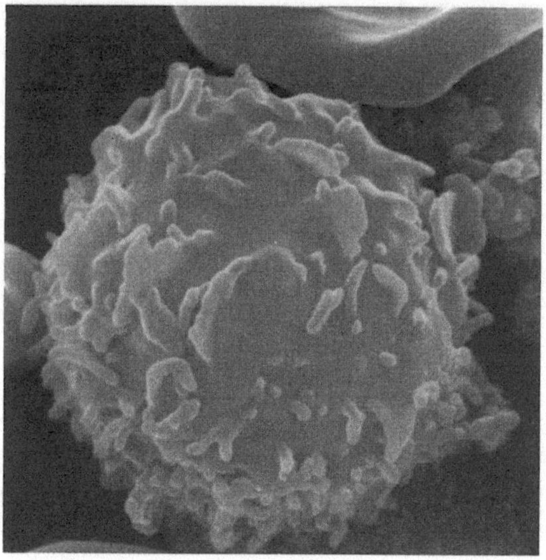

Fig. 13. Close-up of one of the leukemic cells (from the patient with eosinophilic leukemia with ridge-like profiles) (× 10,000)

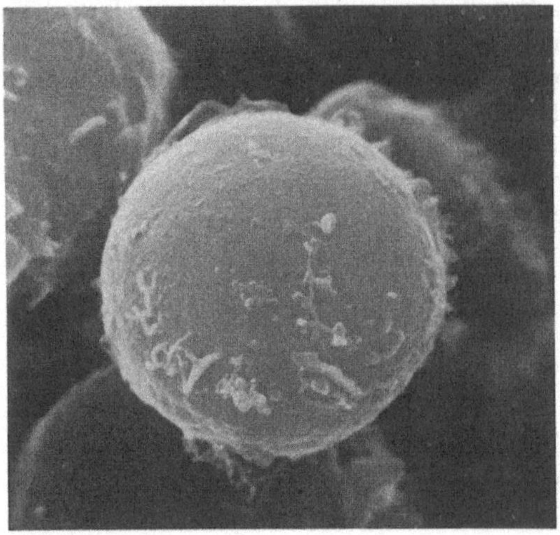

Fig. 14. Cell from the PH-positive K-562 myeloid line showing a few microprojections which are mainly ridge-like profiles (× 7500)

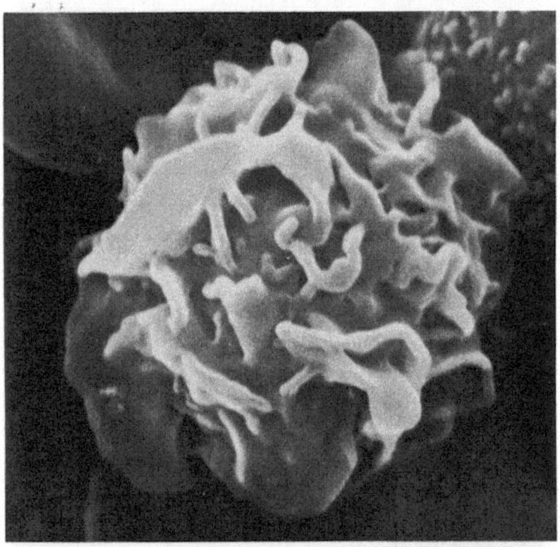

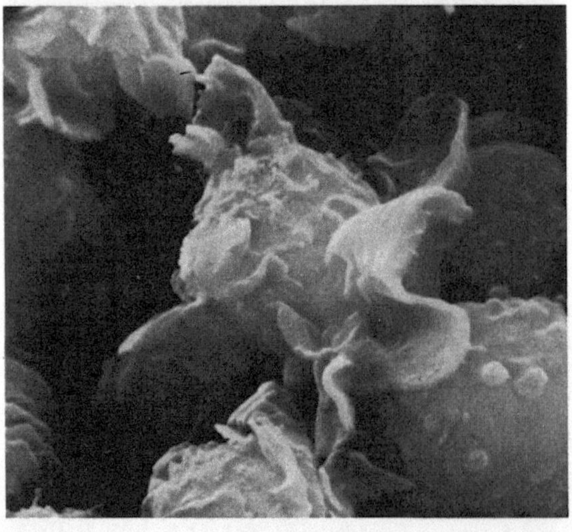

Figs. 15 and 16. Isolated leukemic monoblast from patients with acute monoblastic leukemia, showing well-developed ruffles (× 9600; × 7000)

most reported studies, cases are classified according to the surface morphology of the dominant cell type present. This in itself introduces a problem in the interpretation of findings, which provides a potential source for differences in opinion in this field as these cases are "classified" by different authors using slightly different criteria and definitions of cell surface topography. When the vast majority of cells have the same type of surface architecture, classification is not difficult, but when mixed cell populations of cells are present, the case may be classified according to the "dominant" cell type (over 60%) or as a "mixed" type if approximately equal numbers of two or three cell types are encountered.

Another problem, closely related to the difficulty of defining dominant cell types in mixed cell populations under the SEM is "contamination" of the leukemic population by (nonleukemic) normal leukocytes during separation of the cells to be studied. Even in leukemic patients with high peripheral blood counts, and in particular in cases of CLCL, a proportion of the "enriched" separated population of cells obtained after simple centrifugation or gradient centrifugation using Ficoll-Hypaque will be nonleukemic lymphocytes whose presence no

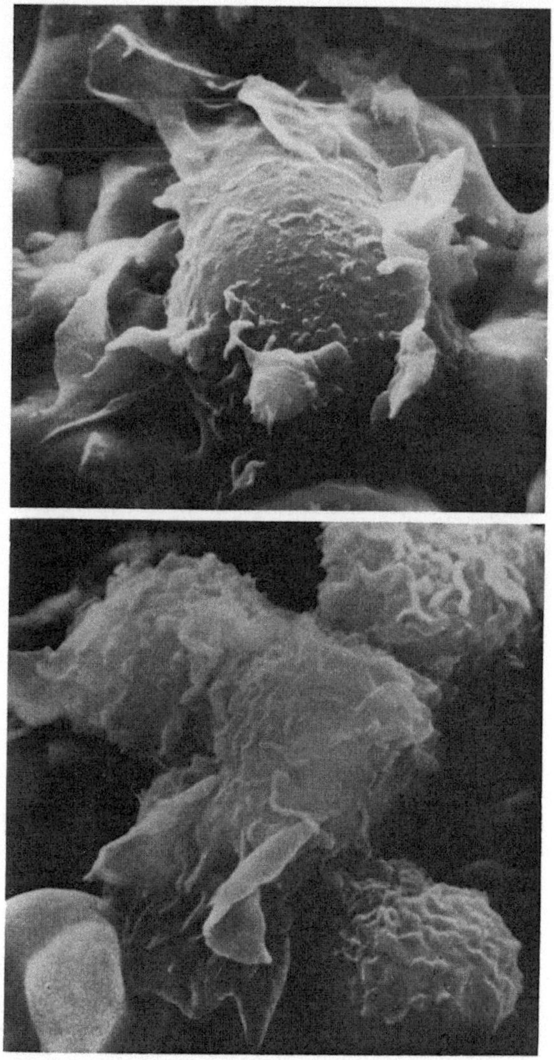

Figs. 17 and 18. Circulating cells from a patient with histiocytic lymphoma in leukemic phase with exaggerated, very well-developed ruffled folds (×6500)

doubt creates difficulties in the final interpretation of SEM results. During the past few years, cells from a large number of cases of acute and chronic leukemia have been studied under SEM [12, 13, 14, 18, 19, 21, 30, 32, 41, 47, 58, 70, 73, 75, 77, 82, 83, 84, 88, 97], primarily in order to recognize the surface architecture of cells of a known type (determined by standard light microscopy and cytochemistry) and to determine whether this relatively new mode of microscopy has anything to contribute to the diagnosis and definition of leukemia.

Our experience over the past 4 years with close to 200 cases of leukemia has been reported in detail in earlier publications [73, 75, 77, 78, 82, 83, 84] and only a summary of these findings will be given here, with additional comments relating to the experiences of others and to differences of opinion in this field. It should be stressed at this point that we have *had little experience with lymphoma cells isolated from organs* and have only examined a few cases of lymphoma in leukemic phase, but many cultured Burkitt and other non-Hodgkin's lymphoma cells. Accordingly, remarks relating to so-called "histiocytic" and lymphocytic lymphoma refer to circulating and cultured cells only and not to cells isolated from the tissues.

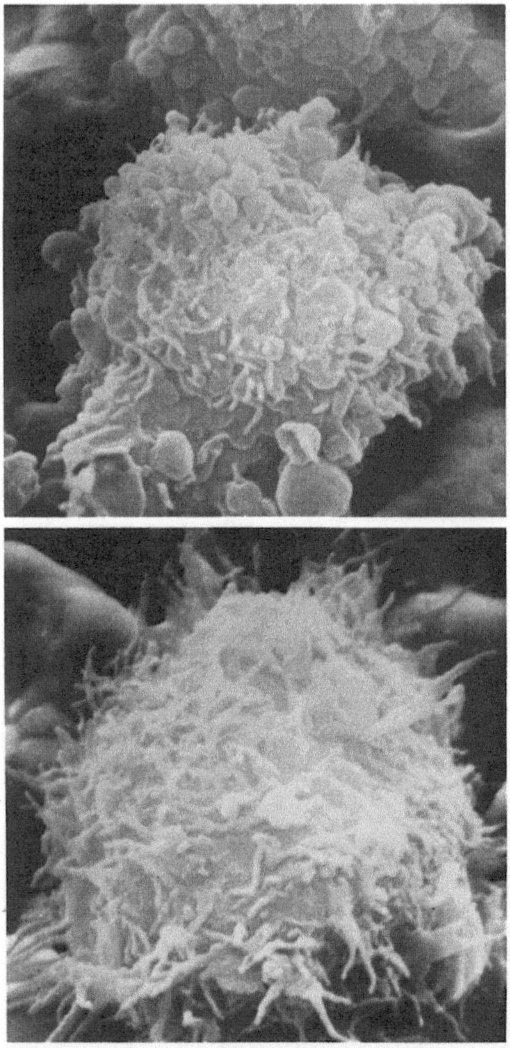

Figs. 19 and 20. Cultured cells from so-called histiocytic cell lines showing ruffles, ridge-like profiles, and blebs (× 9000)

Non-lymphoblastic Leukemias

Acute Myeloblastic, Promyelocytic, and Chronic Myeloid Leukemias (CML)

In all cases examined until now (excluding two cases of blastic crisis in CML), the vast majority of cells had ridge-like profiles or small ruffles [75, 77] (Figs. 10 and 11) resembling mature granulocytes. COLEMAN et al. [19] and GOLOMB and REESE [32] and others have described similar features in their cases. Examination of two cases of eosinophilic leukemia revealed that circulating eosinophils may show a spectrum of surface morphology, including microvilli. However, the vast majority of cells showed small slightly raised ridge-like profiles (Figs. 12 and 13). We have also examined cells from the *K-562 myeloid leukemia cell line* derived from a patient with Philadelphia-positive CML [46] and have shown that the dominant cell in that line was also one which displayed transverse ridge-like profiles (Fig. 14). It is worthwhile recording that leukemic myeloblasts and promyelocytes tended to show a less dense distribution of microprojections, which were also less well-developed when compared with CML cells. This also appears to be the case for the lymphoblastic/lymphocytic leukemias.

Monocytic, Monoblastic, and Myelomonocytic Leukemias

In these cases, the dominant cell type showed well-developed broad-based ruffled folds and prominent ridge-like profiles [13, 32, 75, 77]. No correlation was obtained between the degree of cell differentiation (assessed by light microscopy) and the size of the ruffled folds seen under SEM. A case of myelomonocytosis showed a mixture of cells with ridge-like profiles and ruffles, and it was not possible to distinguish myeloid and monocytic elements. In some cases, exaggerated ruffles (up to a few microns in length) were seen. The similarity between the surface architecture of these cells and tissue macrophages obtained from lymph nodes, spleen, or peritoneum [1, 67, 79, 104] is striking (Figs. 15 and 16).

Thus, it appears that this cell type (monocyte and/or macrophage), like its normal counterpart, is readily distinguishable from normal and leukemic lymphocytes on the basis of surface architecture alone. SEM studies from other laboratories [13, 19, 21, 32] have arrived at similar conclusions. Although *some cases of CLCL* have raised ridge-like profiles and even some small

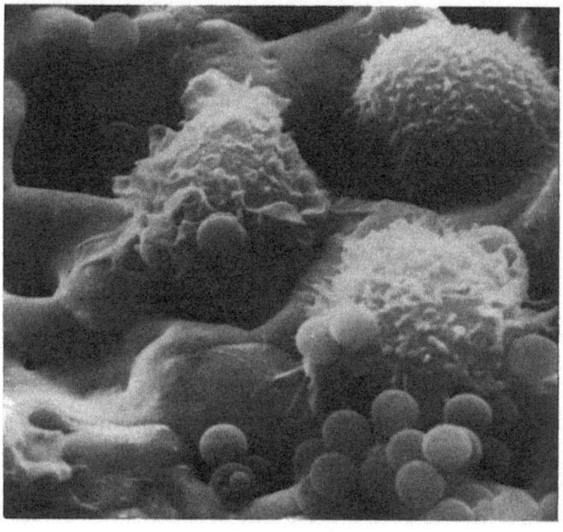

Fig. 21. Hairy cells with surface ruffles and adherent latex beads. On the upper right, there is a lymphocyte with microvilli and no attached latex beads (× 6200)

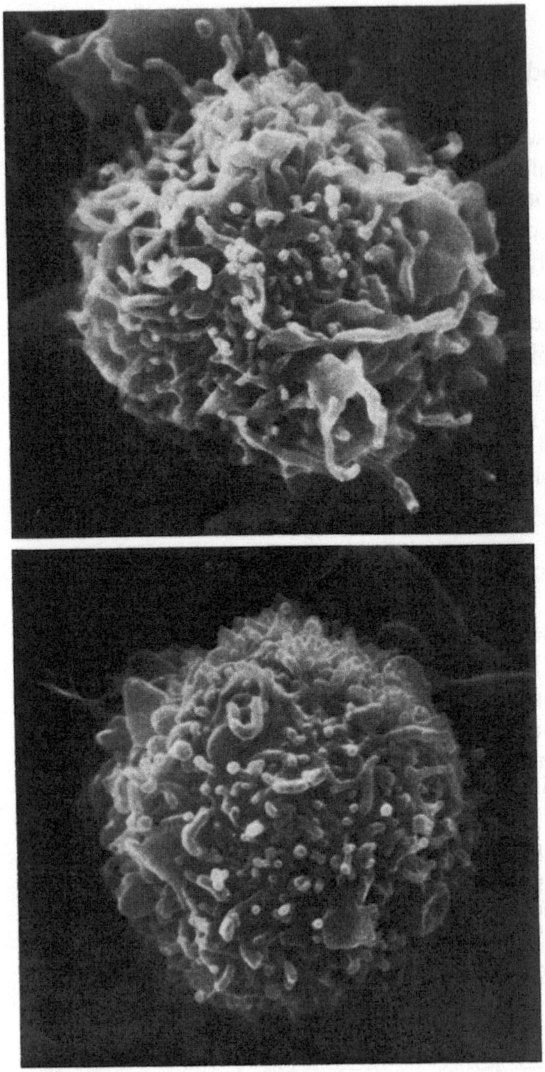

Figs. 22 and 23. Close-up of two hairy cells showing clusters of microvilli and ruffles (× 10,000)

ruffles, one does not encounter very well-developed broad-based ruffles on circulating leukemic lymphocytes. These microprojections, however, do appear on a proportion of cultured lymphoblastoid cells which are nonmalignant in nature and on lymphocytes transformed by phytomitogens.

Histiocytic Lymphoma in Leukemic Phase and Cultured Histiocytic Lymphoma Cell Lines

In the few cases of so-called histiocytic lymphoma in leukemic phase studied by SEM, we have encountered a large proportion of cells with monocyte/macrophage surface features [75, 77], sometimes with an admixture of lymphoid cells with multiple microvilli. In addition, examination of a number of so-called histiocytic lymphoma cell lines [24, 99] has shown a large proportion of cells with prominent surface ruffles, lamellae, and bleb-like excrescences. In

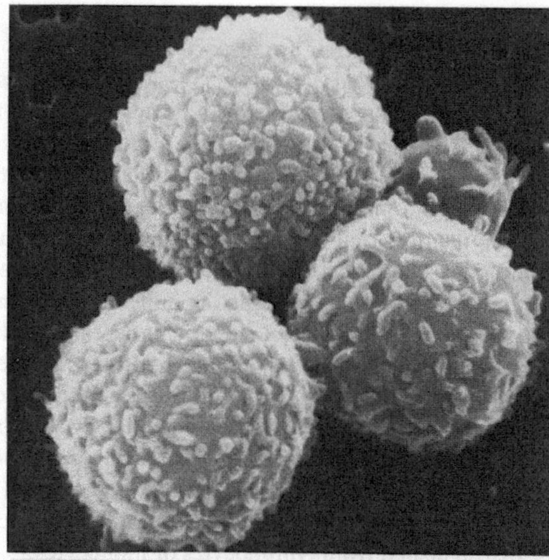

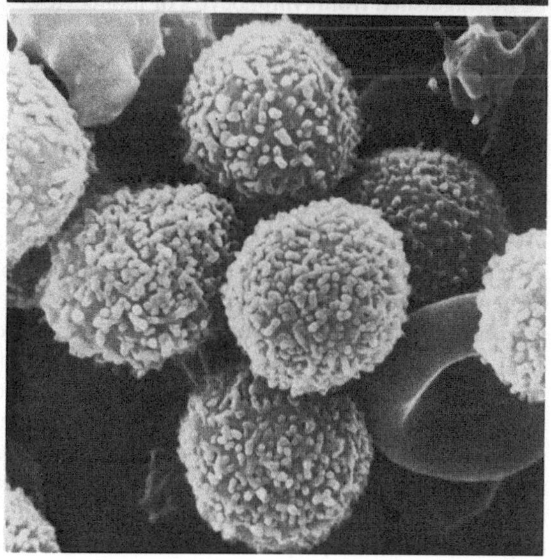

Figs. 24 and 25. Circulating leukemic lymphocytes from a patient with CLCL showing moderate and markedly villous surfaces (×9000; ×6500)

other histiocytic lines, the dominant cell type was a spherical cell with lymphoid features covered with microvilli (Figs. 17–20). These apparently contradictory SEM findings are in keeping with the fact that many of the so-called histiocytic lymphomas are in fact lymphocytic lymphomas. In cases proven to be truly histiocytic in nature (as determined by electron microscopy, histochemistry, and immunological identification, the predominant cell type was invariably one with macrophage/monocyte characteristics [24, 99]. This suggests that histiocytes resemble tissue macrophages and circulating monocytes under SEM and differ in many cases from circulating and tissue lymphocytes.

Hairy Cell Leukemia (Leukemic Reticuloendotheliosis = LRE)

The hairy cells of LRE are of particular interest as there is still much controversy regarding their true nature and derivation [14, 20, 28, 40]. It is still undecided whether these are in fact cells of the monocytic series or phagocytosing B-lymphocytes. We have studied 11 cases of hairy cell leukemia [31, 80], while other workers have also documented their findings on circulating and tissue hairy cells in brief reports [16, 45, 92, 94, 95]. Here there are few real differences of opinion as far as SEM features are concerned. Many circulating hairy cells have surface features that resemble monocytes in that they display ruffles, ridge-like profiles, and can phagocytose latex beads [80] (Fig. 21). Other hairy çells show ruffles and clusters of stub-like microvilli scattered among the ruffles (Figs. 22 and 23), and in this respect hairy cells differ from monocytes or lymphocytes and appear hybrid-like in nature. Others [16] have shown that hairy cells from the spleen differ from those isolated from the peripheral blood and display mainly microvilli, suggesting that the environment modifies their surface morphology. Transmission electron microscopic studies by Burke and co-authors [11] of splenic hairy cells do show that these cells have ruffles and ridges, and so we cannot exclude that some of the hairy cells reported in SEM studies of the spleen were in fact not positively identified as such and represent B-lymphocytes. The hybrid-like appearance of the hairy cell under SEM enables it to be distinguished from lymphocytes or monocytes.

Chronic Lymphocytic Leukemia (CLCL) and Lymphoma in Leukemic Phase (LSL)

We have studied close to 100 cases of CLCL and LSL [73, 77, 97], while other groups [15, 18, 21, 32, 47, 58, 88, 101] have also reported their findings in relatively large series of cases. At the outset, it should be stressed that in the vast majority of our cases cells were not fixed in suspension during their preparation for SEM—this would of course influence the cell surface morphology, particularly in relation to the number of microvilli encountered. Unlike Mathé et al. [21, 58], we did not subclassify our cases of LSL into three types (prolymphocytic, lymphoblastic, or immunoblastic), and thus cannot compare our results directly with those of the above authors. Nevertheless, it is fair to state that by far the majority of cells in CLCL and well-differentiated lymphocytic lymphoma in leukemic phase are spherical with varying numbers of microvilli. A spectrum of surface morphology is frequently seen in these cases, but in most the predominant cell in CLCL is one with moderate to large numbers of microvilli (Figs. 24 and 25). A proportion of cases showed a fairly large number of cells (less than 50%) with relatively few microvilli (Fig. 26), while in 12 cases, cells with few microvilli predominated. These findings are by no means only related to artifact or preparatory techniques as they have been encountered in cells prefixed in suspension [77], by Gourdin and Reyes et al. [34, 91] in their immunoelectron microscopic studies on CLCL, and in regular transmission electron microscopic sections [73]. Similar findings in CLCL were reported by Cohnen et al. [18], Renau-Piqueras [88, 89], Lmabertenghi-Deliliers [47], Tsukada et al. [101], and even in the studies by Catovsky [15] and Mathé and co-workers [58]. Thus, there is little argument relating to the *fact that the most frequent surface microprojections encountered in CLCL are microvilli.* In this respect, it should be stressed that it is difficult to compare different series, as different methodologies are used. Furthermore, not all authors strictly separate cases of CLCL from those of LSL and there may well be subtle differences between these two groups as suggested by Dantchev and Belpomme [21]. In our experience [73], almost all of our cases, including those with few microvilli, were of the B-type. No attempt was made to correlate surface architecture as seen under SEM with the stage of B-cell differentiation determined by immunologic methods and the degree of positive immunofluorescence, but it did appear to us

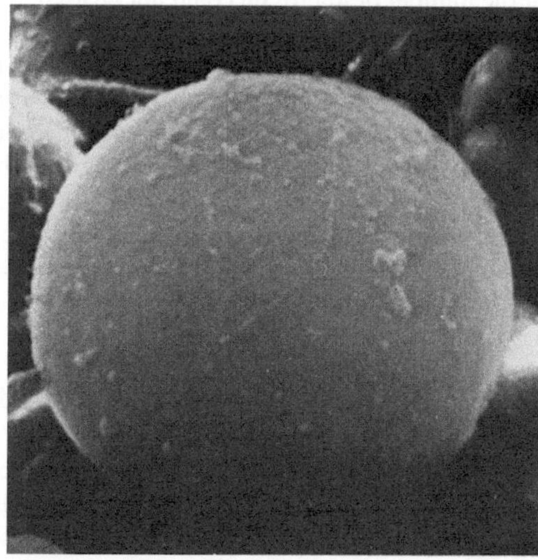

Fig. 26. Close-up of circulating leukemic lymphocyte (fixed in suspension) with relatively large areas of surface devoid of microvilli (× 12,000)

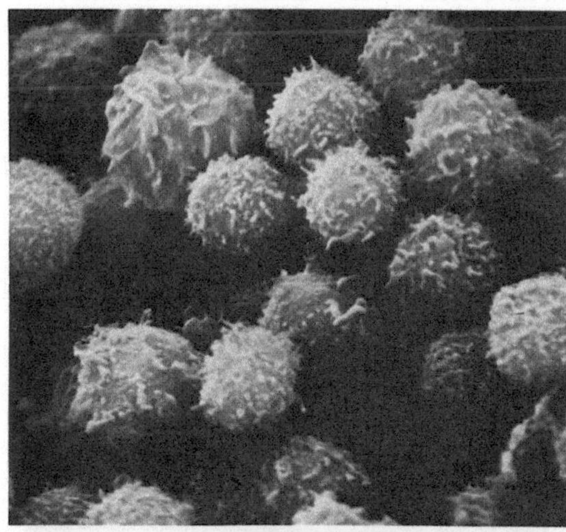

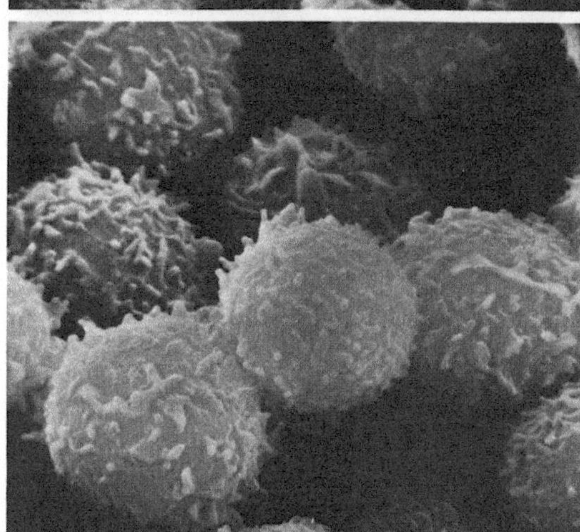

Figs. 27 and 28. *CLCL cells from a case* which showed the *dominant cell type* to be one with *transverse ridge-like profiles* (× 3700). Figure 26 shows another case in which many *CLCL cells with ridges* are evident (× 6500)

that the number of microvilli could not be used to distinguish between leukemic B or T cells or between these cells and those that bore both markers [73, 77, 97]. Similar conclusions were arrived at by BRAYLAN et al. [12] in their study, but they compared cells from lymph nodes, spleen, and peripheral blood which would not be valid in the light of recent data suggesting that the microenvironment alters cells. Furthermore, they compared cells prepared with different methodologies and at varying temperatures. The efforts made by MATHÉ et al. [58] and DANTCHEV and BELPOMME [21] in this respect may be fruitful, and there may well be a correlation between surface morphology and T- or B-cell phenotype when enough cases have been studied.

Cells With Ridge-Like Profiles in CLCL and LSL

In many of our cases of CLCL or LSL, varying proportions of cells with ridge-like profiles were seen, and in a few cases this was the dominant cell type encountered [73, 77] (Figs. 27 and 28). CLCL cells with similar surface features were also encountered by others in their studies [14, 21, 32]. These cells are difficult to distinguish from monocytes or granulocytes in some cases and have been termed "monocytoid" in nature. They may represent subtypes of CLCL cells that still need to be studied more carefully. In cases where they constitute only a minor proportion of the cell population, they may indeed be "contaminating" normal granulocytes and monocytes and may not be part of the leukemic population. In cases where these cells represent a majority, this cannot be a problem of contamination, and they probably represent a subtype of lymphoproliferative disorder. These cases of CLCL and LSL are difficult to classify.

Cultured Burkitt's Lymphoma, Non-Hodgkin's Lymphoma, and Lymphoblastoid Cells (Probably Nonmalignant)

We have examined a large number of cultured Burkitt lymphoma cells [8], most of which are spherical and have varying numbers of microvilli (Fig. 29). Only rare cells show peripheral

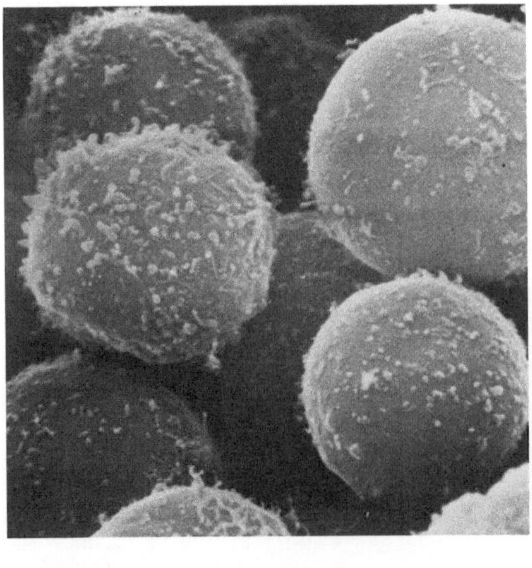

Fig. 29. Spherical cultured Burkitt cells with varying numbers of microvilli (× 7500)

ruffles, ridges, uropods, or blebs. In this respect, Burkitt's lymphoma cells resemble leukemic lymphocytes. Cells from other cultured lymphoblastoid (B) cell lines, that are apparently nonmalignant in nature, show a wider variation of surface morphology and shape (Figs. 30 and 31). Despite this, they also display mainly microvilli, but ridge-like profiles, blebs, ruffles, and uropods are more frequently encountered, as in mitogen-transformed lymphocytes. NILSSON and co-workers [27, 63], who have studied many cell lines of this type using scanning electron electron microscopy and time-lapse cinematography, have postulated that the difference in shape and surface topography between lymphoma and lymphoblastoid cell lines are due to the different growth patterns and motility of these cells in vitro. Burkitt lymphoma cells show mainly surface movement (?via microvilli), while lymphoblastoid cell lines show surface movement and directional locomotion of the entire cell which eventually reflects itself in variations of shape, size, and surface architecture.

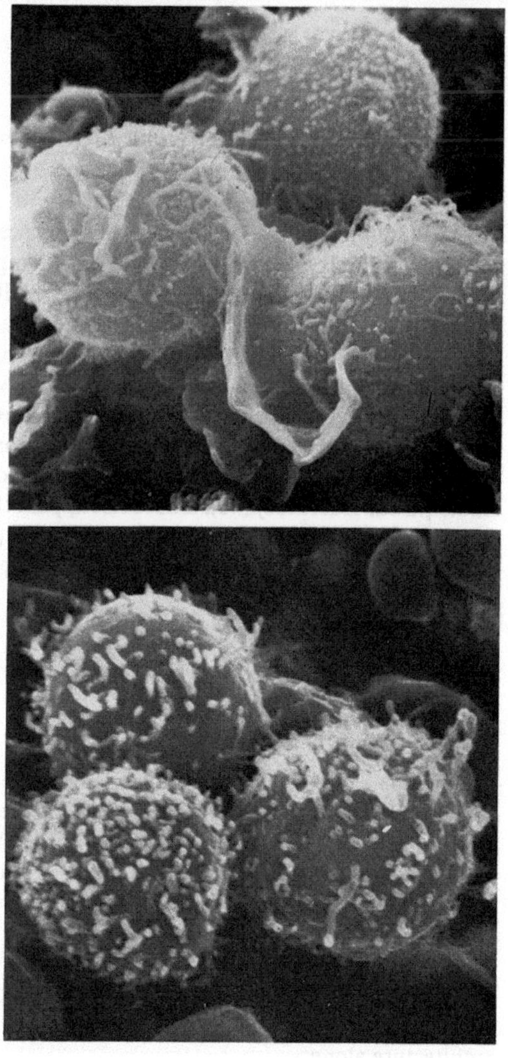

Figs. 30 and 31. Cultured lymphoblastoid cells showing variation in shape and surface architecture. Most cells have microvilli while some have peripheral ruffles (× 8000)

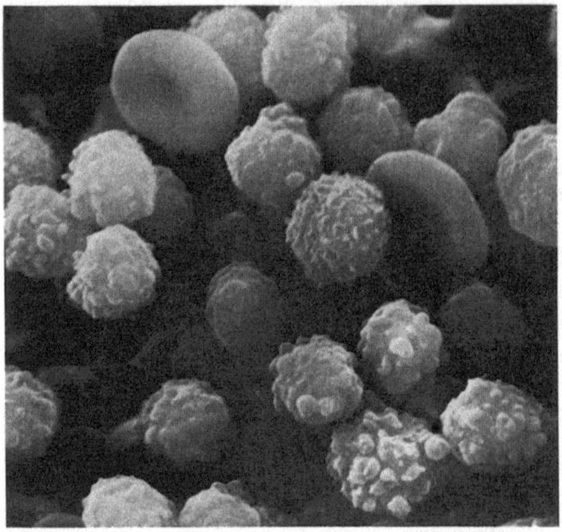

Fig. 32. Circulating leukemic lymphocytes from a *patient with CLCL showing multiple surface blebs* (× 3800)

Plasma Cells, Myeloma Cells, and Bleb Formation on Lymphocytes

Blebs (zeiotic blebs) are seen on a variety of cultured mammalian cells and according to PORTER [86] may be cell-cycle related. Blebs are sometimes seen on cultured lymphoblastoid cells but are rarely encountered on leukemic lymphocytes. We have seen only 1 out of 100 cases of CLCL and LSL in which the predominant cell type had multiple surface blebs (Fig. 32) [73, 77]. In this particular case of CLCL, immunoelectrophoresis was not done, and we could not exclude that the CLCL cells were not plasmacytoid in nature. This is of importance, as in all the cultured myeloma cell lines studied until now by NILSSON et al. [63, 64] and ourselves [48, 84]; large blebs have been shown to be a characteristic feature of this cell type. These blebs appear on the surface of both secreting and nonsecreting myeloma cells and have also been described on circulating plasma cells from cases of plasma cell leukemia [84]. From preliminary studies in our laboratory [48], it does not appear that the blebs contain immunoglobulin, as they also appear on nonsecreting cells. Nor does the appearance of blebs correlate with the cell cycle or growth rate in vitro. Blebs appear to be a consistent and characteristic surface feature of myeloma cells (Figs. 33 and 34).

Sezary Syndrome Cells

In the four cases of Sezary syndrome that we have studied by SEM [82] and in the case described by GOLOMB et al. [30], the abnormal Sezary cells (of T-type) showed variations in size and in the number of microvilli they display. Most cells had moderate to large numbers of microvilli (Fig. 35) while others had few. A proportion of cells were irregular in shape with clusters of short microvilli polarized to one end of the cell (Fig. 36), while others showed uropod-like structures at their periphery (Fig. 37), similar to those described by REYES et al. [91] in their immunoelectron microscopic studies of Sezary cells. Well-developed ruffles were not evident on these cells. It was not possible to distinguish most Sezary cells without polarized uropods from other leukemic lymphocyte or B-derivation on the basis of their surface architecture alone.

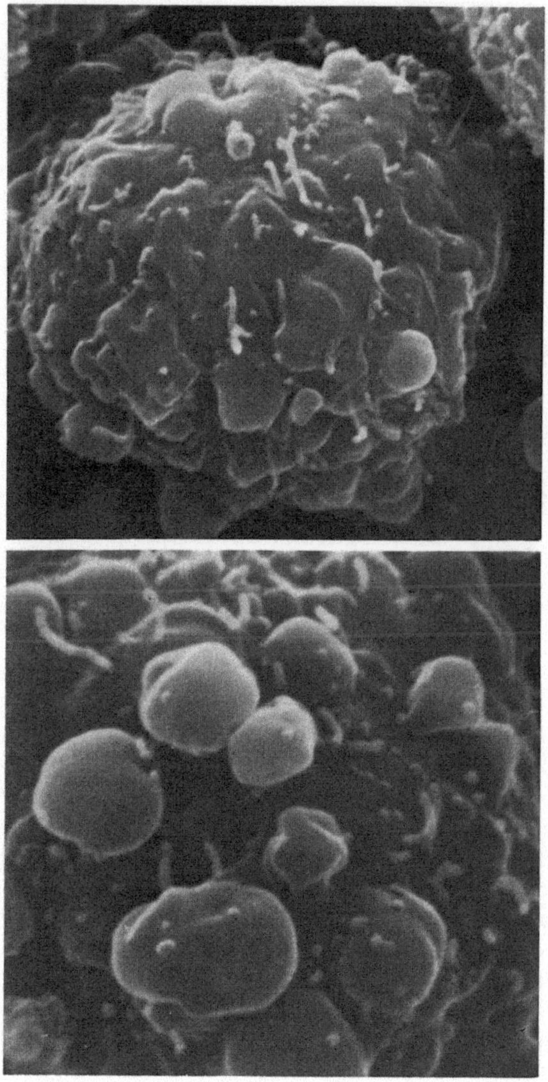

Figs. 33 and 34. Cultured myeloma cell with multiple blebs (× 8800). Close-up of blebs is seen in Figure 34 (× 34,000)

Acute Lymphoblastic Leukemia (ALBL)

In contrast to all the above-described lymphocytes, almost all of the 28 cases of ALBL we examined under SEM showed the dominant cell type to have few microvilli (Figs. 38–40) [77, 83]; cells showed few microvilli irrespective of their mode of preparation for SEM (i.e., with and without prior fixation in suspension). Only a small proportion of cells with moderately or markedly villous surfaces were scattered among a majority of smoother cells. In only 2 of the 28 cases did villous cells predominate. COLEMAN et al. [19], TSUKADA et al. [101], and LAMBERTENGHI-DELILIERS [47] described similar findings in their studies on glass-attached ALBL cells. These results indicate that leukemic lymphoblasts (mostly of the null or T-cell type) generally have less microvilli than CLCL cells. Although JAFFE et al. [41] concluded from

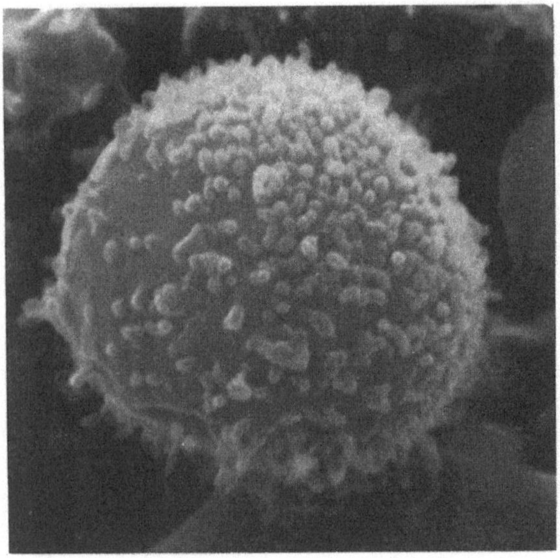

Fig. 35. Circulating Sezary cell with clustered microvilli (× 12,000)

their studies of seven cases on childhood and lymphoblastic lymphoma ALBL that "no consistent surface morphology was observed," they also state that "surface architecture was relatively consistent," and in five of the seven cases "the cells had predominantly smooth surfaces." It should be remembered that they compared cells derived from different sources (bone marrow, blood, lymph nodes, CSF, and pleural fluids) and from different microenvironments which no doubt complicates issues, as VAN EWIJK and co-workers [103] have clearly shown that lymphocytes in tissues have different surface features from those in circulation and should not be compared. Recently, DANTCHEV and BELPOMME [21] have described similar findings to ours in their series of ALBL and null or T-cell lymphosarcomas in which cells with few microvilli dominated, while cells from B-type prolymphocytic disorders were more villous in nature. All these results do suggest that the SEM findings in ALBL may well be consistent and reliable even if different methodologies are used.

In summary, it appears that the circulating *leukemic lymphocytes* and *Sezary cells* show a spectrum of surface morphology with varying numbers of microvilli. Despite some degree of overlapping surface features and the presence of cells with ridge-like profiles, these lymphoid cells characteristically show microvilli. *Leukemic lymphoblasts* may also occasionally show microvilli but more frequently lack them or display only a modest number. Ruffles are rarely encountered in the above cell types. *Plasma/myeloma cells* have characteristic surface blebs and microvilli, while *hairy cells* are readily distinguished from CLCL cells by the presence of a combination of ruffles and clusters of microvilli. *Sezary cells,* although similar to CLCL cells, may exhibit polarized microvilli, which are often in the form of underdeveloped uropods. In some cases of *histiocytic lymphoma,* cells have very well-developed ruffled membranes (and blebs) resembling those seen on monocytes and monoblasts, while in other cases cells are lymphoid in nature and display multiple microvilli. In most cases, *myelo/mono/myelomonocytic cells* are readily distinguished from lymphocytic cells on the basis of their surface architecture and are characterized by raised ridge-like profiles and/or prominent ruffled membranes. SEM is a useful adjunct to other modes of microscopy and may well contribute to the diagnosis of lymphoreticular and leukemic disorders.

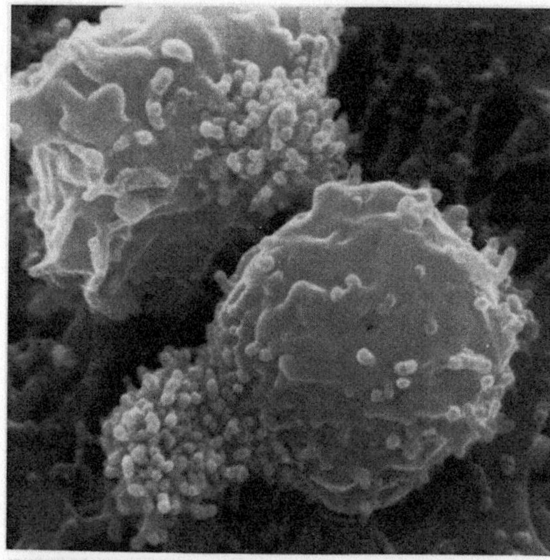

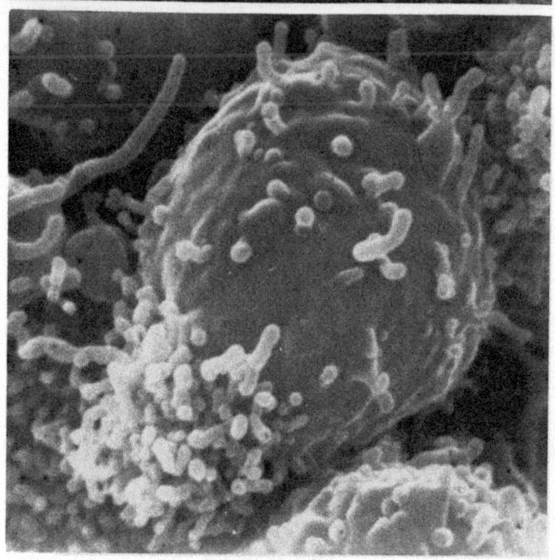

Figs 36 and 37. Circulating Sezary cells with polarized microvilli and small uropods (× 10,000; × 14,000)

Summary

This illustrated review summarizes the current status of knowledge relating to the surface morphology of normal and malignant lymphocytes and other leukocytes, as seen by SEM, with particular emphasis on lymphoreticular disorders. Problems of interpretation of the SEM data and their significance are discussed.

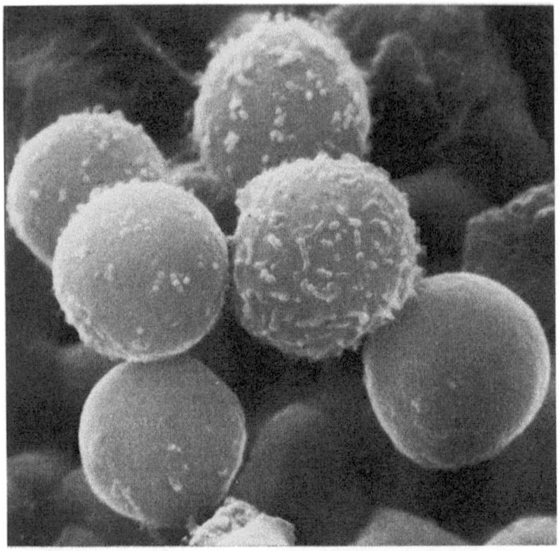

Fig. 38. Circulating ALBL cells, *fixed in cell suspension*, showing that most have few microvilli (× 6500)

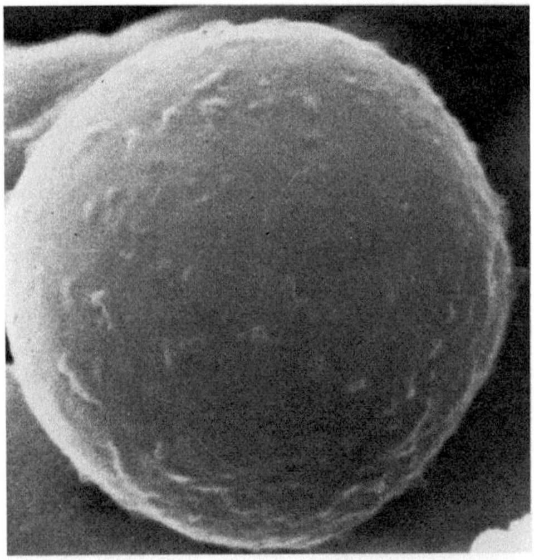

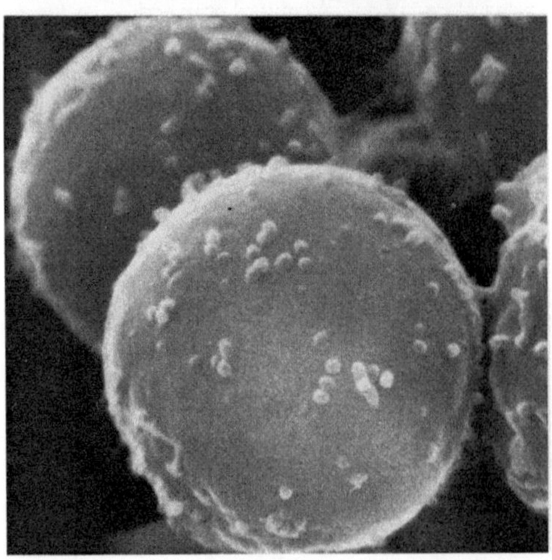

Figs. 39 and 40. Typical surface architecture of the majority of cells in ALBL showing relatively few microvilli (× 9200; × 15,000)

References

1. ALBRECHT, R. M., HINDSDILL, R. D., SANDOK, P. L., MACKENZIE, A. P., SACHS, I. B.: A comparative study of the surface morphology of stimulated and unstimulated macrophages prepared without chemical fixation for scanning electron microscopy. Exp. Cell. Res. *70*, 230 (1972).
2. ALEXANDER, E. L., WETZEL, B.: Human lymphocytes; similarity of B and T cells surface morphology. Science *188*, 732–734 (1975).
3. ALEXANDER, E., SANDERS, S., BRAYLAN, R.: Purported difference between Human T and B cell surface morphology is an artefact. Nature *261*, 239–241 (1976).
4. AMBROS, V. R., CHEN, L. B., BUCHANAN, J. M.: Surface ruffles as markers for studies of cell transformation by Rous sarcoma virus. Proc. Nat. Acad. Sci. USA *72*, 3144–3148 (1975).
5. ANDERSON, T. F.: Techniques for preservation for 3-dimensional structure in preparing specimens for electron microscopy. Trans. N.Y. Acad. Sci. *13*, 130–134 (1951).
6. BARBER, T. A., BURKHOLDER, P. M.: Relation of surface and internal ultrastructure of thymus and bone marrow derived lymphocytes to specimen preparatory technique. In Proceedings of the 8th Annual Scanning Electron Microscopy Symposium, Chicago: ITTRI, 1975, p. 369–378.
7. BAUR, P. S., THURMAN, G. B., GOLDSTEIN, A. L.: Reappraisal of lymphocyte classification by means of surface morphology. J. Immunol. *115*, 1375–1379 (1975).
8. BEN-BASSAT, H., POLLIACK, A., REICHERT, F., FROIMOVICI, M., MITRANI, S., GOLDBLUM, N.: Membrane properties, ultrastructure and surface features of established human hematopoietic cell lines; comparison of lymphoblastoid lymphoma and leukemic cell lines. Cancer *40*, 1481–1491 (1977).
9. BESSIS, M., DEBOISFLEURY, A.: Les mouvements des leukocytes étudiés au microscope électronique à balayage. Nouv. Rev. Fr. Hematol. *11*, 377–400 (1971).
10. BOYDE, A., VESELY, P.: Comparison of fixation and drying procedures for preparation of some cultured cell lines for examination in the SEM. In: Scanning electron microscopy. II. Proceedings of the 5th Annual Scanning Electron Microscope Symposium. JOHARI, D. and CORVIN, J. (Eds), Chicago: ITTRI 1972, p. 265–212.
11. BURKE, J. S., MACKAY, B., RAPPAPORT, H.: Hairy Cell Leukemia (Leukemic reticuloendotheliosis) II. Ultrastructure of the spleen. Cancer *37*, 2267–2274 (1976).
12. BRAYLAN, R., JAFFE, E. S., BURBACH, J. W., FRANK, M. M., JOHNSON, R. E., BERARD, C. W.: Similarities of surface characteristics of neoplastic well differentiated lymphocytes from solid tissues and from peripheral blood. Cancer Res. *36*, 1619–1625 (1976).
13. BRYNES, R. K., GOLOMB, H. M., DESSER, R. K., RECANT, W., REESE, C., ROWLEY, K. J.: Acute monocytic leukemia. Cytologic, histologic, cytochemical ultrastructural and cytogenetic observations. Am. J. Clin. Pathol. *65*, 471–481 (1976).
14. CATOVSKY, D., PETTIT, J. E., GALETTO, J., OKOS, A., GALTON, D. A.: The B-lymphocyte nature of the hairy cell of leukemic reticuloendotheliosis (hairy cell leukemia). Br. J. Haematol. *26*, 29–37 (1974).
15. CATOVSKY, D., FRISCH, B., VAN NOORDEN, S.: B. T. and "Null" cell leukaemias. Electronic cytochemistry and surface morphology. Blood Cells *1*, 115–124 (1975).
16. CATOVSKY, D., FRISCH, B., OKOS, A., VAN NOORDEN, S.: Scanning electron microscopy and the nature of the hairy cell. Lancet *1*, 462–463 (1975).
17. CLARKE, J. A., SALSBURY, A. J., ROWLAND, G. F.: Surface ultrastructure of human leukocytes, macrophages and rat liver cells and of isolated nuclei and nucleoli. Br. J. Haematol. *14*, 533–542 (1968).
18. COHNEN, G., FISCHER, K., LUDWIG, H., BRITTINGER, G.: Surface morphology of normal and chronic lymphocytic leukaemia lymphocytes. Eur. J. Cancer *12*, 199–202 (1976).
19. COLEMAN, M. S., GREENWOOD, M. F., HUTTON, J. J., BOLLUM, S. J., LAMPKIN, B., HOLLAND, P.: Serial observations on terminal deoxynucleotidyl transferase activity and lymphoblast surface markers in acute lymphoblastic leukemia. Cancer Res. *36*, 120–127 (1976).
20. DANIEL, M. TH., FLANDRIN, G.: Fine structure of abnormal cells in hairy cell (tricholeukocytic) leukemia, with special reference to their in vitro phagocytic capacity. Lab. Invest. *30*, 1–8 (1974).
21. DANTCHEV, D., BELPOMME, D.: Critical study of the mononuclear leukocyte morphology based on scanning electron microscopy in normal subjects and in patients with Lymphoid or Monocytoid proliferative disorders. Comparison with the T or B cell membrane phenotypes. Biomedicine (in Press, 1977).
22. DEHARVEN, E., LAMPEN, N., POLLIACK, A., WARFEL, A., FOGH, J.: New observations on methods for preparing cell suspensions for scanning electron microscopy. In Proceedings of the 8th Annual Scanning Electron Microscope Symposium: Chicago: ITTRI 1975, p. 361–367.
23. ENLANDER, D., DREW, L., HOO, R., EVERHART, T. E., SCOTT, T.: The cytopathic effect of Herpes Simplex Virus on HEP-2 cells as shown by scanning electron microscopy. J. Gen. Virol. *25*, 313–316 (1974).

24. Epstein, A., Hun Kim, Pòlliack, A., Levy, R., Dorfman, R., Kaplan, H.: Morphological and functional characterization of seven diffuse histiocytic lymphoma cell lines. Denver: Am. Assoc. Cancer. Res., 1977.
25. Erickson, C. A., Trinkaus, J. P.: Microvilli and blebs as sources of reserve surface membrane during cell spreading. Exp. Cell. Res. *99*, 375–384 (1976).
26. Fagreus, A., Lidman, K., Biberfeld, G.: Reaction of human smooth muscle antibodies with human blood lymphocytes and lymphoid cell lines. Nature *252*, 246–247 (1974).
27. Fagraeus, A., Nilsson, K., Lidman, K., Norberg, R.: Reactivity of smooth muscle antibodies, surface ultrastructure, and mobility in cells of human hematopoietic cell lines. J. Natl. Cancer Inst. *55*, 4–9 (1975).
28. Shu Man Fu, Winchester, R. J., Rai, K. R., Kunkel, H. G.: Hairy cell leukemia—Proliferation of a cell with phagocytic and B-lymphocyte properties. Scand. J. Immunol. *3*, 847–851 (1974).
29. Gamliel, H., Sarov, I., Polliack, A.: Vaccinia virus-induced alterations of surface architecture in human embryonic cells as seen by scanning electron microscopy. Proceedings of the Sixth European Congress on Electron Microscopy, Jerusalem, 1976, p. 404–406.
30. Golomb, H. M., Braylan, R., Reese, C., Variakojis, D., Brynes, R. K., Yachnin, S.: The Sezary syndrom cell: Surface ultrastructural characteristics. Acta Haematol. *54*, 106–114 (1975).
31. Golomb, H. M., Braylan, A., Polliack, A.: "Hairy" cell leukaemia (Leukaemic Reticuloendotheliosis): A scanning electron microscopic study of eight cases. Brit. J. Haematol. *29*, 455–460 (1975).
32. Golomb, H. M., Reese, C.: Surface ultrastructural and marker characteristics of leukemic cells. Proceedings of the 9th Annual Scanning Electron Microscope Symposium, Chicago: ITTRI 1976, p. 41–48.
33. Gormley, I. P., Ross, A.: The morphology of phytohaemagglutinin (PHA) stimulated lymphocytes and permanent cell lines seen by the scanning electron microscope. Eur. J. Cancer *8*, 491–494 (1972).
34. Gourdin, M. F., Reyes, F., Lejonc, J. L., Mannoni, P., Dreyfus, B.: Surface features of cells in human lymphoproliferative disorders. An immunoelectron microscopy study. In: Modern Trends in Human Leukemia. Vol. II Neth, R., Gallo, R. and Spiegelman, S. (Eds). Grune & Stratton 1976.
35. Hale, A. H., Winkelhake, J. L., Weber, M. J.: Cell surface changes and Rous Sarcoma virus gene expression in synchronized cells. J. Cell Biol. *64*, 398–407 (1975).
36. Hammerling, U., Polliack, A., de Harven, E.: (Abstract) Hybrid antibodies in immunoelectron microscopy. Proceedings of the 8th International Congress on Electron Microscopy. Canberra, Australia 1974.
37. Hammerling, U., Polliack, A., Lampen, N., Sabety, M., de Harven, E.: Scanning electron microscopy of tobacco mosaic virus-label lymphocyte surface antigens. J. Exp. Med. *141*, 518–523 (1975).
38. Holmes, K. V.: Scanning electron microscopic studies of virus-infected cells. I. Cytopathic effects and maturation of vesicular stomatitis virus in L2 cells. J. Virol. *15*, 355–362 (1975).
39. Holt, P. J. L., Pal, S. G., Catovsky, D., Lewis, S. M.: Surface structure of normal and leukaemic lymphocytes. I. Effect of mitogens. Clin. Exp. Immunol. *10*, 555–570 (1972).
40. Jaffe, E. S., Shevach, E. M., Frank, M. M., Green, I.: Leukemic reticuloendotheliosis: presence of a receptor for cytophilic antibody. Am. J. Med. *57*, 108–114 (1974).
41. Jaffe, E. S., Braylan, R., Frank, M. C., Green, I., Berard, C. W.: Heterogeneity of immunologic markers and surface morphology in childhood acute lymphoblastic leukemia. Blood *48*, 213–222 (1976).
42. Jerrels, T. R., Hinrichs, C. D. J.: The influence of the medium on the morphology of human peripheral blood rosette forming cells. J. Reticuloendothel. Soc. *13*, 84–94 (1975).
43. Kay, M. M., Belchradsky, B., Yee, K., Vogel, J., Butcher, D., Wybran, J., Fudenberg, H. H.: Cellular interactions. Scanning electron microscopy of human thymus derived-rosette forming lymphocytes. Clin. Immunol. Immunopath. *2*, 301–309 (1974).
44. Kay, M. M. B.: Multiple labelling technique used for kinetic studies of activated human B lymphocytes. Nature *254*, 424–426 (1975).
45. Katayama, I., Schneider, G. B.: Cell surface structure in Hairy Cell Leukaemia. Lancet *1*, 920 (1975).
46. Klein, E., Ben Bassat, H., Neumann, H., Ralph, P., Zeuthen, J., Polliack, A., Vanky, F.: Properties of the K562 cell line derived from a patient with chronic myeloid leukemia. Int. J. Cancer *18*, 421–431 (1976).
47. Lambertenghi-Deliliers, G., Pozzoli, E., Rosso Di San Seconde, V., Francheschini, F., Polli, E.: Surface features of normal and leukaemic lymphocytes under the SEM. Int. Soc. Haematology, Milano, 3–6 September 1975, p. 21.
48. Laskov, R., Reichert, F., Froimovici, M., Avni, M., Polliack, A.: Surface morphology of cultured myeloma cells: Difference between a myeloma cell line producing IgG and its nonproducer variant. Proceedings of the Sixth European Congress on Electron Microscopy, Jerusalem, 1976, p. 379–381.

49. LEVINE, G. D., POLLIACK, A.: The T cell nature of the lymphocytes in the human epithelial thymomas. A comparative, immunologic, scanning and transmission electron microscopic study. Clin. Immunol. Immunopath. *4*, 199–208 (1975).
50. LIN, P. S., COOPER, A. C., WORTIS, H. H.: Scanning electron microscopy of human T cell and B cell rosettes. N. Engl. J. Med. *289*, 548–551 (1973).
51. LIN, P. S., TSAI, S., WALLACH, D. F. H.: Major differences in surface morphology of thymocytes and peripheral lymphocytes as revealed by scanning electron microscopy. In: Erythrocytes, Thrombocytes, Leucocytes. Recent Advances in Membrane and Metabolic Research (GERLACH, MOSER, DEUTSCH, WILMANS (eds)) 1972, p. 438–440.
52. LIN, P. S., WALLACH, D. F. H.: Surface modification of T lymphocyte observed during rosetting. Science *184*, 1300–1301 (1974).
53. LIN, P. S., WALLACH, D. F. H., TSAI, S.: Temperature-induced variations in the surface topology of cultured lymphocytes are revealed by Scanning Electron Microscopy. Proc. Natl. Acad. Sci. U.S.A. *70*, 2492–2496 (1973).
54. LINTHICUM, D. S., SELL, S.: Topography of lymphocyte surface immunoglobulin using scanning electron microscopy. J. Ultrastruct. Res. *51*, 55–68 (1975).
55. LIPSCOMB, M. F., HOLMES, K. V., VITETTA, E. S., HAMMERLING, U., UHR, J. W: Cell surface immunoglobulin XII. Localization of immunoglobulin on murine lymphocytes by immunoelectron microscopy. Eur. J. Immunol. *5*, 255–259 (1975).
56. LOOR, F., HÄGG, LENE-BRITT: The modulation of microprojections on the lymphocytic membrane and the redistribution of membrane-bound ligands, a correlation. Eur. J. Immunol. *5*, 854–865 (1975).
57. MALICK, L. E., LANGENBACH, R.: Scanning electron microscopy of in vitro chemically transformed mouse embryo cells. J. Cell Biology *68*, 654–664 (1976).
58. MATHE, G., BELPOMME, D., DANTCHEV, D., POUILLART, P., SCHLUMBERGER, J. R., LAFLEUR, M.: Leukaemic lymphosarcomas: Respective prognosis of the three types: Prolymphocytic, lymphoblastic (or lymphoblastoid) and immunoblastic. Blood Cells *1*, 25–36 (1975).
59. MICHAELIS, T. W., LARRIMER, N. R., METZ, E. N., BALCERZAK, S. P.: Surface morphology of human leukocytes. Blood *37*, 23–30 (1971).
60. MOLDAY, R. S., DREYER, W. J., REMBAUM, A., YEN, S. P. S.: New immunolatex spheres: visual markers of antigens on lymphocytes for scanning electron microscopy. J. Cell Biol. *64*, 75–98 (1975).
61. NEMANIC, H. K., CARTER, D. P., PITELKA, D. R., WOFSY, L.: Hapten sandwich labelling II. Immunospecific attachment of cell surface markers suitable for scanning electron microscopy. J. Cell Biol. *64*, 311–321 (1973).
62. Newell, D. C., Roath, S., Smith, J. L.: The scanning electron microscopy of normal human peripheral blood lymphocytes. Br. J. Haematol. *32*, 309–316 (1976).
63. NILSSON, K., PONTEN, J.: Classification and biological nature of established human hematopoietic cell lines. Int. J. Cancer *15*, 321–341 (1975).
64. NILSSON, K., KILLANDER, D., KILLANDER, J., MELLSTEDT, H.: Short term tissue culture of two nonsecretory human myelomas: A morphological and functional study. Scand. J. Immunol. /, 819–828 (1976).
65. ORENSTEIN, J. M., SHELTON, E.: Surface topography and interactions between mouse peritoneal cells allowed to settle on an artifical substrate: observations by scanning electron microscopy. Exp. Mol. Pathol. *24*, 201–219 (1976).
66. PADNOS, M.: Differentiation of B and T mouse lymphocytes in cell suspension and smears. Nature *259*, 218–220 (1976).
67. PARAKALL, P., PINTO, J., HAMFIR, J. M.: Surface morphology of human mononuclear phagocytes during maturation and phagocytosis. J. Ultrastruct. Res. *4*, 216–226 (1974).
68. POLLIACK, A., LAMPEN, N., DE HARVEN, E.: Comparison of air drying and critical point drying procedures for the study of human blood cells by scanning electron microscopy. Proceedings of the 6th Annual Scanning Electron Microscopy Symposium, Chicago: ITTRI 1973, p. 529–534.
69. POLLIACK, A., LAMPEN, N., CLARKSON, B. D., DE HARVEN, E., BENTWICH, Z., SIEGEL, F. P., KUNKEL, H. G.: Identification of human B and T lymphocytes by scanning electron microscopy. J. Exp. Med. *138*, 607–624 (1973).
70. POLLIACK, A., LAMPEN, N., DE HARVEN, E.: Scanning electron microscopy of lymphocytes of known B and T derivation. Proceedings of the 7th Annual Scanning Electron Microscope Symposium, Chicago: ITTRI 1974, p. 673–782.
71. POLLIACK, A., FU, S. M., DOUGLAS, S. D., BENTWICH, Z., LAMPEN, N., DE HARVEN, E.: Scanning electron microscopy of human lymphocyte-sheep erythrocyte rosettes. J. Exp. Med. *140*, 146–148 (1974).
72. POLLIACK, A., HÄMMERLING, U., LAMPEN, N., DE HARVEN, E.: Surface morphology of murine B and T lymphocytes: A comparative study by scanning electron microscopy. Eur. J. Immunol. *5*, 32–39 (1975).

73. POLLIACK, A., SIEGAL, F. P., CLARKSON, B. D., SHU MAN FU, WINCHESTER, R., LAMPEN, N., ARCE, J., SIEGEL, M., DE HARVEN, E.: A scanning electron microscopy and immunological study of 84 cases of lymphocyte leukaemia and related lympho-proliferative disorders. Scand. J. Haematol. *15*, 359–377 (1975).
74. POLLIACK, A., TOURAINE, J. L., DE HARVEN, E., LAMPEN, N., HADDEN, J. W.: Scanning electron microscopy of mitogen-transformed human lymphocytes. Isr. J. Med. Sci. *11*, 1285–1298 (1975).
75. POLLIACK, A., MCKENZIE, S., GEE, T., DE HARVEN, E., LAMPEN, N., CLARKSON, E. D.: A scanning electron microscopy study of 34 cases of acute granulocytic, myelomonocytic, monoblastic and histiocytic leukaemia. Am. J. Med. 59, 308–315 (1975).
76. POLLIACK, A., DOUGLAS, S. D.: Surface features of human eosinophils: A transmission and scanning electron microscopic study of a case of non leukemic eosinophilia. Br. J. Haematol. *30*, 303–306 (1975).
77. POLLIACK, A.: Surface morphology of circulating human leukemic cells. Experience with 175 cases of leukemia, as seen by scanning electron microscopy. Proceedings of the 9th Annual Scanning Electron Microscope Symposium Toronto: ITTRI 1976, p. 31–40.
78. POLLIACK, A., DE HARVEN, E.: Surface features of normal and leukaemic lymphocytes as seen by scanning electron microscopy: An Interpretative Review. Clin. Immun. Immunopath. *33*, 412–430 (1975).
79. POLLIACK, A., GORDON, S.: Scanning electron microscopy of murine macrophages. Surface characteristics during maturation, activation and phagocytosis. Lab. Invest. *33*, 469–477 (1975).
80. POLLIACK, A., BRAYLAN, R., GOLOMB, H. M.: Scanning electron microscopy of hairy cells in hairy cell leukemia. Lancet *2*, 1013–1014 (1974).
81. POLLIACK, A., FROIMOVICI, M., FRANKENBURG, S., GERY, I.: Altered surface morphology of concanavalin A transformed thymic lymphocytes as seen by scanning electron microscopy. Biomedicine *24*, 389–395 (1976).
82. POLLIACK, A., DJALDETTI, M., REYES, F., BIBERFELD, P., DANIEL, M. T., FLANDRIN, G.: Surface features of Sezary cells: A scanning electron microscopic study of five cases. Scand. J. Haematol. *18*, 207–213 (1977).
83. POLLIACK, A., FROIMOVICI, M., POZZOLI, E., LAMBERTENGHI-DELILIERS, G.: Acute lymphoblastic leukaemia: A study of 25 cases by scanning electron microscopy. Blut *33*, 359 (1976).
84. POLLIACK, A., NILSSON, K., LASKOV, R., BIBERFELD, P.: Characteristic surface morphology of neoplastic myeloma and plasma cells as seen by scanning electron microscopy. Br. J. Haematol. *39*, 25–30, (1978).
85. PORTER, K. R., KELLEY, E., ANDREWS, P. M.: The preparation of cultured cells and soft tissues for scanning electron microscopy. Proceedings of the 5th Annual Stereoscan Colloquim, Chicago: Kent Cambridge Corp. 1972, p. 1–19.
86. PORTER, K. R., PRESCOTT, D., FRYE, J.: Changes in surface morphology of Chinese hamster ovary cells during the cell cycle. J. Cell Biol. *57*, 815–836 (1973).
87. PORTER, K. R., TODARO, G. J., FONTE, V.: A scanning electron microscopy study of surface features of viral and spontaneous transformants of mouse BALB/373 cells. J. Cell Biol. *59*, 633–642 (1973).
88. RENAU PIQUERAS, J., MARTINEZ RAMON, A., FORTEZA BOVER, G.: Ultrastructura de la Superficie de Los Linfocitos. Humanos. (Monograph) Valencia: 1976.
89. RENAU PIQUERAS, J.: Morphological differences in human peripheral blood lymphocytes. A freeze-etching and scanning electron microscopic study. Acta Haematologica *59*, 19–24 (1978).
90. REVELL, P. A., SWETTENHAM, K. V., SORETIRE, E. A.: Populations of guinea pig lymphocytes displayed by Nomarski microscopy. Lancet *1*, 394 (1974).
91. REYES, F., LEJONC, J. L., GOURDIN, M. R., MANNONI, P., DREYFUS, B.: The surface morphology of human B lymphocytes as revealed by immunoelectron microscopy. J. Exp. Med. *141*, 392–410 (1975).
92. ROATH, S., NEWELL, D. G.: Cell surface characteristics in hairy cell leukemia. Lancet *1*, 283–284 (1975).
93. RUBIN, R. W., EVERHART, L. P.: The effect of cell-to-cell contact on the surface morphology of Chinese hamster ovary cells. J. Cell Biol. *57*, 837–844 (1973).
94. SCHNITZER, B., HAMMACK, W. J.: B lymphocyte nature of hairy cells in hairy cell leukemia. Lancet *2*, 649 (1974).
95. SCHNITZER, B., MEAD, M. L.: Nature of the hairy cell. Lancet *1*, 805 (1975).
96. SCIORRA, L., ECKERT, C.: Distinguishing T and B lymphocytes by light microscopy and Nomarski optics. Lancet *2*, 1526 (1974).
97. SIEGAL, F. P., VOSS, R., AL-MONDHIRY, H., POLLIACK, A., HANSEN, J. A., SIEGAL, M., GOOD, R. A.: Association of a chromosomal abnormality with lymphocytes having both T and B markers in a patient with lymphoprolifarative disease. Am. J. Med. *60*, 157–166 (1976).
98. SULLIVAN, A. K., ADAMS, L. S., SILKE, I., JERRY, L. M.: "Hairy" B cells and "Smooth" T cells. Letter to the Editor. N. Engl. J. Med. *290*, 689 (1974).

99. SUNDSTRÖM, C., NILSSON, K.: Establishment and characterization of a human histiocytic lymphoma cell line (U-937), Int. J. Cancer *17*, 567–577 (1976).
100. TOURAINE, J. L., HADDEN, J. W., POLLIACK, A., TOURAINE, F., HADDEN, E. M., GOOD, R. A.: Sous population de lymphocytes T humains répondant aux mitogens et aux stimulations allogéniques. In: Transplantation and Clinical Immunology, Lyon: Simep Editions 1975, p. 122–137.
100. TOURAINE, J. L., HADDEN, J. W., POLLIACK, A., T
101. TSUKADA, M., HANAMURA, K. EGUCHI, M.: Scanning electron microscopic study of peripheral blood lymphocytes, thymic cells and acute lymphoblastic leukemic cells in children. Acta. Haematol. Jpn. *39* (1), 43–52 (1976).
102. VILA, J. M., TAUB, R. N.: Nomarski Optics and T and B markers. Lancet, Apr. 26, 977 (1975).
103. VAN EWIJK, W., BRONS, N. H. C., ROZING, J.: Scanning electron microscopy of homing and recirculating lymphocyte populations. Cell. Immunol. *19*, 245–261 (1975).
104. WARFEL, A. H., ELBERG, S. S.: Macrophage membranes viewed through a scanning electron microscope. Science *170*, 446–447 (1970).
105. WETZEL, B., ERICKSON, B. W., JR., LEVIS, W. R.: The need for positive identification of leukocytes examined by SEM. Proceedings of the 6th Annual Scanning Electron Microscopy Symposium, Chicago: ITTRI 1973, p. 535–541.
106. WETZEL, B., CANNON, G. B., ALEXANDER, E. L., ERICKSON, B. W., JR., WESTBROOK, E. W.: A critical approach to the scanning electron microscopy of cells in suspension. Proceedings of the 7th Annual Scanning Electron Microscopy Symposium, Chicago: ITTRI 1974, p. 581–588.

Scanning Electron Microscopy Morphology of Mononuclear Leukocytes in Normal Subjects and in Patients With Lymphoid and Monocytoid Neoplasias

D. DANTCHEV

During our experience with scanning electron microscopy, we have examined four different types of cells [5, 6, 7, 8, 9]:

1. Thymus cells and bursa of Fabricius cells
2. Peritoneum free histiocytes and fixed activated macrophages
3. Normal blood mononuclear cells
4. Mononuclear leukemia and malignant lymphoma cells.

Scanning was used in accordance with the critical dry point method as described previously [5, 6, 13]. Always using the same technique, without aspiration, and under the same experimental conditions, our results were constant and reproducible. All samples were simultaneously studied by immune marker tests: E-, EA-, and EAC-rosettes and membrane immunofluorescence [2, 3, 4, 7, 8]. This paper summarizes the results of our inventory of the different mononuclear cells.

Results

Thymus Cells and Bursa of Fabricius Cells

We confirmed the conclusion reached by previous authors [10, 13, 16] that thymus cells are round and smooth; we also observed that their surface is slightly undulated (Fig. 1). Fabricius bursa cells are also round but covered with regular short villosities (Fig. 2).

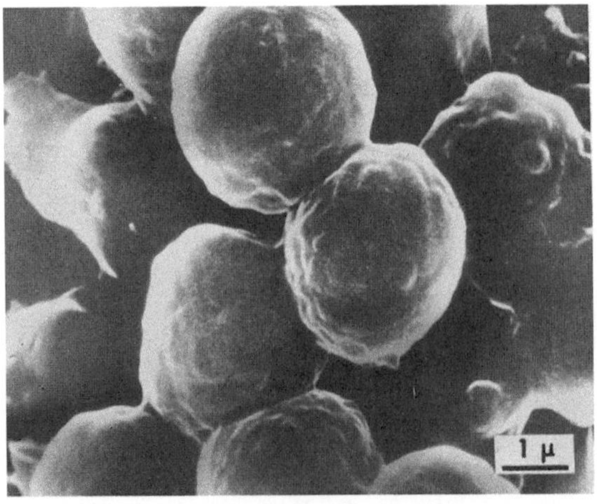

Fig. 1. Normal mouse thymus cells

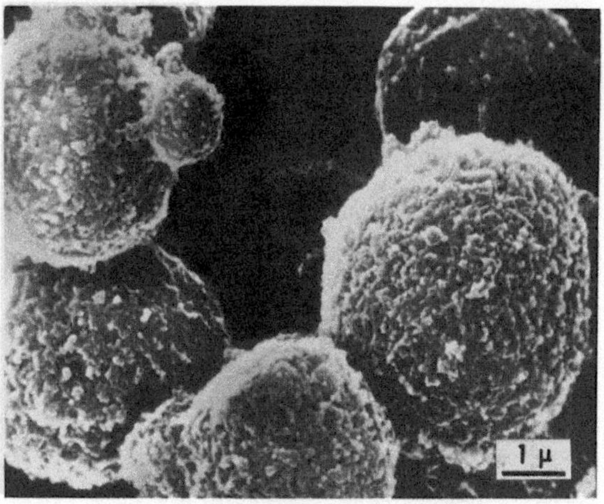

Fig. 2. Normal chicken bursa Fabricius cells

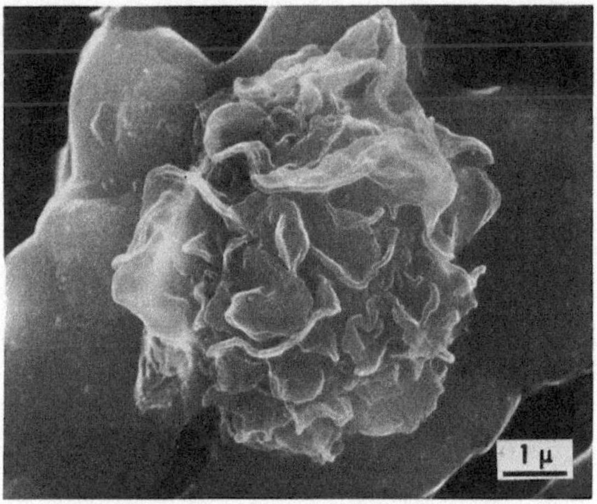

Fig. 3. Normal mouse peritoneal histiocyte

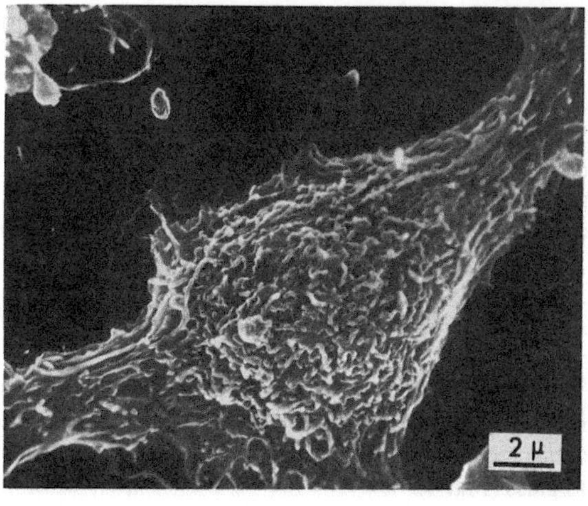

Fig. 4. Activated peritoneal macrophage

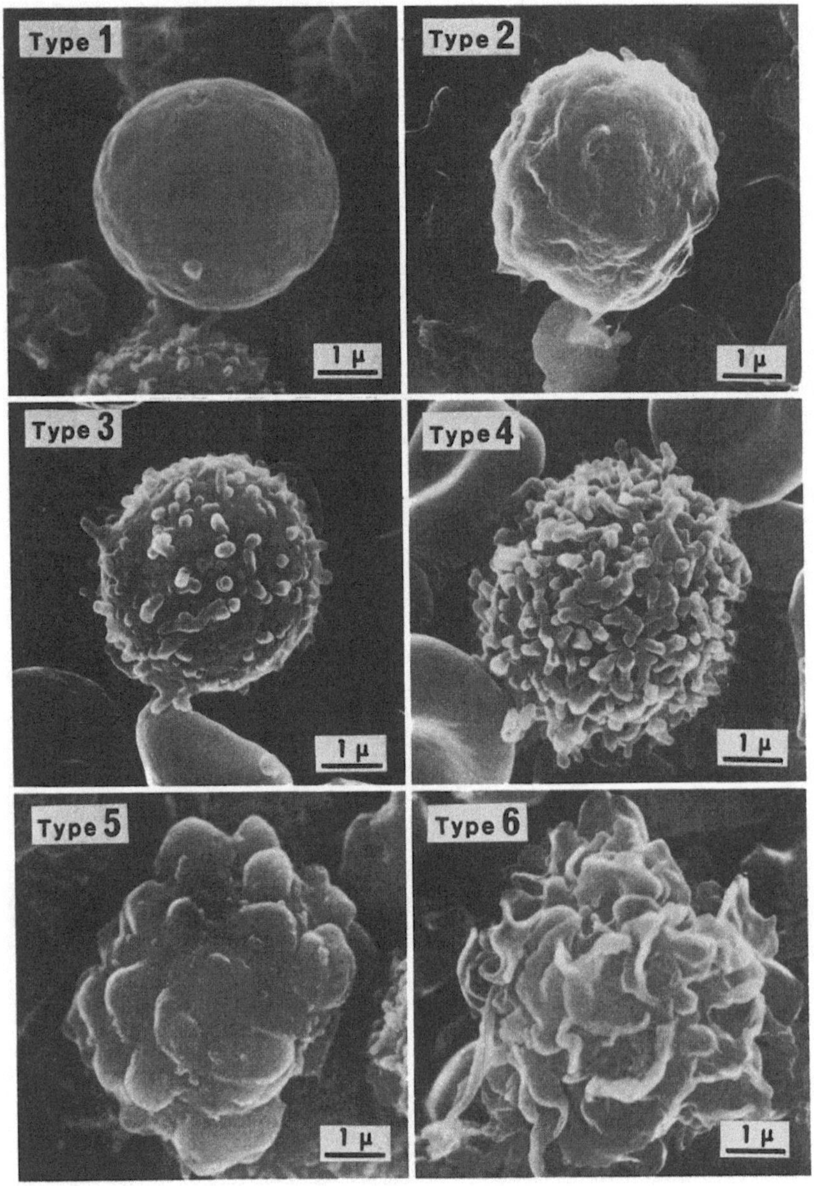

Fig. 5. The six main types of mononuclear cell surfaces. Type 1: Completely smooth surface. Type 2: Smooth-undulated surface. Type 3: Slightly villous surface. Type 4: Extremely villous surface. Type 5: Blebs covered surface. Type 6: Ruffled surface with ridge-like profiles. Types 1, 2, 3, and 4 correspond to different lymphocytes, type 5 to plasma cells, and type 6 to monocytoid cells

Peritoneum-Free Histiocytes and Fixed Activated Macrophages

The peritoneum-free histiocytes or inactive macrophages have a ruffled membrane and ridge-like profiles as do blood monocytes (Fig. 3). The peritoneum-fixed and activated macrophages, subjected to in vivo BCG treatment, are very different, with a rather villous surface and adhere to glass (Fig. 4).

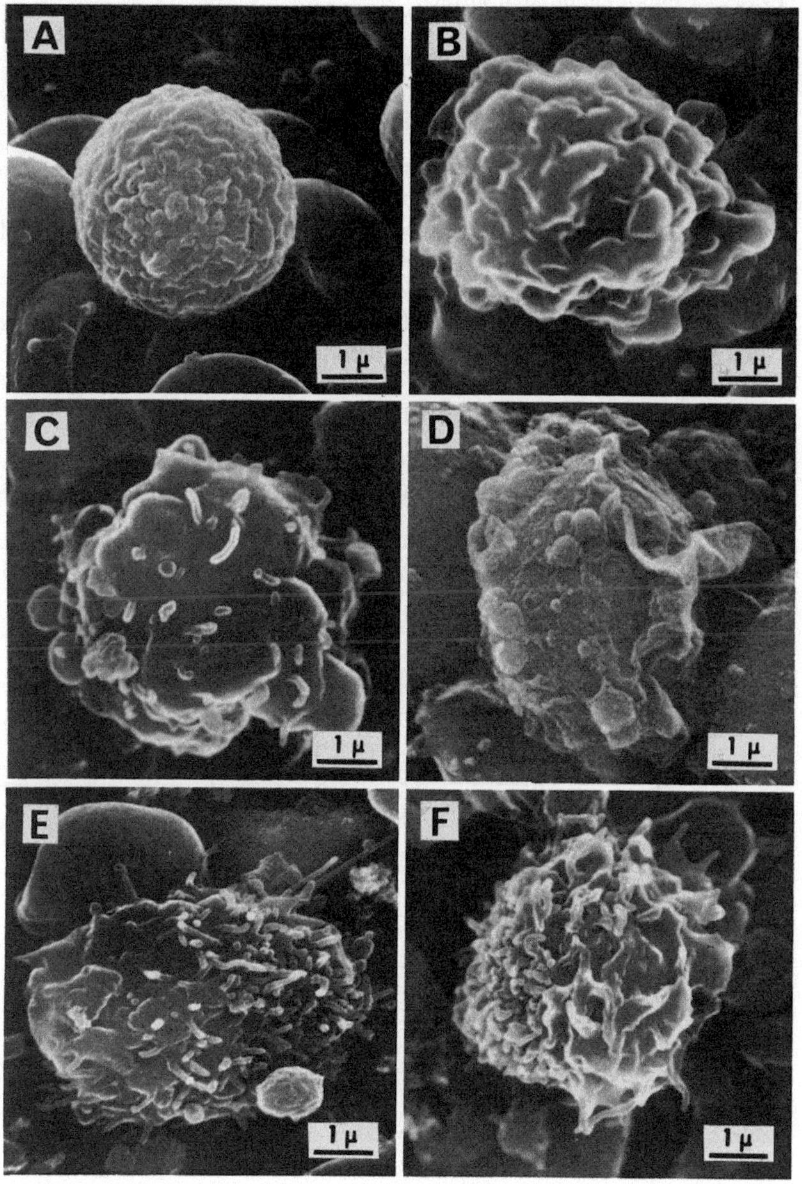

Fig. 6. Intermediate and hybrid forms. (A) Intermediate form between types 2 and 3. (B) Intermediate form between types 2 and 5. (C) Intermediate form between types 3 and 6. (D) Intermediate form between types 1, 5, and 6. (E) Hybrid form from types 2 and 4. (F) Hybrid form from types 4 and 6

Normal Blood Mononuclear Cells

When we have examined the blood of 12 subjects presumed to be normal and of one patient with toxoplasmosis and another with mononucleosis, we found a much more complex population as far as scanning was concerned. According to our observations, there are at least six main types of mononuclear cells, as seen in Fig. 5:

Type 1: a completely smooth surface

Type 2: a smooth undulated surface
Type 3: a slightly villous surface
Type 4: an extremely villous surface
Type 5: a surface covered with blebs
Type 6: a ruffled surface with ridge-like profiles

In addition, there are intermediate and hybrid cell forms, as shown in Figure 6:
A: an intermediate form between types 2 and 3 (undulated and villous)
B: an intermediate form between types 2 and 5 (undulated and bleb-covered surfaces)
C: a form between types 3 and 6 (villous and ridge-like profiles)
D: a form between types 1, 5, and 6 (smooth, bleb, and ridge-like profiles)
E: a hybrid form from types 2 and 4 (undulated at one pole and villous at the other)
F: a hybrid form from types 4 and 6 (villous at one pole and ridge-like at the other)
These atypical forms are usually rare in normal blood, but interesting in pathologic tissue.
Table 1 shows the percentages by scanning electron microscopy of different mononuclear cell

Table 1. Percentage of different circulating mononuclear cell types under scanning electron microscopy (SEM) in 12 subjects presumed normal

SEM types	Type 1 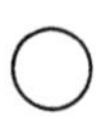	Type 2 	Type 3 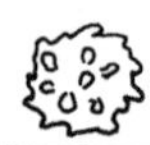	Type 4 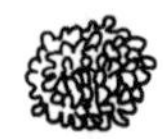	Type 5 	Type 6 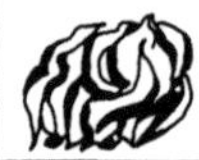
Mean % values	3	1	50	37	0.2	9
	4		87			

Percentage of T- and B-lymphocytes, peroxidase-positive cells (monocytes), and null cells in the peripheral blood of 12 subjects presumed normal

Mononuclear cells	T-lymphocytes	B-lymphocytes	Peroxidase positive cells	Null cells
Mean % values	60	15	13	12

Table 2. List of neoplastic lymphomononuclear disorders examined by scanning electron microscopy and immune markers

A. Chronic disorders:
- 26 cases of chronic lymphoid leukemia (CLL)
- 4 cases of hairy cell leukemia (HCL)
- 3 cases of multiple myeloma (Kahler's disease)
- 2 cases of primary macroglobulinemia (Waldenström's disease)
- 1 case of primary chronic monocytoid leukemia (CMoL)

B. Acute disorders:
- 30 cases of typical acute lymphoid leukemia (ALL)
- 4 cases of primary immunoblastic acute lymphoid leukemia (IALL)
- 2 cases of acute monoblastoid leukemia (AMoL)
- 34 cases of non-Hodgkin's lymphoma including 31 leukemic
- 12 cases of Hodgkin's disease
- 1 case of mycosis fungoides

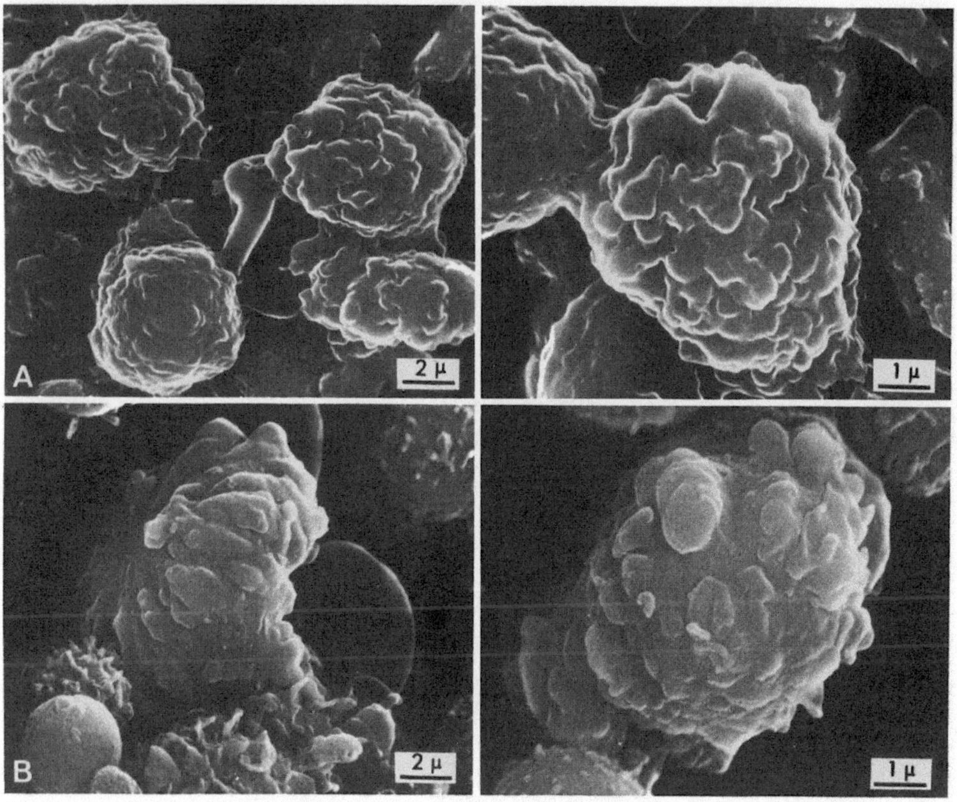

Fig. 7. (A) Primary macroglobulinemia (Waldenström disease). (B) Multiple myeloma (Kahler disease)

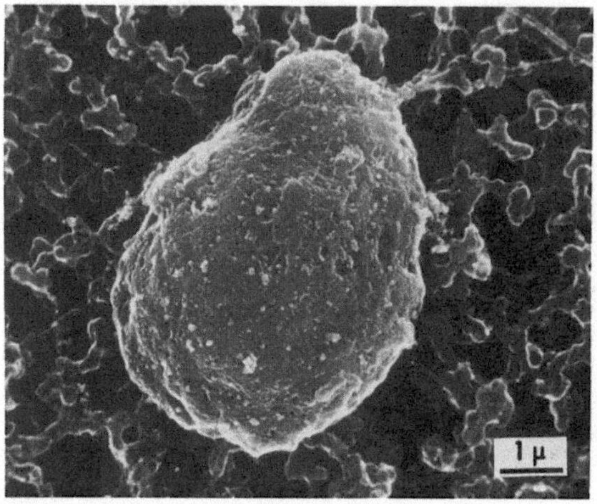

Fig. 8. Mycosis fungoides cell

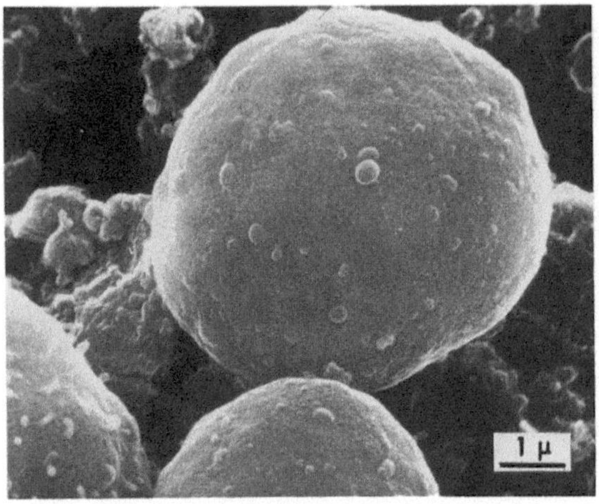

Fig. 9. Reticulosarcoma cells

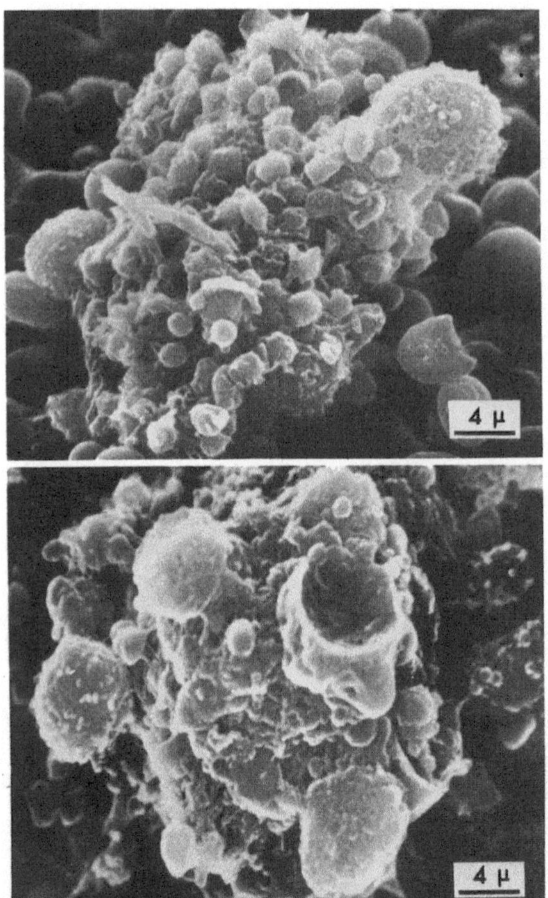

Fig. 10. Hodgkin's disease. Two examples of presumed Reed-Sternberg cells

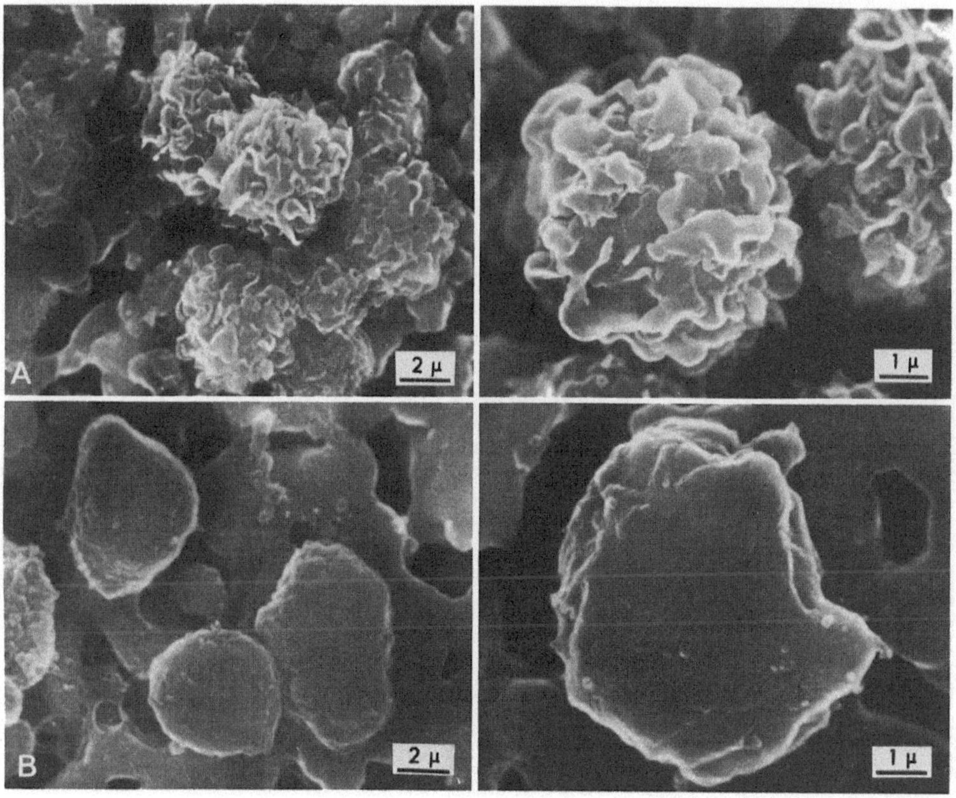

Fig. 11. (A) Chronic monocytoid leukemia. (B) Acute monoblastic leukemia

types in the blood of normal subjects and the corresponding immunologic data for T, B, null, and peroxidase-positive cells or monocytes [8, 9]. Comparison of these results shows that in normal blood, villous cells (types 3 and 4) are the most frequent (87%) and that there are only 4% of smooth cells (types 1 and 2). On the other hand, immunologic tests showed 60% of T cells, which implies that most T cells are just as villous as B cells. During the workshop held in Montpellier in June, 1976 on the different techniques of separation and characterization of human lymphocytes, we were able to study, by scanning, different lymphocyte populations isolated by many specialists, and our results confirmed this view.

Finally, in normal circulating blood, there is no correlation between the scanning aspect and immune markers, and most T cells are as villous as B cells [1, 8, 9]. This may either be due to functional or metabolic phenomena, frequently present in the blood, or to changes in scanning aspects caused by the different techniques used to separate cell population during the Montpellier Workshop. Whatever the reason, the T- or B-nature of a lymphocyte in normal blood cannot be identified on the basis of scanning electron microscopy alone.

Mononuclear Leukemia and Malignant Lymphoma Cells

Examination of mononuclear cell leukemias and lymphomas proved more rewarding. We examined the cells of patients with the different diseases listed in Table 2 and obtained two

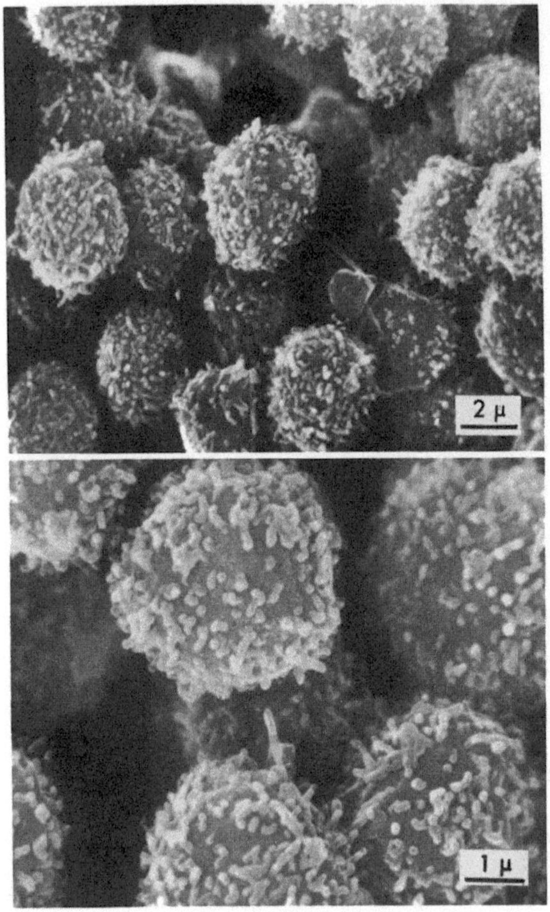

Fig. 12. B-cell chronic lymphoid leukemia

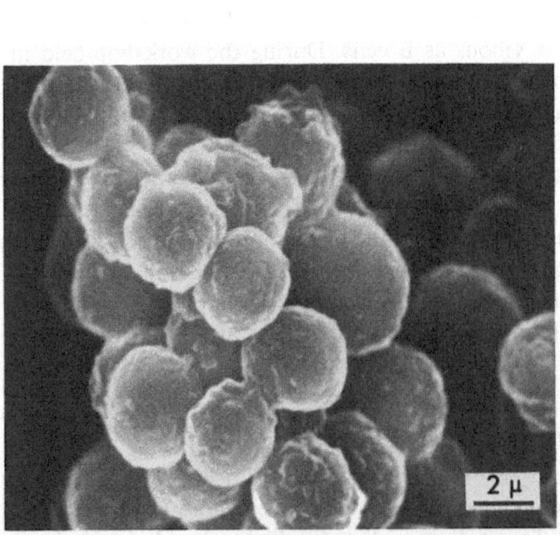

Fig. 13 (Legend see p. 103)

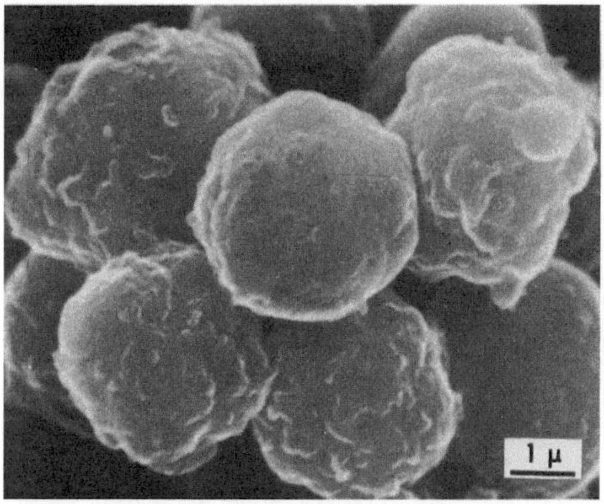

Fig. 13. T-cell chronic lymphoid leukemia

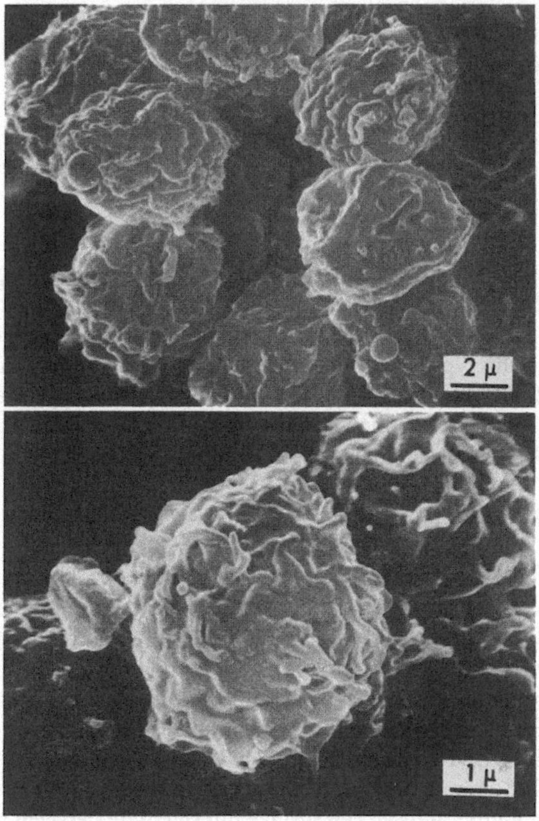

Fig. 14. Null cell hairy cell leukemia

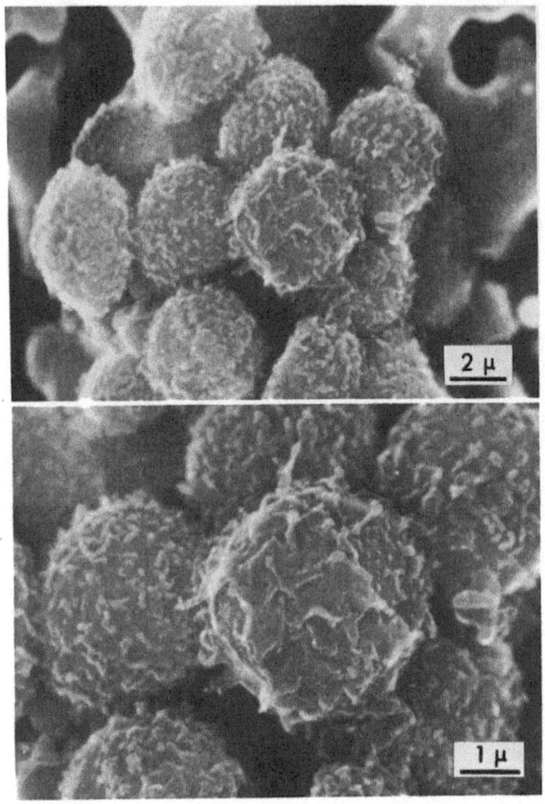

Fig 15. B-Cell hairy cell leukemia

kinds of data. The first kind concerned the scanning aspects of certain cells that had not yet been described when our study was published [8]. These cells are:

1. Plasma cells, which have a characteristic bleb-covered surface. Figure 7 shows some cells of this type (type 5 in our classification) in primary macroglobulinemia and multiple myeloma.
2. Mycosis fungoides cells, which are round or pear-shaped with smooth or smooth-undulated surfaces, as shown in Figure 8.
3. Reticulosarcoma cells in lymphoid and bone reticulosarcomas, which are large and generally have a smooth surface (Fig. 9).
4. Reed-Sternberg cells, which have a surface densely covered with blebs and in close contact with numerous lymphocytes (Fig. 10).

The second kind of data are surprising. Contrary to normal blood, in which there is no correlation between the scanning aspect and immune markers, in mononuclear cell neoplasias, there is a good correlation between the scanning aspect and both cytochemical and immune markers [8, 9, 15]. Figure 11 shows monocytoid neoplasias: a chronic monocytic and an acute monoblastic leukemia. Lymphoid neoplasias also showed a good correlation between the immune markers and the scanning aspects, as seen in Figures 12–17.

In B- and T-chronic lymphoid leukemia, the cells are more or less villous in the B-case (Fig. 12) and smooth or slightly undulated in the T (Fig. 13). In a case of null cell hairy cell leukemia, scanning showed cell surface intermediate between undulated and ridge-like profiles (Fig. 14). In a B-cell hairy cell leukemia, scanning showed forms with cell surfaces intermediate between villous and ridge-like profiles (Fig. 15). Figure 16 shows three cases of acute lymphoid leukemia:

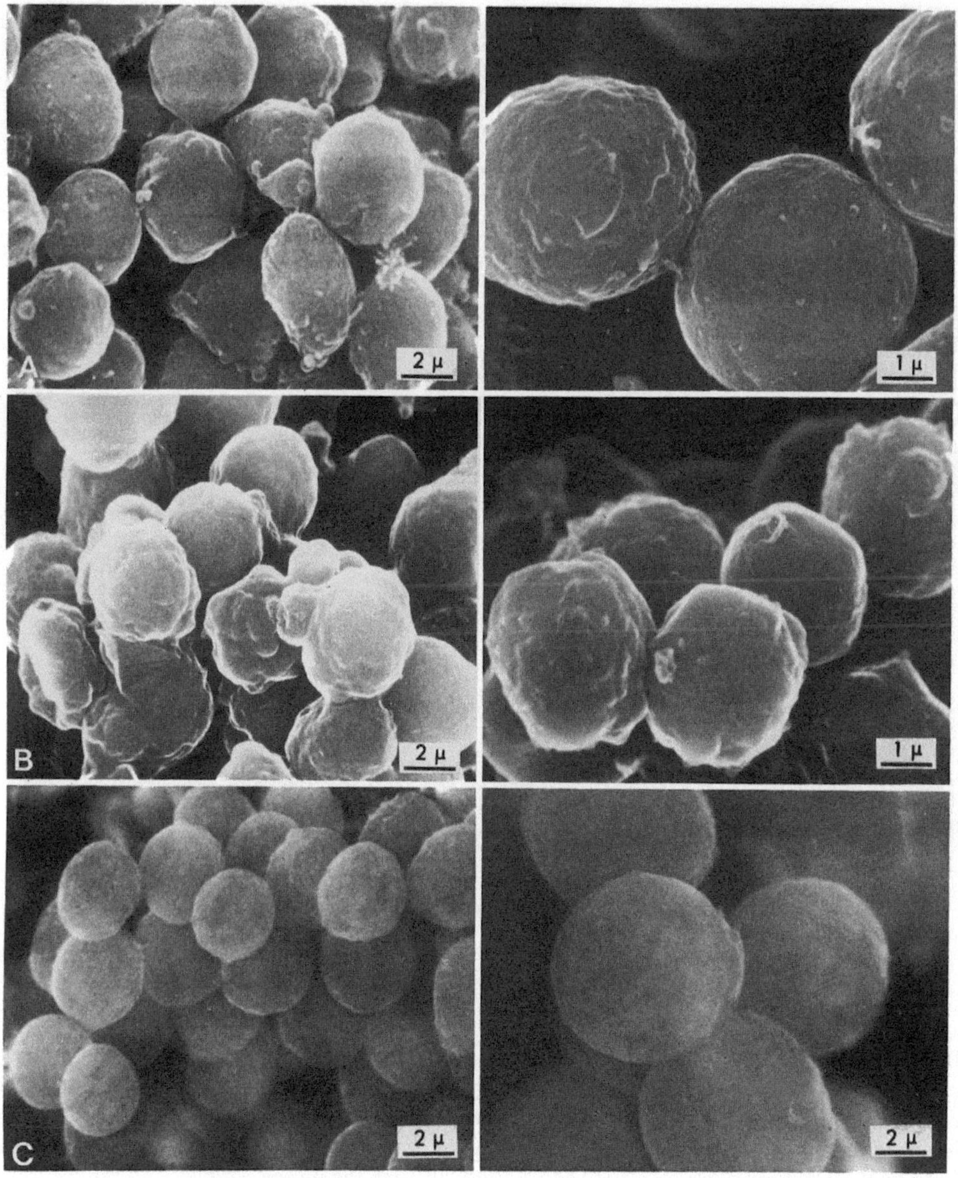

Fig. 16. (A) T-cell macrolymphoblastic acute leukemia. (B) T-cell prolymphocytic acute leukemia. (C) Null cell prolymphocytic acute leukemia

T-macrolymphoblastic, T-prolymphocytic, and null prolymphocytic, according to the WHO classification [11]. In these and almost all our other cases of acute lymphoid leukemia, scanning showed a smooth or smooth-undulated surface. Figure 17 shows four types of lymphosarcomas or malignant lymphomas: null lymphoblastic lymphosarcoma with a very smooth cell surface, T-immunoblastic lymphosarcoma with a very smooth but slightly undulated surface, B-prolymphocytic or centrofollicular cell lymphoma with few villosities, and B-prolymphocytic lymphoma with an extremely villous cell surface.

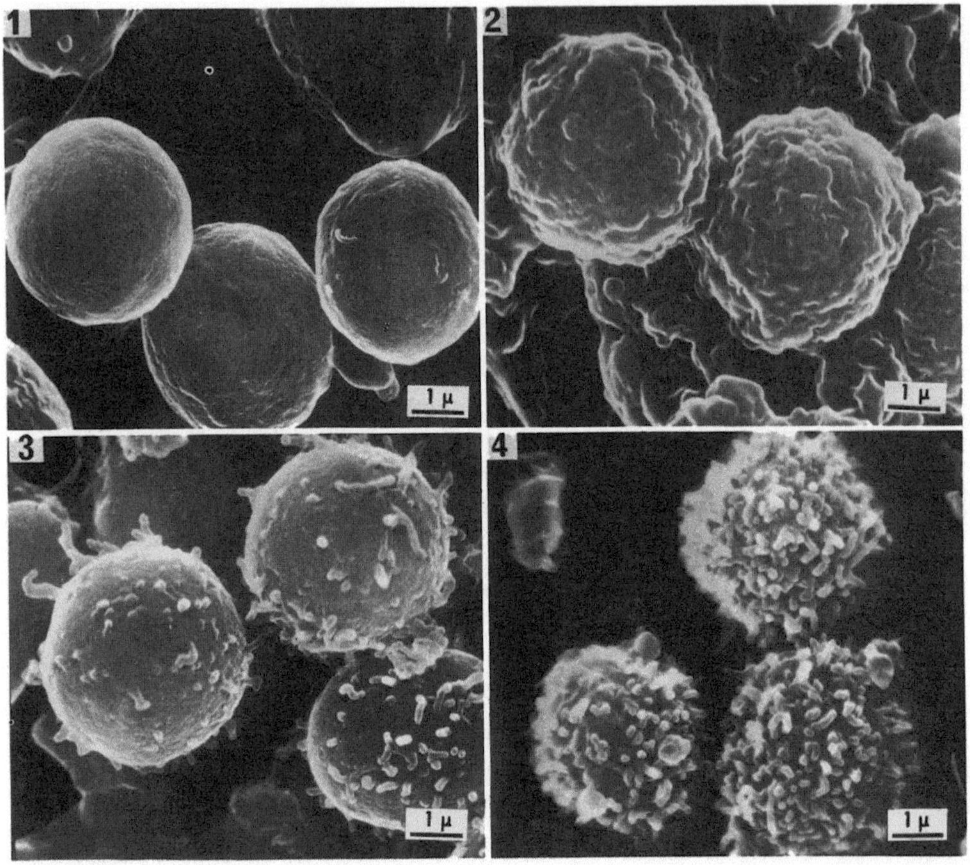

Fig. 17. Non-Hodgkin's hematosarcomas (lymphomas): (1) Null cell lymphoblastic lymphoma. (2) T-cell immunoblastic lymphoma. (3) B-cell prolymphocytic lymphoma. (4) B-cell prolymphocytic lymphoma.

In conclusion, even though scanning electron microscopy is not acceptable as a valid method of distinguishing between the various types of lymphocytes in normal blood, it does seem to be of interest for identifying mononuclear cell neoplasias. The scanning technique allows specific identification of malignant proliferation among monocytes, plasma cells, and mycosis fungoides. Our study revealed a good correlation between the immune typing and the scanning aspects of lymphoid neoplasias such as chronic lymphoid leukemia, acute lymphoid leukemia, and malignant lymphoma. However, as regards this last observation, our results must now be confirmed by other groups, and we hope they will succeed in correlating the scanning aspect of the cells with more markers than we used in our study.

References

1. ALEXANDER, E. L., WETZEL, B.: Human lymphocytes: Similarity of B and T cell surface morphology. Science *188*, 732 (1975).
2. BELPOMME, D., LELARGE, N.: Caractérisation immunologique et cytochimique des lymphocytes et monocytes: Nécessité d'une batterie de tests. In: Les Techniques de Séparation et d'Identification des Lymphocytes Humains. Séminaire technologique, Montpellier, 12–15 May 1976. Paris: I.N.S.E.R.M. 1976, Vol. LVII, p. 75.
3. BELPOMME, D., PONVERT, D., MATHE, G.: Une nouvelle méthode d'exploration des lymphocytes et monocytes par leurs marqueurs de membrane: son intérêt en pathologie. In: Rencontre Biologique. Paris: Expansion Scientifique Française 1975, p. 25.
4. BELPOMME, D., DANTCHEV, D., JOSEPH, R., SANTORO, A., FEUILHADE DE CHAUVIN, F., LELARGE, N., GRANDJON, D., PONTVERT, D., MATHE, G.: Classification of leukemias and hematosarcomas based on cell membrane markers and scanning electron microscopy. In: Clinical Tumor Immunology. WYBRAN, J. (ed.) Oxford: Pergamon Press 1976, p. 131.
5. DANTCHEV, D.: Sémiologie des cellules mononuclées étudiées par la microscopie électronique à balayage. In: Les Techniques de Séparation et d'Identification des Lymphocytes Humains. Séminaire technologique, Montpellier, 12–15 May 1976. Paris: I.N.S.E.R.M. 1976a, Vol. LVII, p. 273.
6. DANTCHEV, D.: Revised semiology of the different mononuclear cells under scanning electron microscopy. In: Recent Results in Cancer Research. Berlin-Heidelberg-New York: Springer Verlag 1976b, p. 8.
7. DANTCHEV, D.: Apports de la Microscopie Electronique à Balayage dans l'Etude des Plasmocytes et Cellules Plasmocytoïdes du Myélome Multiple et de la Macroglobulinémie Primaire. Rencontre Biologique. Paris: Expansion Scientifique Française 1977, p. 21.
8. DANTCHEV, D., BELPOMME, D.: Critical study of the mononuclear leucocyte morphology based on scanning electron microscopy in normal subjects and in patients with lymphoid or monocytoid proliferative disorders. Comparison with the T, B or null cell membrane phenotypes. Biomedicine *26*, 202 (1977).
9. DANTCHEV, D., BELPOMME, D., MATHE, G.: Etude critique de la sémiologie morphologique des leucocytes mononucléés normaux et pathologiques à l'aide de la microscopie électronique à balayage. Corrélation avec les marqueurs immunologiques des surfaces cellulaires. In: Entretiens de Bichat 1976, Rencontre biologique. Paris: Expansion Scientifique Française 1976, p. 13.
10. LIN, P. S., WALLACH, F. H., TSAI, S.: Temperature induced variations in the surface topology of cultured lymphocytes are revealed by scanning electron microscopy. Proc. Natl. Acad. Sci. U.S.A. *70*, 2492 (1973).
11. MATHE, G., RAPPAPORT, H.: Histological and Cytological Typing of the Neoplastic Diseases of the Haematopoietic and Lymphoid Tissues. Genève: WHO: Internat. Histological Classification of Tumors, n°14.
12. POLLIACK, A.: Surface features of circulating human leukemic cells: experience with 175 cases of leukemia examined by scanning electron microscopy. In: Proceeding of the Workshop on Advance in Biomedical Applications of the S.E.M., Chicago: I.T.T., Res. Inst. 1976, Part V.
13. POLLIACK, A., LAMPEN, N., CLARKSON, B. D., DE HARVEN, E., BENTWICH, Z., SIEGAL, F. P., KUNKEL, H. G.: Identification of human B and T lymphocytes by scanning electron microscopy. J. Exp. Med. *138*, 607 (1973a).
14. POLLIACK, A., LAMPEN, N. DE HARVEN, E.: Comparison of air drying and critical point drying procedures for the study of human blood cells by scanning electron microscopy. In: Proceedings of 6th Annual Scanning Electron Microscopy Symposium. Chicago: I.T.T. Res. Inst. 1973b, p. 535.
15. POLLIACK, A., SIEGAL, F. P., CLARKSON, B. D., FU, S. M., WINCHESTER, R. J., LAMPERT, N., SIEGAL, M., DE HARVEN, E.: A scanning electron microscopy and immunological study of 84 cases of lymphocytic leukemia and related lymphoproliferative disorders. Scand. J. Haematol. *15*, 359 (1975).
16. POLLIACK, A., FROIMOVICI, M., FRANKENBURG, S., GERY, I.: Altered surface morphology of concanavalin A transformed thymic lymphocytes as seen by scanning electron microscopy. Biomedicine *24*, 389–395 (1976).

Cytochemistry: An Aid to the Diagnosis and Classification of the Acute Leukemias

D. Catovsky, Maureen O'Brien, and M. Cherchi

The correct diagnosis and classification of the acute leukemias relies very often on the accurate recognition and characterization of the blast cell population. Romanowsky-stained blood and bone marrow films permit this in most cases if the features of differentiation are well developed. When this is not so, cytochemical methods may demonstrate features not apparent on conventional stains, thus providing an indication of the degree of cell maturation. An important step towards a uniform nomenclature and a more objective classification was provided by the joint proposals of the FAB group [1]. The FAB workers recognized two main groups of acute leukemia: those showing myeloid differentiation (AML) and the "lymphoblastic" leukemias (ALBL). Most categories of AML (M2, M3, M4, M6) can be recognized on Romanowsky-stained films alone. For M1 and M5, in which signs of maturation of the blast cells are less obvious, cytochemical tests may be essential.

In myeloblastic leukemia with minimal maturation (M1), for example, the demonstration of the peroxidase and/or Sudan black reaction defines those cases without difficulty. Primary granules in myeloblasts and early promyelocytes are relatively large, and evidence of enzyme activity can almost always be seen by light microscopy (LM). Very rarely, the enzyme is localized exclusively in the membranes of the nuclear envelope, Golgi apparatus, and endoplasmic reticulum (ER) and is thus demonstrable by transmission electron microscopy (TEM) only [2]. It may be less easy to recognize blasts with monocytic differentiation (M5) because the sequence of the development of the cytoplasmic enzymes is less well-known than in M1. This is illustrated by the following studies.

Ultrastructure and Cytochemistry of Acute Leukemia (M5)

Studies on the early development of monocytic differentiation in normal bone marrow suggest that this is associated with the presence (as in myeloblasts) of peroxidase activity in the primary granules [10]. However, because the peroxidase reaction is often negative in monocytic leukemia, we decided to look at other monocyte enzymes as well in order to determine the sequence and timing of their appearance in the cell cytoplasm. Ten patients with M5 leukemia were studied by the techniques shown in Table 1. According to the degree of maturation, three types of cases were observed (Table 2).

1. Four patients had very immature or poorly differentiated blast cells with a round nucleus with few or no electron-dense granules by TEM; the only positive cytochemical reactions were NASA and acid phosphatase.
2. In two patients, there was some morphological evidence of monocytic differentiation (promonocytes); the peroxidase reaction was positive in the small cytoplasmic granules at TEM level (Fig. 1), while under LM it was negative; moderate lysozyme activity was demonstrated in some of the cells; both patients were positive for acid phosphatase and NASA.

Table 1. Monocytic leukemia—methods used

1. *Morphology* (*LM*) (May-Grünwald-Giemsa)
2. *Cytochemistry*
Peroxidase
Sudan black B
Naphthol AS-acetate esterase ($\pm$ NaF)
Acid phosphatase
3. *Lysozyme*
Cytobacterial test
Serum levels
4. *Electron microscopy* (*TEM*)
Morphology (lead—uranyl acetate stain)
Peroxidase (Graham-Karnovsky)

3. In the last four cases, the cells were more mature both morphologically and cytochemically (Table 2). An illustrated description of these stages of monoblast-monocyte maturation as seen by TEM has been given elsewhere [4]. The present study demonstrates three points:
   a) That NASA and acid phosphatase enzyme activities appear earlier than the granules which contain peroxidase and lysozyme—they are thus probably the earliest differentiation features of monoblasts. The near absence of lysosomal granules under TEM suggests that these early enzymes are probably not associated with granules at this stage.
   b) That cases of poorly differentiated M5 leukemia may sometimes be wrongly classified as ALBL (L2 type) unless the NASA $\pm$ NaF and acid phosphatase reactions (particularly the former) are performed routinely; even TEM may not show in such cases as clear evidence of monocyte differentiation as these two cytochemical reactions.
   c) That peroxidase and lysozyme seem to appear later, at a time when morphologically (both under LM and TEM) evidence for monocytic differentiation is already apparent.

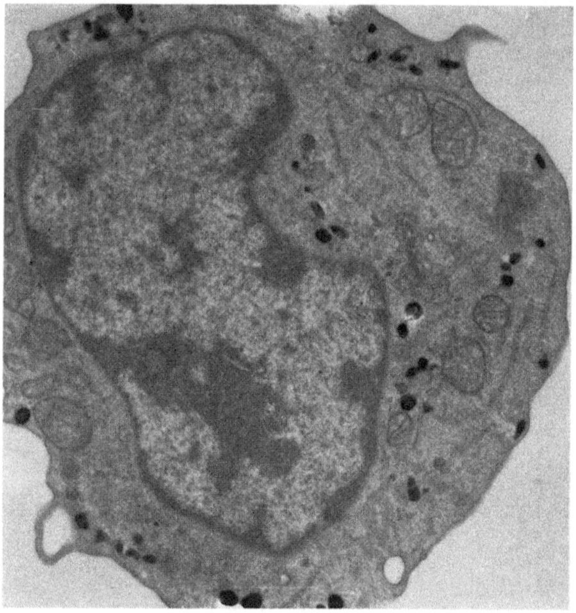

Fig. 1. Electron photomicrograph of a leukemic promonocyte in M5 leukemia. All the small cytoplasmic granules are positive with the peroxidase reaction. Note areas of condensed nuclear chromatin, which are characteristic of this intermediate degree of differentiation, and the active Golgi apparatus. (Graham-Karnovsky technique; lead citrate stain $\times$ 20,000)

Table 2. Correlation between ultrastructural and cytochemical features in acute monocytic leukemia

Light microscopy (LM)[a]	Ultrastructure (TEM) (*4*)	Peroxidase LM-TEM		Lysozyme (Cytobacterial-serum)	NASA (NaF sensitive)	Acid phosphatase
M5—poorly differentiated	Blasts with round nuclei. Few or no granules. Long ER	–	–	–	+/++	+/++
M5—poorly differentiated or differentiated	Monocytoid nucleus with variable maturation; active Golgi; granules (19–20)	–	+	+	++	++
M5—differentiated	Mature monocytoid nucleus. Abundant small granules (15–30)	+	++	++	++	++

[a] FAB classification (1).

Acute Lymphoblastic Leukemia

ALBL was defined in the FAB classification [1] on the basis of morphology and on the absence of myeloid differentiation by cytochemical criteria. Within ALBL we have observed that the PAS reaction is positive in two-thirds of cases only and that the reaction does not seem to correlate with any morphological type. A positive reaction, therefore, cannot be considered as essential for the diagnosis of ALBL as has been generally thought. When considered in relation to the type of ALBL assessed by immunological markers, the PAS reaction is typically negative in B-ALBL (Burkitt-type); it is positive in 50% of cases of T-ALBL, and positive in the highest proportion (about 70%) in null ALBL, both in children and adults. On the other hand, studies of the acid phosphatase reaction have shown that T-lymphoblasts (T-ALBL) are characterized by a strong paranuclear reaction localized to the Golgi zone [3, 5, 6, 11, 12]. We have now completed a double-blind study on material from the UKALL trials (co-ordinated by Dr. H. E. M. Kay) in which fresh samples of blood and bone marrow were sent by the participating centers to Dr. M. F. Greaves's laboratory (Imperial Cancer Research Fund) for immunological typing (B- and T-markers and anti-ALBL serum) [7, 8] and unfixed bone marrow and blood films were sent to us for cytochemical testing (May-Grünwald-Giemsa, peroxidase and acid phosphatase). One hundred and six cases have been studied; a positive peroxidase reaction excluded four cases of myeloblastic leukemia (M1). (This was important because the acid phosphatase was also positive in these cases.) The results of the acid phosphatase reaction were recorded as *positive* when the majority of blasts (> 65%) showed the characteristic localized strong reaction, *negative* when no cells reacted or up to 30% showed a weak reaction, and *intermediate* when 30%–60% of blasts showed a moderate to strong reaction. The *intermediate* reaction was seen in four cases only; for the analysis they were considered as *positives*. The acid phosphatase reaction was correlated with the immunological cell marker test as follows.

1. Null ALBL (negative B- and T-markers): two cases out of 85 (4.7%) were positive. When only null ALBL cases which were positive with the anti-ALBL serum were considered, all 64 were negative.
2. T-ALBL (positive T-markers): 15 out of 19 cases (79%) were positive and four were negative. It is interesting that two of the latter were cases in which, in addition to the positive T-cell markers, the reaction with the anti-ALBL serum was weakly positive, suggesting that the cells possessed a special type of surface phenotype not found in most T-ALBL cases. The difference between the null ALBL and T-ALBL cases was statistically highly significant ($p < 0.001$; Chi square test).

Conclusions

The results of our studies using a battery of routinely performed cytochemical methods are summarized in Table 3. It should be noted that:

1. in some categories of AML (M2, M3, M4, and M6), cytochemistry is not essential for the diagnosis and it is largely confirmatory,
2. in M1 and M5, cytochemical tests may be essential in order to exclude some types of ALBL (e.g., L2), and
3. that the acid phosphatase reaction in ALBL is relevant once cytochemical reactions for myeloid enzymes have been proved to be negative. This reaction should not replace the testing for surface markers, but it has the advantage that a positive reaction can still be demonstrated on slides up to 1 month old and that it may be valuable in T-ALBL cases with a low percentage of E-rosettes or in cases showing simultaneously receptors for sheep RBC and complement [9, 12].

Table 3. Cytochemical methods as aids in the classification of acute leukemia

Cytochemical reaction	Acute myeloid leukemia[a]						Acute lymphoblastic leukemia		
	M1	M2	M3	M4	M5	M6	Null ALBL	T-ALBL	B-ALBL
Peroxidase	+	++	++	++	−/+	+[b]	−	−	−
Sudan	+	++	++	++	−/+	+[b]	−	−	−
NASA (NaF sensitive)	−	−	−	+	++	−	−	−	−
Acid phosphatase	±	+	+	+	++	±[b]	−/±	++	−
Lysozyme	−	−	−	+/++	+/++	−	−	−	−

[a] FAB Classification [1].
[b] Positive in myeloblasts not in erythroid precursors.

References

1. Bennett, J. M., Catovsky, D., Daniel, Marie-Thérèse, Flandrin, G., Galton, D. A. G., Gralnick, H. R., Sultan, C. (FAB-Co-operative group): Proposals for the Classification of the Acute Leukaemias. Br. J. Haematol. *33*, 451–458 (1976).
2. Bessis, M., Maigné, J.: Le diagnostic des variétés de leucémies aigues par la réaction des peroxydases au microscope electronique. Rev. Eur. Etud. Clin. Biol. *6*, 691–698 (1970).
3. Brouet, J. C., Valensi, F., Daniel, Marie-Thérèse, Flandrin, G., Preud'homme, J. L., Seligmann, M.: Immunological classification of acute lymphoblastic leukemias: evaluation of its clinical significance in a hundred patients. Br. J. Haematol. *33*, 319–327 (1976).
4. Catovsky, D.: Morphological recognition of lymphocytes and macrophages. In: Recent Results in Cancer Research. Mathé, G., Florentin, I., Simmler, M-C. (eds.) Berlin: Springer-Verlag 1976, Vol. LVI, pp. 1–7.
5. Catovsky, D., Galetto, J., Okos, A., Miliani, E., Galton, D. A. G.: Cytochemical profile of B and T leukaemic lymphocytes with special reference to acute lymphoblastic leukaemia. J. Clin. Pathol. *27*, 767–771 (1974).
6. Catovsky, D., Frisch, B., Van Noorden, Susan: B, T and "Null" cell leukaemias. Electron Cytochemistry and Surface Morphology. Blood Cells *1*, 115–124 (1975).
7. Greaves, M. F., Brown, G., Rapson, N. T., Lister, T. A.: Antisera to acute lymphoblastic leukaemia cells. Clin. Immunol. Immunopathol. *4*, 67–84 (1975).
8. Greaves, M. F., Janossy, G., Roberts, M., Rapson, N. T., Ellis, R. B., Chessels, J., Lister, T. A., Catovsky, D.: Membrane phenotyping: diagnosis, monitoring and classification of acute 'lymphoid' leukaemias. In: 'Immunological Diagnosis of Leukemias and Lymphomas'—(Haematology and Blood Transfusion). Thierfelder, S., Rodt, H., Thiel, E. (eds.) Berlin: Springer-Verlag 1977, Vol. XX, pp. 61–75.
9. Jaffe, E. S., Braylan, R. R. C., Frank, M. M., Green, I., Berard, W.: Heterogeneity of Immunologic Markers and Surface Morphology in Childhood Lymphoblastic Lymphoma. Blood *48*, 213–222 (1976).
10. Nichols, B. A., Bainton, D. F., Farquhar, M. G.: Differentiation of monocytes. Origin, nature and fate of their azurophil granules. J. Cell Biol. *50*, 498–515 (1971).
11. Ritter, J., Gaedicke, G., Winkler, K., Beckman, H., Landbeck, G.: Possible T-cell origin of lymphoblasts in acid phosphatase positive Acute Lymphatic Leukaemia. Lancet *1975/ii*, 75.
12. Stein, H., Petersen, N., Gaedicke, G., Lennert, K., Landbeck, G.: Lymphoblastic lymphoma of convoluted or acid phosphatase type—a tumor of T precursor cells. Int. J. Cancer *17*, 292–295 (1976).

Dynamic Morphology of Human Lymphoid Leukemias

G. HAEMMERLI, H. FELIX, and P. STRÄULI

In descriptions of scanning electron micrographs of normal and leukemic white blood cells, little thought has been given to the fact that surface morphology and shape are a function of cell motility and, thus, subject to frequent changes. Consideration of these facts necessitates the combination of scanning electron microscopy (SEM) with microcinematography (MCM) under identical experimental conditions. BESSIS and DE BOISFLEURY [1, 2] were the first to utilize this approach for studies on white cell movements. We have applied the two methods for the analysis of cell populations from human acute and chronic leukemia and for two transplantable rat leukemias [3, 4].

For the interpretation of static morphology, obtained by SEM, in relation to the behavior of living cells, recorded by MCM, we use the term dynamic morphology [3]. The concurrent application of the two methods allowed us to make the following observations (Figs. 1–12):

1. Leukemia cells *do not flatten on a glass surface*. They are either spherical or polarized.
2. *Spherical leukemia cells* are nonlocomotive but display on-spot motility. "On-spot motility" refers to cell movements not connected with a net translocation of the whole cell. On-spot motility is an individual and not a generic feature of spherical leukemia cells. Accordingly, SE micrographs of leukemic populations show considerable variation in surface architecture of the pertinent cells. In our experience, the range of this variation in different populations does not fall into distinct patterns. Therefore, dynamic morphology is an unsuitable method for categorization of spherical leukemia cells.
3. *Spherical cells of the monocytoid series* are an exception, as they can be classified. Their surface is characterized by prominent folds (Fig. 3).
4. *Polarized cells* are locomotive or in preparation for locomotive activity. Such cells have an anterior and posterior or a free and attached part that can be well distinguished. There is a difference in the polarized structure of blast cells (Figs. 4 and 7), promyelocytes (Figs. 5 and 6), and myelocytes (Figs. 8 and 9), and also of granulocytes and lymphocytes. Provided these cell types had been fixed while engaged in locomotion, their characteristic shapes allow recognition by SEM.
5. *Polarized blast cells of different origin*—lymphoid, myeloid, or unclassifiable—cannot be distinguished by dynamic morphology (Figs. 10–12). Their mode of locomotion is so similar that it is justified to speak of a "blast pattern of locomotion" [5]. Surface architecture, superimposed on the similar overall shape of all moving blast cells, is again of an individual rather than a generic nature and, thus, cannot be used for classification.

When we apply dynamic morphology to lymphoid leukemias (Figs. 13–24), SEM reveals that spherical cells of the same population can have different surface features: some have shorter microvilli, some longer, some ridges or small folds. The amount of microvilli is also subject to variation. This is illustrated by two examples, an acute lymphatic leukemia (Figs. 13–15) and a chronic lymphatic leukemia (Figs. 16–19). Because of this variation in surface morphology of cells occurring in the same population, SEM, under our experimental conditions, cannot distinguish one lymphatic population from the other.

Leukemic cell populations can contain polarized cells in varying amounts. We know from cinematography that in most cases the polarized configuration is equivalent to locomotion.

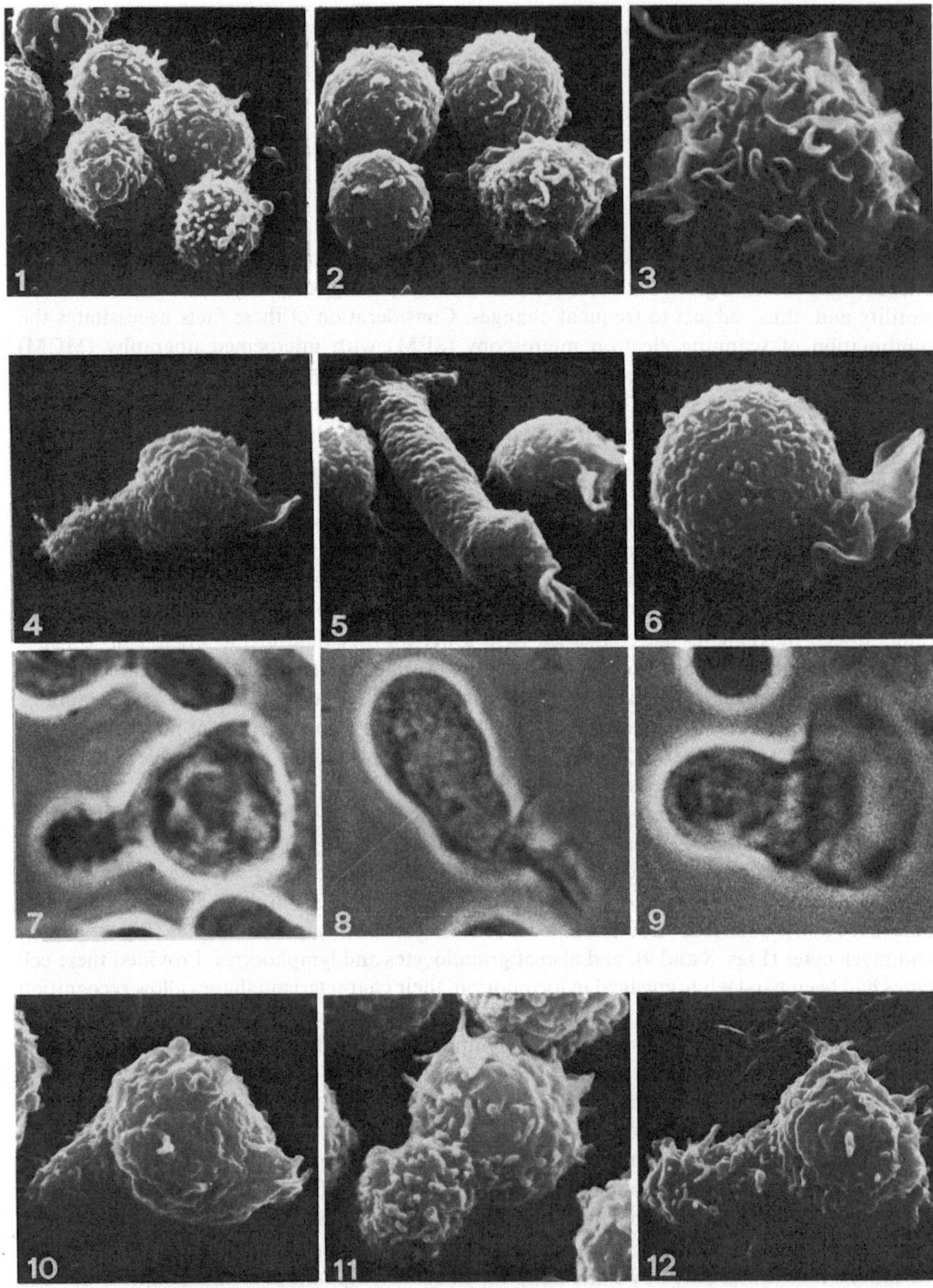

Plate 1. Principles of dynamic morphology of leukemia cells. Figures 1–12:
Fig. 1. Leukemic population from a patient with AML. Note the difference in surface morphology of the spherical cells. SEM: × 3000;
Fig. 2. Leukemic population from a patient with ALL. The variation in surface extensions is evident. SEM: × 3000;
Fig. 3. Monocytoid cell from AMML. In contrast to the spherical cells in Figures 1 and 2, monocytoid cells have characteristic large folds. SEM: × 4800;

Locomotive blast cells have a distinct anterior and posterior part with regard to the direction of movement. While the anterior part is often characterized by the production of larger or smaller cytoplasmic extensions, the posterior part can be called a tail. Cells from a patient with ALL in locomotive configuration are presented in Figures 19–21. The phase contrast photographs from a time-lapse sequence (Figs. 19 and 21) represent locomotive cells that moved with a speed of ~ 1 and 1.5 μm, respectively.
The surface architecture of spherical and polarized cells is somewhat different (Fig. 22). While the body of the polarized cell shows more ridge like cytoplasmic extensions, the microvilli seem to be concentrated on the tail. Similar features are shown for two further cells from the same population from a case of ALL (Figs. 23 and 24).

Conclusions

Surface morphology and cellular configuration can be well described by SEM. However, the additional use of cinematography has the advantage of relating such descriptions to the functional state of the cell. We know from time-lapse films that all living cells, under appropriate experimental conditions, are motile. Motility comprises two types of cellular activity: movements not connected with translocation of the whole cell and locomotion. The first type, on-spot motility, is the expression of surface activities consisting of the projection and retraction of cytoplasmic extensions. The two modes of cellular motility imply that shape and surface morphology continuously undergo changes of varying degrees and thereby reflect the momentary kind of activity in which the cells were engaged at the moment of fixation. This could explain the differences in size, number, shape, and distribution of surface extensions on spherical cells from the same lymphoid population. As such differences occurred in most of the leukemic populations included in our survey, we believe that a classification based on surface morphology is not feasible.
In our experience, the polarized form of lymphatic leukemia cells represents, in most instances, locomotive blast cells. However, blast cells from the myeloid series have the same configuration. For this reason, the generic nature of polarized blast cells has to be determined by conventional hematologic methods.

Acknowledgments

The authors gratefully acknowledge the skilled technical assistance of Miss S. BAUMGARTNER and Miss B. ARNOLD. Blood samples were generously supplied by the Department of Internal Medicine from the University of Zürich. The study was supported by the Swiss Cancer League, Credit No. FOR.075 AK. 75 (5), and by the Zürich Cancer League.

Plate 1 (continued)

Fig. 4. Blast cell from AML in a polarized shape. Note the typical configuration with the distinct anterior part and the tail that allows recognition of the direction of movement. SEM: × 3300;

Fig. 5. Promyelocyte from AML in a polarized shape. The elongated form and the cytoplasmic folds at the anterior end are characteristic of locomotive promyelocytes. SEM: × 3000;

Fig. 6. Myelocyte from AML in a pseudopolarized shape, given by the large veils at the front part. Note that the body is completely round. SEM: × 6000;

Figs. 7–9. A blast cell (Fig. 7), a promyelocyte (Fig. 8), and a myelocyte (Fig. 9) from a patient with AML, all engaged in locomotion. The similarity in shape, if compared to the same cell types presented in SEM (Figs. 4–6), is evident. Fig. 7. Phase contrast × 7200; Fig. 8. Phase contrast × 2300; Fig. 9. Phase contrast × 7200;

Figs. 10–12. Blast cells in the polarized configuration from patients with AML. ALL, and an unclassified leukemia. Although individual cells show variations in their surface features, the similar overall shape, together with the identical mode of locomotion, prevents classification. Fig. 10. SEM: × 5400; Fig. 11. SEM: × 5400; Fig. 12. SEM: × 4800

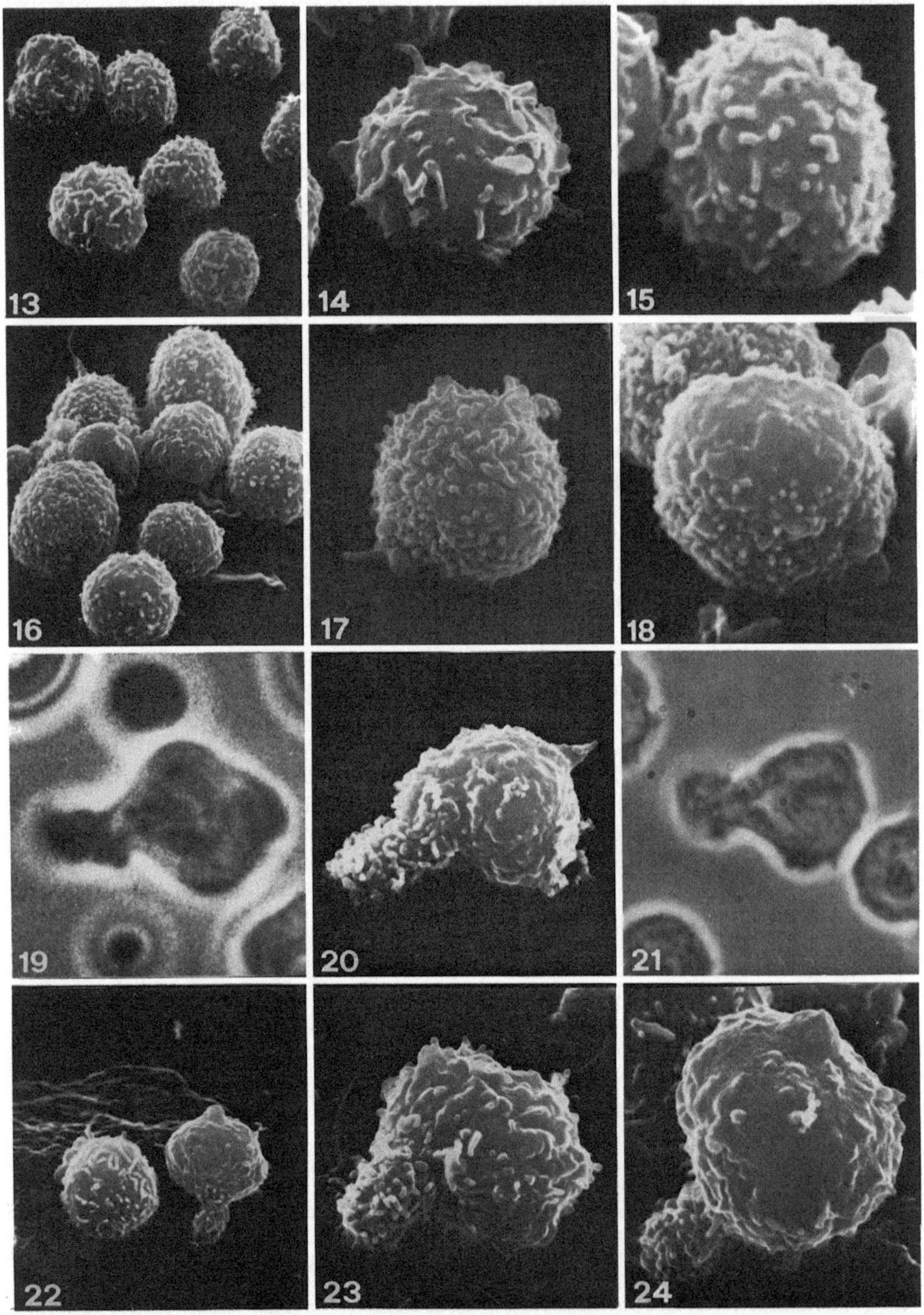

Plate 2. Dynamic morphology applied to lymphoid leukemia cells. Figures 13–24:
Figs. 13–15. Leukemic blast cells in the spherical shape from a patient with ALL. Note the difference in surface morphology of individual cells within the population. Fig. 13. SEM: × 2700; Fig. 14. SEM: × 6000; Fig. 15. SEM: × 8600;

References

1. BESSIS, M., DE BOISFLEURY, A.: Les mouvements des leucocytes étudiés au microscope électronique à balayage. Nouv. Rev. Fr. Hermatol. *11*, 377–400 (1971).
2. BESSIS, M., DE BOISFLEURY, A.: A catalogue of white blood cell movements. Blood Cells *2*, 365–410 (1976).
3. FELIX, H., HAEMMERLI, G., STRÄULI, P.: Atlas of Dynamics of Leukemia Cells: A Comparative Study by Scanning Electron Microscopy and Microcinematography. Berlin-Heidelberg-New York: Springer-Verlag 1978.
4. HAEMMERLI, G., FELIX, H.: Motility of acute human leukemia cells: A study by time-lapse cinematography and scanning electron microscopy. Blood Cells *2*, 415–430 (1976).
5. HAEMMERLI, G., FELIX, H.: Dynamics of leukemia cells. Film, color, sound, duration: 12 min. (1977).

Plate 2 (continued)

Figs. 16–18. Similar variations in surface features of spherical cells in the population of a patient with CLL. Fig. 16. SEM: × 3000; Fig. 17. SEM: × 6000; Fig. 18. SEM: × 6500;
Figs. 19–21. Polarized cells from ALL with their distinct anterior and posterior part (tail). Note the similarity in overall shape of the cell in the SE micrograph (Fig. 20) and the locomotive cells in the phase contrast photographs (Figs. 19 and 21) taken from time-lapse film sequences. Fig. 19. Phase contrast × 8300; Fig. 20. SEM: × 1730; Fig. 21. Phase contrast × 7200;
Figs. 22–24. Cells from a patient with ALL. Compared to the spherical cell (Fig. 22), the more heterogenous aspect of the surface extensions of the polarized cells (Figs. 22–24) is evident. Fig. 22. SEM: × 3000; Fig. 23. SEM: × 5400; Fig. 24. SEM: × 7200

Histiocytic and/or Reticulum Cell Neoplasias

C. NEZELOF and F. JAUBERT

It is now well-established that the histiocytes and/or macrophages in the tissues are the representatives of a distinctive system: the mononuclear phagocyte system (MPS) [27, 28]. It is of interest to recall that the cells belonging to that system originate from the bone marrow and migrate to the peripheral tissues, where most of them are normally unable to multiply [28]. This mobility and widespread distribution account for the disseminated character of most of the tumoral or reactive proliferations originating from MPS.

The MPS cell, from the bone marrow monoblast to the peripheral macrophage, has a very variable configuration. So the usual morphologic criteria, i.e., the size and the shape of the cell and its nucleus are of little use for its identification [7]. Nevertheless, the behavior of the MPS cell, especially the histiocyte, its mobility, its adherence to glass, its ability to phagocytose large particles, its enzymic equipment (nonspecific esterase, acid phosphatase), and the presence of membrane receptors are peculiar to it and provide some concrete criteria for identification [27]. Thus, the histiocytic origin of a tumoral process can be identified if two of the criteria, listed in Table 1, are present in the tumoral cells. In fact, very few tumoral processes fulfil these criteria. It now appears necessary to discuss the histogenesis of the tumors that have in the past been regarded as histiocytosarcomas or reticulosarcomas on the basis of morphologic features, i.e., the size of the cell, the shape of the nucleus, and the reticulin pattern on the silver staining [16, 30].

The identification of a histiocytic neoplasia implies two steps. First, the identification of the real tumoral character of the cellular proliferation. All the numerous varieties of reactive histiocytosis are to be excluded (Table 2). Secondly, the identification of the true histiocytic nature of the neoplastic cell, using the criteria listed in Table 1. From a topographic point of view, the histiocytic neoplasias can be separated into two groups: 1) the disseminated forms, which include the malignant histiocytosis, the histiocytosis X, and 2) the localized forms, which include the histiocytic lymphomas, some so-called reticulum cell sarcomas, and malignant histiocytofibromas (Table 3).

Disseminated Histiocytosis

Malignant Histiocytosis

Since the initial description by CAZAL in France [6] and SCOTT and ROBB SMITH in England [22] under the names of malignant reticulosis or histiocytic medullary reticulosis, the main clinicopathologic features of the malignant histiocytosis have been well-established. Various names have been given to this condition, including: aleukemic reticulosis, histiocytic reticulosis, and histiocytic leukemia. RAPPAPORT proposed the term malignant histiocytosis, now widely accepted, to describe a disorder characterized by a "systemic, progressive invasive

Table 1. Mononuclear phagocyte system: histiocyte-macrophage

Morphology	
Cellular pleomorphism	
Variable geometry cell	
Indented nucleus	
Formation of some polycaryocytes	
Lipid storage	
Adherence to glass	
Enzymic equipment	
Non-specific esterase	+++
Acid phosphatase	+++
Intracellular immunoglobulin = 0	
Surface receptors	
C_3	++
Fc	++
Immunodependent erythrophagocytosis	

Table 2. Reactive histiocytosis

Chronic infections
Intracellular organisms
Immune deficiencies
Chronic granulomatous disease
Hemophagocytic familial reticulosis
Histiocytosis associated with GVH
Unknown etiology
Adenomegalic cytophagic histiocytosis (Rosai disease)

Table 3. Histiocytic tumoral processes

DISSEMINATED HISTIOCYTOSIS
Malignant histiocytosis
Histiocytic reticulosis
Histiocytic medullary reticulosis
Reticulum cell leukemia
Histiocytosis X
Letterer-Siwe disease
Hand-Schüller-Christian disease
Eosinophilic granuloma
LOCALIZED FORMS
Histiocytic lymphomas (?)
Diffuse
Nodular
Reticulum cell sarcoma (?)
Malignant histiocytofibromas

proliferation of morphologically atypical histiocytes" [5, 21]. More than 100 cases have been reported in the literature. The paper published by WARNKE and co-workers [29] based on the study of 29 cases presented a good survey of the disease. The main clinical manifestations include fever, rapid deterioration of the general condition, lymphadenopathy, and enlargement of the spleen and the liver. Anemia, leukopenia, and thrombocytopenia are frequently noted [8].

Our results based on seven cases observed in children, are in many ways similar to those of WARNKE, except for the frequency of bone (3/7) and soft part (3/7) localizations (Table 4). The histologic diagnosis in many cases was difficult and was missed at the first examination in one-third of the specimens that are more often skin biopsies, liver needle biopsies, or bone marrow material than lymph node biopsies.

The cellular proliferation is made up of large atypical cells. They are not cohesive and mitotic figures are frequent. Plasma cells and eosinophils are present in many cases. Multinucleate cells, resembling in some instances Sternberg cells, are sometimes observed. In some cases, particularly in the bone marrow, areas of necrosis are present.

Finding erythrophagocytosis by tumoral cells is often difficult (Fig. 1) and is not as helpful as it is commonly said to be. Demonstration of a nonspecific esterase and acid phosphatase activity in the cytoplasm of some cells, mainly the multinucleate ones, provides support for the diagnosis. Electron microscopy studies are not very helpful. They show large undifferentiated cells with a thick nuclear membrane. Despite repeated studies, no X bodies (Langerhans granules) were observed. However, some evidence of erythrophagocytic activity can be picked out in some cases.

Few immunologic studies have been reported on this material. The pathologic material is usually very limited and grows with difficulty in tissue culture. Our own assays on three cases were unsuccessful. However, some cases have been reported in which the presence of C_3 and Fc membrane markers have been demonstrated [10].

Histiocytosis X

In our experience, histiocytosis X is a good illustration of a tumoral or pseudotumoral process of histiocytic origin. More precisely, it represents the proliferation of a differentiated type of a subpopulation of the histiocytomacrophage lineage: the Langerhans cell system. Histiocytosis X (HX) includes various clinical disorders: Letterer-Siwe disease, Hand-Schüller-Christian disease, and eosinophilic granuloma. HX is mainly a childhood disease and is a sporadic condition. It mainly involves the bones. Its course is in most cases chronic and benign [17]. HX is associated with the local or disseminated proliferation of a distinctive cell. The HX cell appears to be a differentiated element, having abundant cytoenzymic equipment and an ultrastructural marker: the *X body* [1, 2].

On optical examination the HX cells are large. The nucleus is deeply indented and contains few very small nucleoli. Mitotic figures are scarce. The cytoplasm is abundant, eosinophilic, and often contains vacuoles, some of them loaded with lipid material. It is important to underline that the HX cells are not cohesive, exhibiting probably in this way a membrane inhibition. Lymphocytes, plasma cells, and mainly eosinophils are abundant and give the lesion a very variable and heterogeneous appearance. Electron microscopy discloses the presence of a pentalaminar ultrastructure, which is frequently connected with the plasma membrane or the

Table 4. Malignant histiocytosis in children (7 cases)

Fever	7
Splenomegaly	6
Hepatomegaly	6
Anemia	6
Leukopenia	5
Thrombocytopenia	5
Lymphadenopathies	3
Skin nodules	3
Bone lesions	3

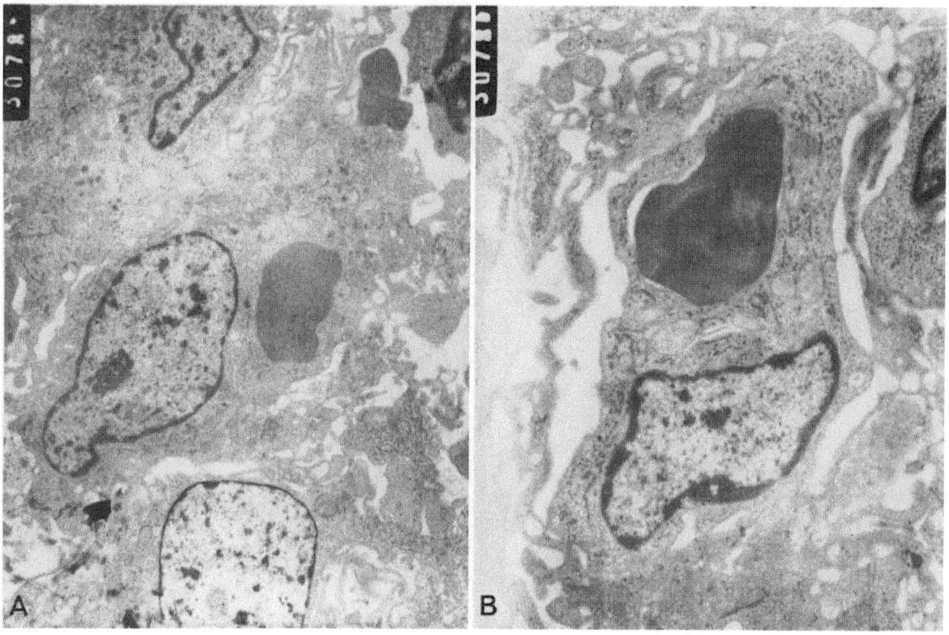

Fig. 1. Malignant histiocytosis: the mononuclear cells involved exhibited a spontaneous erythrophagocytic activity in specimens processed for electronmicroscopy. (A) A large mononuclear cell has engulfed an erythrocyte (× 5000). (B) A little one exhibits the same phagocytic activity. There are no X bodies (× 8000)

membranous structure of the cytoplasma. This pentalaminar structure, discovered 10 years ago by F. BASSET in a case of pulmonary histiocytosis, is present in all forms and all localizations of histiocytosis X. We called it the X body, and we regarded it as a very good marker of HX [1]. Tissue cultures on HX material were carried out for 10 years. Eosinophilic granulomas are a very suitable material for in vitro explantation because they are homogeneous and contain a great number of HX cells. A satisfactory growth can be obtained in two out of three cases. HX cells containing HX bodies can still be observed several months after the explanation. A very peculiar feature is the occurrence of large polycaryocytes by the 7th–10th day of the culture. They contain a great number of nuclei, and their cytoplasm is always loaded with large lipidic vacuoles. Although we think that they originate from the fusion of HX cells, we have never been able to find one X body in these polycaryocytes [18]. This fact leads us to think that the X body represents a temporary membranous structure indicating a level of cellular differentiation. This concept may explain the absence of this pentalaminar structure in young or anaplastic cells and in old and lipid-loaded elements. The tissue culture material provides an opportunity for making additional investigations on the behavior of HX cells (Fig. 2).

Under the scanning electron microscope, the HX appears as an actively moving cell with a bumpy surface and many cytoplasmic processes on the inflated part of the cell, resembling the external appearance of an alveolar macrophage.

Cytochemical investigations show that the HX cells, particularly the polycaryocytes, are strongly positive with acid phosphatase, nonspecific esterase, and NAD and NADP diaphorase [2]. This activity mainly involves the mitochondrion- and lysosome-related enzymes and does not differ from the activity of the common macrophage. The accumulation of lipids within the cytoplasm is commonly observed in old chronic forms. It is thought to be related to some phagocytic activity or degenerative process. However, we think that the fat storage is partially the result of an active synthesis since there is an elective labeling of HX cells after the introduction into the culture medium of certain labeled precursors.

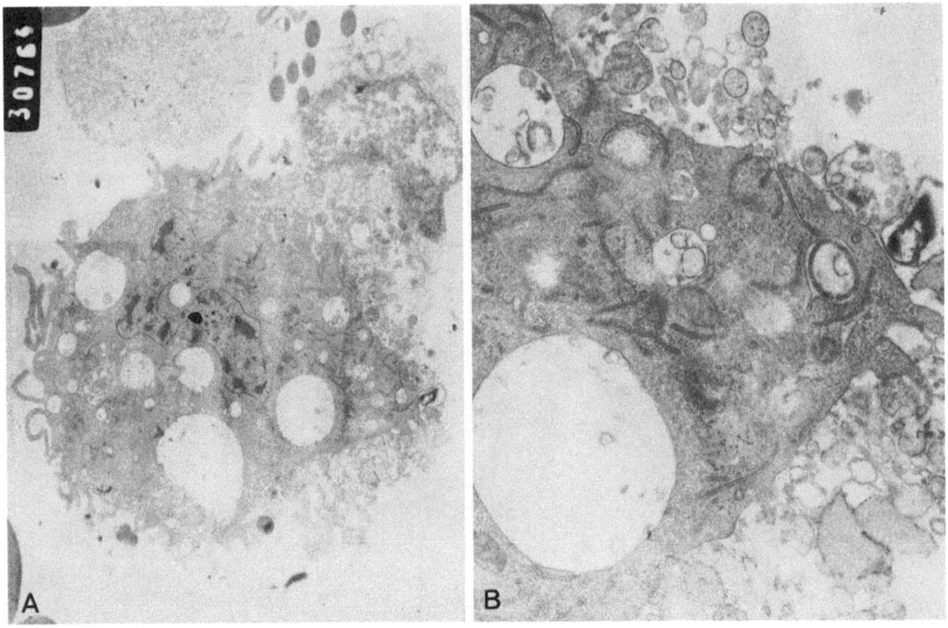

Fig. 2. Histiocytosis X: induced phagocytosis on cell suspension incubated for 20 min at 37°C with opsonized latex particle and processed for electronmicroscopy. (A) A small histiocyte exhibits an intense phagocytic activity (× 8000) (B) At higher magnification, the X body relationship to the phagocytic vesicle and cell plasma membrane was evident (× 20,000)

These investigations have shown that the HX cells do not incorporate thymidine and mevalonate (which is a precursor of cholesterol) but incorporate a small amount of acetate and palmitate. They avidly take up a great number of choline, serine, and glycerol molecules, which are known to build more complex lipid substances, such as triglycerides and phospholipids.
Cultures on a collagen film result in the rapid digestion of this material, confirming the definite lytic activity of the HX cells which can be related to the destructive behavior of the disease. In our study, incubation of HX cells in patient's serum or in AB serum with the simultaneous use of fluorescein-conjugated antihuman globulin revealed surface immunoglobulins on the plasma membrane. They appear as a discontinuous punctuate ring similar, if not identical, to the surface immunofluorescence pattern of monocytes or macrophages after exposure to various blood sera [19]. Incubation of HX cells with chicken-nucleated red blood cells coated with antichicken rabbit serum leads to the formation of rosettes which indicates the presence of FC receptors [19]. The use, under the same conditions, of EAC cells also results in rosetting and reveals the presence of C_3 receptors on the surface of HX cells. This rosetting appears to be the first step of an active erythrophagocytosis which is de facto immunodependent. It is probably important to stress that the small HX cells show a greater erythrophagocytic activity than the large ones. The polycaryocytes are not able to engulf any red blood cells [19].
Comparison of the morphology and the behavior of HX cells and common macrophages shows nothing but similarities. We believe that the HX cells belong to the MPS. However, the presence of the pentalaminar ultrastructure makes the HX cell and the common macrophage very different. It is now established that a similar, if not identical, structure is present in the cytoplasm of the Langerhans cell of the epidermis and it has been named the Langerhans body [4]. The origin and function of the Langerhans cell have been discussed at length, but it seems from recent studies that the Langerhans cell is of mesenchymal origin and may be involved in skin hypersensitivity reactions [3, 23, 24, 25].

Assuming that the X bodies and Langerhans bodies are identical structures labeling a distinct cell lineage, we postulated that:

1. The histiocytosis X is a well-differentiated proliferative process whose stem cell belongs to the Langerhans cell system.
2. The Langerhans cell system is a distinct subpopulation of the mononuclear phagocyte system, which originates in the bone marrow and normally and spontaneously homes to the epithelial surfaces where it exerts some epidermoclastic and immunologic functions [20, 24, 25].
3. The tumoral process, called histiocytosis X, may involve the whole system and more frequently a limited part of this system (Table 5).

This histogenetic concept integrates most of the morphologic and functional data presently known about the HX cells and the Langerhans cells. It accounts for the frequency and early appearance of bone and mucocutaneous localizations and, together with the well-differentiated character of the cellular proliferation, might explain the intrinsically benign course of the disease.

Localized Forms

Diffuse and nodular varieties of malignant histiocytic lymphomas have been recognized for a long time. The individualization of those histiocytic tumors was established on a morphologic

Table 5. Langerhans histiocytic lineage

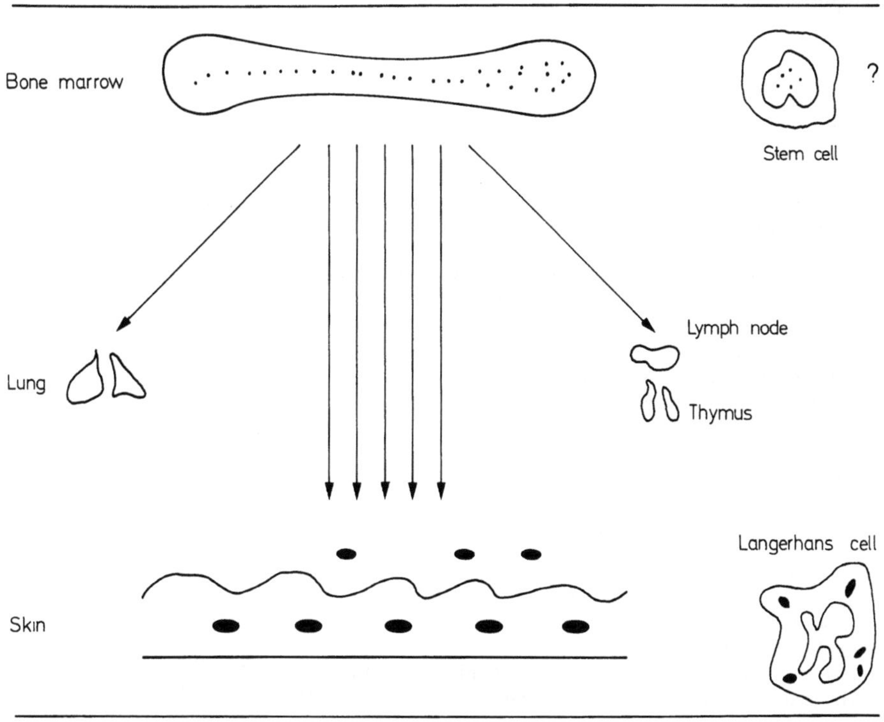

basis and the assumption was made that the histiocytic cell and its associate, the reticulum cell, could represent a multipotent local stem cell belonging to the Aschoff reticuloendothelial system.

This histogenetic concept accounted for the multifocal character and the cellular pleomorphism of the histiocytic neoplasias. However, from a great number of various investigations, the following data have been established:

1. The classic concept of the Aschoff reticuloendothelial system is no longer valid [27].
2. The ability of the peripheral histiocyte to divide is very poor, making this cell a poor candidate for any tumoral process.
3. The reticulum cell represents at present a very heterogeneous group of cells which rather confusedly includes centrofollicular dentritic cells, interdigitate reticulum cells, immature fibroblasts and histiocytes, and some probably true reticulum cells [11, 26]. Thus, in the interest of clarity it seems wise at present to put the term reticulum sarcoma aside.
4. The germinal centers of the lymphoid follicles are made up of pleomorphic and actively dividing cells and may represent, therefore, the likely source of some previously unidentified pleomorphic lymphomas [12, 13, 14, 15].
5. A great number of lymphoid cells, either spontaneously or under appropriate stimulation, are able to multiply and transform into large basophilic cells. These cells, often named immunoblasts, can mimic the undifferentiated histiocytes and subsequently represent an important source of confusion [9].

For all these reasons, it appears that in the past the real incidence of the histiocytic lymphomas was considerably overestimated. From the survey of previously recognized histiocytic lymphomas, it appears today more accurate to classify a good number of them as immunoblastosarcomas, follicular center cell lymphomas, or convoluted cell lymphomas [12, 14]. However, since the Kupffer cell sarcoma does exist, there is certainly still a place in malignant lymphomas for some true histiocytic sarcomas. But the histiocytic origin of the unusual lymphomas has to be substantiated by unequivocal cytochemical, ultrastructural, and immunologic data.

References

1. Basset, F., Nezelof, C.: Présence en microscopie electronique de structures filamenteuses originales dans les lésions pulmonaires et osseuses de l'histiocytose. Etat actuel de la question. Bull. Mem. Soc. Med. Hop. Paris *117*, 413 (1966).
2. Basset, F., Nezelof, C.: L'histiocytose X. Microscopie electronique, culture in vitro et histoenzymologie. Discussion à propos de 21 cas. Rev. Fr. Etud. Clin. Biol. *14*, 31 (1969).
3. Bock, P.: The mesenchymal origin of Langerhans cells. J. Submicrosc. Cytol. *4*, 271 (1972).
4. Breathnach, A. S.: The cell of Langerhans. Int. Rev. Cytol. *18*, 1 (1965).
5. Byrne, G. E., Rappaport, H.: Malignant histiocytosis. Monograph on cancer research 145. Malignant Diseases of the hematopoietic system. Gann *15*, 145 (1973).
6. Cazal, P.: Aspects cliniques et hématologiques de la reticulose maligne. Acta Haematol. (Basel) *7*, 65 (1952).
7. Cohn, Z. A., Belinda, B.: The differentiation of mononuclear phagocytes. Morphology, cytochemistry and biochemistry. J. Exp. Med. *121*, 153 (1965).
8. Dao, C., Schmitt, T., Diebold, J., Bilski-Pasquier, G., Bousser, J.: Histiocytose de Scott et Robb Smith. Nouv. Presse Med. *23*, 1725 (1975).
9. Habeshaw, J. A., Stuart, A. E.: Cell receptor studies on seven cases of diffuse malignant lymphoma (reticulum cell sarcoma). J. Clin. Pathol. *28*, 289 (1975).
10. Hansen, J. A., Good, R. A.: Malignant disease of the lymphoid system in immunological perspective. Hum. Pathol. *5*, 567 (1974).
11. Kaiserling, E., Lennert, K.: Die interdigitierende Reticulumzelle in menschlichen Lymphknoten. Eine specizifische Zelle der thymusabkangigen Region. Virchows. Arch. [Zell pathol.] *16*, 51 (1974).

12. LENNERT, K.: Follicular lymphoma: a special entity of malignant lymphomas. First meeting of the European Division of the International Society of Hematology 1971, POLLI, E. E., MAIOLO, A. T. (eds.) Milan: p. 108.
13. LENNERT, K., STEIN, H., KAISERLING, E.: Cytological and functional criteria for the classification of malignant lymphomata. Br. J. Cancer *31*, supl. 11, 29 (1975).
14. LUKES, R. J., COLLINS, R. D.: Immunologic characterization of human malignant lymphomas. Cancer *34*, 1488 (1974).
15. LUKES, R. J., COLLINS, R. D.: A functional approach to the classification of malignant lymphomas. Recent Results Cancer Res. *46*, 18 (1974).
16. MATHE, G., GERARD-MARCHANT, R., TEXIER, J. L., SCHLUMBERGER, J. R., BERUMEN, L., PAINTRAND, M.: The two varieties of lymphoid tissue "reticulo-sarcomas" histiocytic and histioblastic types. Br. J. Cancer *24*, 687 (1970).
17. NEZELOF, C.: L'histiocytose X. Rev. Fr. Etud. Clin. Biol. *2*, 22 (1966).
18. NEZELOF, C., BASSET, F., ROUSSEAU, M. F.: Histiocytosis X. Histogenetic arguments for a Langerhans cell origin. Biomedicine *18*, 365 (1973).
19. NEZELOF, C., DIEBOLD, N., ROUSSEAU MERCK, M. F.: Ig surface receptors and erythrophagocytic activity of histiocytosis X cells in vitro. J. Pathol. (1977) (in press).
20. PRUNIERAS, M.: Interactions entre les cellules de l'epiderme. Rev. Fr. Etud. Clin. Biol. *13*, 743 (1968).
21. RAPPAPORT, H.: Tumors of the Hematopoietic System. Atlas of Tumor Pathology, sect. III, fasc 8. Washington, D.C.: Armed Forces Institute of Pathology 1966.
22. SCOTT, R. B., ROBB SMITH, A. H. T.: Histiocytic medullary reticulosis. Lancet 1939/II, 194.
23. SHELLEY, W. R., LENNART, Juhlin: Langerhans cells form a reticuloepithelial trap for external contact antigenes. Nature *261*, 46 (1976).
24. SILBERBERG, I., BAER, R. L., ROSENTHAL, S. A.: The role of Langerhans cells in contact allergy. An ultrastructural study in actively induced contact dermatitis in guinea pigs. Acta Derm. Venereol. (Stockh.) *54*, 321 (1974).
25. SILBERBERG-SINAKIN, I., THORBECKE, G. J., BAER, R. L., ROSENTHAL, S. A., BEREZOWSKY, V.: Antigen-bearing Langerhans cells in skin, dermal lymphatics and in lymph nodes. Cell. Immunol. *25*, 137 (1976).
26. STUART, A. E., DAVIDSON, A. E.: The human reticular cell: morphology and cytochemistry. J. Pathol. *103*, 41 (1971).
27. VAN FURTH, R.: The origin and turnover of promonocytes, monocytes and macrophages in normal mice. In: Mononuclear Phagocytes. (ed.) VAN FURTH, R. Oxford: Blackwell 1970, p. 151.
28. VAN FURTH, R., THOMPSON, J.: Review of the origin and kinetics of the promonocytes, monocytes and macrophages and a brief discussion of the mononuclear system. Ann. Inst. Pasteur *120*, 337 (1971).
29. WARNKE, R. A., HUN, Kim, DORFMAN, R.: Malignant histiocytosis (histiocytic medullary reticulosis). Cancer *35*, 215 (1975).
30. YAO SHI FU, GABBIANI, G., KAYE, G. I., LATTES, R.: Malignant soft tissue tumors of probable histiocytic origin (malignant fibrous histiocytomas). General considerations and electron microscopic and tissue culture studies. Cancer *35*, 176 (1975).

Conclusions of the First Session: Correlations Between Current Morphologic Categorizations

G. T. O'Conor and L. H. Sobin

Morphology continues to be the principal basis for the identification of the non-Hodgkin's lymphomas. Although immunologic markers provide essential information relating to function, which may indeed be another logical basis for classification, one must accept that the initial diagnosis, the accurate estimation of extent of disease, and the determination of prognosis are all dependent on evaluation of histologic and cytologic characteristics.

Despite what appears to be continuing and unresolvable controversy over the classification of malignant lymphomas, it should be emphasized that this is largely a matter of terminology. There is, in fact, today more accord than discord. Significant progress has been made and there is remarkable agreement in the recognition and characterization of the important disease entities within this group of neoplasms. If the natural history of specific disease entities is appreciated, the actual terms assume less importance, as does the method of classification, be it according to architectural pattern, cell type, behavior, or function.

Nodularity is now generally accepted as an indication of tumor origin from germinal centers, and this architectural pattern has considerable prognostic significance. Tumors of the same cell type, based on morphologic criteria, can also be diffuse but usually have a more malignant behavior. Lymphoblastic tumors with or without convoluted nuclei are recognized as a distinct group, and immunoblastic has been widely adopted as a descriptor for those tumors composed of large cells with deeply basophilic (pyroninophilic) cytoplasm and believed to be derived from B- or T-lymphocytes transformed by antigenic stimulus. Further, it is now agreed that most tumors formerly designated as histocytic lymphomas or reticulum cell sarcomas are, in fact, neoplasms of large lymphoid cells. It is suggested that the older terms might well be suppressed and such tumors be designated according to the appropriate terms within the lymphoid series. Reticulosarcoma has been proposed in the WHO International Classification [4] to refer to those relatively rare tumors composed of large cells which cannot be identified as of lymphoid origin and which, because of certain morphologic and cytochemical features, might be derived from the dendritic cells or other elements of the supporting reticuloendothelial network.

Although there is now reasonable agreement on concepts, the plethora of terms for the same entities among the non-Hodgkin's lymphomas and their arrangement into numerous classifications unfortunately continues to cause a degree of consternation and frustration. It is, therefore, important, and perhaps now is the opportune time, to attempt to find common acceptable terms in order to allay the confusion which does to some extent impede clinical studies. An alternative is a glossary of common terms or a conversion table which would permit "translation" and facilitate international comparisons. We have chosen to present the latter as part of the Chairmen's Summary. Table 1 provides equivalent terms to the WHO International Histological Classification of Tumors [5] in which each entity is defined and illustrated. It is believed that this table is a reasonable representation of principles and concepts which have been published and which were presented at the Colloquium.

Table 1. Comparative list of terms for non-Hodgkin's lymphomas

WHO [4]	RAPPAPORT [5]	Kiel [2]	British Lymphoma Study Group [1]	LUKES-COLLINS [3]
1. Nodular lymphosarcoma	Malignant lymphoma, nodular	Follicular lymphoma	Follicular lymphoma	
Prolymphocytic			Follicle cell	Follicular center cell, follicular
Cleaved or Noncleaved cells – small cell	Lymphocytic, well-differentiated	Centroblastic-centrocytic	Small	Cleaved or Noncleaved cells – small cell
Cleaved or Noncleaved cells – mixed cell	Mixed lymphocytic, poorly differentiated		Mixed	
Cleaved or Noncleaved cells – large cell	Histiocytic		Large	Cleaved or Noncleaved cells – large cell
2. Diffuse lymphosarcoma	Malignant lymphoma, diffuse	Diffuse lymphoma	Diffuse lymphoma	
(a) Lymphocytic	Lymphocytic, well-differentiated	Lymphocytic	Lymphocytic, well-differentiated	Small lymphocyte
(b) Lymphoplasmacytic	Lymphocytic with plasmacytoid features	Lymphoplasmacytoid (immunocytic)		Plasmacytoid lymphocyte
(c) Prolymphocytic				Follicular center cell, diffuse
Cleaved or Noncleaved cells – small cell	Lymphocytic, poorly differentiated	Centrocytic	Lymphocytic, intermediate differentiation (small follicle cell)	Cleaved or Noncleaved cells – small cell
Cleaved or Noncleaved cells – mixed cell	Mixed cell	Centroblastic-centrocytic	Mixed small lymphoid and undifferentiated large cell	
Cleaved or Noncleaved cells – large cells		Centroblastic	Undifferentiated large cell	Cleaved or Noncleaved cells – large cell
(d) Lymphoblastic Convoluted Nonconvoluted	Lymphoblastic Convoluted Nonconvoluted	Lymphoblastic Convoluted Nonconvoluted	Lymphocytic poorly differentiated	Convoluted lymphocyte
(e) Immunoblastic	Immunoblastic	Immunoblastic	Undifferentiated large cell	Immunoblastic sarcoma
(f) Burkitt's tumor	Burkitt's type	Burkitt's type	Undifferentiated large cell	Follicular center cell, small cell, noncleaved
Reticulosarcoma	Histiocytic		True histiocytic	Histiocytic

References

1. Bennett, M. H., Farrer-Brown, G., Henry, K., Jeliffe, A. M.: Classification of non-Hodgkin's lymphomas. Lancet *1974/ii*, 405–406.
2. Gerard-Marchant, R., Hamlin, I., Lennert, K., Rilke, F., Stansfeld, A. G., Van Unnik, J. A. M.: Classification of non-Hodgkin's lymphomas. Lancet 1974/ii, 406–408.
3. Lukes, R. J., Collins, R. D.: Immunological characterization of human malignant lymphomas. Cancer *34*, 1488–1503 (1974)
4. Mathe, G., Rappaport, H., O'Conor, G. T., Torloni, H.: Histological and cytological typing of neoplastic diseases of hematopoietic and lymphoid tissues. Geneva. WHO International Classification of Tumours. No. 14, 1976.
5. Rappaport, H.: Tumors of the hematopoietic system. In: Atlas of Tumor Pathology, sect. 3, fasc. 8. Washington, D.C.: Armed Forces Institute of Pathology 1966.

Part II

Membrane Markers and Immunologic Categorization

Human T-Derived Lymphoproliferative Diseases

J. C. BROUET, J. L. PREUD'HOMME, G. FLANDRIN, and M. SELIGMANN

Introduction

A T-derived origin of malignant human lymphoid cells was first demonstrated in patients affected with Sezary's syndrome [6, 9]. During the past few years, the study of membrane markers considered specific for B- or T-lymphocytes on neoplastic cells from a number of patients has delineated several malignancies characterized by T- derived cells.

The methods used for the identification of B- and T-lymphocytes in our laboratory have been given in detail elsewhere [13, 39]. B-lymphocyte markers included the detection of membrane bound Ig by direct immunofluorescence [39], the presence of a receptor for the Fc fragment of IgG detected by aggregates or immune complexes (although other cells such as monocytes, myeloid cells, and a subset of T-lymphocytes also possess this marker), and the reactivity of cells with an heteroantiserum to human B cells [13]. T cells were characterized by the formation of spontaneous rosettes with sheep erythrocytes (E-rosettes) and their ability to react with rabbit heteroantisera obtained by immunization with peripheral T cells, fetal thymocytes [13], or fetal brain [8].

Sezary's Syndrome

Sezary's syndrome is characterized by a diffuse erythrodermia, pruritus, and abnormally large cells, which may be found in the skin and blood. These cells have a large nucleus, which is round or oval, folded, and grooved with heavily clumped chromatin and a characteristic ultrastructural cerebriform profile [42, 45]. This typical Sezary cell was observed in one-third of our patients. In the other cases, the small cell variant [31] of the Sezary cell was recognized. Cytochemical studies may be helpful for the diagnosis of the Sezary cell. These cells have a strikingly high content of β-glucuronidase and acid phosphatase [20]. Lymphocytes with many fine granules scattered throughout the cytoplasm, as seen in normal controls, were absent or very rare.

The immunologic data obtained in patients with Sezary syndrome are listed in Table 1. In all these cases, there was a high ($\geqslant 60\%$) percentage of Sezary cells in cell suspensions. The Sezary cells formed E-rosettes and were killed by a conveniently absorbed rabbit antiserum to peripheral T cells. It is important to note that the percentage of E-rosettes may be low, i.e., not all Sezary cells formed rosettes, and that only three to five sheep erythrocytes may be bound to the positive Sezary cells; this number is lower than that observed with most normal T-lymphocytes under the same technical conditions. It is thus necessary to study these cells with several T-lymphocyte markers: in our experience, Sezary cells were susceptible in all cases to killing by an anti-T-cell antiserum, even in those cases where few cells formed E-rosettes.

It is noteworthy that in many patients the absolute number of circulating B-lymphocytes was

Table 1. Membrane markers in 12 cases of Sezary syndrome

Abnormal circulating cells		SIg	*Aggr.* IgG	*Rosette-forming cells*	*Cells killed by anti-T*
Morphology	%	%	%	%	%
Large	60	2	–	90	—
Large	39	4	3	75	88
Large	98	0	0	80	—
Large and small	60	0	0	62	70
Large and small	91	3	2	30	60
Small	71	6	5	60	70
Small	60	9	6	10	—
Small	53	1	2	75	68
Small	84	1	1	40	—
Small	46	1	–	87	55
Small	41	3	2	65	—
Small	60	2	2	66	—

very low. However, these patients showed no hypogammaglobulinemia nor unusually high incidence of infections. Circulating normal T cells are also much reduced in number; for instance in certain patients with large Sezary cells, the number of residual normal lymphocytes may be as low as $100/mm^3$. It is conceivable that the traffic of T cells in Sezary patients is grossly abnormal.

The demonstration of the T-cell nature of Sezary cells had several implications. The lymphoid nature of the cell, which was much disputed in the past, was definitely assessed. The morphologic diagnosis of the small variants of the Sezary cell was supported by the immunologic studies, which in all cases demonstrated their T-nature. Finally, the mycosis fongoides cells were shown to be of T-origin [19, 47], leading to a uniform concept of these cutaneous lymphomas. However, a word of caution upon the diagnostic significance of the Sezary cell is needed. We studied two patients with chronic lymphocytic leukemia (CLCL) without erythrodermia in whom a small percentage of leukemic lymphocytes had the morphologic and ultrastructural features of Sezary cells; in both cases, all leukemic cells were of B-cell origin and carried a monoclonal surface Ig.

T-Derived Chronic Lymphocytic Leukemia

Only a few cases of T-derived CLCL have been reported until recent years [5, 17, 46]. It is of interest that three of these cases have been observed in Japan where CLCL is an uncommon disorder. However, T-CLCL may not be as rare as previously thought since we have recently diagnosed 23 consecutive cases of T-CLCL, 11 of which have been reported [10]. Four of these patients had no peculiar features except for a high leukocyte count and two had the prolymphocytic type of leukemia (which is more often of B-origin in our experience). The 19 other patients exhibited quite unusual clinical and hematologic features which suggest that we are presumably dealing with a distinct entity. All our recent patients were labeled as probable T-derived CLCL on the basis of this peculiar clinicohematologic presentation, and immunologic studies confirmed this assumption in all cases. In these patients, the blood and bone marrow invasion by the leukemic T cells was moderate but definite. These lymphocytes had a high content of lyzosomal enzymes and peculiar cytoplasmic azurophil granules were readily apparent in 14 cases. Other features were massive splenic involvement in 11 cases, skin involvement in nine cases (without any cytologic or histologic features of the Sezary syndrome), and severe neutropenia in nine cases. Lymph node biopsies in three cases showed a heavy infiltration of T-dependent areas with a relative sparing of germinal centers.

A panel of surface markers was used to establish the T-cell nature of the leukemic cells from these patients. In some cases, only a small percentage of the leukemic lymphocytes were able to form E-rosettes, a finding similar to that previously recorded for Sezary cells. The use of different antisera against T-cell antigens showed striking variation from patient to patient. Whereas normal blood lymphocytes and the cells from eight patients reacted equally well with antisera to peripheral T cells and to fetal thymocytes, leukemic cells from the other patients reacted strongly with only one of these two antisera (more frequently with the antiserum to thymocytes). An antiserum to human brain which reacts only with a subset of peripheral T cells [8] stained most or all leukemic lymphocytes in nine cases but gave negative results in the six other cases studied. These differences provide suggestive evidence for the homogeneity of this population of leukemic T-lymphocytes for which no monoclonal marker is yet available. Cytogenetic studies also favor the monoclonal origin of these leukemic cells [5].

The need to use several markers for B- and T-lymphocytes in the study of CLCL is illustrated by the ambiguous results of the study of leukemic cells which may be observed in some cases. The lymphocytes from five of our patients exhibited monotypic SmIg and also formed E-rosettes with sheep erythrocytes. In one case, the leukemic cells proved to be B cells with SmIgM possessing antibody activity against the Forssman antigen [7]. In two other cases, the SmIg were shown to be exogeneous and the T-cell origin of the leukemic cells was confirmed by the reactivity with an antiserum against human T cells [40]. However, in the two last cases, the SmIg appeared to be actual cell products and the leukemic cells could represent a malignant clone expressing an aberrant cell surface phenotype. Another case [24] was described in which the leukemic cells synthesized SmIg, bound sheep erythrocytes, bore a receptor for complement, and were killed by heteroantisera to T cells. Although in this latter case the percentage of cells positive for these markers varied during the course of the disease, an overlap between several markers for B and T cells was found on a large number of proliferating cells.

T-Derived Acute Lymphoblastic Leukemia (ALBL)

The study of membrane markers in patients with ALBL revealed that in 25% of the cases the leukemic cells were T-derived, whereas in the majority of ALCL cases the leukemic cells were devoid of the usual B- or T-lymphocyte membrane markers [2, 13, 15, 28, 41]. The immunologic diagnosis of T-ALBL may be difficult since E-rosette formation may be restricted to a small proportion of blast cells. The use of antisera to T cells is, therefore, critical in these patients. Several characteristics of the T-derived ALBL cells are much more similar to those of normal thymocytes than to those of peripheral T-lymphocytes. The formation of E-rosettes occurs at both 4° and 37°C, whereas the more mature peripheral blood T cells fail to form rosettes at 37°C [4]. These blast cells react with certain antisera to thymocytes that have been previously absorbed by peripheral T cells [34]. They also contain a precipitating antigen which is found in thymocytes and not in peripheral T cells [18]. Some antisera to T-derived ALBL cells enable one to demonstrate antigenic determinants, which are shared by these cells, and thymocytes but which are absent on peripheral T cells [40]. Finally, these T-derived blast cells contain terminal deoxynucleotidyl transferase (TDT), an enzyme normally found in high quantities in thymocytes but lost as the cells further mature to peripheral T-lymphocytes [32].

The "non-T–non-B" ALBL cells are characterized by several positive findings which enable one to distinguish them from T-derived ALBL cells: the presence of membrane-bound Ia-like antigens revealed by alloantisera or heteroantisera [3, 21, 40, 44], the detection of Nacetylhexosaminidase [22], and the presence of at least two distinct kinds of leukemia-associated antigens [13, 16, 37]. The "leukemia-specific" antigen revealed by rabbit homologous antisera and described by GREAVES [16] is found on the blast cells of 69% of the patients with non-B–non-T ALBL [23]. The antigen shared by CLCL cells and thymocytes is found on the blast cells from 90% of these patients [13].

The question of the true cellular origin of non-T–non-B ALBL remains unsettled at present. Several findings have led to the suggestion that it may derive from an immature bone marrow thymocyte precursor. Another possibility is that non-T–non-B ALBL may arise from an undifferentiated pluripotential stem cell. Terminal deoxynucleotidyl transferase is present in the blast cells of most cases of non-T–non-B ALBL. Some antisera to human thymus antigens show reactivity with the blast cells of many cases of non-T–non-B ALBL [13, 18, 29, 35]. It should, however, be stressed that the results obtained with some antisera to thymic cells should be carefully interpreted when evaluating the possible T-origin of leukemic cells since they may show a wide pattern of reactivity with all ALBL and acute myeloblastic leukemia (AMBL) cells [13, 36]. On the other hand, some authors have suggested that the presence of Ia-like antigens, as mentioned above, may reflect a B-cell origin of non-B–non-T ALBL cells. This hypothesis seems unlikely since the majority of AMBL cells are also positive for these Ia-type antigens [3, 22, 40]; as well as normal precursors of the granulocytic line.

Correlations between the immunologic characteristics of the blast cells and a number of clinical and hematologic parameters were worked out in the two major groups of patients with ALBL [2, 13, 27, 28, 41, 43].

We have found no difference in the distribution for age and sex between patients with T-derived and non-T–non-B ALBL. This is at variance with the reports of other investigators [23, 41] who found that T-derived ALBL predominantly affects boys over 5 years of age. However, similarly to these and other investigators [23, 29, 41, 43], we found that T-derived ALBL were statistically more often characterized by high blast cell blood counts, a tumoral disease, and the presence of a thymic mass. These characteristics applied to cases with a low percentage of E-rosetting blasts and positive reactions with the antiserum to T cells (see above), as well as to E-rosette-positive cases. The above parameters, which are more frequently found in T-derived ALBL, are well-known poor risk factors. It is, therefore, not surprising that several groups have reported a poor prognosis in children affected with T-derived ALBL [23, 41, 43]. In our series, with a follow-up of 3–45 months, there is no statistically significant difference in the actuarial survival curves between the two main subgroups of ALBL. The complete remission rate was similar in T-derived ALBL and non-T–non-B ALBL patients. Lasting complete remissions were more frequent in the non-T–non-B group, but the difference is not significant at present. Meningeal relapses were more frequent in patients with T-derived ALBL. In contrast to some of the other studies, our series includes both children and adults, and in most instances the dose schedule of the chemotherapeutic regimens was adjusted according to the known bad risk factors, independently of the immunologic typing. Future studies on large groups of patients should aim at determining whether the membrane phenotype of the leukemic cells represents per se an important prognostic factor and whether a different approach to therapy should be considered at the time of diagnosis according to it.

Non-Hodgkin's Lymphomas

Immunologic studies have helped to define a subgroup of childhood lymphomas which was previously included in the diffuse poorly differentiated lymphocytic lymphomas and which is now often denominated "childhood lymphoblastic lymphomas" [38]. The proliferating cells may have a convoluted appearance, but this feature is not constant. A strong positivity for acid phosphatase is usually found in blast cells. The presence of an anterior mediastinal mass in many of these children has indicated a possible thymic origin for these tumors. The expression of T-lymphocyte markers on the neoplastic cells has been demonstrated in many cases [26, 27]. Leukemia develops rapidly in many of these patients and this group of lymphomas may be closely related to the T-derived subgroup of ALBL.

Non-Hodgkin's lymphomas in adults are mostly of B-cell origin [1, 11, 25, 30, 33]. Cells from rare cases of poorly differentiated lymphocytic lymphomas and of so-called "histiocytic" lymphomas have T-cell markers [1, 12]. The prognostic significance of T-markers in these patients is still unknown.

Concluding Remarks

The study of membrane markers in various human T-cell neoplasias allowed us to lump together some diseases which were previously considered as separate entities. For instance, the T-nature of abnormal cells of Sezary syndrome, mycosis fungoides, and lymphomatoid papulosis led to a unified concept of cutaneous lymphomas. T-derived ALBL and lymphoblastic lymphomas of children share several clinical, morphologic, and cytochemical features and may well represent a single disease. On the other hand, in a given disease such as CLCL or ALBL, there is a subgroup of patients whose leukemic cells are of T-origin and who share several distinctive clinical or hematologic features such as high WBC and mediastinal tumors in T-derived ALBL or moderate lymphoid infiltration, splenomegaly, and cytoplasmic azurophilic granules in leukemic cells in the subgroup of T-CLCL. It is of interest that cutaneous lesions may be observed preferentially in these T-cell malignancies, suggesting a preferential homing of neoplastic T cells in the skin.

The monoclonal nature of these T-cell proliferations is supported by indirect evidence. The leukemic clones may arise from distinct subpopulations of T cells, as shown by their different reactivity with serious antisera to T cells; Sezary cells were shown to involve only helper T cells [14]; the responsiveness of leukemic cells to various mitogens or allogeneic cells is variable from patient to patient. More formal proof of the monoclonality of these malignant T cells was obtained by cytogenetic studies.

We lack markers of differentiation in order to define the situation of these leukemic T-cell clones along the maturation pathway of normal T cells. However, the results obtained from several studies with antisera specific for thymocytes or peripheral T cells and from the study of TDT as a biochemical marker for immature thymocytes clearly showed that one is dealing in some cases with cells resembling prethymic cells (non-T–non-B ALBL?), thymic cells (T-derived ALBL), or mature T cells (T-CLCL or Sezary syndrome). Investigation of such patients may prove to be particularly helpful in the definition of human T-cell subsets with distinct markers and functions.

References

1. Aisenberg, A. C., Long, J. C.: Lymphocyte surface characteristics in malignant lymphoma. Am. J. Med. *58*, 300–306 (1975).
2. Belpomme, D., Mathe, G., Davies, A. J. S.: Clinical significance and prognostic value of the T-B immunological classification of human primary acute lymphoid leukaemias. Lancet *1977/i*, 555–558.
3. Billing, R., Rafizadeh, B., Drew, I., Hartman, G., Gale, R., Terasaki, P.: Human B lymphocyte antigens expressed by lymphocytic and myelocytic leukemia cells. J. Exp. Med. *144*, 167–178 (1976).

4. Borella, L., Sen, L.: E receptors on blasts from untreated acute lymphocytic leukemia (ALL): comparison of temperature dependence of E rosettes formed by normal and leukemic lymphoid cells. J. Immunol. *114*, 187–190 (1975).
5. Brody, J. L., Burningham, R. A., Nowell, P. C., Rowlands, D. T., Freiberg, G. F., Daniele, R. P.: Persistent lymphocytosis with chromosomal evidence of malignancy. Am. J. Med. *58*, 547–552 (1975).
6. Broome, J. D., Zucker-Franklin, D., Weiner, M. S., Bianco, S., Nussenzweig, V.: Leukaemic cells with membrane properties of thymus derived (T) lymphocytes in a case of Sezary's syndrome: morphologic and immunological studies. Clin. Immunol. Immunopathol. *1*, 319–329 (1973).
7. Brouet, J. C., Prieur, A. M.: Membrane markers on chronic lymphocytic leukemia cells: a B cell leukemia with rosettes due to antisheep erythrocytes antibody activity of the membrane bound IgM and a T cell leukemia with surface Ig. Clin. Immunol. Immunopathol. *2*, 481–487 (1974).
8. Brouet, J. C., Toben, H. R.: Characterization of a subpopulation of human T lymphocytes reactive with an heteroantiserum to human brain. J. Immunol. *116*, 1041–1044 (1976).
9. Brouet, J. C., Flandrin, G., Seligmann, M.: Indications for the thymus derived nature of the proliferating cells in six patients with Sezary's syndrome. N. Engl. J. Med. *289*, 341–344 (1973).
10. Brouet, J. C., Flandrin, G., Sasportes, M., Preud'homme, J. L., Seligmann, M.: Chronic lymphocytic leukaemia of T cell origin. An immunological and clinical evaluation in eleven patients Lancet *1975/ii*, 890–893.
11. Brouet, J. C., Preud'homme, J. L., Seligmann, M.: Lymphocyte membrane markers in B cell proliferations and human non-Hodgkin's lymphomas. In: Clinical Tumor Immunology. Wybran, J., Staquet, M. (eds) Oxford: Pergamon Press 1976a pp. 123–130.
12. Brouet, J. C., Preud'homme, J. L., Flandrin, G., Chelloul, N., Seligmann, M.: Membrane markers in so called "histiocytic" lymphomas. J. Natl. Cancer Inst. *56*, 631–633 (1976b).
13. Brouet, J. C., Valensi, F., Daniel, M. T., Flandrin, G., Preud'homme, J. L., Seligmann, M.: Immunological classification of acute lymphoblastic leukaemias, evaluation of its clinical significance. Br. J. Haematol. *33*, 319–328 (1976c).
14. Broder, S., Edelson, R. L., Lutzner, M. A., Nelson, D. L., MacDermott, R. P., Drum, M. E., Goldman, C. K., Meade, B. D., Waldmann, T. A.: The Sezary syndrome. A malignant proliferation of helper T cells. J. Clin. Invest. *58*, 1297–1306 (1976).
15. Brown, G., Greaves, M. F., Lister, T. A. Rapson, N., Papamichael, M.: The expression of human T and B lymphocyte cell surface markers on leukaemic cells. Lancet *1974/ii*, 753–755.
16. Brown, G., Capellaro, D., Greaves, M.: Leukemia-associated antigens in man. J. Natl. Cancer Inst. *55*, 1281–1289 (1975).
17. Catovsky, D., Galetto, J., Okos, A., Galton, D. A. G., Wiltshaw, E., Staphopoulos, G.: Prolymphocytic leukaemia of B and T cell type. Lancet *1973/II*, 232–234.
18. Chechik, B. E., Pyke, K. W., Gelfand, E. W.: Human thymus/leukemia-associated antigen in normal and leukemic cells. Int. J. Cancer *18*, 551–556 (1976).
19. Edelson, R. L., Kirkpatrick, C. H., Shevach, E. M., Schein, P. S., Smith, R. W., Green, I., Lutzner, M.: Preferential cutaneous infiltration by neoplatis thymus derived lymphocytes. Ann. Intern. Med. *80*, 685–692 (1974).
20. Flandrin, G., Brouet, J. C.: The Sezary cell: cytologic, cytochemical and immunologic studies. Mayo Clin. Proc. *49*, 575–583 (1974).
21. Fu, S. M., Winchester, R. J., Kunkel, H. G.: The occurrence of the HL-B alloantigens on the cells of unclassified acute lymphoblastic leukemias. J. Exp. Med. *142*, 1334–1338 (1975).
22. Greaves, M., De Gicco, D., Janossy, G.: Membrane phenotypes of human leukaemic cells. In:. Topics in Hematology (Siseno, F. Takaku et S. Irino, eds) Excerpta Medica, Amsterdam–Oxford, pp. 319–327 (1977).
23. Greaves, M., Roberts, M., Janossy, G., Pain, C.: Membrane antigens and the immuno-diagnosis of human leukaemia. In: Topics in Hematology (Siseno, F. Takaku et S. Irino, eds) Excerpta Medica, Amsterdam-Oxford, pp. 684–690.
24. Hsu, C. C. S., Marti, G. E., Schrek, R., Williams, R. C.: Lymphocytes bearing B and T cell markers in patient with lymphosarcoma cell leukemia. Clin. Immunol. Immunopathol. *3*, 385–395 (1975).
25. Jaffe, E. S., Shevach, E. M., Sussman, E. H., Frank, M., Green, I., Berard, C. W.: membrane receptor sites for the identification of lymphoreticular cells in benign and malignant conditions. Br. J. Cancer *31*, suppl. II, 107–120 (1975).
26. Jaffe, E. S., Braylan, R. C., Frank, M. M., Green, I., Berard, C. W.: Heterogeneity of immunologic markers and surface morphology in childhood lymphoblastic lymphoma. Blood *48*, 213–222 (1976).
27. Kaplan, J., Mastrangelo, R., Peterson, W. D.: Childhood lymphoblastic lymphoma, a cancer of thymus derived lymphocytes. Cancer Res. *34*, 521–525 (1974).
28. Kersey, J. H., Sabad, A., Gajl-Peczalska, K. J., Hallgren, H. M., Yunis, E. J., Nesbit, M. E.: Acute lymphoblastic leukaemia cells with T (thymus-derived) lymphocytes markers. Science *182*, 1355–1356 (1973).

29. KERSEY, J. H., NESBIT, M. E., HALLGREN, H., YUNIS, E. J., GAJL-PECZALSKA, K. J.: evidence for origin of certain childhood acute leukemias and lymphomas in thymus-derived lymphocytes. Cancer *36*, 1348–1352 (1975).
30. LEECH, J. H., GLICK, A. D., WALDRON, J. A., FLEXNER, J. M., HORN, R. G., COLLINS, R. D.: Malignant lymphomas of follicular center cell origin in man. I. Immunologic studies. J. Natl. Cancer Inst. *54*, 11–20 (1975).
31. LUTZNER, M. A., EMERIT, I., DUREPAIRE, R., FLANDRIN, G., GRUPPER, C., PRUNIERAS, M.: Cytogenetic, cytophotometric and ultrastructural study of large cerebriform cells of the Sezary syndrome and description of a small-cell variant. J. Natl. Cancer Inst. *50*, 1145–1162 (1973).
32. MCCAFFREY, R., HARRISON, T. A., PARKMAN, R., BALTIMORE, D.: Terminal desoxynucleotidyl transferase activity in human leukemic cells and in normal human thymocytes. N. Engl. J. Med. *292*, 775–780 (1975).
33. MATHE, G., BELPOMME, D., DANTCHEV, D., POUILLART, P.: Progress in the classification of lymphoid and/or monocytoid leukemias and of lympho and reticulosarcomas (non Hodgkin's lymphomas). Biomedicine *22*, 177–185 (1975).
34. MILLS, B., SEN, L., BORELLA, L.: Reactivity of antihuman thymocyte serum with acute leukemic blasts. J. Immunol. *115*, 1038–1044 (1975).
35. MINOWADA, J., TSUBOTA, T.: Comparative study on surface and antigen markers between human leukemic lymphoid cell lines and fresh leukemic lymphocytes. In: Topics in Hematology (Siseno, F. Takaku et S. Irino, eds) Excerpta Medica, Amsterdam–Oxford, pp. 328–332.
36. MOHANAKUMAR, T., METZGAR, R. S.: Human thymus leukemia related antigen(s). Detection by a non human primate antiserum. Cell. Immunol. *12*, 30–36 (1974).
37. MOHANAKUMAR, T., METZGAR, R. S., MILLER, D. S.: Human leukaemia cell antigens: serologic characterization with xenoantisera. J. Natl. Cancer Inst. *52*, 1435–1444 (1974).
38. NATHWANI, B. N., KIM, H., RAPPAPORT, H.: Malignant lymphoma, lymphoblastic. Cancer *38*, 964–983 (1976).
39. PREUD'HOMME, J. L., LABAUME, S.: Detection of surface immunoglobulins on human cells by direct immunofluorescence. In: In Vitro Methods in Cell-Mediated and Tumor Immunity. BLOOM, B. R., DAVIDS, J. R. (eds) New York: Academic Press 1976, pp. 155–169.
40. SCHLOSSMANN, S. F., CHESS, L., HUMPHREYS, R. E., STROMINGER, J. L.: Distribution of la-like molecules on the surface of normal and leukemic human cells. Proc. Natl. Acad. Sci. U.S.A. *73*, 1288–1292 (1976).
41. SEN, L., BORELLA, L.: Clinical importance of lymphoblasts with T markers in childhood acute leukaemia. N. Engl. J. Med. *292*, 828–832 (1975).
42. TASWELL, H. F., WINKELMANN, R. K.: Sezary syndrome: a malignant reticulemic erythroderma. J. Am. Med. Assoc. *177*, 465–472 (1961).
43. TSUKIMOTO, I., WONG, K. Y., LAMPKIN, B. C.: Surface markers and prognostic factors in acute lymphoblastic leukemia. N. Engl. J. Med. *294*, 245–248 (1976).
44. WERNET, P.: Human la-type antigens: Methods of detection, aspects of chemistry and biology, markers for disease states. Transplant. Rev. *30*, 271–298 (1976).
45. WINKELMANN, R. K.: T-cell erythroderma (Sezary syndrome). Arch. Dermatol. *108*, 205–206 (1973).
46. YODOI, J., TAKATSUKI, K., MASUDA, T.: Two cases of T cell chronic lymphocytic leukaemia in Japan. N. Engl. J. Med. *290*, 572–573 (1974).
47. ZUCKER-FRANKLIN, D., MELTON, J. W., QUAGLIATA, F.: Ultrastructural immunologic and functional studies on Sezary: a neoplastic variant of thymus derived (T) lymphocytes. Proc. Natl. Acad. Sci. U.S.A. *71*, 1877–1881 (1974).

Immunologic Markers of Non-Hodgkin's Lymphomas

C. W. BERARD, E. S. JAFFE, R. C. BRAYLAN, R. B. MANN, and K. NANBA

Malignant lymphomas have to date been diagnosed and classified on solely morphologic grounds. For clinicopathologic studies of the non-Hodgkin's lymphomas, the classification of RAPPAPORT [29], with current modifications (Table 1) [4, 7, 20, 27], has proved to be both widely applicable and valuable. In recent years, however, advances in understanding of the physiology and immunology of the lymphoreticular system have led to increasing recognition of these tumors as neoplasms of the immune system [4, 5, 7, 20]. The purpose of this paper is to give a brief summary, based primarily on our own data, of the immunologic and salient cytochemical features of the neoplastic cells of some of these disorders.

Table 1. Classification of non-Hodgkin's lymphomas

Nodular (follicular) lymphomas
Lymphocytic, poorly differentiated
Mixed lymphocytic-histiocytic
Histiocytic
Diffuse lymphomas
Lymphocytic, well-differentiated
Lymphocytic, intermediate differentiation
Lymphocytic, poorly differentiated
Mixed lymphocytic-histiocytic
Histiocytic
Undifferentiated, Burkitt's type
Undifferentiated, pleomorphic (non-Burkitt's)
Lymphoblastic
Unclassified

The malignant cells have been studied in suspension for spontaneous rosette (E) formation with sheep red blood cells, receptors for complement (EAC), receptors for cytophilic antibody (IgGEA), and surface immunoglobulins (SIg) using both polyvalent and monovalent antisera. All suspensions were subsequently evaluated on stained cytocentrifuge preparations for precise morphologic identification of rosetted and nonrosetted cells. EAC and IgGEA were also applied to frozen sections (FS) of the tumors to assess the topographic distributions of the rosetted cells. In addition, we have used enzyme histochemical techniques on FS and cytochemical reactions on cytocentrifuge preparations to identify selected hydrolytic enzymes.

Nodular (Follicular) Lymphomas

These tumors are now generally acknowledged to be composed of neoplastic follicular B-lymphocytes [4, 5, 7, 18, 20, 23, 24]. They represent, both in pattern and in cytology, malignant counterparts of normal germinal centers. The term "histiocytic" in the RAPPAPORT classification [29] is a misnomer based on older morphologic concepts, since all of the neoplastic cells in any nodular (follicular) lymphoma belong to a single clone of B cells with strong complement receptors and bright-staining monoclonal SIg (Table 2). In frozen sections, the EAC-rosetted cells can often be observed to be exquisitely localized within the neoplastic nodules [7, 18]. These large and small follicular B cells probably represent kinetic variants within a single neoplastic population. The tumors usually contain an impressive admixture of normal-appearing T cells (mean 37.6% in Table 2), but their significance remains at present speculative [20].

Table 2. Nodular (follicular) lymphomas. Summary of surface markers (49 specimens from 36 individuals)

EAC	48/49 Strong rosettes	
SIg	31/32 Bright staining	
	Monoclonal	15/15
	IgM (with either κ or λ)	13/15
	IgD (with and without IgM)	2/5
E mean 37.6%. No demonstration on tumor cells		

Diffuse Lymphomas

Lymphocytic, Well-Differentiated

The neoplastic cells of well-differentiated lymphocytic lymphomas (WDLL) have in our experience (Table 3) [8] B-cell markers identical to those commonly observed on the cells of chronic lymphocytic leukemia (CLL) [2, 3, 8], although CLL of T-cell type (and with some distinctive features) has been reported in a small percentage of cases [10]. In contrast to the neoplastic cells of nodular (follicular) lymphomas, the cells of WDLL bear only small quantities of SIg [2, 8] and exhibit a qualitative or quantitative deficiency in complement receptors [8]. For the latter reason, the tumors manifest poor or no binding of EAC in frozen tissue sections. In these characteristics, they most resemble the small lymphocytes of the medullary cords of normal lymph nodes.

Table 3. Comparison of surface markers in chronic lymphocytic leukemia vs. well-differentiated lymphocytic lymphoma

	(14 cases)		(14 cases)
SIg	Weakly positive (faint staining)	*SIg*	Weakly positive (faint staining)
EAC	Weakly positive in suspension	*EAC*	Weakly positive in suspension Absent or poor binding in FS
E	Reduced	*E*	Reduced

Lymphocytic, Intermediate Differentiation

Lymphocytic lymphomas of intermediate differentiation have pathologic [4, 7] and immunologic [20] features intermediate between those of WDLL and nodular (follicular) lymphomas of the poorly differentiated lymphocytic type (NPDL). They are usually diffuse in pattern, but they may have a subtle vague nodularity. The component cells are small with scant cytoplasm and coarsely clumped chromatin. Nuclei, however, vary in shape from round to somewhat indented or "cleaved." In our study of six cases (Table 4), all were of B-lymphocytic type, with monoclonal SIg usually of the IgM heavy chain class. The surface fluorescence was readily detectable and intermediate in intensity between that of WDLL and NPDL. The cells exhibited moderately avid complement receptors and bound EAC not only in suspension but also on frozen tissue sections. E-rosette forming cells were generally few except in case 6, in which the lymph nodes and spleen were both only focally involved by the malignant proliferation.

Table 4. Six lymphocytic lymphomas of intermediate differentiation

Case No.	Tissue	E[a]	EAC	IgGEA	SIg	Clon.	EAC-FS	ALP
1	LN	16	80	6	80	MDk	++++	+
2	LN	21	64	7	50	Gk	+++	−
3	LN	6	76	16	55	MDk	++	−
4	LN	25	50	7	61	Mλ	++++	−
5	LN	17	85	17	85	Mk[b]	++	+
	LN	19	86	36	90	MDk	++	+
6	LN	76	18	2	15	Mk	+++	+
	SPL	63	23	16	34	Mk	+++	+

[a] Results are expressed as % positive cells.
[b] Not studied for IgD.
LN: lymph node; SPL: spleen; Clon: clonality; EAC-FS: rosette formation on frozen tissue sections; ALP: surface alkaline phosphatase activity.

The neoplastic cells of three of the six cases had surface membranes positive for alkaline phosphatase (ALP) activity [26]. In our laboratory, such ALP activity has been identified, in a broad screen of non-Hodgkin's lymphomas and lymphocytic leukemias, only in a minority of NPDL, and in one out of seven Burkitt's tumors. In normal lymph nodes studied similarly, ALP was found on the surface membranes of follicular-cuff lymphocytes but not on lymphoid cells in other areas [26]. By histology, immunologic markers, and ALP activity, these tumors thus seem to represent a distinct entity. They recapitulate (and perhaps even originate from) B cells of the follicular lymphoid cuffs and thus manifest features at the interface between NPDL and WDLL.

Histiocytic

Diffuse large cell lymphomas termed histiocytic in the Rappaport classification [29] have attracted increasing interest with regard to their diverse immunologic markers [1, 6, 7, 11, 13, 17, 23, 28]. Table 5 details our data from a study of the neoplastic cells from 17 patients with such tumors. Morphologically, 13 of these cases were clearly classified as diffuse histiocytic while 4 might have been designated as either histiocytic or undifferentiated pleomorphic (non-Burkitt's). B-lymphocytic markers were demonstrable in 11 of the 17 tumors (cases 5–15), but there was marked variation in the numbers of markers detected and in the percentages of malignant cells manifesting individual markers. The most consistent marker in all thoroughly studied cases was SIg, with a monoclonal pattern in all tumors evaluated with monovalent antisera. In none of these 11 cases did the neoplastic cells contain notable hydrolytic enzyme activity [20]. Six of these 11 large cell lymphomas occurred in patients with previous nodular lymphomas. All six manifested retention of B-cell markers, as has been reported also in blastic

Table 5. Diffuse histiocytic lymphoma

Case No.	Tissue	SIg	Clon.	EAC	IgGEA	E	NSE	Markers identified
1	LN	ND	—	21	17	28	0	——
2	Colon	ND	—	16	0	3	0	——
3	PB	10	—	12	17	13	0	——
4	Ascites	5	—	9	9	1	0	——
5	SPL	50	—	50	8	47	0	SIg EAC
6	BM	95	Mk	7	93	10	0	SIg EA
7	LN	62	k	32	10	20	0	SIg EAC
8	Bowel	63	Mk	38	0	20	0	SIg EAC
9	LN	98	Mk	29	19	2	0	SIg EAC
10[a]	LN	75	—	14	19	5	0	SIg (EAC)[b] (EA)[b]
11[a]	LN	92	—	43	12	11	0	SIg EAC
12[a]	LN	NS	—	50	ND	NS	0	EAC
13[a]	LN	40	—	80	ND	6	0	SIg EAC
14[a]	SPL	41	Mk	39	50	59	0	SIg EAC EA
	LN	45	Mk	64	41	55	0	SIg EAC EA
15[a]	PB	85	Mk	17	21	2	0	SIg (EAC)[b] (EA)[b]
16	LN	15	—	NS	NS	85	±	E
17	Bone	0	—	33	19	2	++	(EAC)[b] (EA)[b] NSE

[a] Previous diagnosis of nodular lymphoma.
[b] Indicates marker present on less than 25% neoplastic cells.
LN: lymph node; PB: peripheral blood; SPL: spleen; BM: bone marrow; ND: not done; NS: not satisfactory; Clon: clonality; NSE: nonspecific esterase.

transformation of CLL [9], in Richter's syndrome [11], and in large cell lymphoma supervening on Waldenström's macroglobulinemia [11].

Of the six tumors without B-cell markers, one (case 16) had features consistent with a T-cell lymphoma. The cells were SIg-negative and formed E-rosettes. Unfortunately, they could not be evaluated for specific rosetting with EAC and IgGEA since they formed E-rosettes at both 37° and 4°C. They thus formed E-rosettes not only with E but also with EAC and IgGEA. These neoplastic cells lacked demonstrable enzyme activity [20], but within the tumor there were numerous benign-appearing macrophages with diffuse cytoplasmic positivity for hydrolytic enzymes.

The malignant cells in one (case 17) of the 17 tumors exhibited markers consistent with origin from true histiocytes. A small proportion formed rosettes with EAC or IgGEA and they were devoid of SIg. In addition, the neoplastic cells rosetting with EAC and IgGEA actually phagocytosed the bound erythrocytes, a phenomenon restricted in our experience to cells of the monocyte-macrophage series. The cells were large and bizarre, with abundant deeply staining cytoplasm, oval to lobulated vesicular nuclei, and basophilic macronucleoli. Their cytoplasm was diffusely and strongly positive not only for α-naphthyl acetate esterase but also for acid phosphatase, β-glucuronidase, and naphthyl-ASD-acetate esterase (not inhibited by sodium fluoride). They exhibited a positive but somewhat weaker activity for α-naphthyl butyrate esterase [20]. This tumor occurred in a 14-year-old and, unlike the other cases, appeared to be primary in bone (clavicle).

In the remaining four cases (cases 1–4), no immunologic markers were detected, but two (cases 1 and 2) were not studied for SIg. The malignant cells of cases 3 and 4 were positive for acid phosphatase and α-naphthyl acetate esterase. β- Glucuronidase activity was also demonstrable in the cells of case 4. The staining pattern, unlike that in cells of the monocyte-macrophage series, was not diffuse. Rather, it was seen as discrete punctate dots, in one case confined to the Golgi area. Such enzyme activity has been observed in both normal and neoplastic lymphocytes, particularly in T-cell tumors [10, 31], but the cells of these two cases did not form E-rosettes. Case 4 was also assayed for terminal deoxynucleotidyl transferase (TdT) and was devoid of detectable TdT activity [14]. Case 3 had plasmacytoid features, both with light microscopy and ultrastructurally [15]. Mature plasma cells and myeloma cells have been reported to contain acid phosphatase activity. Unlike normal or malignant plasma cells, however, the neoplastic cells of case 3 did not contain demonstrable intracytoplasmic immunoglobulin.

Undifferentiated, Burkitt's Type

We have recently reported our results of studies of American patients with lymphomas histologically and cytologically typical of Burkitt's tumor [25]. In eight cases, the neoplastic cells were evaluated for immunologic membrane markers and for hydrolytic enzymes. In addition, a retrospective review was performed on 47 biopsies and 17 autopsies of such patients to assess patterns of involvement by tumor in lymph nodes, spleens, and Peyer's patches. In all cases studied, the malignant cells bore monoclonal SIg of the IgM heavy chain class. A minority of the cells rosetted with EAC and IgGEA. They contained little or no detectable hydrolytic enzyme activity. Like Burkitt's tumor in Africans, histologically identical tumors in American patients thus consist of B-lymphocytes. Moreover, in ten biopsies and two autopsies, it was possible to find germinal centers selectively involved by Burkitt's tumor. These neoplastic cells may be related to some B-lymphocytes of normal germinal centers.

Lymphoblastic

Lymphoblastic lymphomas (LBL) are now recognized to be distinctive tumors closely related if not identical to acute lymphoblastic leukemia of T-cell type [12, 14, 18, 19, 21, 22, 27, 30, 31, 32]. Table 6 summarizes the clinical, immunologic, and enzymic features of nine cases studied in our laboratory. The neoplastic cells were in all cases devoid of SIg and receptors for IgGEA. E-rosettes were formed by variable percentages of the malignant cells in five cases. EAC-rosettes around neoplastic cells were also detected in five cases. In individual cases, there was rosette formation with either, both, or neither of the E- and EAC-reagents. We have previously noted the presence of complement receptors in LBL [19]. The reported identification of such receptors on fetal thymocytes [16] renders this observation easier to rationalize and is consistent with the thymus-related nature of these neoplasms.

Table 6. Membrane surface markers and cytochemical findings in nine lymphoblastic lymphomas

Case No.	Age Sex	Med	Source	E[a]	EAC	IgGEA	SIg	AP[b]	BG	TdT
1	12 F	+	PB	7	85+	3	8	ND	ND	ND
2	23 M	+	PB	10	9	4	8	ND	ND	ND
3	22 M	+	PB	80+	70+	8	0	ND	ND	ND
4	18 M	+	BM	3	4	1	0	ND	ND	ND
5	19 M	+	LN	7	30+	1	0	50^{M}	80^{M}	+
6	18 M	+	PF	32+	34+	1	1	55^{M}	18^{M}	+
7	30 F	+	PF	23+	16+	1	0	100^{P}	99^{P}	+
8	23 M	+	PF	63+	N	1	0	94^{P}	99^{P}	+
9	60 M	−	Skin	20+	9	N	0	ND	63^{M}	±
		−	PB	6	3	0	ND	62^{M}	18^{M}	−
						2				

[a] Results are expressed as % positive cells; + indicates marker identified on neoplastic cells.
[b] Percent of neoplastic cells positive for enzymes AP (acid phosphatase) or βG β-glucuronidase).
M: Multigranular reaction product; P: punctate perinuclear reaction product; PB: peripheral blood; BM: bone marrow; LN: lymph node; PF: pleural fluid; Med: mediastinal mass; ND: not determined; N: negative for receptors; TdT: terminal deoxynucleotidyl transferase.

Regardless of surface markers, acid phosphatase (AP) and β-glucuronidase (βG) were present in all cases studied for these enzymes. Among the cases, there was some variation in the percentages of positive cells and in the pattern of reactivity (punctate vs. multigranular). Assays for TdT were unequivocally positive in four cases and borderline in the fifth (case 9) [14, 20]. Case 9, a 60-year-old man, had unusual features both clinically and pathologically. The tumor presented in the skin and remained apparently confined to the skin for 2 years. He subsequently became leukemic (WBC 80,000/mm^3) and malignant cells were demonstrated in the cerebrospinal fluid. Although the patient never developed a mediastinal mass, both the leukemic progression and the meningeal involvement are characteristic features of LBL.

Summary

The neoplastic cells of non-Hodgkin's lymphomas frequently manifest markers identifiable on normal cells of the lymphoreticular system. *Nodular (follicular) lymphomas* of all three subtypes in the RAPPAPORT classification are neoplasms of follicular B-lymphocytes. Both in pattern of growth and in cellular composition they are malignant counterparts of normal germinal centers, their cytologic variation probably being attributable to kinetic diversity. *Well-differentiated lymphocytic lymphomas* also have B-cell markers, but immunologically they differ from follicular B-lymphocytes and more closely resemble small lymphocytes of the medullary cords of normal lymph nodes.

Lymphocytic lymphomas of intermediate differentiation seem to represent a third distinctive form of B-cell malignancy, with features similar to B-cells of normal follicular lymphoid cuffs. Conceptually, they appear to be at the interface between nodular lymphomas of poorly differentiated lymphocytic type and diffuse lymphomas of well-differentiated lymphocytic type. The cells of American cases of *Burkitt's tumor*, like those of African cases, also bear B-lymphocytic markers. Evidence from a retrospective morphologic study of 47 cases has suggested a possible relationship between the malignant cells and some B-lymphocytes of normal germinal centers.

Among 17 large cell lymphomas termed *histiocytic* in the RAPPAPORT classification, 11 bore markers indicative of B-lymphocytic origin. In 4 of the 17 cases no definite markers were demonstrable, but rare tumors of neoplastic T cells (1/17) or true histiocytic nature (1/17) were identified. *Lymphoblastic lymphomas* consistently lack SIg or receptors for IgGEA, but they are somewhat heterogeneous with respect to expression of receptors for E and/or EAC. Acid phosphatase, β-glucuronidase, and terminal deoxynucleotidyl transferase serve to link these tumors to T-lymphoblasts and the cells of T-cell ALL.

Evidence to date indicates that immunologic, cytochemical, and functional studies of the cells of non-Hodgkin's lymphomas may have important implications for advancing present understanding of the etiology, pathogenesis, clinical manifestations, and optimal therapy of these tumors.

Acknowledgements

The authors are grateful to Ms. Sheila SANDERS, Mrs. Eileen SUSSMAN, and Mr. Edward SOBAN for their expert technical assistance and to Dr. Michael M. FRANK of the National Institute of Allergy and Infectious Diseases for providing the sheep red blood cell reagents employed in these studies.

References

1. Aisenberg, A. C., Long, J. C.: Lymphocyte surface characteristics in malignant lymphoma. Am. J. Med. *58*, 300–306 (1975).
2. Aisenberg, A. C. Wilkes, B.: Lymphosarcoma cell leukemia: the contribution of cell surface study to diagnosis. Blood *48*, 707–715 (1976).
3. Aisenberg. A. C., Bloch, K. J., Long, J. C.: Cell-surface immunoglobulins in chronic lymphocytic leukemia and allied disorders. Am. J. Med. *55*, 184–191 (1973).
4. Berard, C. W.: Chapter 15. Reticuloendothelial system: an overview of neoplasia. In: International Academy of Pathology Monograph No. 16: The Reticuloendothelial System. Rebuck, J. W., Berard, C. W., Abell, M. R. (eds) Baltimore: Williams and Wilkins 1975, pp. 301–317.
5. Berard, C. W., Gallo, R. C., Jaffe, E. S., Green, I., De Vita, V. T.: Current concepts of leukemia and lymphoma: etiology, pathogenesis, and therapy. Ann. Intern. Med. *85*, 351–366 (1976).
6. Bloomfield, C. D., Kersey, J. H., Brunning, R. D., Gajl-Peczalska, K. J.: Prognostic significance of lymphocyte surface markers in adult non-Hodgkin's malignant lymphoma. Lancet *1976/ii*, 1330–1333.
7. Braylan, R. C., Jaffe, E. S., Berard, C. W.: Malignant lymphomas: current classification and new observations. In: Pathology Annual 1975. Sommers, S. C. (ed) New York: Appleton-Century-Crofts 1975, Vol. X, pp. 213–270.
8. Braylan, R. C., Jaffe, E. S., Burbach, J. W., Frank, M. M., Johnson, R. E., Berard, C. W.: Similarities of surface characteristics of neoplastic well-differentiated lymphocytes from solid tissues and from peripheral blood. Cancer Res. *36*, 1619–1625 (1976).
9. Brouet, J. C., Preud'homme, J., Seligmann, M.: Blast cells with monoclonal surface immunoglobulin in two cases of acute blast crisis supervening in chronic lymphocytic leukemia. Br. Med. J. *1974/IV*, 23–24.
10. Brouet, J. C., Flandrin, G., Sasportes, M., Preud'homme, J. L., Seligmann, M.: Chronic lymphocytic leukemia of T-cell origin. Immunological and clinical evaluation in eleven patients. Lancet *1975/ii*, 890–893.
11. Brouet, J. C., Preud'homme, J. L., Flandrin, G., Chelloul, N., Seligmann, M.: Brief communication: Membrane markers in "histiocytic" lymphomas (reticulum cell sarcomas). J. Natl. Cancer Inst. *56*, 631–633 (1976).
12. Coccia, P. F., Kersey, J. H., Gajl-Peczalska, K. J., Krivit, W., Nesbit, M. E.: Prognostic significance of surface marker analysis in childhood non-Hodgkin's lymphoproliferative malignancies. Am. J. Hematol. *1*, 405–417 (1976).
13. Davey, F. R., Goldberg, J., Stockman, J., Gottlieb, A. J.: Immunologic and cytochemical cell markers in non-Hodgkin's lymphomas. Lab. Invest. *35*, 430–438 (1976).
14. Donlon, J. A., Jaffe, E. S., Braylan, R. C.: Terminal deoxynucleotidyl transferase activity in malignant lymphomas. N. Engl. J. Med. *297*, 461–464 (1977).
15. Fisher, R. I., Jaffe, E. S., Braylan, R. C.: Immunoblastic lymphadenopathy: evolution into a malignant lymphoma with plasmacytoid features. Am. J. Med. *61*, 553–559 (1976).
16. Gatien, J. G., Schneeberger, E. E., Merler, E.: Analysis of human thymocyte subpopulations using discontinuous gradients of albumin: precursor lymphocytes in human thymus. Eur. J. Immunol. *5*, 312–317 (1975).
17. Habeshaw, J. A., Stuart, A. E.: Cell receptor studies on seven cases of diffuse histiocytic malignant lymphoma (reticulum cell sarcoma). J. Clin. Pathol. *28*, 289–297 (1975).
18. Jaffe, E. S., Shevach, E. M., Frank, M. M., Berard, C. W., Green, I.: Nodular lymphoma: evidence for origin from follicular B lymphocytes. N. Engl. J. Med. *290*, 813–819 (1974).
19. Jaffe, E. S., Braylan, R. C., Frank, M. M., Green, I., Berard, C. W.: Heterogeneity of immunologic markers and surface morphology in childhood lymphoblastic lymphoma. Blood *48*, 213–222 (1976).
20. Jaffe, E. S., Braylan, R. C., Nanba, K., Frank, M. M., Berard, C. W.: Functional markers: a new perspective on malignant lymphomas. Cancer Treat. rep. *61*, 953–962 (1977).
21. Kaplan, J., Mastrangelo, R., Peterson, W. D.: Childhood lymphoblastic lymphoma, a cancer of thymus-derived lymphocytes. Cancer Res. *34*, 521–525 (1974).
22. Kersey, J., Sabad, A., Gajl-Peczalska, K. J.: Neoplastic cells from childhood lymphoblastic leukemia and lymphoma with T and B lymphocyte markers. Am. J. Pathol. *74*, 64A (1974).
23. Leech, J. H., Glick, A. D., Waldron, J. A., Flexner, J. M., Horn, R. G., Collins, R. D.: Malignant lymphomas of follicular center cell origin in man. I. Immunologic studies. J. Natl. Cancer. Inst. *54*, 11–21 (1975).
24. Levy, R., Warnke, R., Dorfman, R. F., Haimovich, J.: The monoclonality of human B-cell lymphomas. J. Exp. Med. *145*, 1014–1028 (1977).

25. MANN, R. B., JAFFE, E. S., BRAYLAN, R. C., NANBA, K., FRANK, M. M., ZIEGLER, J. L., BERARD, C. W.: Non-endemic Burkitt's lymphoma. A B-cell tumor related to germinal centers. N. Engl. J. Med. *295*, 685–691 (1976).
26. NANBA, K., JAFFE, E. S., BRAYLAN, R. C., SOBAN, E. J., BERARD, C. W.: Alkaline phosphatase-positive malignant lymphoma. A subtype of B-cell lymphomas. Am. J. Clin. Pathol. *68*, 535–542 (1977).
27. NATHWANI, B. N., KIM, H., RAPPAPORT, H.: Malignant lymphoma, lymphoblastic. Cancer *38*, 964–983 (1976).
28. PETER, C. R., MACKENZIE, M. P.: T or B cell origin of some non-Hodgkin's lymphomas. Lancet *1974/ii*, 686–689.
29. RAPPAPORT, H.: Tumors of the hematopoietic system. In: Atlas of Tumor Pathology. sect. III, fasc. 8. Washington, D.C.: Armed Forces Institute of Pathology 1966.
30. SEN, L., BORELLA, L.: Clinical importance of lymphoblasts with T markers in childhood acute leukemia. N. Engl. J. Med. *292*, 828–832 (1975).
31. STEIN, H., PETERSEN, N., GAEDICKE, G., LENNERT, K., LANDBECK, G.: Lymphoblastic lymphoma of convoluted or acid phosphatase type—a tumor of T precursor cells. Int. J. Cancer *17*, 292–295 (1976).
32. TSUKIMOTO, I., WONG, K. Y., LAMPKIN, B. C.: Surface markers and prognostic factors in acute lymphoblastic leukemia. N. Engl. J. Med. *294*, 245–248 (1976).

Categorization of Non-Hodgkin's Hematosarcomas (Lymphomas) According to T- and B-Cell Markers: Its Value for Diagnosis and Prognosis

D. Belpomme, B. Caillou, N. Lelarge, I. Botto, E. Pujade Lauraine, L. Denaro, R. Gerard-Marchant, A. J. S. Davies, and G. Mathé

Non-Hodgkin's hematosarcomas (NHHS) or non-Hodgkin's "lymphomas" are the objects of so many different morphologic microscopic classifications [12, 17, 23, 24, 26, 27, 31, 33, 34, 36, 38, 39] that it is almost impossible for clinicians from different centers to compare their observations and therapeutic results. Until the time that an international classification can be accepted by all pathologists, we propose that a categorization using cell membrane markers is helpful for diagnosis and prognosis in these disorders, as in acute lymphoid leukemias [8, 10]. The object of this paper is to summarize the preliminary data given by such categorization of 100 cases of NHHS, with particular reference to its value for prognosis, correlation with the clinical presentation of the disease, and comparison with the WHO microscopic classification [34]. A further paper will be devoted to a computer multiparametric analysis of those cases [11].

Methods and Patients

Methods

Neoplastic cells from the 100 cases under investigation were analyzed for the presence of T- and B-cell markers using several immunologic and cytochemical tests. The various cell markers and their technical backgrounds are listed in Table 1. Neoplastic cells tested originated from

Table 1. Various cell markers and their technical backgrounds[a]

Markers	Tests	Interpretation
E	SRBC spontaneous rosettes	T-cell lineage
Human T-lymphocyte antigen (HTLA)	Anti.T.cell sera	T-cell lineage
Thymus leukemia antigen (TL)	Anti.T.cell sera	T-cell lineage
Acid phosphatase		T-cell lineage
MIg	Direct immunofluorescence after in vitro incubation of cells	B-cell lineage
FcAg-IgG	EA	Monocyte B (?), T (?)
C_3	EAC	Monocyte B (?), T (?)
Ia-like specificities	Heterologous B-cell antisera; Alloantisera	B, Monocyte, myeloid cells
Terminal deoxynucleotidyl transferase (TDT)		All except B
Lysosomal hexoaminidase		Null ALL antigen positive cases
?	Null cell antisera and others	

[a] From WHO Technical Report, Munich 1976, modified 1977 [45].

Table 2. Material submitted to immunologic markers study and cytohistologic study

	Lymph nodes	Bone marrow ± blood	Spleen	Skin	Pleural abdominal dffusion	Digestive tract	Breast
Immunologic marker study	50	37[a]	4	3	3	2	1
Cytohistologic study	80	13	0	1	0	3	1
	18 early leukemic lymphosarcomas (Lymph nodes, Bone marrow ± blood, Spleen)						

[a] 19 cases of secondary leukemic lymphosarcomas investigated.

solid tissues in 60 cases, abnormal bone marrow and peripheral blood in 37 cases, and pleural abdominal effusion in three cases (Table 2). Immunologic cell typing was performed on bone marrow and peripheral blood rather than on solid tissues in the case of leukemic lymphosarcomas. In all instances, neoplastic cells were purified using the Ficoll-Hypaque gradient method [2, 6, 7, 45], and particular attention was paid to morphologic examination before assuming that purified mononuclear cells were of neoplastic origin.

Patients

The 100 patients in this study were followed in Villejuif. This series of patients differs from that reported by MISSET et al. in this issue, since the cases collected in the present report were only those from which a sample was sent to our laboratory for immunologic cell typing. The ages of the patients ranged from 2–72 years (mean age = 37.6). There were 21 females and 69 males. Categorization of the cases according to the WHO classification is given in Table 3. One sees that there are four so-called reticulosarcoma (RS) cases and 95 so-called lymphosarcomas (LS).

Table 3. 100 cases of non-Hodgkin's hematosarcomas (lymphomas) according to the WHO classification

	Lymphocytic	Lymphoplasmocytic	Prolymphocytic	Lymphoblastic	Immunoblastic	Reticulosarcomas	Others (2)
Nodular			13				
Diffuse	4	3	26	29	20	4	1
Total	4	3	39	29	20	4	1[a]

[a] Lymphoepithelial (LENNERT)?

Results

Immunologic Categorization

In 52 cases, between 30% and 95% of the mononuclear cell population exhibited positive B-cell markers, but no T-cell markers and they were, accordingly, classified as B-cell lymphosarcomas (LS) (Table 4). In 32 of these 52 cases, monoclonality of the lymphoid proliferation emerged from the ability of the neoplastic cells to synthesize monoclonal membrane immunoglobulin determinants, the majority of which were of the IgM κ or λ types in vitro (Table 5). In 14 other cases, the B-cell origin of the neoplastic cells was ascertained by detection of membrane Ig

Table 4. T-B membrane phenotypes in 100 cases of non-Hodgkin's hematosarcomas

Observations	Interpretation	No. of cases
mIg (+), FcAgIg (±), C_3 (+), E (−)	B	52
mIg (−), FcAgIg (±), C_3 (?), E (+)	T	16
mIg (−), FcAgIg (±), C_3 (±), E (−)	Null	32
	Total	100

mIg = membrane immunoglobulins (synthetized by cells) detected by direct membrane immunofluorescence test after in vitro procedures; FcAgAc = Fc receptors for antigen-antibody complexes detected by EA-rosettes test; C_3 = activated C_3 complement receptors detected by EAC-rosettes test; E = spontaneous E-rosette test using sheep red blood cells; ± = some cases negative, some positive.

using a polyvalent antiserum, but the monoclonal characterization was not possible as the cell samples contained too few cells. In the three remaining cases, a mixed immunofluorescênce pattern was observed, even after in vitro incubation procedures. Finally, when the percentage of positive fluorescent mononuclear cells was less than 50% and in cases where the neoplastic origin of the majority of cells could not be assessed on the standpoint of morphology, monoclonality was sought since normal B cells could have been mixed with the pathologic cells in some preparations. In 16 patients, between 60% and 90% of the mononuclear cell population exhibited T-cell markers but no B-cell markers. These cases were accordingly classified as T-cell LS. In the remaining 32 patients, between 30% and 90% of the mononuclear cells had neither T- nor B-membrane markers, using both the sheep red blood cell spontaneous rosette test and the direct membrane immunofluorescence test. These cases, which we attempted to further characterize using other techniques, were classified as "null" cell NHHS. The membrane phenotypes of the 100 cases studied are summarized in Table 4.

Further Characterization of Null Cell Hematosarcomas

A variety of means was used to further characterize the cases determined as null on their membrane markers. It was not possible to apply all tests to all cases. Of 11 cases tested for Fc and C_3 receptors, three proved positive, which could indicate a derivation from the B-cell series. Two out of five tested gave an acid phosphatase-positive reaction perhaps showing affinity with the T-cell series [35]. None of six tested were positive with an anti-T-cell antiserum although three E-rosette-positive cases used as control were positive with the same antiserum [25]. Furthermore, 4 out of 24 cases were associated with pericellular reticulin fibrils which perhaps indicates their origin from reticulum cells (Table 6).

Prognosis Significance of the Immunologic Categorization

Figure 1, which represents the survival curves dealing with the three immunologic groups of NHHS, shows that T-cell LS are associated with a poorer prognosis than either B-cell LS or null

Table 5. Membrane immunologic determinants of neoplastic cells in B-cell lymphosarcomas[a]

	Igmk[b]	IgMλ[b]	IgGk	IgGλ	κ
No of cases	17	7	6	1	1
Percentage of evaluable cases	53%	22%	19%		

[a] 32 cases evaluable for monclonality.
[b] Associated monoclonal IgD in 50% of cases.

Table 6. Detailed study of null large cell diffuse non-Hodgkin's hematosarcomas

Markers[a]	Observations	Interpretation
Presence of Fc and C_3 receptors	3/11 (27%)	B-lymphocytes ? Histiomonocytes ?
Acid phosphatase positivity	2/5	T ? (pre-T ?) lymphocytes ?
Brain T-cell antigen (s)	0/6	
Reticulin positivity	4/24 (16%)	Reticulum cells ?
Permanent cell cultures[b]	Several lines derived from null cell lymphoma and having some B-cell characteristics	B- or pre-B-lymphocytes but not proven monoclonality of the in vitro established B-cell population

[a] See text and Table 1.
[b] D. BELPOMME et al. (to be published).

cell NHHS. The median survival was still not reached in either the group of patients with B-cell LS or with null cell NHHS after 50-months follow-up, whereas the median survival was 10 months in the group of patients with T-cell LS. However, the survival plateau reached by the B-cell LS was 80% at 18 months, while the survival plateau reached by the null cell NHHS was only 65% at 22 months (The difference is not statistically significant). Finally, these results suggest that cases of B-cell LS, whether diffuse or nodular, as well as the diffuse null cell cases, have a significantly better prognosis than diffuse T-cell LS.

Correlation Between Immunologic Categorization and Clinical Presentation

The 16 patients with T-cell LS as well as the 32 patients with null cell NHHS were found to be significantly younger than the 52 patients with B-cell LS. The mean age was 29.7 years (2–54 years for the group of patients with T-cell LS and 27 years (5–55 years for the group of null cell

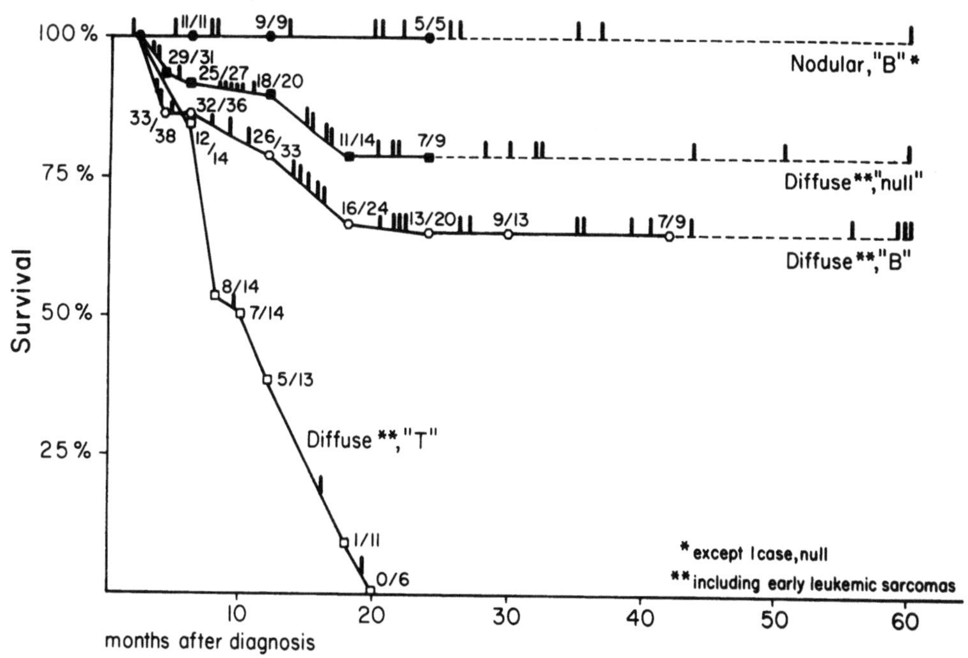

Fig. 1. Survival of patients with non-Hodgkin's hematosarcomas according to histology and T- and B-cell markers (direct curves)

NHL, while the mean age was 46.6 years (7–72 years) for the group of patients with B-cell LS. There was a male predominance in both groups of patients having T-cell LS or B-cell LS when compared to the group of patients with null cell NHHS. The sex ratio was 75% and 73% for the T-cell and B-cell groups respectively, and only 59% for the null cell group (Table 7). Clinical staging analysis revealed that cases in the B-cell group tended to have a less voluminous tumoral presentation, whereas both the T-cell and the null cell groups had a more disseminated presentation at the first examination. At the first presentation, 81% of the patients were staged as III and IV in both the T-cell and null cell groups. Only 68% of patients in the B-cell group had similar staging (Table 7). Mediastinal masses were found in 43% of the patients with T-cell LS, 3% with B-cell LS, and 12% with null cell NHL. Abdominal presentations of the disease were observed in each immunologic group with a similar frequency 12%–19%. However, skin localizations were found more frequently in the T-cell group (18%) than in either the B-cell group (5%) or the null cell group (3%). The percentage of leukemic conversion was similar in both T-cell and null cell groups with values of 56% and 43%, respectively, but lower in the B-cell group with a value of 34%.

Delay of leukemic conversion after diagnosis was significantly longer in the B-cell group than in either the T-cell or null cell groups. This delay reached 11.8 months (1–49 months) in the B-cell group, while T-cell and null cell groups were characterized by a mean value of 4.2 and 4.1 months (0.5–10 and 0.5–24 months, respectively) (Table 8).

Correlation Between Immunologic Categorization and WHO Microscopic Classification

In 100 cases of the series were available for morphologic categorization since the WHO classification is based on cytologic as well as on histologic examination of cells. Table 9 shows that the 16 T-cell cases were composed of ten cases of the lymphoblastic type (62%), three cases

Table 7. Clinical presentation of non-Hodgkin's lymphomas according to the T-B immunologic classification

	T	B	Null
Age (years)	29.7[a] 2–54[b]	46.6 7–72	27 5–55
% Males	75%	73%	59%
Clinical staging			
% I	6%	7%	6%
% ii	12%	23%	12%
%III	25%	32%	31%
% IV	56%	36%	50%

[a] Mean value. [b] Range.

Table 8. Clinical presentation of non-Hodgkin's lymphomas according to the T-B immunologic classification

	T	B	Null
% Mediastinal mass	43%	3%	12%
% Abdominal presentation	12%	19%	15%
% Skin localization	18%	5%	3%
% Leukemic conversion	56%	34%	43%
Delay (months)	4.2[a] 0.5–10[b]	11.8 1–49	4.1 0.5–24

[a] Mean value. [b] Range.

of the immunoblastic type (18%), and two cases of the prolymphocytic type. One case was, in addition, difficult to classify according to the criteria recorded in the WHO Reference Center for neoplastic diseases of hematopoietic and lymphoid tissues [34]. This case probably corresponds to the lymphoepitheloid variety described by LENNERT [24] (table 9). On the other hand, the 52 B-cell cases included, as shown in Table 10, 30 cases classified as prolymphocytic (58%), 14 cases classified as immunoblastic (27%), three cases as lymphocytic, three cases as lymphoplasmocytic, and two cases as lymphoblastic. Finally, the 32 so-called null cell NHHS included 17 cases of the lymphoblastic type (55%), seven cases of the prolymphocytic type (22%), three cases of the immunoblastic type, and one case of the lymphocytic type. In addition, the four cases of so-called reticulosarcoma were included in this group of null cell NHHS (Table 11).

From this study it was also found that prolymphocytic LS was associated with a B-cell type in 76% of the cases (30/39) and with a null cell type in 17% of the cases (7/39). There were only two T-cell prolymphocytic LS (5%) in this series. All nodular NHL, except one case (1 out of 13 nodular cases), were found to be of the B-cell type (12 cases). The case of nodular NHL with no detectable B-cell membrane markers was classified as null. On the other hand, diffuse NHL included all T-cell cases (16 cases), 77% of the B-cell cases (40 cases), and 96% of the null cell cases (all cases except for 1 out of 31 cases). Lymphoblastic LS were, in contrast, found to be of the null cell type in 58% of the cases (17/29) and of the T-cell type in 34% of the cases (10/29). Blastic cells from the null cell cases were morphologically, as well as immunologically, difficult to distinguish from those of typical null cell primary ALL. There were only two B-cell lymphoblastic LS (6%) in this series. Immunoblastic LS were of the B-cell type in 70% of the

Table 9. 16 cases of T-cell lymphosarcomas: correlation with the WHO classification

	Prolymphocytic	Lymphoblastic	Immunoblastic	Lymphoepithelioid[a]
No. of T-cell cases	2	10	3	1
Percentage of T-cell cases in each cytohistologic group	2/39 (5%)	10/29 (34%)	3/20 (15%)	

[a] LENNERT.

Table 10. 52 cases of B-cell lymphosarcomas: correlation with the WHO classification

	Lymphocytic[a]	Lymphocytoplasmocytic[a]	Prolymphocytic[b]	Lymphoblastic[a]	Immunoblastic[a]
No. of B-cell cases	3	3	30	2	14
% of B-cell cases in each cytohistologic group	3/4	3/3	30/39 (76%)	2/29 (6%)	14/20 (70%)

[a] All cases diffuse. [b] 12 nodular, 18 diffuse.

Table 11. 32 cases of so-called null cell hematosarcomas: correlation with the WHO classification[a]

	Lymphocytic	Prolymphocytic	Lymphoblastic	Immunoblastic	Reticulosarcoma (WHO)
No. of null cell cases	1	7	17	3	4
% of null cell cases in each cytohistological group	1/4	7/39 (17%)	17/29 (58%)	3/20 (15%)	4/4 (100%)

[a] All diffuse except one prolymphocytic case, nodular.

cases (14/20) as well as of the T-cell type in 15% of the cases (3/20). In three cases (15%) immunoblastic cells were associated with a lack of detectable T- and B-membrane markers and therefore classified as null cells (Table 11).

Finally, these results suggest that T-cell LS are mainly lymphoblastic in type, whereas B-cell LS are mostly of the prolymphocytic or the immunoblastic type (Table 10). On the other hand, the group of null cell NHL is particularly heterogeneous since this group not only includes a majority of cases of null cell lymphoblastic LS, but also cases of prolymphocytic LS, immunoblastic LS, and four cases of reticulosarcoma; the clinical presentation and the survival characteristics of these last four cases are summarized in Table 12. The survival characteristics of all cases studied for both the immunologic and cytohistologic parameters of classification are presented in Figures 2, 3, and 4.

Table 12. Clinical, cytohistologic, and immunologic presentation of reticulosarcomas (four cases)

Sex (F/M)	Age (years)	Cytologic and histologic characteristics		Immunologic T- and B-membrane phenotype	Clinical localizations		Duration of first remission	Survival[a]
3/1	38.6 (21–53)	Large "blastic" cells	4/4	Null 4/4	Lymph nodes	3/4	8, 12, 15, >36	2 patients living[b]
		Diffuse	4/4		Bones	2/4		2 patients died[c]
		Reticulin fibrils	4/4		Lung	1/4		
		Phagocytic neoplastic cells	1/4		Skin	1/4		

[a] See Figure 4. [b] At 16 and 36 months. [c] At 11 and 15 months.

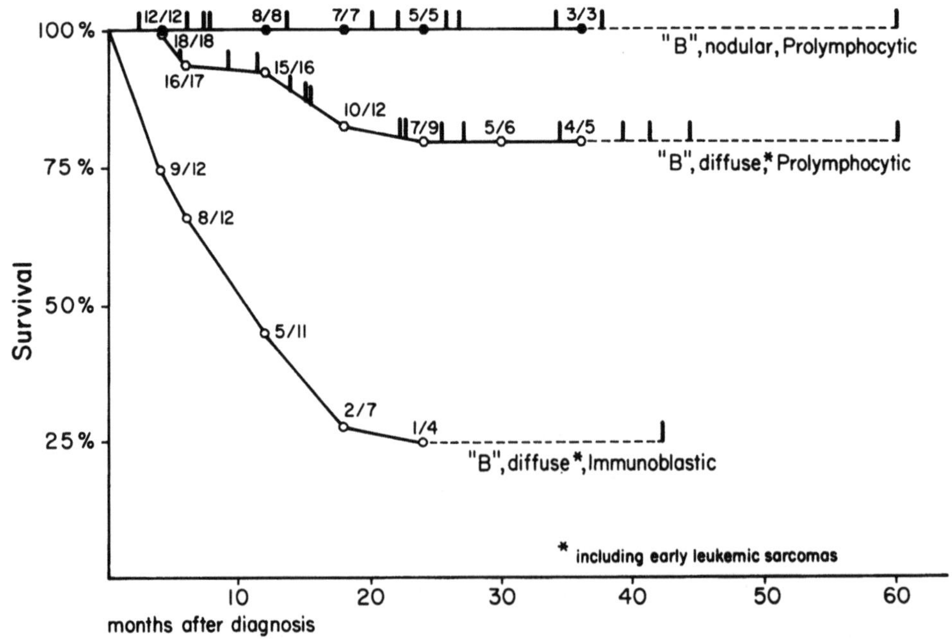

Fig. 2. Survival of patients with B-cell lymphosarcomas according to the WHO cytohistologic categorization (direct curves)

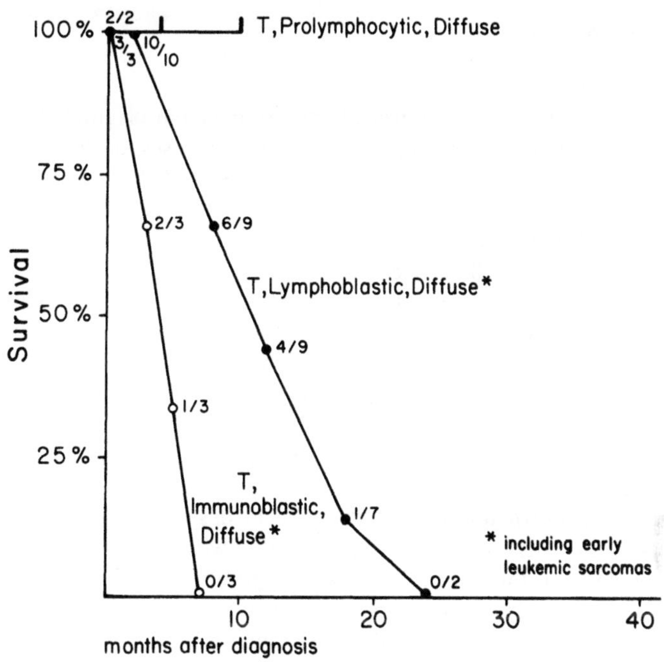

Fig 3. Survival of patients with T-cell lymphosarcomas according to the WHO cytohistologic categorization (direct curves)

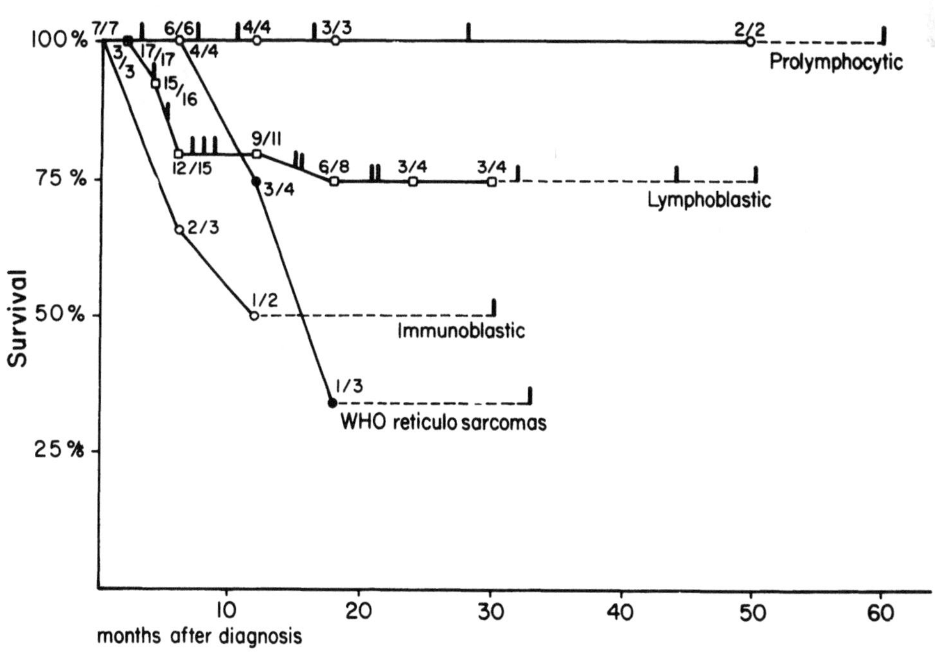

Fig. 4. Survival of patients with so-called null cell hematosarcomas according to the WHO cytohistologic categorization (direct curves)

Discussion

In this study, we have confirmed and extended our original observations showing that NHHS are of the B-cell type in approximately 55% of cases, of the T-cell type in 15% of cases, and of the non-T–non-B cell type in 30% of cases [3, 4, 5, 6, 7, 8]. These data concur with those reported by several groups [1, 14, 15, 16, 18, 20, 38, 43]. A conclusion from the present investigation is that T-cell LS are associated with a significantly poorer prognosis than either B-cell LS or null cell NHHS.

We have shown in a previous paper that primary T-cell ALL is also of poor prognosis [8], as has been confirmed by several investigators (see 10). Thus, it seems that malignant T-cell disorders, whatever their hematologic presentation, are of poor prognosis. Our data suggest that T-cell LS are associated with: 1) a male predominance, 2) the youngest mean age in comparison with that found in the group of B-cell LS, and 3) clinical features including mediastinal mass and tumoral skin localizations. This particular clinical picture agrees with that described in some studies [13, 21, 22, 28, 29, 41, 42].

It is also worth noting that the clinical description of the mediastinal leucosarcomatosis reported by STERNBERG [44], as associated with a very poor prognosis, was similar to that of only 43% of the T-cell LS cases suggesting that immunologic markers provide further information which could not be derived from simple clinical examination. These clinical observations, as well as the demonstration of the T-cell nature of the neoplastic cells of these particular LS, suggest that human T-cell LS may, in fact, correspond to the murine AKR leukemic lymphoma model which has been demonstrated to be of thymic origin and that human T-cell LS may, therefore, have a similar thymic origin [19, 30].

In contrast to T-cell LS, B-cell LS was found to be associated with a better prognosis, since the majority of patients in our series are still living after 50-months follow-up. These results are perhaps not surprising since B-cell LS tends to be associated at the first examination with a less disseminated presentation of the disease than either the T-cell LS or the null cell NHHS and the delay of leukemic conversion is significantly longer for B-cell LS than for either T-cell LS or null cell NHHS. Furthermore, the majority of nodular LS, which we know to be associated with a better prognosis than diffuse LS [39], were found to be of the B-cell type. In addition, B-cell LS included a majority of prolymphocytic types, a group of LS which have been demonstrated to be associated with the best prognosis, when compared to the other cytohistologic types [30, 31, 32].

Our results showing that B-cell LS have a good prognosis whatever their nodular or diffuse histologic presentation disagrees with the observations of some authors, who suggest that B-cell LS is associated with a poor prognosis [13]. This discrepancy may be related to difference in the age of patients since our series included not only children but also a number of adults. It could, in addition, be related to the collection of more immunoblastic cases within the reported series since, in contrast to prolymphocytic B-cell LS, immunoblastic B-cell LS is associated with a very poor prognosis [32, 33] (see Fig. 2).

Null cell NHHS have been found to be associated with a prognosis of similar range to diffuse B-cell LS. This group of so-called null cell disorders have, however, been found to be morphologically and immunologically heterogeneous. Since this observation supports the concept that this group probably covers different physiologic and clinical entities, survival data concerning it should be interpreted with caution (see Fig 4). It is interesting to note, however, that this group of null cell NHHS includes two types of disorders, according to the WHO classification. In 87% of the cases, null cell NHHS have been morphologically classified as "lymphosarcoma" and all the cytologic types of LS (i.e., the prolymphocytic, lymphoblastic, and immunoblastic types) have been found to be represented in this group. We wonder if these so-called "null cell LS" may not, in fact, correspond to true LS, in which lymphoid neoplastic cells are characterized by a lack (or a loss) of either the T- or B-cell membrane markers. This can result from different "functional" antigenic membrane modifications (or modulations) associated with the malignant phenotype. In 13% of the cases, however, null cell NHHS have been morphologically classified as reticulosarcomas. The question of whether these disorders are truly derived from neoplastic histiocytes or reticulum cells still remains a matter of controversy or speculation, since there is no good marker for the histiocytic cells or reticulum cell lines. Our finding based on morphologic and clinical observations suggests that these cases may represent a distinct entity within the framework of NHHS.

Finally, an interesting result of the present investigation is that by using T-B membrane markers, it is possible to distinguish several groups of NHHS which have a different prognostic significance. This distinction does not appear a priori directly related to morphology, since the different immunologic groups were found to be relatively heterogeneous in terms of cytology and histology. The routine use of both the immunologic and morphologic parameters of classification of NHHS thus appears useful in distinguishing groups of patients with different prognoses: such distinction may prove well worthwhile if different treatments are indicated. It is what we intend to prove in further studies based on computer multiparametric analysis [11].

Acknowledgments

The authors would like to express their gratitude to Mrs. Marie-Dominique Goujon and Mrs. Micheline Bérardet for their efficient technical assistance and Mrs. Ximena Benavente and Mrs. Fenella Riseley for their help in the preparation of this manuscript.

This study was supported by a Grant from INSERM A.T.P., 10.74.31, Décision N° 13; and by a Grant from a DGRST 77.7.0039.

References

1. Aisenberg, A. C., Lung, J. C.: Lymphocyte surface characteristics in malignant lymphomas. Ann. J. Med. *58*, 300 (1975).
2. Aiuti, F.: Identification, enumeration and isolation of B and T lymphocytes from human peripheral blood. Report of W.H.O. I.A.R.C., sponsored Workshop on human B and T cells. Scand. J. Immunol. *3*, 521 (1974) (London 15–17 July 1974).
3. Belpomme, D., Dantchev, D., Joseph, R., Santoro, A., Feuilhade de Chauvin, F., Grandjon, D., Mathe, G.: Cell membrane markers of T and B lymphocytes and monocytes in leukemias and hematosarcomas. In: Biological Characterization of Human Tumors. Amsterdam: Excerpta Medica ICS 375 1976, P. 298.
4. Belpomme, D., Dantchev, D., Joseph, R., Santoro, A., Feuilhade de Chauvin, F., Lelarge, N., Grandjon, D., Pontvert, D., Mathe, G.: Classification of leukemias and hematosarcomas based on cell membrane markers and scanning electron microscopy. In: Clinical Tumor Immunology. Wybran, J. (ed.) Oxford and New York: Pergamon Press, 1976, p. 131.
5. Belpomme, D., Lelarge, N., Feuilhade de Chauvin, F., Joseph, R., Mathe, G.: An immunological classification of leukemias and hematosarcomas based on cell membrane markers with special reference to null-cell disorders. In: Lymphocytes, Macrophages and Cancer. Mathé, G., Florentin, I., Simmler, M. C., (eds.) Heidelberg New York: Springer-Verlag, 1976c, p. 98.
6. Belpomme, D., Dantchev, D., Karima, A. M., Lelarge, N., Joseph, R., Caillou, B., Lafleur, N., Mathé, G.: Search for correlations between immunological and morphological criteria used to classify lymphoid leukemias and non-Hodgkin's hematosarcomas with special reference to scanning electron microscopy and T and B membrane markers. In "Lymphocytes, Macrophages and Cancer". Mathé, G., Florentin, I., Simmler, M. C., (eds.) Heidelberg New York: Springer-Verlag, 1976d, p. 131.
7. Belpomme, D., Lelarge, N., Joseph, R., Mathé, G.: An immunological classification of leukemias and hematosarcomas based on cell membrane markers with special reference to null cell disorders. Eur. J. Cancer *13*, 311 (1977a).

8. BELPOMME, D., MATHÉ, G., DAVIES, A. J. S.: Clinical significance and prognostic value of the T-B immunological classification of human primary acute lymphoid leukaemias. Lancet 1977b. I, 555.
9. BELPOMME, D., LELARGE, N., MATHÉ, G., Davies, A. J. S.: Etiological, clinical and prognostic significance of the T-B immunological classification of primary acute lymphoid leukaemias and non-Hodgkin's lymphomas. In: "Immunological Diagnosis of Leukemias and Lymphomas". THIERFELDER, S., RODT, H., THIEL, E. (eds.). Heidelberg New York: Springer-Verlag 1977c, p. 33.
10. BELPOMME, D., MATHÉ, G., DAVIES, A. J. S.: Prognostic value of the T-B immunological classification of human primary acute lymphoid leukaemias: a further report (in preparation).
11. BELPOMME, D., CAILLOU, B., AMAR, H., LELARGE, N., GEREARD MARCHANT, R., FLAMANT, R., RAPPAPORT, H., DAVIES, A. J. S., MATHÉ, G.: A T-B immunological classification of non-Hodgkin's lymphomas: its clinical significance, prognostic value and relationship with other classifications. (To be published).
12. BENNETT, M. H., FARRER-BROWN, G., HENRY, K., JELIFFE, A. M.: Classification of non-Hodgkin's lymphomas. Lancet 1974 I, 1295.
13. BLOOMFIELD, C. D., KERSEY, J., BRUMMING, R. D., GAJL-PECZALSKA, K.: Prognostic significance of lymphocyte surface markers in adult non-Hodgkin's malignant lymphomas. Lancet 1976 II, 1330.
14. BRAYLAN, R. G., JOFFE, E. S. BERARD, C. W.: Malignant lymphomas Current classification and new observations SOMMERS, S. C. (ed.) In: Pathology Annual. New York: Appleton Century Crofts, 1975 p. 213.
15. BROUET, J. C., LABAUME, S., SELIGMAN, M.: Evaluation of T and B lymphocyte membrane markers in human non-Hodgkin malignant lymphomata. Br. J. Cancer *31*, 121 (1975).
16. BROUET, J. C., PREUD'HOMME, J. L., FLANDRIN, G., CHELLOUL, N. SELIGMAN, M.: Membrane markers in "Histiocytic" lymphomas (Reticulin cell sarcomas). J. Natl. Cancer Inst. *56*, 631 (1976).
17. DORFMAN, R. F.: The non-Hodgkin's lymphomas. In: "The Reticulo-Endothelial System". REBUCK, J. W., BERARD, C. W., ABELL, M. R., (eds.) Baltimore: Williams and Wilkins 1975, p. 262.
18. GAJL-PECZALSKA, J., BLOOMFIELD, C. D., COCCIA, P. F., SOSIN, H., BRUNNING, R. D., KERSEY, J. H.: B and T cell lymphomas analysis of blood and lympho-nodes in 87 patients. Am J. Med. *59*, 674 (1975).
19. GROSS, L.: Effect of thymectomy on development of leukemia in CH mice inoculated with "passage" virus. Proc. Soc. Exp. Biol. *100*, 325 (1959).
20. JAFFE, E. S., SHEVACH, E. M., FRANK, M. M., VERAUD, C. W., GREEN, I.: Nodular lymphoma: evidence for origin from follicular B-lymphocytes. N. Engl. J. Med. *290*, 813 (1974).
21. KAPLAN, J., MASTRANGELO, R., PETERSON, W. D.: Childhood lymphoblastic lymphoma, a cancer of thymus-derived lymphocytes. Cancer Res. *34*, 521 (1974).
22. KERSEY, J., NESBIT, M., HALLGRER, H., SABAD, A., YUNIS, E., GAJL-PECZALSKA, K.: Evidence for origin of certain childhood acute lymphoblastic leukemias and lymphomas in thymus derived lymphocytes. Cancer *36*, 1348 (1975).
23. LENNERT, K., STEIN, H., KAISERLING, E.: Cytological and functional criteria for the classification of malignant lymphoma. Br. J. Cancer *31*, suppl. 2, 29 (1975).
24. LENNERT, K., MOHRI, N., STEIN, H., KAISERLING, E.: The histopathology of malignant lymphoma. Br. J. Haematol. *31*, 193 (1975b).
25. LOISILIER, J., BURTIN, P., BELPOMME, D., et al.: Characterization of lymphoid cells by an anti.T heteroserum. (In preparation).
26. LUKES, R. J., COLLINS, R. D.: Immunologic characterization of human malignant lymphomas. Cancer *34*, 1488 (1974).
27. LUKES, R. J., COLLINS,R. D.: A functional classification of malignant lymphomas. In: "The Reticulo-Endothelial System." REBUCK, J. W., BERARD, C. W., ABELL, M. R. (eds.) Baltimore: Williams and Wilkins 1975, p. 213.
28. LUTZNER, M., EDELSON, R., SCHEIN, P., GREEN, I., KIRKPATRICK, C., AHMED, A.: Cutaneous T-cell lymphomas: the Sezary syndrome mycosis fungoïdes and related disorders. Ann. Intern. Med. *83*, 534 (1975).
29. MANN, R. B., JAFFE, E. S., BRAYLAN, R. C., EGGLASTON, J. C., RANSOM, L., KIZE, H., BERARD, C. W.: Immunologic and morphologic studies of T-cell lymphoma. Am. J. Med. *58*, 307 (1975).
30. MATHÉ, G. BELPOMME, D.: T and B lymphocytic nature of leukemias and lymphosarcomas: a new but still uncertain parameter for their classification. Biomedicine *20*, 81 (1974).
31. MATHÉ, G., BELPOMME, D., DANTCHEV, D., POUILLART, P.; Progress in the classification of lymphoid and/or monocytoid leukemias and of lympho- and reticulosarcomas (non Hodgkin's lymphomas). Biomedicine *22*, 177 (1975).
32. MATHÉ, G., BELPOMME, D., DANTCHEV, D., POUILLART, P., SCHLUMBERGER, J. R. LAFLEUR, M.: Leukemic lymphosarcomas: respective prognosis of the three types: prolymphocytic, lymphoblastic and immunoblastic. Blood Cells *1*, 25 (1975b).
33. MATHÉ, G., BELPOMME, D., DANTCHEV, D., KHALIL, A., AFIFI, A. M., TALEB, N., POUILLART, P., SCHWARZENBERG, L., HAYAT, M., DE VASSAL, F., JASMIN, C., MISSET, J. L., MUSSER, M.: Immunoblastic lymphosarcomas: A cytological and clinical entity? Biomedicine *22*, 473 (1975c).

34. MATHÉ, G., RAPPAPORT, H., O'CONNOR, G. T., TORLONI, H.: Histological and cytological typing of neoplastic diseases of haematopoietic and lymphoid tissues. World Health Organization, Geneva, 1976.
35. MICHEAU, C., BELPOMME, D.: Comparision between membrane markers and enzyme markers in 26 cases of non-Hodgkin's malignant lymphomas. (In the same volume).
36. NATHWANI, B. N., KIM, H., RAPPAPORT, H.: Malignant lymphoma, lymphoblastic. Cancer *38*, 964 (1976).
37. PETER, C. R., MACKENZIE, M. R., GLASSY, F. J.: T or B cell origin of some non-Hodgkin's lymphomas. Lancet 1974 II, 686.
38. RAPPAPORT, H.: Tumors of the hematopoietic systems. In: Atlas of Tumor Pathology. Section 3, Fasc. 8, Washington: Armed Forces Institute Pathology 1966.
39. RAPPAPORT, H., WINTER, W. J., HICKS, E. B.: Follicular lymphoma A reevaluation of its position in the scheme of malignant lymphoma, based on a survey of 253 cases. Cancer *9*, 792 (1956).
40. SCHEDAL, I., FINK, P. C., BODENBERGER, H., DEICHER, H.: Monoclonal lymphoid cell surface immunoglobulins with tumor specific determinant in lymphosarcoma. Clin. Immunol. Immunopathol. *5*, 74 (1976).
41. SMITH, J. L., BARKER, C. R., KLEIN, G. P., COLLINS, R. D.: Characterization of malignant mediastinal lymphoid neoplasm (Sternberg Sarcoma) as thymic in origin. Lancet 1973 I, 74.
42. STATHOPOULOS, G., DAVIES, A. J. S., PAPAMICHAIL, M., HOLBOROW, E. J., WITSHAW, E.: Origin of malignant cells in lymphoma apparently originating in anterior mediatinum. Lancet 1974 I, 927.
43. STEIN, H., LENNERT, K., PARWARESCH, M. R.: Malignant lymphomas of a cell type. Lancet 1972 II, 855.
44. STERNBERG, C.: Leukosarcomatose und myeloblastenleokämie. Br. Pathol. *61*, 75 (1916).
45. W.H.O./International union of immunological societies: Immunological diagnosis of leukemia and lymphoma. Technical Report. BELPOMME, D., BORELLA, L., BRAYLAN, R., GREAVES, M., HERBERMAN, R., HITZIG, W., KERSEY, J., PETROV, R., RITTS, R., SELIGMAN, M., SOBIN, L., THIERFELDER, S., TORRIGIANI, G. Report of a Meeting Held in Munich, Oct. 31, 1976. Br. J. Haematol. (To be published).

Demonstration of Immunoglobulin Production by Tumor Cells in Non-Hodgkin's and Hodgkin's Malignant Lymphomas and Its Significance for Their Classification[1]

H. STEIN, C. S. PAPADIMITRIOU, H. BOUMAN, K. LENNERT, and J. FUCHS[2]

Introduction

A tumor classification should be both reliable and reproducible. Each type of tumor differentiated by the classification should be uniform in cellular origin and clinical, pathoanatomic, prognostic, and therapeutic features. Since it has become obvious that a lymphoma classification based on morphology alone does not fulfill all of these criteria, we attempted to elucidate the cellular origin of lymphatic neoplasms by means of a combined investigation of morphologic properties and immunologic characteristics. On the basis of these studies, we revised the current concepts for classifying non-Hodgkin's lymphomas. This revised concept was called the Kiel classification [12]. Table 1 presents the latest revision of the Kiel classification. In this paper, we shall describe the most common immunoglobulin-(Ig-) producing lymphoma types of the Kiel classification and the most important immunochemical and immunologic findings that led to the differentiation of these entities. We shall also present some recent immunohistochemical findings in Hodgin's lymphomas. In contrast to non-Hodgkin's lymphomas, which are usually monoclonal proliferations from the beginning, or at least from the time of first biopsy, our findings provide evidence that Hodgin's disease is a primary, polyclonal B-cell proliferation that tends to develop into a monoclonal neoplasm.

Material and Methods

Determination of Ig in the Tissue Extracts of Biopsies and in Sera

Lyophilized biopsy tissue was suspended in saline and homogenized with a micropotter. The homogenate was centrifuged at 105,000 *g* for 1 h. The supernatant was completely pipetted off. In the present study, this saline supernatant was not used for Ig assays. The pellet was resuspended with a saline Tris buffer containing 0.5% NP40 (Nonidet P40, Shell Co., United States) and 0.5% sodium deoxycholate, homogenized, and centrifuged at 105,000 g for 1 h. The resulting supernatant was examined for its concentration of IgM, IgG, IgA, and albumin by radial immunodiffusion using Hyland low-level immunoplates (Hyland, United States). The Ig content of the tissue extracts was expressed as a ratio of IU Ig/mg albumin. The Ig concentration of the sera was also measured with radial immunodiffusion.

Isoelectric Focusing (IEF)

IEF was performed on polyacrylamide plates as described by KARLSON et al. [18]. The IgM was rendered suitable for IEF by reducing it to a monomer and introducing carboxymethyl groups

1 This work was supported by the Deutsche Forschungsgemeinschaft SFB 111/C3, C7, D2.
2 In collaboration with the "Kiel Lymphoma Study Group".

Table 1. Kiel classification of non-Hodgkin's lymphomas

Low-grade malignancy	High-grade malignancy
ML lymphocytic	ML centroblastic
B-CLL	primary
T-CLL	secondary
Prolymphocytic leukemia (B or T)	
Hairy-cell leukemia	ML lymphoblastic
Mycosis fungoides and Sézary's syndrome	B-lymphoblastic, Burkitt type and others
T-zone lymphoma	T-lymphoblastic, convoluted-cell type and others
ML lymphoplasmacytic/-cytoid (LP immunocytoma)	Unclassified
	ML immunoblastic (B, T, or unqualified)
ML plasmacytic (plasmacytoma)	
ML centrocytic	
ML centroblastic/centrocytic	
follicular	
follicular and diffuse	
diffuse	
with or without sclerosis	

ML: malignant lymphoma.

into the molecule [4]. The whole extracts and sera were applied to the plates. After the run, the IgM fraction was made visible by incubating the plates with ^{125}iodine-labeled pure anti-IgM antibodies prepared by affinity chromatography.

Surface Ig (SIg)

Surface Ig was demonstrated on viable suspended cells using either horseradish peroxidase-coupled or fluorescein-coupled anti-Ig antibodies in the direct procedure as formerly described [34, 35, 44].

Cytoplasmic Ig (CIg)

In a few cases, we demonstrated CIg in cytocentrifuge slides of fixed washed cells by means of fluorescein-coupled anti-Ig antibodies as described by Vossen [44]. In a larger series, CIg was demonstrated on paraffin sections using the enzyme-bridge method of Sternberger et al. [40] as modified by Taylor [41].

Complement Receptors

Complement receptors were demonstrated using trypsinized sheep erythrocytes (E) coated with IgM antibodies (A) and whole complement (C) components. To specify the two complement receptor subtypes, EAC_{3b} was prepared according to the method of Borsos and Rapp [3], using functionally pure complement components (Cordis, United States). EAC_{3b} was converted into EAC_{3d} by incubating EAC_{3b} in purified C_3 inactivator (Cordis, United States). EAC_{3b} was used only when it showed strong hemagglutination with human erythrocytes. EAC_{3d} was applied only when it was completely immune adherence-negative with human erthrocytes but strongly positive with germinal center cells. The binding of EAC intermediates was demonstrated on frozen sections and on suspended cells in the form of rosettes.

Results and Discussion

Quantitative determination of Ig in extracts of 179 lymphoma biopsies and corresponding sera revealed an overall increase in Ig in 63% of cases, whereas the serum Ig level was increased in 6.1% (Fig. 1). The increased Ig class was mostly IgM. The rate of Ig increase varied from just significant to 80-fold above the normal range. In comparison, the highest increase in serum Ig was only up to ten times above the normal mean.

To determine what kind of morphology is combined with a high tissue and/or serum Ig level, we compared the tissue and serum Ig values with the cytology of the lymphomas. During this study, we observed no correlation between morphology and serum Ig, but we did find a rather good correlation between morphology and tissue IgM (Fig. 1).

Lymphoplasmacytoid Immunocytoma (LP Immunocytoma) and Chronic Lymphocytic Leukemia (CLL)

The most frequently and the most highly increased tissue IgM values were found in a lymphoma group [20, 21, 33, 38, 39] which, until recently, was not present in other classification schemes of human lymphomas but did appear under classifications of murine lymphomas [26, 27]. This lymphoma group is characterized by proliferation of small lymphoid cells (lymphocytes and/or

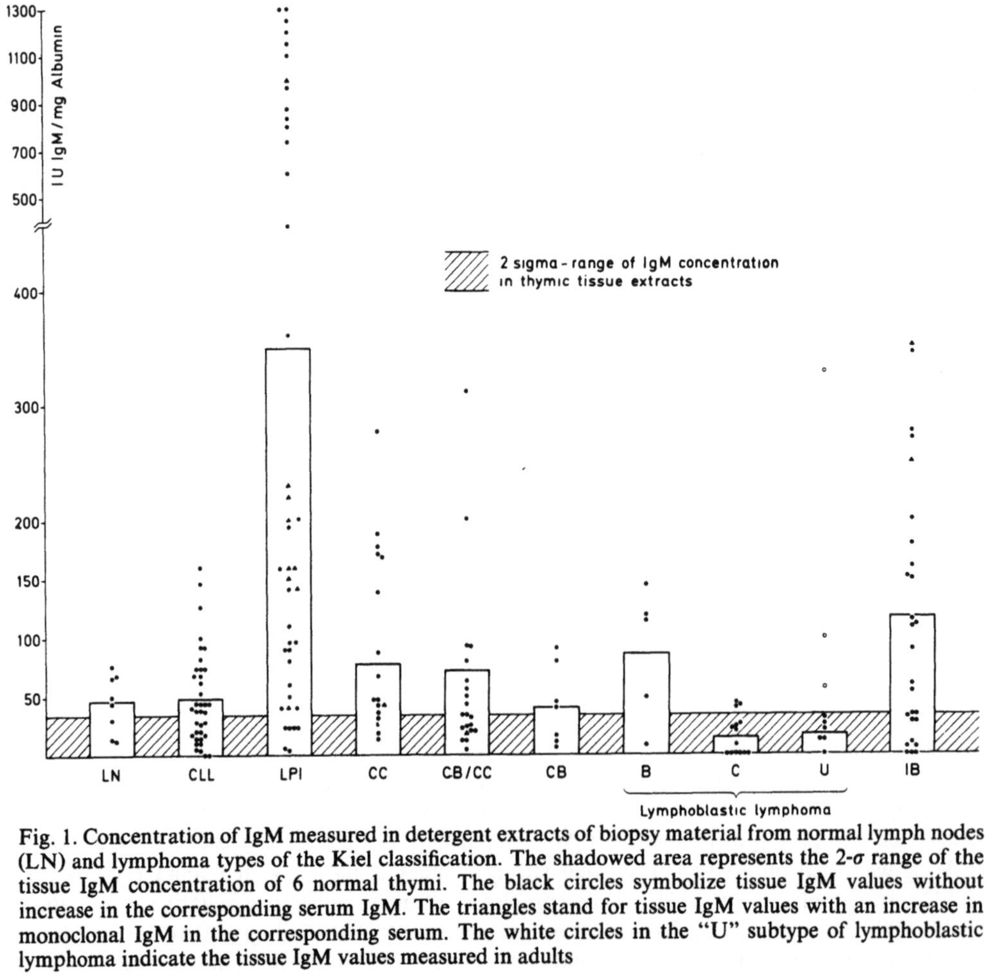

Fig. 1. Concentration of IgM measured in detergent extracts of biopsy material from normal lymph nodes (LN) and lymphoma types of the Kiel classification. The shadowed area represents the 2-σ range of the tissue IgM concentration of 6 normal thymi. The black circles symbolize tissue IgM values without increase in the corresponding serum IgM. The triangles stand for tissue IgM values with an increase in monoclonal IgM in the corresponding serum. The white circles in the "U" subtype of lymphoblastic lymphoma indicate the tissue IgM values measured in adults

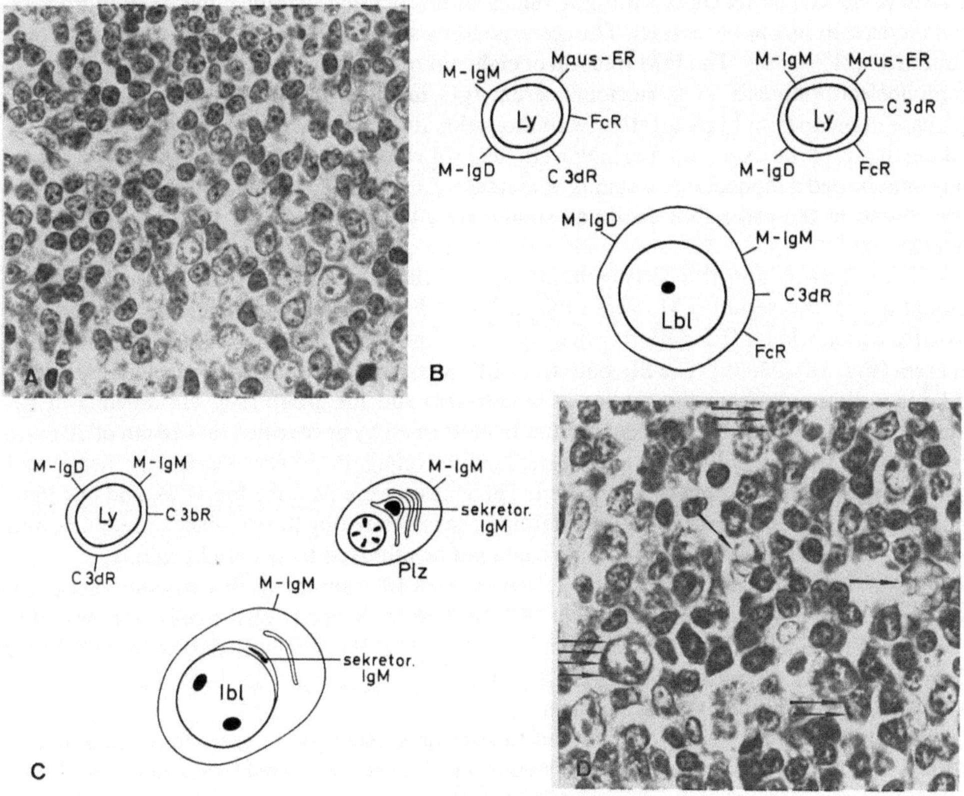

Fig. 2. (A) Histologic picture of B-CLL. This neoplasm consists of lymphocytes, which predominate in number, and larger cells. The latter are morphologically clearly different from immunoblasts and centroblasts (= large, noncleaved germinal center cell). They are called lymphoblasts by LENNERT. Giemsa's stain (× 840);
(B) Schematic drawing of the cells which proliferate in B-CLL and their most frequent surface markers. Ly: lymphocyte; Lbl: lymphoblast; M-IgM (M-IgD): membrane-bound IgM (IgD); Maus-ER: receptor for mouse erythrocytes; FcR: receptor for the Fc part of IgG; C3dR: receptor for the complement fragment C3d;
(C) Schematic drawing of the cells which proliferate in lymphoplasmacytoid immunocytoma and their most frequent functional parameters. Ly: lymphocyte; Ibl: immunoblast; Plz: plasma cell; sekretor. IgM: secretory IgM;
(D) Histologic picture of lymphoplasmacytoid immunocytoma. 1 arrow: Russell body-like material; 2 arrows: plasma cell; 3 arrows: plasmablast; 4 arrows: immunoblast; lymphocytes not marked. Giemsa's stain. (× 840)

centrocytes), lymphocytes, blasts (immunoblast-like and/or centroblast[1]-like cells), plasmablasts and/or plasmacytoid cells (Fig. 2D). Russell body-like material is often present and therefore of diagnostic significance. This is especially valid for PAS globules located in the nucleus. Because of the cellular composition described, we proposed the term lymphoplasmacytoid lymphoma, and LP immunocytoma for short, for this lymphoma group [20, 21, 38]. In contrast, CLL lymphoma tissue is composed of lymphocytes and a few larger cells, but real immunoblasts, plasmablasts, and plasmacytoid cells are lacking (Fig 2A).

As Fig. 1 illustrates, IgM was significantly increased in 37 out of 43 cases (86%). In two cases, IgM was increased together with IgA, in one case together with IgG, and in yet another case with IgA and IgG. In 15 (35%) cases, the IgM values were 20–80 times higher than the mean

1 Proposed term for the large, noncleaved germinal center cell.

thymic value. Of the six cases with IgM values within the thymic range, two showed a 15–18-fold increase in IgA in the extract. The corresponding serum IgM values were increased in only 7 out of 43 (21%) cases. The IgM fraction of eight out of nine cases proved to be monoclonal in immunoelectrophoresis. A monoclonal serum IgG increase was not found in any case; an increase in monoclonal IgA together with monoclonal IgM occurred in one case.

Interestingly, of the cases with the highest tissue IgM values (about 20–80 times above normal), only one showed a monoclonal serum IgM increase. All other eight increased serum IgM values were found in the cases that exhibited significantly but not markedly increased tissue IgM values (Fig. 1).

The tissue extracts and the corresponding sera of 18 cases with increased tissue IgM, but normal or reduced serum IgM, were subjected to IEF. The tissue IgM from all but one case revealed a monoclonal IEF pattern, whereas the serum IgM pattern was of monoclonal type in all cases (Fig. 3B) [33, 39]. The SIg pattern of LP immunocytoma with a monoclonal serum Ig spike is well-known from the studies of SELIGMANN and his group [30]. SIg labeling of LP immunocytomas without monoclonal serum Ig performed by us revealed that 18 out of 20 cases were positive using a polyvalent anti-Ig-rhodamine conjugate. In seven cases, the heavy and light chain type of the SIg was determined. Three cases were positive for μ-, δ-, and one light chain type. Four cases showed a mixed staining characterized by the presence of μ-, γ-, λ-, and κ-chains. In one case, the mixed staining could not be removed by overnight culture.

Using two-color fluorescence, we studied three cases of LP immunocytoma without a serum Ig spike for the simultaneous occurrence of SIg and CIg. A majority of the cells from all three cases bore SIgM, whereas CIgM was found in only 4–20% of the cells. Some, but not all, of the CIg-positive cells were also positive for SIg. The light chain types on the surface and in the cytoplasm were identical in all three cases.

Application of the enzyme-bridge method to paraffin sections of 43 cases in order to detect intracytoplasmic light chains provided results in 27 cases that could be evaluated. In 18

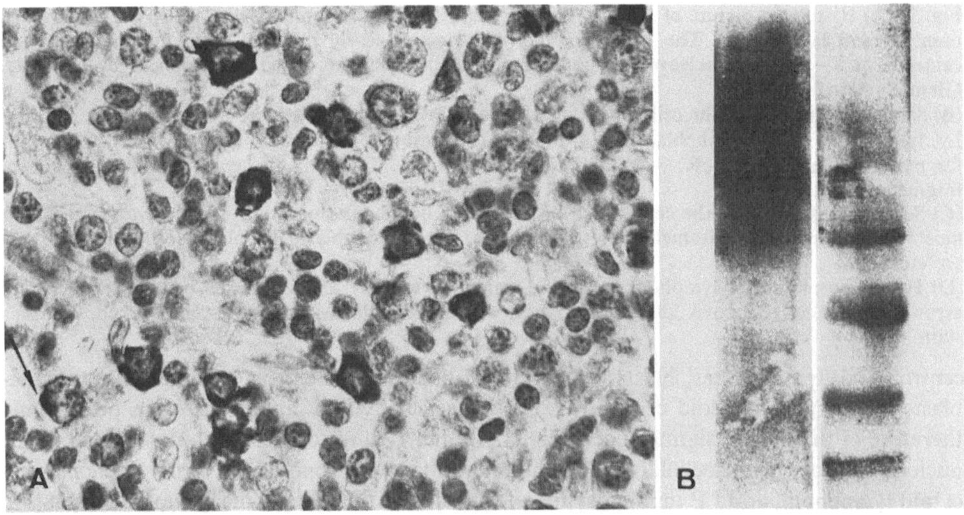

Fig. 3. (A) Paraffin section of a lymphoplasmacytoid immunocytoma immunostained for λ. Many positively immunostained lymphoplasmacytoid cells are scattered between the lymphocytes. Arrow = positively stained blast. A similar immunostaining was achieved with anti-IgM serum, whereas anti-κ, anti-IgG, and anti-IgA sera did not stain tumor cells but only some reactive plasma cells that were near or in the capsule of the lymph node. Counterstain hematoxylin. (× 840);

(B) Autoradiograph of reduced and carboxymethylated isoelectrofocused IgM. On the left, homogenate from a hyperplastic tonsil. On the right, homogenate from biopsy material of lymphoplasmacytoid immunocytoma cases, the enzyme-bridge staining revealed a clear predominance of plasmacytoid cells and/or PAS-positive globules reacting for one light chain type (Fig. 3A). In nine cases, plasmacytoid cells that were positive for κ- or λ- chains were found in approximately equal numbers, suggesting their reactive nature. In seven cases, the κ- and λ-positive plasmacytoid cells stained predominantly positive for γ-chains. These cases apparently do not represent LP immunocytoma, but are CLL cases with a marked infiltration by reactive plasma cells. However, in two of the λ- and κ-positive cases, the tumor cells stained unquivocally positive for μ-, λ-, and κ-chains. The tissue extract of one of these cases was subjected to IEF. The fraction with μ- chain antigenicity exhibited a monoclonal pattern. Unfortunately, we have not as yet developed this IEF plate with an anti-κ or anti-λ serum.

From the data presented we conclude that:

1. Lymphomas with lymphoplasmacytoid cytology are distinguished from other non-Hodgkin's lymphomas by a particularly large amount of monoclonal tissue Ig in the extract, indicating a high rate of Ig synthesis in most cases.

2. Demonstration of Ig by means of labeled anti-Ig antibodies revealed special immunologic conditions that are not found in other non-Hodgkin's lymphomas except Waldenström's macroglobulinemia. In LP immunocytoma, three groups of differently labeled cells were detected: 1) cells positive for SIg but negative for CIg, 2) cells positive for SIg and CIg, and 3) cells negative for SIg but positive for CIg.

SIg is not destined for secretion; it remains fixed to the cell membrane as a receptor molecule. Functionally, SIg is therefore nonsecretory Ig. In contrast, CIg is destined for secretion and is therefore called secretory Ig. Accordingly, the corresponding producer cells are called nonsecretory and secretory B cells, respectively. Applying this functional terminology, LP immunocytoma is defined as a proliferation of both nonsecretory and secretory B cells. In contrast, B-CLL in every case, centrocytic lymphoma, centroblastic/centrocytic lymphoma, centroblastic lymphoma, and lymphoblastic lymphoma of Burkitt's type are, as a rule, proliferations of nonsecretory B cells, while plasmacytoma is a purebred proliferation of secretory B cells.

3. Because of the presence of secretory B cells in LP immunocytoma, one would expect the serum—as in plasmacytoma—to reveal an increase in the same Ig class as that detected in the cytoplasm. However, only approximately 20% of the cases revealed a serum Ig spike indicating that the secretory mechanism of the secretory cells (plasmacytoid cells) is blocked in a majority of cases. This explains why large amounts of Russell body-like material occur in many lymphomas without changes in the serum Ig level.

There is, however, no fundamental difference between LP immunocytoma with and that without a serum Ig spike. When the serum Ig spike is of the IgM class, the neoplasm is identical with Waldenström's macroglobulinemia. In other words, Waldenström's macroglobulinemia is a minor variant of LP immunocytoma that produces IgM and is capable of releasing the produced IgM into the blood. Considering these findings, it appears to us to be justifiable to regard LP immunocytoma as an entity and to separate it from other lymphoma types, especially from B-CLL.

Table 2 and Figure 2 summarize the morphologic and immunologic findings in CLL and LP immunocytoma. To make a clear distinction, we prefer to define B-CLL as a purebred proliferation of CIg-negative, nonsecretory B cells that do not—in contrast to LP immunocytoma—transform into plasma cells. Accordingly, all CLL cases with intracytoplasmic inclusions in the form of globules or crystals described in the literature are actually LP immunocytomas, since these cytoplasmic inclusions represent secretory Ig as revealed by their envelope of ergastoplasm and their reactivity with anti-Ig sera. After removal of all cases with intracytoplasmic inclusions, our CLL series showed no cases with a monoclonal serum Ig increase.

LP immunocytoma and CLL differ not only in cellular composition and absence or presence of CIg but also in the expression of complement receptor subtypes. Whereas a vast majority of B-

Table 2. Morphologic and immunologic differences between CLL and LP immunocytoma

	CLL	LP immunocytoma
Proliferating cells		
Lymphocytes	+	+
Immunoblasts	+ (atypical)	+ (or centroblasts)
Plasmablasts	−	+
Plasmacytoid cells	−	+
Cells containing PAS+ globular inclusions	−	+
Cells containing ergastoplasm	−	+
Surface Ig	+	+
Cytoplasmic Ig	−	+
Tissue Ig	slightly ↑	greatly ↑
Monoclonal serum Ig	−	+ in 20% of cases
C 3b receptors	−	+
C 3d receptors	+	+

CLL cases bore only the receptor for C_{3d} [28, 29], the nonsecretory cells of LP immunocytoma carried a receptor for C_{3b} and C_{3d} in 9 out of 13 cases and a receptor for C_{3b} alone in 1 out of 13 cases. Four cases did not express any complement receptors. From reactive lymphatic cells present in peripheral lymphatic tissue, we could demonstrate receptors for both C_{3b} and C_{3d} on the germinal center cells including the cells of the follicle mantle. The B cells between the germinal centers (interfollicular area) carried merely a receptor for C_{3b} in most instances or no complement receptors at all in some instances. That means germinal center cells are characterized by the presence of the receptors for both C_{3b} and C_{3d}. The B cells of the interfollicular area, of which a majority belong to the plasma cell reaction cell series, often possess a receptor for C_{3b}. These findings suggest that LP immununocytoma cells originate from a B-subset different from that from which CLL cells are derived. Regarding this, LP immunocytoma seems to be closely related to the cell series of the two antigen-induced B-cell reactions, viz.: the germinal center cell reaction, and less frequently, the plasma cell reaction. In contrast, CLL apparently originates from a B cell of an early differential or maturation stage in which it has not yet had contact with an antigen.

There are also differences between LP immunocytoma and CLL in clinical behavior. The most important differences, found in a retrospective study [31], are listed in Table 3. So-called B-symptoms as well as joint pain and Coombs-positive anemia occurred more often in LP immunocytoma than in CLL. In CLL, the absolute and relative blood counts were more frequently and more highly increased.

At the time of diagnosis, the bone marrow was infiltrated in all cases of B-CLL, whereas only 70% of the cases of LP immunocytoma showed bone marrow infiltration. It appears likely that CLL cells either primarily originate in the bone marrow or infiltrate the bone marrow

Table 3. Clinical differences between CLL and LP immunocytoma

	CLL % (n)	LP immunocytoma % (n)
Fever	19.2 (52)	42 (80)
Weakness, poor physical condition	55 (66)	71 (80)
No appetite, loss of weight	26.3 (38)	48 (80)
Joint pain	12.5 (56)	35 (80)
Coombs-positive hemolytic anemia	Seldom	Sometimes
Increase in peripheral blood lymphocytes >20,000/µl	50 (65)	7.8 (76)
Bone marrow involved at time of diagnosis	100 (52)	70 (80)
Primary extranodal development of tumor	Seldom or never	Sometimes

immediately after their genesis in lymphatic tissue outside the bone marrow. In other words, the B-CLL cell has a great homing propensity toward bone marrow. In contrast, LP immunocytoma cells unusually seem to originate primarily in lymph nodes, or in some instances, only in the spleen [31, 43]. Sometimes, LP immunocytoma originates extranodally, for instance as a solitary lesion in the eye or its region, the skin, lung, intestine, brain, muscles, etc. [31]. We have evidence that LP immunocytoma is by far the most common lymphoma to arise outside the well-organized lymphatic tissue. For survival data, see BRITTINGER et al. in this volume.

Germinal Center Cell Tumors

In the Kiel classification, we distinguish between three subtypes of germinal center cell lymphomas.

1. A germinal center cell lymphoma that imitates the germinal center structure and even retains its cytologic spectrum, i.e., the large germinal center cell (centroblast) and the small germinal center cell (centrocyte) proliferate in a follicular growth pattern (Fig. 4A). Since the cytologic composition of follicular lymphoma proved to be constant, in contrast to the follicular growth pattern (transitions from follicular to diffuse pattern occur; in approximately 5% of the cases the follicular growth pattern is primarily missing), the term centroblastic/centrocytic lymphoma was proposed [12, 20]. A further reason for our proposal of a cytologically based term is that there are two other germinal center cell-derived lymphoma types (described below) that also sometimes show a follicular growth pattern,
2. A germinal center cell lymphoma that shows, with rare exceptions, a diffuse growth pattern and consists of a purebred proliferation of the small germinal center cells (centrocytes) (Fig. 4D); thus, the term centrocytic lymphoma.
3. A germinal center cell lymphoma that shows either a follicular or a diffuse growth pattern. The main proliferating cells resemble the large germinal center cell (Fig. 4C); thus, the term centroblastic lymphoma.

These three germinal center cell-derived lymphomas differ in clinical signs and prognosis. Survival data are given by BRITTINGER et al. in this volume.

Centroblastic/Centrocytic Lymphoma (CB/CC)

The mean tissue IgM value of 21 CB/CC cases was relatively, but significantly, higher than that of normal thymi and also higher than that of CLL (Fig 1). This indicates that the Ig synthesis of CB/CC is not very high in most cases. However, in two cases, the IgM concentration of the tissue extract was 20 times higher than that measured in the thymus. Many cells from these two cases contained PAS-positive Russell body-like material, indicating synthesis of secretory IgM. In the sera of all but one of the 21 cases, no monoclonal serum Ig increase was found.

The SIg analysis we performed showed SIg on most of the cells of all 15 CB/CC cases. IgM was the predominant heavy chain class. Recently, we investigated two cases for the simultaneous presence of IgM and IgD by means of two-color fluorescence. In the one case, IgD was present on 40% and in the other on 90% of the cells bearing IgM. The cells of infantile tonsils, which are rich in germinal centers, also exhibited IgM and IgD in a high percentage.

In contrast to LEECH et al. [19] we observed in many cases a mixed staining for light chains on freshly drawn cells. After overnight culture, the staining for one light chain predominated in all cases studied. The staining of fixed smears of CB/CC cells with fluorescein-labeled antibodies revealed in most cases only occasional cells whose cytoplasm reacted positively for the same heavy and light chains as detected on the surface. However, cases with many CIg-positive tumor cells showed that the CB/CC cells can undergo transformation from nonsecretory

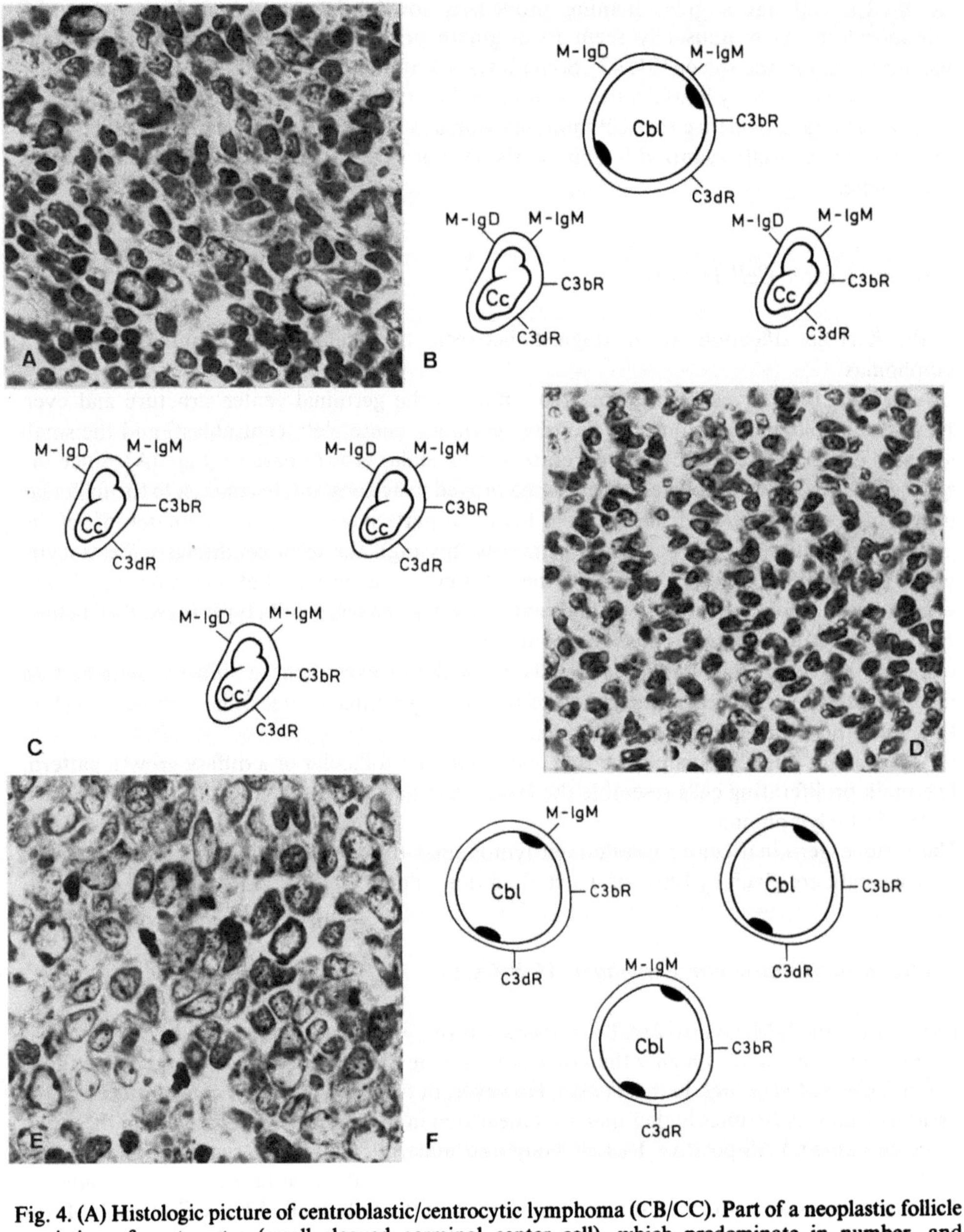

Fig. 4. (A) Histologic picture of centroblastic/centrocytic lymphoma (CB/CC). Part of a neoplastic follicle consisting of centrocytes (small cleaved germinal center cell), which predominate in number, and centroblasts (large noncleaved germinal center cell). At the lower margin, follicular mantle lymphocytes. Giemsa stain. (× 840);

(B) Schematic drawing of the cells that predominantly proliferate in CB/CC and their characteristic surface markers. Cbl: centroblast; Cc: centrocyte; M-IgM (M-IgD): membrane-bound IgM (IgD); C3bR (C3dR): receptor for the complement fragment C3b (C3d);

(C) Schematic drawing of the cells that proliferate in centrocytic lymphoma (CC) and their characteristic surface markers;

(D) Histologic picture of CC. Note the purebred proliferation of small cleaved cells resembling reactive centrocytes. Centroblasts are absent. Giemsa stain. (× 840);

(E) Histologic picture of centroblastic lymphoma (CB). The tumor consists of a nearly purebred proliferation of large noncleaved cells with marginally located nuclei, similar to reactive centroblasts. Only a few centrocytes are scattered among the neoplastic centroblasts;

differentiation to secretory differentiation. These are borderline cases to LP immunocytoma. Although Ig assays proved the B-cell nature of typical follicular lymphoma, they were not able to yield decisive evidence as to whether follicular lymphomas develop unrelated to germinal center cells or whether follicular lymphomas are the neoplastic equivalents of germinal center structures. In this context, complement receptor studies have especially provided evidence for the latter concept. JAFFE et al. [14] found six cases and we observed 15 out of 16 cases [32] in which the cells of the neoplastic nodules expressed complement receptors like the cells of reactive germinal centers. Recently, we were able to demonstrate that the cells of neoplastic nodules of seven cases bore both complement receptor subtypes, i.e., receptors for C_{3b} and C_{3d}. Reactive germinal center cells were also found to carry both complement receptor subtypes [33]. Thus, there is complete congruence in the expression of complement receptor subtypes between follicular lymphoma cells and the cells of reactive germinal centers.

Centrocytic Lymphoma (CC)

As Figure 1 shows, the mean tissue IgM content of 16 cases was significantly higher than that found in CLL, CB/CC, and lymphoblastic lymphoma other than Burkitt's type, lower than that of LP immunocytoma and immunoblastic lymphoma, and as high as in lymphoblastic lymphoma of Burkitt's type. Regarding the single values, 13 out of 16 cases revealed a significant Ig increase and six showed a particularly high increase. With one exception, the serum IgM fraction consisted of monoclonal IgM/κ but was not increased above the normal range.

In our experiments, SIg was present in a high percentage of the cells of all cases of CC. The predominant heavy chain class was IgM, followed by IgD. In addition to μ-chains, γ-chains were detected in 4 out of 12 cases. Labeling for light chains did not provide clear-cut results, since the cells from 5 out of 14 cases stained for both light chain types. Overnight culture performed in two cases removed the stainability of the surface membrane for one light chain, indicating that the mixed staining pattern on freshly drawn cells was due to passively absorbed Ig. The staining for CIg in three representative cases of CC was completely negative, as demonstrated by labeling fixed cells of cytocentrifuge slides of washed suspended tumor cells with fluorescein-coupled anti-Ig antibodies. The cells of all nine cases studied carried complement receptors. In two cases, we specified the complement receptor subtypes. In both cases, most of the cells bore the C_{3b} and C_{3d} receptors, like reactive centrocytes. Thus, reactive centrocytes and centrocytic lymphoma cells correspond in morphology, the occurrence of SIg, and complement receptor subtypes, indicating a close relationship between these cells.

Centroblastic Lymphoma (CB)

Ig analysis of tissue extracts revealed a significant increase in four out of seven cases. The increased Ig class was always IgM. The mean IgM value of seven cases was relatively low but significantly higher than that of thymus (Fig. 1). The serum Ig levels of all cases studied were either within or below the normal range. Until now, we have had the opportunity to label only two cases for SIg. IgM was detected on the cells of one case and IgG on the cells of the other

---

Fig. 4 (continued)
(F) Schematic drawing of the cells that proliferate in centroblastic lymphoma (CB). As on reactive centroblasts, both complement receptor subtypes should be present on the neoplastic centroblasts. However, so far, we have demonstrated complement receptors only with EAC prepared with whole mouse serum as complement source in two out of four cases

case. In two out of the four cases investigated, EAC adhered to the frozen sections in a nodular pattern.

The immunologic data obtained are compatible with our view that this tumor type is closely related to reactive large germinal center cells (centroblasts) [20, 21, 32]. Our view was primarily based on the morphologic resemblance of centroblastic lymphoma cells to reactive centroblasts and on the observation of frequent transformation of CB/CC into CB [32]. The primary CB were formerly often classified as (large cell) lymphoblastic lymphoma, reticulum cell sarcoma, histiocytic lymphoma, or malignant lymphoma, undifferentiated, and the secondary CB as reticulosarcoma, histiocytic lymphoma, or more recently as large cell malignant lymphoma [6].

Lymphoblastic Lymphoma, Burkitt's Type

The Ig concentration was analyzed in five European cases; one case was EBV-positive with nuclear acid hybridization [2]. A significant increase in IgM was detected in four cases, three of which showed a great increase. In two cases analyzed, the light chain associated with μ-chains proved to be of κ-type. Thus, the tissue Ig assay results are consistent with those of SIg labeling reported by other authors. The results of both methods indicate that lymphomas with Burkitt's-type morphology are lymphomas of the B-cell type. In two out of three Burkitt's-type lymphomas, we detected complement receptors. The morphologic resemblance of Burkitt's and Burkitt's-type lymphoma cells with cells of germinal centers of an early developmental stage and the detection of C_{3d} receptors in all Burkitt's lymphomas and Burkitt's lymphoma-derived cell lines [45] suggest that lymphomas with Burkitt's-type morphology are neoplasms of a certain subtype of germinal center cells.

Lymphoblastic Lymphoma Other Than Burkitt's Type

Ig assays provided only little aid toward elucidating the nature of the lymphomas and leukemias comprised in this group. The markers that helped to classify acute lymphatic leukemia (ALL) cells are discussed by others in detail in this volume. Whether the data obtained for ALL can be fully transferred to nonleukemic lymphoblastic lymphoma remains to be determined. Data from other studies and our own investigations suggest, however, that the convoluted cell type of lymphoblastic lymphoma is usually identical with the immunologic T-type. The morphologically unclassified type of the Kiel classification seems to be highly heterogeneous. It probably includes the immunologically unqualified cases, some cases of T-type, as well as all common ALL antigen-positive cases and all B-types other than Burkitt's type.

Immunoblastic Lymphoma (IBL)

The most frequently increased and the most highly increased tissue Ig values, following those found in LP immunocytoma, were observed in the lymphoma group that is termed malignant lymphoma, histiocytic according to the Rappaport classification, reticulum cell sarcoma according to the former European classifications, and immunoblastic lymphoma according to the Kiel classification [12, 20, 21, 32, 33, 37]. As has been repeatedly stated [20, 21, 36, 38, 39], the IgM values of our tissue extraction studies were not consistent with the assumption that these lymphoma cells are of reticulocytic or histiocytic origin. Significantly increased amounts of Ig were detected in 16 out of 27 (59%) cases. The predominant Ig class was IgM. IgM was increased in eight cases alone, in two cases together with IgG, and in one case with IgA. Of four extracts studied, one contained significantly increased amounts of IgM and IgD. Eight cases in this series showed no increase in tissue Ig. The increase in tissue IgM in nearly 60% of the cases suggests Ig synthesis by the so-called reticulum sarcoma cells and thus their B-cell origin in more than half of the cases.

The B-cell nature of the so-called reticulum cell sarcoma was further substantiated by our SIg assay [33]. Cells from all but one of the six cases studied were SIg positive. IgM was predominant in four cases and IgG was the main Ig class in one case. The Ig staining was clearly restricted to one light chain type in three cases. We did not look for the presence of SIgD. MORRIS and DAVEY [23] studied a series of seven diffuse histiocytic lymphomas for the presence of SIg and found only one devoid of SIg. Other authors found a positive labeling for SIg in less than half of the cases they studied [6, 7].

The frequent objection that the increased amounts of Ig measured in the tissue extracts and the surface Ig detected were not produced by the tumor cells but might have been passively absorbed Ig (autoantibodies or immunocomplexes) had been refuted by our IEF studies [4, 33, 39]. The increased tissue IgM of five cases showed, without exception, a monoclonal IEF pattern like that seen in Figure 5D. The IEF pattern of IgM from the corresponding sera was polyclonal in all five cases. The monoclonality of the tissue IgM of the so-called reticulosarcomas is a strong argument in favor of the production of the Ig by the tumor cells. The absence of

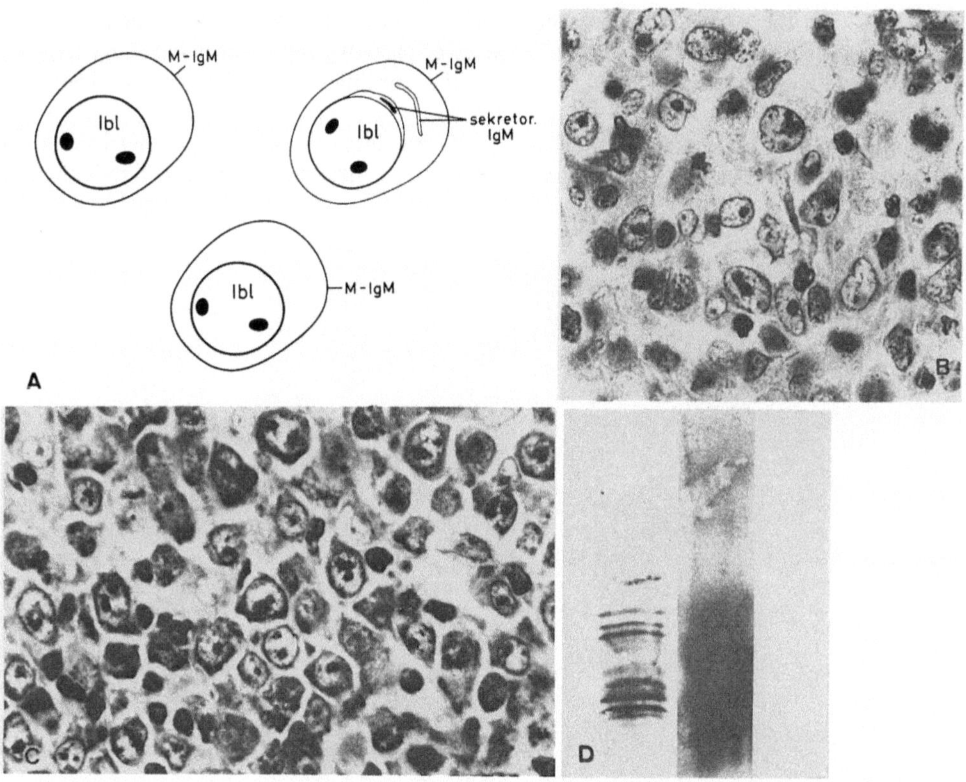

Fig. 5. (A) Schematic drawing of the cells that proliferate in most (60%) of the so-called reticulum cell sarcomas (RCS) or histiocytic lymphomas (HL) corresponding to B-type immunoblastic lymphomas (IB) of the Kiel classification. Ibl: immunoblast; M-IgM: membrane-bound IgM; sekretor. IgM = secretory IgM;

(B) Paraffin section of a so-called RCS or HS or IB stained with H and E. (× 840);

(C) Paraffin section of the same case stained with Giemsa. (× 840);

(D) Autoradiograph of reduced and carboxymethylated isoelectrofocused IgM. On the left, homogenate from the tissue extract of so-called RCS or HL or IB; on the right, corresponding serum

serum IgM increase and the polyclonal serum IgM IEF pattern indicate that the cells of this lymphoma usually did not secrete the produced Ig.

Using the enzyme-bridge method on paraffin sections, we observed a positive CIg staining of the blast-like tumor cells in nearly half of the cases (Fig. 6). Our findings are consistent with the staining results of TAYLOR [41], who found CIg staining in 67% (n=31). With one exception, the CIg staining of the lymphoma cells of our series was restricted to one light chain. The significance of the mixed light chain staining of the one case in our series remains to be determined. However, mixed staining seems to be the exception and not the rule in the so-called reticulosarcoma. The data collected clearly indicate that majority of the so-called reticulosarcomas are Ig producers.

Because of the great morphologic similarity between the immunoblasts of the plasma cell reaction and the so-called reticulum cell sarcomas [20, 32, 33, 37], we assume that most of these lymphomas are actually proliferations of B-immunoblasts. The differentiation of the immunoblast-like tumor cells in some cases toward plasmablasts substantiates this interpretation. The immunologic findings also favor this concept. Reactive immunoblasts have, like the so-called reticulum cell sarcoma cells, Ig on the surface and within the cytoplasm.

In some cases of so-called reticulosarcomas, there was morphologically a greater similarity of the reticulum cell sarcoma cells to particularly large centroblasts of the germinal centers than to reactive immunoblasts [32]. Furthermore, complement receptors could be demonstrated with EAC_{3d} in these cases. The presence of EAC_{3d} in peripheral lymphatic tissue is highly characteristic of germinal center cells. These cases probably represent particularly large-cell centroblastic lymphomas and should be grouped accordingly under the germinal center cell lymphomas.

It appears that in unselected series, up to 40% of reticulum cell sarcomas did not have any of the known B- or T-characteristic markers. The nature of these non-B and non-T reticulum cell

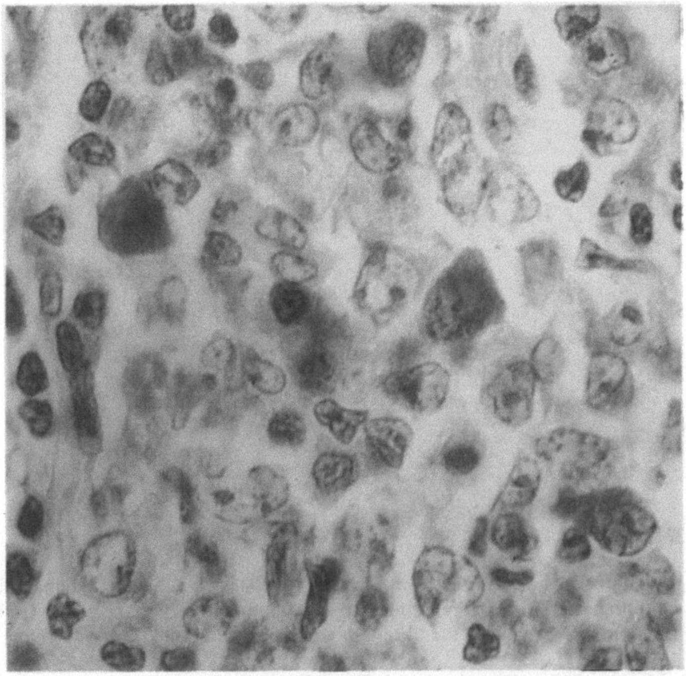

Fig. 6. Paraffin section of a so-called reticulum cell sarcoma (RCS) or histiocytic lymphoma (HL) equivalent to the B-type immunoblastic lymphoma (IB) of the Kiel classification immunostained for λ. Counterstain hematoxylin. (× 840)

sarcomas remains to be determined. However, the absence of the markers does not exclude their lymphatic origin. So-called reticulum cell sarcomas with T-cell properties are repeatedly reported but seem to be infrequent [6, 7]. It is notable that all cases except one of our present series did not show a staining for nonspecific esterase.

Hodgkin's Disease

Conventional morphologic studies did not elucidate the origin of Hodgkin's (H) and Sternberg-Reed (SR) cells. The same was true for the immunologic surface marker studies. The results have been controversial. The lack of large amounts of nonspecific esterase and acid phosphatase in H and SR cells spoke for an origin from cells other than histiocytes [5, 8].

Strong evidence for a B-cell origin of H and SR cells came from the detection of Ig in the cytoplasm of these cells using the enzyme-bridge method [10, 11, 41, 42]. However, it is very striking that TAYLOR [41, 42] and GARVIN et al. [10, 11] observed in most specimens of Hodgkin's disease κ- as well as λ-positive H and SR cells. CIg staining restricted to one light chain was observed in only very few cases. The mixed light chain staining suggests that Hodgkin's disease usually represents a polyclonal proliferative disease. Since such a polyclonal cell proliferation is quite unusual and contradicts the concepts of unicellular origin of neoplasms, we investigated a larger number of specimens [25]. We found in 68 out of 87 cases

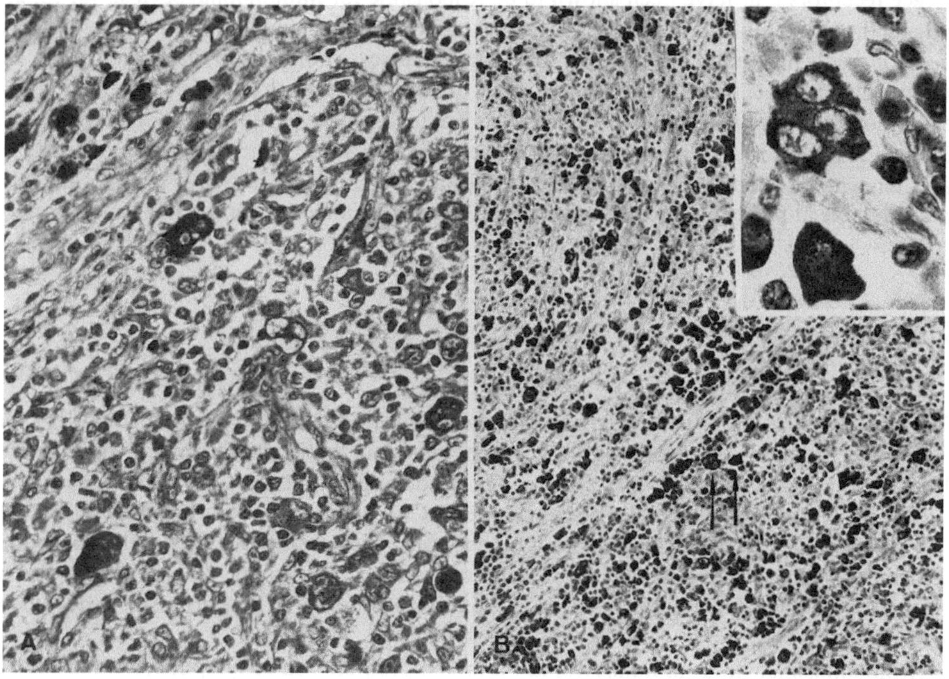

Fig. 7. (A) Hodgkin's disease, nodular sclerosing type. Part of a nodule. Positively stained reactive plasma cells (upper left) are accumulated around the nodule. Some Sternberg-Reed cells are strongly immunostained for κ, whereas others show only a faint or no staining. Immunostaining for λ gave similar results. Counterstain hematoxylin. (× 310);
(B) Hodgkin's disease, lymphocyte depleted type. Nearly all of the numerous Hodgkin and Sternberg-Reed cells are strongly stained for κ. The immunostaining for λ was completely negative. Arrows: Hodgkin's cell (right) and Sternberg-Reed cell (left), which are shown in the inset at a higher magnification. Counterstain hematoxylin. (× 125, inset × 846)

a positive staining pattern of H and SR cells; most commonly these cells stained for IgG, followed by IgD. With five exceptions, the specimens of all cases contained κ- and λ-chain-positive H and SR cells (Fig. 7A), a finding consistent with the data of the literature. The five cases whose H and SR cells stained for only one light chain belonged to the lymphocyte-depleted type (Fig. 7B), i.e., the cases with the poorer prognosis. Of considerable significance was one case: the first biopsy of this case showed both κ- and λ-chain-positive H and SR cells with a predominance of λ-chain-positive cells. In the subsequent biopsy obtained three months later, only λ-chain-positive H and SR cells were present. This transition from polytypic to monotypic CIg staining was paralleled by a change of the histologic type, from nodular sclerosing to lymphocyte-depleted type.

The B-cell origin of H and SR cells is suggested by the presence of δ-chains in these cells in many cases, the occurrence of cases in which H and SR cells showed restricted light chain staining, and the absence of lysozyme-positive H and SR cells in the cases studied by TAYLOR [42]. The possibility that the CIg was phagocytosed Ig cannot be excluded, since it is known that in long-lasting immune reactions and infections the produced antibodies may show restricted heterogeneity [24]. The CIg of the numerous (reactive) plasma cells usually present in the granulomatous tissue, however, was not restricted to the same heavy and light chains as those detected in the H and SR cells [25].

In our surface marker studies, H and SR cells did not react with EAC_{3b}, EAC_{3d}, or IgG-EA, nor did they show immunophagocytosis, whereas the lymphocytes present in the same suspensions included a large proportion of cells that formed rosettes with EAC_{3b}, EAC_{3d}, and IgG-EA. These findings indicate that the H and SR cells of the cases we studied lacked the surface receptors that have been shown to be responsible for immunophagocytosis [9, 13, 22] and that the H and SR cells of our cases were incapable of easily inducible immunophagocytosis. The supposedly malignant cell clones from Hodgkin's disease obtained in suspension [1, 15, 16] and monolayer cell cultures [17] show distinctly different features that are consistent with a B-cell or monocytoid cell origin, respectively. Our findings appear to support the hypothesis that Hodgkin's disease is a primary, polyclonal B-cell proliferation, which in only a minority of cases tends to develop into a monoclonal neoplasm. Nevertheless, we wish to stress that the data available at present do not allow a definite conclusion about the origin of H and SR cells.

Summary

Combined application of morphologic, immunochemical, and immunologic methods has led to a reinterpretation of non-Hodgkin's lymphomas and to the establishment of the Kiel classification. In the present paper, the main Ig-producing entities are considered. These are:

1. Chronic lymphocytic leukemia of the B-type (B-CLL)—a proliferation of lymphocytes and a few so-called prolymphocytes and lymphoblasts. The mean tissue IgM value is slightly increased; the serum IgM level is normal or reduced. The tumor cells bear SIg, and a majority of them have a receptor for C_{3d} but always lack CIg and are usually devoid of receptors for C_{3b}.
2. Lymphoplasmacytoid immunocytoma—a mixed proliferation of lymphocytes and centrocytes, blast cells, plasma cells, or plasmacytoid cells. The tissue Ig content is most often (91%) and most highly increased in this group, whereas the serum Ig level is increased in only 20% of the cases. The tissue IgM of 17 cases was shown to be monoclonal by IEF. Most tumor cells have SIg and a variable number CIg. The tumor cells bear both complement receptor subtypes, only a receptor for C_{3b}, or no complement receptors at all.
3. Centroblastic/centrocytic lymphoma—usually a follicular proliferation of abundant small germinal center cells (centrocytes) and some large germinal center cells (centroblasts). The

tumor cells bear SIg and both complement receptor subtypes. The C_{3b}- and C_{3d}-positive cells are located in the follicles, as in nonneoplastic lymphatic tissue.

4. Centrocytic lymphoma—a purebred, diffuse proliferation of the small germinal center cells (centrocytes). These cells bear SIg and receptors for C_{3b} and C_{3d} but usually lack CIg.
5. Centroblastic lymphoma—a proliferation of the large germinal center cells (centroblasts).
6. Lymphoblastic lymphoma of Burkitt's type.
7. Immunoblastic lymphoma—a diffuse proliferation of large basophilic cells resembling immunoblasts. The tissue IgM content is increased in 60% of the cases. It proved to be monoclonal with IEF in all five cases studied. The cells of five cases with increased tissue Ig content bore SIg. Nearly half of the cases studied showed CIg.

Besides non-Hodgkin's lymphomas, paraffin sections of 87 biopsies from Hodgkin's disease were investigated for CIg in Hodgkin's and Sternberg-Reed cells. These cells stained positively in 68 cases, most often for IgG, followed by IgD. In five cases of the lymphocyte-depleted type, the staining of the Hodgkin's and Sternberg-Reed cells was restricted to one light chain type.

References

1. BOECKER, W. R., HOSSFELD, D. K., GALLMEIER, W. M., SCHMIDT, C. G.: Clonal growth of Hodgkin's cells. Nature (Lond.) *258*, 235–236 (1975).
2. BORNKAMM, G. W., STEIN, H., LENNERT, K.,RÜGGEBERG, F., BARTELS, H., ZUR HAUSEN, H.: Attempts to demonstrate virus-specific sequences in human tumors. IV. EB viral DNA in European Burkitt lymphoma and immunoblastic lymphadenopathy with excessive plasmocytosis. Int. J. Cancer*17*, 177–181 (1976).
3. BORSOS, T., RAPP, H. J.: Immune hemolysis: A simplified method for the preparation of EAC/4 with guinea pig or human complement. J. Immunol. *22*, 263–268 (1967).
4. BOUMAN, H., LÜSEBRINK, W. D., HAVSTEEN, B., STEIN, H.: Discrimination between monoclonal and heterogeneous immunoglobulin M by isoelectric focusing and radioautography. Febs Letters *64*, 201–203 (1976).
5. BRAUNSTEIN, H., FREIMAN, D. G., THOMAS, W., GALL, E. A.: A histochemical study of the enzymatic activity of lymph nodes. II. Further investigation of normal and hyperplastic lymph nodes. Cancer *15*, 130–138 (1962).
6. BRAYLAN, R. C., JAFFE, E. S., MANN, R. B., FRANK, M. M., BERARD, C. W.: Surface receptors of human neoplastic lymphoreticular cells. In: Immunological Diagnosis of Leukemias and Lymphomas. Haematology and Blood Transfusion. THIERFELDER, S., RODT, H., THIEL, E. (eds.) Berlin – Heidelberg – New York: Springer 1977, Vol. XX, pp. 47–53.
7. BROUET, J. C., PREUD'HOMME, J. L., FLANDRIN, G., CHELLOUL, N., SELIGMANN, M.: Membrane markers in 'histiocytic' lymphomas (reticulum cell sarcomas). J. Natl. Cancer Inst. *56*, 631–633 (1976).
8. DORFMAN, R. F.: Enzyme histochemistry of normal, hyperplastic and neoplastic lymphoreticular tissues. In: Symp. Lymph. Tumours in Africa, Paris 1963. ROULET, F. C. (ed.) Basel – New York: Karger 1964, pp. 304–326.
9. EHLENBERGER, A. G., NUSSENZWEIG, V.: The role of membrane receptors for C3b and C3d in phagocytosis. J. Exp. Med. *145*, 357–371 (1977).
10. GARVIN, A. J., SPICER, S. S., PARMLEY, R. T., MUNSTER, A. M.: Immunohistochemical demonstration of IgG in Reed-Sternberg and other cells in Hodgkin's disease. J. Exp. Med. *139*, 1077–1083 (1974).
11. GARVIN, A. J., SPICER, S. S., MCKEEVER, P. E.: The cytochemical demonstration of intracellular immunoglobulin in neoplasm of lymphoreticular tissue. Am. J. Pathol. *82*, 457–478 (1976).
12. GERARD-MARCHANT, R., HAMLIN, I., LENNERT, K., RILKE, F., STANSFIELD, A. G., VAN UNNIK, J. A. M.: Classification of non-Hodgkin's lymphomas. [Letter to the Editor] Lancet 1974 II, 406–408.
13. HUBER, H., POLLEY, M. J., LINSCOTT, W. D., FUDENBERG, H. H., MÜLLER-EBERHARD, H. J.: Human monocytes: distinct receptor sites for the third component and for immunoglobulin G. Science *162*, 1281–1283 (1968).
14. JAFFE, E. S., SHEVACH, E. M., FRANK, M. M., BERARD, N. C., GREEN, I.: Nodular lymphoma – evidence for origin from follicular B lymphocytes. N. Engl. J. Med. *290*, 813–819 (1974).
15. KADIN, M. E.: In vitro study of multinucleated cells in Hodgkin's disease. Natl. Cancer Inst. Monogr. *36*, 211–217 (1973).

16. Kadin, M. E., Asbury, A. K.: Long term cultures of Hodgkin's tissue. A morphologic and radioautographic study. Lab. Invest. *28*, 181–184 (1973).
17. Kaplan, H. S., Gartner, S.: "Sternberg-Reed" giant cells of Hodgkin's disease: Cultivation in vitro, heterotransplantation and characterization as neoplastic macrophages. Int. J. Cancer *19*, 511–525 (1977).
18. Karlsson, C., Davies, H., Öhman, J., Andersson, U. B.: LKB multiphor. I. Analytical Thin Layer Gel Electrofocusing in Polyacrylamide Gel. Application Note, LKB Produkter AB, Bromma, Sweden, March 1973.
19. Leech, J. H., Glick, A. D., Waldron, J. A., Flexner, J. M., Horn, R. G., Collins, R. D.: Malignant lymphomas of follicular center cell origin in man. I. Immunologic studies. J. Natl. Cancer Inst. *54*, 11–21 (1975).
20. Lennert, K., Mohri, N., Stein, H., Kaiserling, E.: The histopathology of malignant lymphoma. Br. J. Haematol. *31* (Suppl.), 193–203 (1975a).
21. Lennert, K., Stein, H., Kaiserling, E.: Cytological and functional criteria for the classification of malignant lymphomata. Br. J. Cancer *31*, (Suppl. II), 29–43 (1975b).
22. Mantovani, B., Rabinovitch, M., Nussenzweig, V.: Phagocytosis of immune complexes by macrophages. Different roles of the macrophage receptor sites for complement (C3) and for immunoglobulin (IgG). J. Exp. Med. *135*, 780–792 (1972).
23. Morris, M. W., Davey, F. R.: Immunologic and cytochemical properties of histiocytic and mixed histiocytic-lymphocytic lymphomas. Am. J. Clin. Pathol. *63*, 403–414 (1974).
24. Natvig, J. B., Kunkel, H. G.: Human immunoglobulins: classes, subclasses, genetic variants, and idiotypes. Adv. Immunol. *16*, 1–59 (1973).
25. Papadimitriou, C. S., Stein, H., Lennert, K.: The complexity of immunohistochemical staining pattern of Hodgkin and Sternberg-Reed cells—demonstration of immunoglobulin, albumin, α_1-antichymotrypsin and lysozyme. Int. J. Cancer *21*, 531–541 (1978).
26. Rask-Nielsen, R., Gormsen, H.: Spontaneous and induced plasma cell neoplasia in a strain of mice. Cancer *4*, 387–397 (1951).
27. Rask-Nielsen, R. Gormsen, H.: On the occurrence of plasma cell leukemia in various strains of mice. J. Natl. Cancer Inst. *16*, 1137–1147 (1956).
28. Ross, G. D., Polley, M. J.: Specificity of human lymphocyte complement receptors. J. Exp. Med. *141*, 1163–1180 (1975).
29. Ross, G. D., Polley, M. J., Rabellino, E. M., Grey, H. M.: Two different complement receptors on human lymphocytes. One specific for C3b and one specific for C3b inactivator-cleaved C3b. J. Exp. Med. *138*, 798–811 (1973).
30. Seligmann, M., Preud'Homme, J. -L., Brouet, J. -C.: B and T cell markers in human proliferative blood diseases and primary immunodeficiencies, with special reference to membrane bound immunoglobulins. Transplant. Rev. *16*, 85–113 (1973).
31. Stacher, A., Waldner, R., Theml, H. (Kieler Lymphomgruppe): Klinik der malignen non-Hodgkin-Lymphome entsprechend der Kieler Klassifikation: Lymphoplasmozytoides Lymphom (LPL) und chronisch lymphatische Leukämie (CLL). In: Maligne Lymphome und monoklonale Gammopathien. Hämatologie und Bluttransfusion. Löffler, H. (ed.) München: Lehmanns 1976, Vol. XVIII, pp. 199–209.
32. Stein, H.: Klassifikation der malignen Non-Hodgkin-Lymphome aufgrund gemeinsamer morphologischer und immunologischer Merkmale zwischen normalen und neoplastischen lymphatischen Zellen. Immunol. Infekt. *4*, 52–69, 95–109 (1976).
33. Stein, H.: The immunologic and immunochemical basis for the Kiel Classification. In: Malignant Lymphomas Other than Hodgkin's Disease. Lennert, K., in collaboration with Stein, H., Mohri, N., Kaiserling, E., Müller-Hermelink, H. K. New York – Heidelberg – Berlin: Springer 1978, pp. 529–657.
34. Stein, H., Drescher, S.: Darstellung von Oberflächen-IgM an Blutlymphozyten mit der Immuno-Peroxydase-Methode. Blut *26*, 35–42 (1973).
35. Stein, H., Kaiserling, E.: Surface immunoglobulins and lymphocyte-specific surface antigens on leukaemic reticulo-endotheliosis cells. Clin. Exp. Immunol. *18*, 63–71 (1974).
36. Stein, H., Lennert, K., Parwaresch, M. R.: Malignant lymphoma of B-cell type. Lancet 1972 II, 855–857.
37. Stein, H., Kaiserling, E., Lennert, K.: Evidence for B-cell origin of reticulum cell sarcoma. Virchows Arch. (Pathol. Anat.) *364*, 51–67 (1974a).
38. Stein, H., Kaiserling, E., Lennert, K.: Lympho-Plasmocytoid Immunocytoma—a New Entity of Human Non-Hodgkin's Lymphoma. (Lecture) 10. Int. Congr. Int. Acad. Path. Hamburg, Abstract Book No. 122, 1974b, p. 58.
39. Stein, H., Bouman, H., Lennert, K., Fuchs, J., Havsteen, B.: Isoelectric focusing pattern of IgM and surface markers in non-Hodgkin's lymphomas. In: Immunological Diagnosis of Leukemias and Lymphomas. Haematology and Blood Transfusion. Thierfelder, S., Rodt, H., Thiel, E. (eds.) Berlin – Heidelberg – New York: Springer 1977, Vol XX, pp. 315–327.

40. STERNBERGER, L. A., HARDY JR., P. H., CUCULIS, J. J., MEYER, H. G.: The unlabeled antibody enzyme method of immunohistochemistry. Preparation and properties of soluble antigen-antibody complex (horseradish peroxidase-anti-horseradish peroxidase) and its use in identification of spirochetes. J. Histochem. Cytochem. *18*, 315–333 (1970).
41. TAYLOR, C. R.: The nature of Reed-Sternberg cells and other malignant "reticulum" cells. Lancet 1974 II, 802–807.
42. TAYLOR, C. R.: An immunohistochemical study of follicular lymphoma, reticulum cell sarcoma and Hodgkin's disease. Eur. J. Cancer *12*, 61–67 (1976).
43. THEML, H., BURGER, A., KEIDITSCH, E., ENNE, W., EGGERT, K., DIETZFELBINGER, H., GRÄFF, L., ZSIDA, L.: Klinische Beobachtungen zur Charakterisierung des splenomegalen Immunocytoms (in press).
44. VOSSEN, J.: The Development of the B Immune System in Man. Rotterdam: Proefschrift 1975.
45. YEFENOF, E., KLEIN, G., JONDAL, M., OLDSTONE, M. B.: Surface markers on human B- and T-lymphocytes. IX. Two-colour immunofluorescence studies on the association between EBV receptors and complement receptors on the surface of lymphoid cell lines. Int. J. Cancer *17*, 693–700 (1976).

Immunoglobulin Production in Lymphoma Cells: An Immunoelectron Microscopy Study

F. REYES, M. F. GOURDIN, J. P. FARCET, J. BRETON-GORIUS, and B. DREYFUS

Introduction

Studies of surface markers in lymphoproliferative disorders have provided important help in the understanding of the nature of involved cells. Among available assays, the detection of surface immunoglobulins (SIg) has been shown to be essential for the identification of B-lymphocytes [5]. However, there is a possibility that cells of the B-lymphocyte series express few or no SIg as they produce and secrete intracellular immunoglobulins (Ig) [3]. Therefore, the absence of SIg does not preclude a cell, at certain maturation stages, from being of B-derivation. Immunoelectron microscopy (IEM) using conjugated anti-Ig antibodies has been used in recent years. Satisfactory results have been obtained more easily in detecting surface rather than intracellular components. This has been generally taken as evidence of the poor penetration of conjugates into fixed cells [for more detailed discussion, see [2]]. As a matter of fact, using IEM and peroxidase-conjugated anti-Ig antibodies, we initially found that in chronic lymphocytic leukemia (CLL) proliferating small lymphocytes strongly reacted at the surface without any intracellular staining, just as normal human small B-lymphocytes [4]. However, in more recent studies including various samples from patients with lymphomas, we found that penetration of conjugates was readily achieved, resulting in an intracellular specific staining.

Material and Methods

Samples

The following three samples were examined: blood lymphocytes from a patient with CLL (patient 1), marrow cells from a patient with a previously known α-chain disease and who developed an acute leukemic picture with unusual features (manuscript in preparation) (patient 2), and blood lymphocytes from a patient with CLL and massive lymph node enlargement, hypogammaglobulinemia, and small amounts of κ-light chain in the urine (patient 3).

Preparation of Specimens for IEM

This was carried out as described previously [4].

Anti-Ig Antibodies

They were purified for hyperimmune sera and rendered monospecific for heavy and light chains by appropriate immunoadsorption, as already described [1, 4].

Results

Patient 1

As illustrated in figure 1, blood lymphocytes exhibited a strong and diffuse surface staining outlining all the membrane. A monoclonal pattern of SIg was demonstrated in that case by anti-γ and anti-κ antibodies. It is to be noted that no intracellular staining was detectable in lymphocytes.

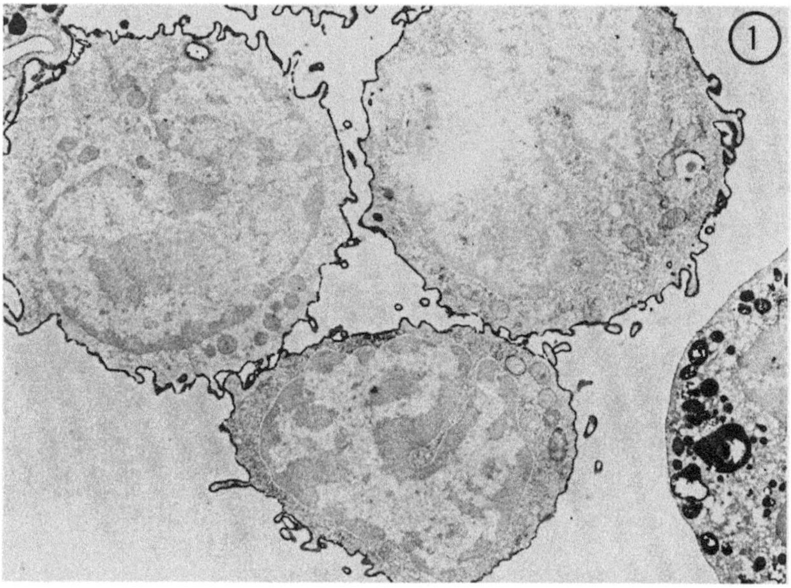

Fig. 1. Blood lymphocytes in patient 1 with CLL. The surface of lymphocytes is diffusely stained by peroxidase coupled anti-γ antibodies. Cells were also stained by anti-κ but not by anti-λ or anti-μ antibodies. The cytoplasm of lymphocytes is free of dense reaction product. Part of two contaminating polymorphs is seen; these cells are recognized by the presence of myeloperoxidase-containing granules. (× 8000)

Patient 2

In this case of α-chain disease, marrow cells were negative with all reagents except anti-α antibodies. Surprisingly, no surface labeling was found; the absence of detectable SIg was also confirmed by immunofluorescence (kindly performed by Dr. J. L. Preud'Homme). However, an intracellular specific staining was found in 95% of the marrow cells. These blast cells were characterized by the presence of varying amounts of endoplasmic reticulum (ER) profiles, which were positively stained by anti-α antibodies (Fig. 2), in some cases including the perinuclear cisternae. The Golgi complex was negative. Some cells contained simultaneously positive and negative ER strands.

Patient 3

A specific dense intracellular staining was found with anti-κ antibodies. Most cells had no surface labeling. They had, however, a diffuse cytoplasmic staining (Fig. 3); this aspect was not due to the staining of the ER or the Golgi complex (which appeared free of reaction product) but of the remaining cytoplasmic structures (i.e., dispersed ribosomes). Controls with anti-λ antibodies were negative and clearly showed that the diffuse staining did not result from nonspecific adsorption of conjugates into damaged cells.

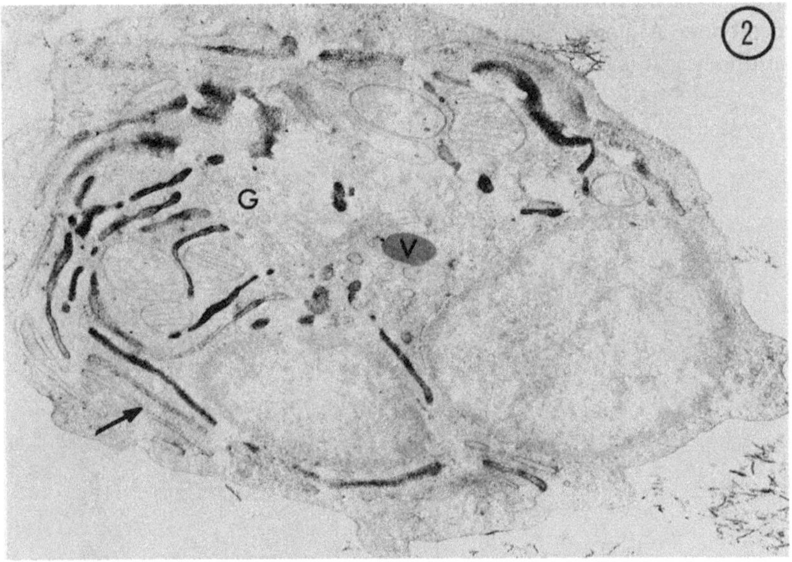

Fig. 2. Marrow blast cell in patient 2 with α-chain disease. The surface of this cell has no detectable SIg. The cyctoplasm contains several ER cisternae positively stained by anti-α antibodies and also a few negative cisternae (arrow). The large Golgi area (G) is unstained. v is a lipid-containing vacuole, similar to those found in normal transformed lymphocytes. ($\times$ 10800)

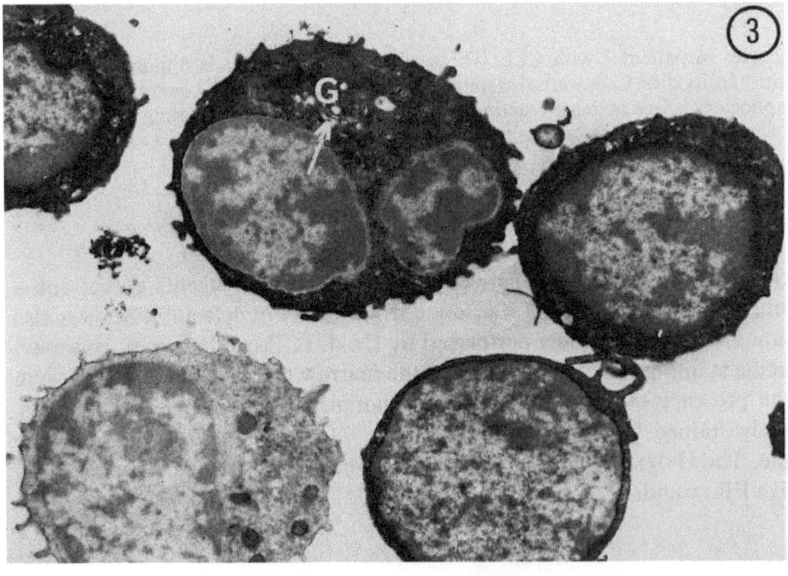

Fig. 3. Blood lymphocytes in patient 3 with tumoral CLL and hypogammaglobulinemia. Four lymphocytes are heavily stained by anti-κ antibodies; the staining is diffuse in the cytoplasm leaving negative ER (arrow) and Golgi complex (G). Lower left is a normal looking lymphocyte whose cytoplasm is free of staining; its surface is lightly labeled. ($\times$ 8000)

Discussion

These results demonstrate that both SIg and intracellular Ig can be detected by a simple IEM method in which a fixed cell suspension is reacted with peroxidase-coupled antibodies. They establish that conjugates made of entire antibody molecules and peroxidase do penetrate into fixed cells. It must be recalled that in our method the prior fixation of cells excludes a possible endocytosis of the conjugate.

As shown in patient 2, the precise localization of the specific staining in ER cisternae proves that the detected Ig are newly synthesized proteins that have been packed before being secreted by the cells. In this patient as in others we recently studied this method enabled us to identify B-immunoblasts, i.e., large cells with minute amounts of synthesized Ig and no detectable SIg (manuscript in preparation). These findings emphasize the possible underestimation of B cells in some cases, when only studied by surface markers.

In addition, the present IEM method allows one to discriminate between different pathways of Ig synthesis, as shown in patients 2 and 3. The diffuse ribosomal staining was a striking feature in patient 3, strikingly different from the ER staining generally expected in synthesizing B cells. Further work is needed to determine whether such a phenotype is an acquired abnormality due to disease or whether it represents the counterpart of some normal transitional steps of maturing B cells.

References

1. Gourdin, M. F., Reyes, F., Lejonc, J. L., Mannoni, P., Dreyfus, B.: Surface features of cells in human lymphoproliferative disorders. In : Modern Trends in Human Leukemia. II. Neth, R., Gallo, R.C., Mannweiler, K., Moloney, W.C. (eds.) Munich: J. F. Lehmans Verlag 1976, p. 207.
2. Kuhlmann, W. D., Avrameas, S., Ternynck, T.: A comparative study for ultrastructural localization of intracellular immunoglobulins using peroxidase conjugates. J. Immunol. Methods *5*, 33–48 (1974).
3. McConnell, I., Hurd, C. M.: Receptors for Fc of IgG and complement (C_3b) on immunoglobulin-bearing, antigen-binding and antibody-secreting cells. Immunology *30*, 825–833 (1976).
4. Reyes, F., Lejonc, J. L., Gourdin, M. F., Mannoni, P., Dreyfus, B.: The surface morphology of human B lymphocytes as revealed by immunoelectron microscopy. J. Exp. Med. *141*, 392–410 (1975).
5. Seligmann, M., Preud'Homme, J. L., Brouet, J. C.: B and T cell markers in human proliferative blood disease and primary immuno-deficiencies, with special reference to membrane bound immunoglobulin. Transplant Rev. *16*, 85–113 (1973).

Biochemical Markers in Hodgkin's Disease and Non-Hodgkin's Lymphoma

J. A. CHILD, E. H. COOPER, S. ILLINGWORTH, and T. S. WORTHY

Introduction

It has been known for many years that the concentration of a number of plasma proteins may be subject to acute change, for example, following surgical trauma [6, 7, 26]; hence the term 'acute phase' reactant protein (APRP). Many of these proteins are glycoproteins travelling electrophorectically in the α-region and are made in the liver. The biological function of only some of them is fully understood and their metabolism also requires elucidation. All of them are detectable in the plasma of healthy subjects with the notable exception of C-reactive protein, which is usually absent. The study of these proteins, encouraged by improved specificity in measurement, has been extended to a variety of disease states not necessarily limited to acute phenomena. An important observation is that dissociated increases of particular APRPs have a discriminant function; for example, while in neoplastic invasion of the liver, α_1-antitrypsin and α_1-acid glycoprotein are both increased, there is dissociation in hepatitis and cirrhosis [10, 11]. The study of ulcerative colitis and Crohn's disease has illustrated the value of studying a protein profile in which as many as eight proteins are estimated [16]. Investigation of protein profiles in various types of malignant disease [2, 4, 5, 15, 17, 18] suggests that they may be of value in several ways: they show promise in terms of the staging of some diseases, they can be of value in the early warning and monitoring of metastatic disease, and they may be able to discriminate between inflammatory/infective and neoplastic processes.

Would application of APRP profiles to the lymphomas be of comparable or even greater value? Currently, the best and most logical management of the lymphomas requires precise histopathological identification coupled with accurate staging before treatment is started. However, even assuming that these requirements are met, there may remain doubts as to the extent and activity of the disease process, especially in non-Hodgkin's lymphoma, because of the limitations of currently available techniques. In subsequent management, it may be impossible to reassess the disease state accurately by non-invasive investigation. The well-known difficulty in patient follow-up is the lack of objective measurement to confirm the often subjective clinical impression. Although it *may* be possible to identify progressive improvement and complete remission, 'partial remission', 'partial response' and 'resistant disease' are labels frequently used with little or no scientific basis. There is a need for indicators which will accurately reflect response and be of help in deciding, for example, whether and when a particular therapy should be continued or replaced by an alternative. Various haematological and biochemical measurements have been used in the attempt to monitor the lymphomas [8, 9, 13, 19, 20, 23, 24, 25]. These 'markers' or 'biological signs' are listed in Table 1. The serum copper, caeruloplasmin, and the erythrocyte sedimentation rate (ESR) have been shown to correlate reasonably well with disease activity and/or the extent of disease [8, 19, 20, 25]. Individually, these indices are non-specific. The ESR has the merit of being a simple routine investigation and some reliance has been put on it, although it has been known for many years that the ESR represents a complex interplay of factors, not least the haematocrit and the levels of acute phase reactants, especially fibrinogen. In terms of protein changes, false positives and negatives are known to be frequent [12].

Table 1. A selection of 'markers' of disease previously applied to the lymphomas

Biochemical indices
Metals
Iron
Copper
Zinc
Transport proteins
Transferrin
Ferritin
Caeruloplasmin
Haptoglobin
Enzymes
Alkaline phosphatase
Lysozyme
γ
Glutamyl transpeptidase
Haematological indices
White blood cell counts
Erythrocyte sedimentation rate
Leucocyte alkaline phosphatase

We have revisited the problem. In adopting a profile of APRPs as a possible source of valuable indices, we were well aware that looked at individually they have far less value. Considered as a profile, however, they represent highly structured systems with considerable discriminant properties. From our group's preliminary studies in patients with solid tumours [4, 17, 18], it was thought that longitudinal studies of APRP profiles comprising α_1-antitrypsin (AT), α_1-antichymotrypsin (ACT), α_1-acid glycoprotein (AGP), and C-reactive protein (CRP) (Table 2) might be of considerable value in the lymphomas. Preliminary work established that this APRP profile could reflect disease activity and have predictive value in terms of clinical course. This paper represents our experience to date.

Patients and Methods

Forty seven patients with Hodgkin's disease and 32 patients with non-Hodgkin's lymphoma were investigated. Diagnosis and staging (as appropriate) were by standard methods; most of the patients with Hodgkin's disease were staged according to the Ann Arbor classification [1]. Serum samples were obtained at out-patients visits, or as appropriate, during in-patient care and stored at $-20°C$ until analysed. The following acute phase reactant proteins were measured: α_1-antitrypsin (AT), α_1-antichymotrypsin (ACT), α_1-acid glycoprotein (AGP), and C-reactive protein (CRP) by single radial immunodiffusion (Mancini technique) using antisera and standards obtained from BEHRINGWERKE, A. G., Marburg/Lahn, W. Germany [17].

Vertical Studies

In both major groups, measurement of APRPs in patients with active disease and in remission were carried out. The designation 'active' disease, while chiefly applying to untreated patients and patients at relapse, also included some being treated although showing suboptimal response or no response clinically. The designation 'remission' in both groups of patients was applied

Table 2. A selection of APRPs[a]

Acute phase reactant proteins
Transport proteins
Haptoglobin
Caeruloplasmin
Antiproteases
α_1-Antitrypsin
α_1-Antichymotrypsin
Intertrypsin
Steroid binding
α_1-Acid glycoprotein
Function uncertain
C-reactive protein
Blood clotting
Fibrinogen

[a] Those underlined were measured in this study.

only to those judged to be clinically disease-free (based on physical examination and standard investigation). In both instances, authenticated infective episodes were excluded. The principal subgroup with Hodgkin's disease comprised patients with stages IIIb and IV.

Longitudinal Studies

Although many of the patients included in the vertical studies have had serial measurements of APRPs over months, and in some cases years, five patients (Figs. 1–5) have been selected to illustrate in more detail certain features of the APRP profile. It is apparent that AGP and ACT measurements produce the same general pattern, although not very closely correlated ($r = 0.46$ in Hodgkin's disease, $r = 0.66$ in non-Hodgkin's lymphoma). A three APRP profile (of AT, ACT, and CRP) has been used to illustrate changes in all but one of these patients (T.B.).

Results

The mean values for AT, ACT, and AGP and the *median* (with range) for CRP in a control group of blood donors and in-patients with Hodgkin's disease (stage IIIb and IV) and non-Hodgkin's lymphoma are given in Tables 3 and 4, respecitvely. The results of analysis of variance between and within the groups are also presented in the Tables. They confirm the significance of the elevations of APRPs. The increases in all four APRPs are more marked in active Hodgkin's disease than active non-Hodgkin's lymphoma. CRP is frequently absent from normal plasma, is not a continuous variant, and its values may not, therefore, be analysed in the same way as for the other APRPs.

Considering a smaller group with Hodgkin's disease (stages I, II, and IIIa) separately (11 with active disease and 6 in remission), the APRPs were as follows for active disease and remission respectively: AGP 1.9 ± 0.9 and 0.8 ± 0.3, AT 4.7 ± 1.2 and 2.7 ± 0.9, ACT 0.90 ± 0.34 and 0.54 ± 0.18. Considered together with the data obtained in the patients with more extensive disease, this suggests that active Hodgkin's disease produces responses that are not stage dependent.

Table 3. Results of acute phase reactant protein measurements in Hodgkin's disease, stages IIIb and IV (active disease and remission), with values obtained in 40 healthy blood donors

Hodgkin's disease	CRP mg/l	AGP g/l	AT g/l	ACT g/l
Active n=32	33[a] 0–198	1.9±0.8[b]	5.7±2.5	1.03±0.36
Remission n=19	5 0–9	1.0±0.3	3.5±0.7	0.58±0.18
Blood donors n=40	2 0–6	0.6±0.1	2.7±0.4	0.42±0.65
Analysis of variance[c] F 2=88	—	62	33	60

[a] Median (range).
[b] Mean ± SD.
[c] All F values $p<0.001$.

Table 4. Results of acute phase reactant protein measurements in non-Hodgkin's lymphoma (active disease and remission) with values obtained in 40 healthy blood donors

Non-Hodgkin lymphoma	CRP mg/l	AGP g/l	AT g/l	ACT g/l
Active n=31	7[a] 0–105	1.5±0.7[b]	4.4±1.9	0.85±0.31
Remission n=15	4 0–11	0.9±0.3	3.1±0.8	0.52±0.10
Blood donors n=40	2 0–6	0.6±0.1	2.7±0.4	0.42±0.65
Analysis of variance[c] F 2=83	—	35	21	48

[a] Median (range).
[b] Mean ± SD.
[c] All F values $p<0.001$.

The longitudinal APRP profiles in three patients with Hodgkin's disease and two patients with non-Hodgkin's lymphoma are shown in Figures 1–5. The comments on these illustrative cases indicate how the APRP profile can be interpreted. It is of considerable interest that patient T.B. (Fig. 5) developed multi-focal leuco-encephalopathy and that extremely high titres (up to 1:20,480) of haemagglutination inhibition antibodies to BK virus (a member of the SV40 group) were detected in sera dating from 14 months before death (Fig. 6). Any relationship between reaction to virus, the leuco-encephalopathy, and the very "noisy" APRP profile during this period is still speculative.

Discussion

Previous studies of APRP profiles in malignant disease have held out the promise of their being valuable in monitoring the extent and activity of disease [2, 3, 17, 18]. In this study we have presented evidence that indicates that APRPs reflect disease activity in both Hodgkin's and non-Hodgkin's lymphoma and that, particularly when considered as a profile of three to four indices in longitudinal study, they have potential value in the management of these diseases. In vertical studies, the timing of sampling is to some extent arbitrary and the comparisons are

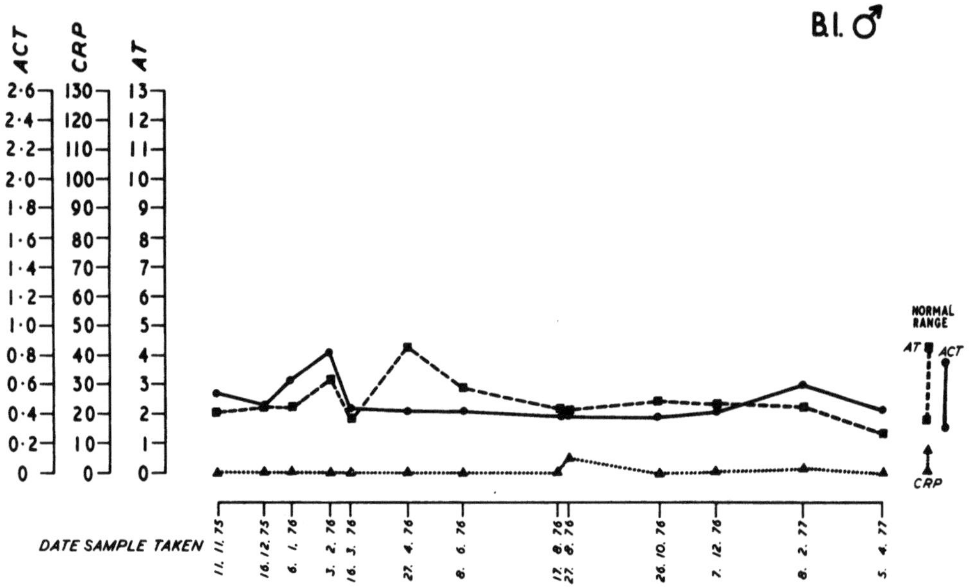

Fig. 1. B. I. age 25. Mixed lymphocytic histiocytic lymphoma; diagnosed September, 1974. Disease probably confined to soft tissues right leg and iliac and inguinal nodes (although ultra-sound raised possibility of more extensive disease). Treatment: small dose of radiotherapy, six courses CHOP. Clinically disease-free—complete remission. *Profile*; continuing stability with no significant elevations—consistent with the clinical assessment. (Typical of complete remission in both Hodgkin's disease and non-Hodgkin's lymphoma)

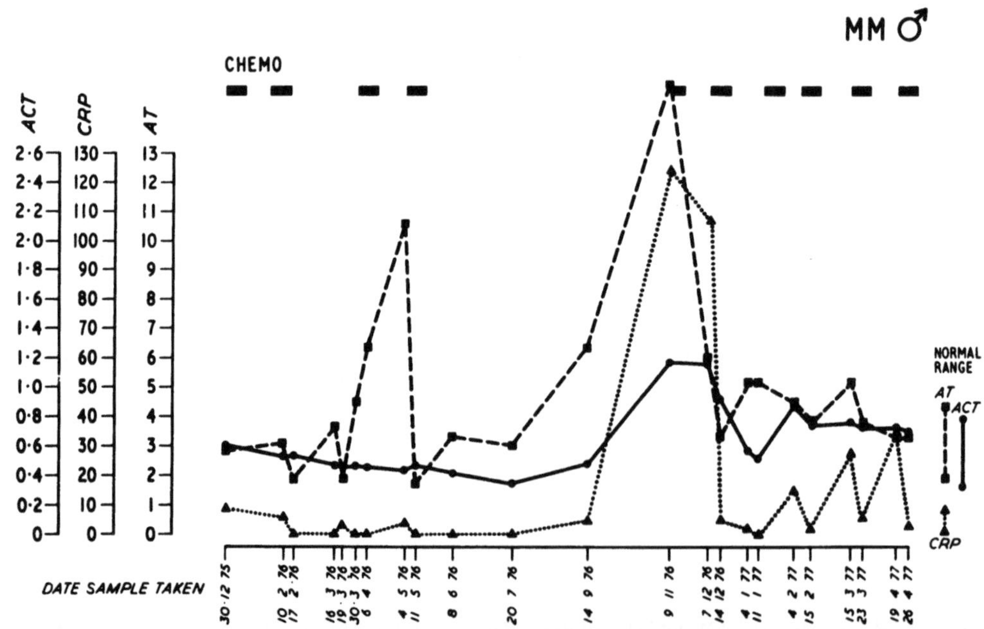

Fig. 2. M.M. age 33. Hodgkin's disease, diagnosed April 1975. CS IVA. PS IV H + M + D +; nodal histopathology: lymphocyte predominant. Treatment: ten courses MOPP. Nodal relapse, September, 1976. Subsequent treatment: five courses of MOPP. Recent evidence to suggest probable marrow relapse. *Profile*: apart from the obvious marked elevation of APRPs coinciding with the recent relapse, there is an increasing lability in the profile, particularly of the C-reactive protein. Our clinical suspicion that the disease is no longer controlled by therapy is reinforced

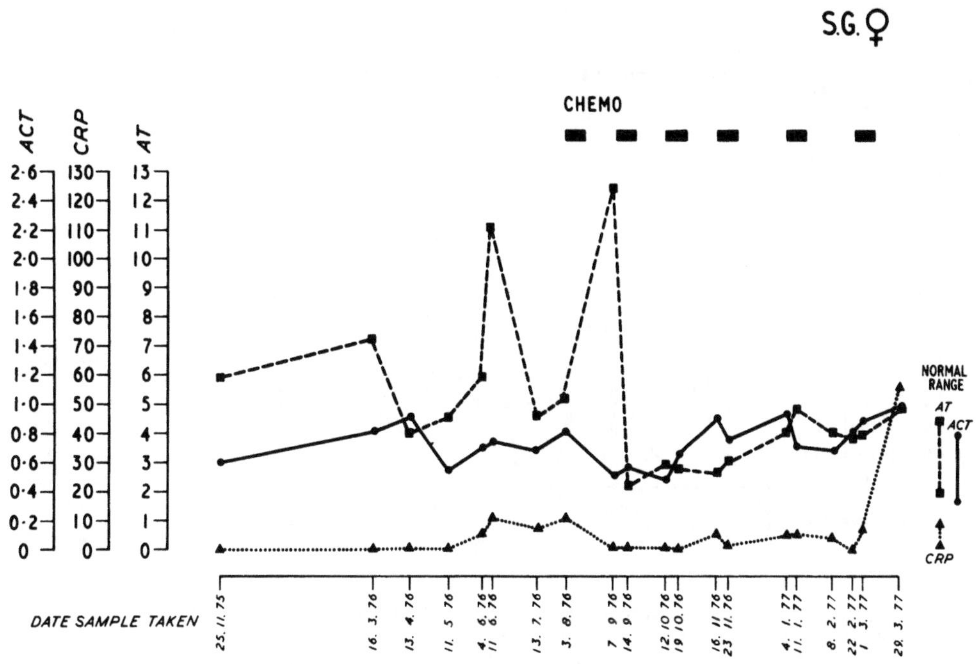

Fig. 3. S.G. age 57. Hodgkin's disease, diagnosed November, 1955. ? CS IIA; nodal histopathology: nodular sclerosing. Treatment: courses of radiotherapy above and below diaphragm. No nodal relapse since 1970. Recent relapse indicated by severe B-symptoms. Subsequent treatment: six courses MOPP with rapid clinical improvement and resolution of symptoms. *Profile*: shows considerable instability during the relapse period. A more 'orderly' profile follows the institution of chemotherapy, although C-reactive protein now appears to be increasingly labile

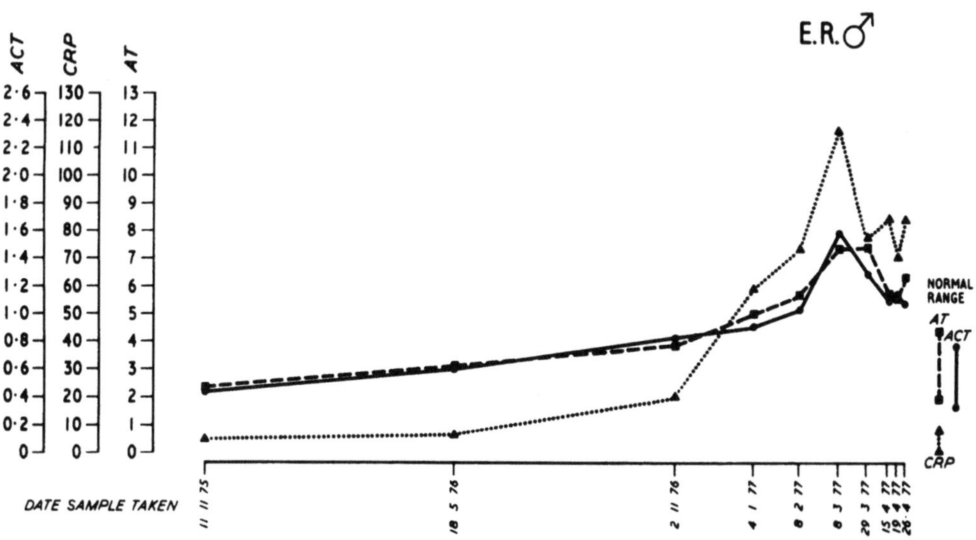

Fig. 4. E.R. age 53. Diffuse undifferentiated NHL, diagnosed 1968. treatment: radiotherapy (neck, abdomen, iliac, and inguinal); relapses treated by chemotherapy. Recent relapse: systemic symptoms, hepatomegaly (biopsy negative). Current treatment: CHOP. *Profile*: Initially very stable. Synchronous elevation with relapse is followed by instability which contrasts quite markedly with the previous consistent pattern. This supports the clinical supposition of active, as yet, uncontrolled disease

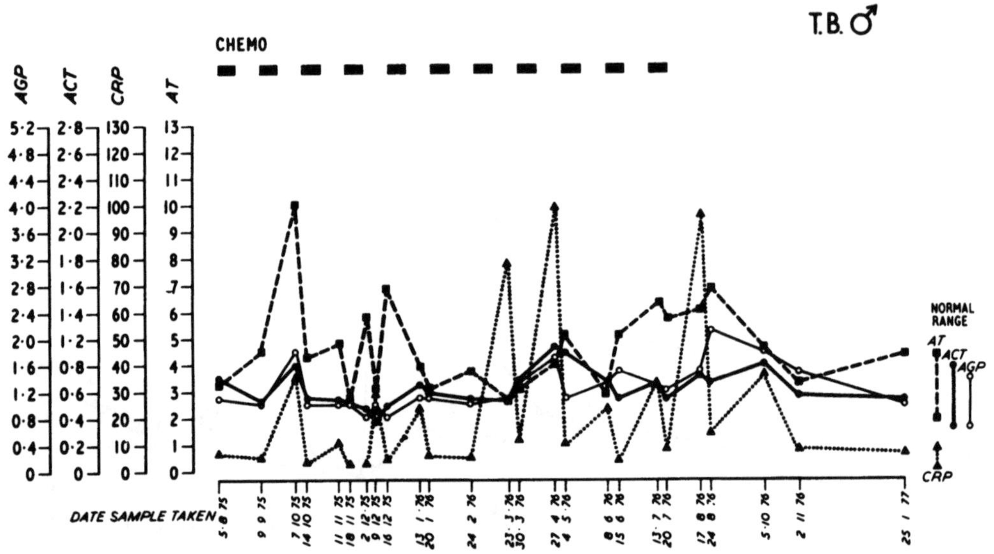

Fig. 5. T.B. age 31. Hodgkin's disease, diagnosed July, 1974. CS IIIB PS III N + H − S − M −; nodal histopathology: mixed cellularity. Initial treatment: six courses MOPP. Relapse: nodal and systemic symptoms, July, 1975. Subsequent treatment: MOPP (three courses) then MOPP + Bleomycin (nine courses). 'Partial' remission only. Developed leuco-encephalopathy: died. *Profile*: a most erratic unstable profile with asynchrony and no suggestion of modification by chemotherapy. Appears to reflect the 'resistant' disease

not necessarily between the zenith of activity and true remission in all cases. However, they did confirm that striking changes in APRPs are to be expected when disease is active and encouraged a continuous surveillance of our patients by longitudinal measurements. From these, it would appear that the stable APRP profile is characteristic of the cure or prolonged remission. Loss of this stability seems to be a characteristic feature of relapsing disease. We have given examples to illustrate that both subtle and obvious relapses are reflected in disturbance of the APRP profile, and it is apparent that serial estimation of APRPs in profile can provide lead time in the diagnosis of relapse. The poorly controlled, non-responding disease also produces a recognisable disturbance and may give warning to the clinician of practical value in management. It is hoped that continuing analysis of APRP profiles will help us to characterize events in the course of these disease states, be they extension or regression of disease, infective or non-specific; the patterns of rates of change of APRP values and synchronous or asynchronous variation of the individual proteins with time may provide key information.

Increased understanding of Hodgkin's disease coupled with therapeutic advances have made the cure of this disease a reality [14]. However, there is still much to be achieved in terms of treatment of advanced disease, and undoubtedly the meticulous assessment of the extent and activity of disease will be important in the further improvement of prognosis.

Although the changes in APRPs individually, collectively, and in profile appear slightly less striking in non-Hodgkin's lymphoma—as in the case of other markers [9, 23]—the potential value, where staging and assessment of disease activity can be so difficult, is probably much greater. We believe that further study of plasma protein profiles, not necessarily the array of APRPs adopted in the present investigation, will prove rewarding. β_2-Microglobulin [22] and α_2-macroglobulin seem logical candidates for assessment. Finally, as the liver is a frequent site of involvement, it would appear sensible to include in any battery of indices a sensitive indicator of hepatic function. Serum γ-glutamyl transpeptidase is the most useful [3, 21, 27], although its interpretation (especially when moderately raised) may be full of subtle nuances.

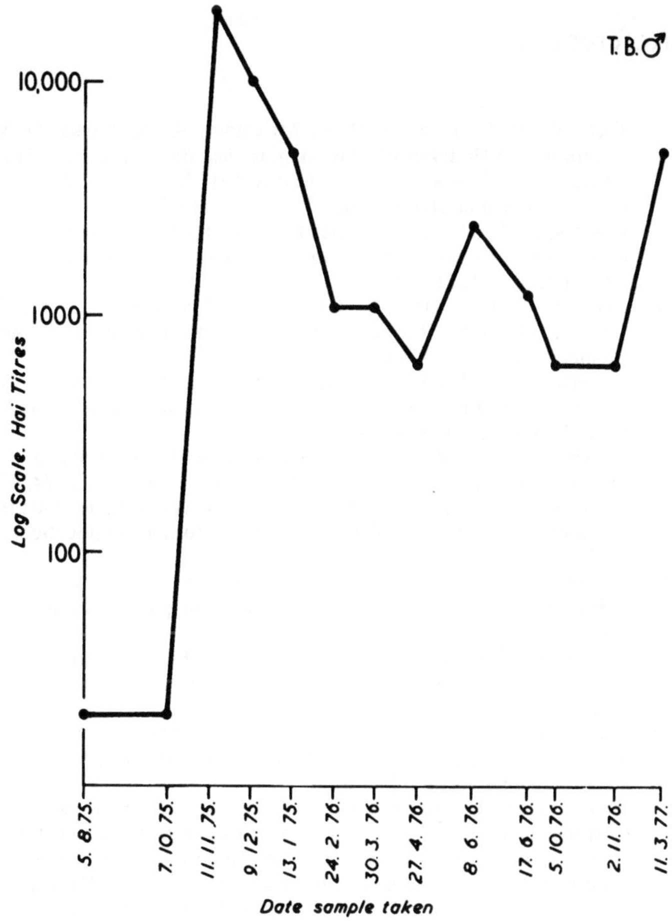

Fig. 6. Haemagglutination inhibition titres to BK virus in patient with Hodgkin's disease (T.B.). (Virus Reference Laboratory, Colindale, London)

Summary

Vertical studies indicate that, in general, acute phase reactant proteins (APRP) reflect disease activity in both Hodgkin's disease and non-Hodgkin's lymphoma. Longitudinal studies of the selected APRP profile demonstrate the following:

1. The stable profile is characteristic of remission.
2. Considerable elevation of APRPs coincides with relapsed disease.
3. An unstable profile is a feature of relapsing disease and may give early warning of relapse.
4. Patients responding inadequately to treatment frequently have unstable APRP profiles.

Acknowledgements

The work was supported by a grant of the Yorkshire Regional Cancer Organisation. Professor E. H. Cooper is supported by the Yorkshire Cancer Research Campaign. The authors are grateful to their colleagues, Dr. B. E. Roberts and Dr. J. Stone, for their involvement in management of some of the patients.

References

1. Carbone, P. P., Kaplan, H. S., Musshoff, K., Smithers, D. W., Tubiana, M.: Report of the Committee on Hodgkin's disease staging classification. Cancer Res. *31*, 1860–1861 (1971).
2. Child, J. A., Roberts, B. E., Illingworth, S., Cooper, E. H.: Acute phase reactant proteins in chronic leukaemia. Biomedicine *27*, 188–189 (1977).
3. Cooper, E. H., Turner, R., Steele, L., Neville, A. M., Mackay, A. M.: The contribution of serum enzyme and carcinoembryonic antigen to the early diagnosis of metastatic colorectal cancer. Br. J. Cancer *31*, 111–117 (1975).
4. Cooper, E. H., Turner, R., Geekie, A., Munro Neville, A., Goligher, J. C., Graham, N. G., Giles, G. R., Hall, R., MacAdam, W.A.F.: Alpha-globulins in the surveillance of colorectal cancer. Biomedicine *24*, 171–178 (1976a).
5. Cooper, E. H., Turner, R., Milford-Ward, A., Neville, A. M.: Multiparametric tests in the monitoring of cancer. In: Cancer Related Antigens. Franchimont, P. (*ed.*) Amsterdam–New York–Oxford: North-Holland 1976b, pp. 179–186.
6. Crockson, R. A., Payne, C. J., Ratcliff, A. P., Soothill, J. F.: Time sequence of acute phase reactive proteins following surgical trauma. Clin. Chim. Acta *14*, 435–441 (1966).
7. Fischer, C. L., Gill, C., Forrester, M. G., Nakamura, R.: Quantitation of "Acute-phase proteins" postoperatively—Value in detection and monitoring complications. Am. J. Clin. Pathol. *66*, 840–846 (1976).
8. Foster, M., Fell, L., Pocklington, T., Akinsete, F., Dawson, A., Hutchison, J. M. S., Mallard, J. R.: Electron spin resonance as a useful technique in the management of Hodgkin's disease. Clin. Radiol. *28*, 15–22 (1977a).
9. Foster, M., Dawson, A., Pocklington, T., Fell, L.: Electron spin resonance measurements of blood caeruloplasmin and iron transferrin levels in patients with non-Hodgkin's lymphoma. Clin. Radiol. *28*, 23–28 (1977b).
10. Giusti, G., Piccinino, F., Sagnelli, E., Pasquale, G.: Differential diagnosis between benign and malignant biliary tract obstruction. Discriminative usefulness of some clinical and laboratory data. Acta Hepatogastroenterol. (Stuttg.) *22*, 374–379 (1975).
11. Hiramatsu, S., Kojina, J., Okada, T. T., Inai, S., Ohmori, K.: The serum protein profile in chronic hepatitis, cirrhosis and liver cancer. Acta Hepatogastroenterol. (Stuttg.) *23*, 177–182 (1976).
12. Hutchinson, R. M., Eastham, R. D.: A comparison of the erythrocyte sedimentation rate and plasma viscosity in detecting changes in plasma proteins. J. Clin. Pathol. *30*, 345–349 (1977).
13. Jacobs, A., Worwood, M.: Ferritin: clinical aspects. In: Iron Metabolism and its Disorders. Kief, H. (*ed.*) Amsterdam—Oxford: Excerpta Medica 1975, Vol. III, pp. 90–95.
14. Kaplan, H. S.: Hodgkin's disease and other human malignant lymphomas: Advances and Prospects—G.H.A. Clowes Memorial Lecture. Cancer Res. *36*, 3863–3878 (1976).
15. Koj, A.: "Acute-phase reactants." In: The Structure and Function of Plasma Proteins. Allison, A. C. (ed.) New York: Plenum Press 1975, Vol. I, pp. 73–132.
16. Milford-Ward, A.: Personal communication.
17. Milford-Ward, A., Cooper, E. H., Turner, R., Anderson, J. A., Neville, A. M.: Acute-phase Reactant Protein Profiles: an aid to monitoring large bowel cancer by CEA and serum enzymes. Br. J. Cancer *35*, 170–178 (1977).
18. Neville, A. M., Cooper, E. H.: Biochemical monitoring of cancer. Ann. Clin. Biochem. *13*, 283–305 (1976).
19. Pagliardi, E., Giangrandi, E.: Clinical significance of the blood copper in Hodgkin's disease. Acta Haematol. (Basel) *24*, 201–212 (1960).
20. Ray, R. G., Wolf, P. H., Kaplan, H. S.: Value of laboratory indicators in Hodgkin's disease: Preliminary Results. Natl. Cancer Inst. Monogr. *36*, 315–323 (1973).
21. Roberts, B. E., Child, J. A., Cooper, E. H., Turner, R., Stone, J.: An evaluation of the usefulness of serum gamma glutamyl transpeptidase levels in the management of haematological neoplasia. Acta Haematol. (Basel) *59*, 65–72 (1978).
22. Shuster, J., Gold, P., Poulik, M. D. L.: β_2-Microglobulin levels in cancerous and other disease states. Clin. Chim. Acta *67*, 307–313 (1976).
23. Simmons, A. V., Spiers, A. S. D., Fayers, P. M.: Haematological and clinical parameters in assessing activity in Hodgkin's disease and other malignant lymphomas. Q. J. Med. (New Series) *42*, 111–124 (1973).
24. Teillet, F., Boiron, M., Bernard, J.: A reappraisal of clinical and biological signs in staging of Hodgkin's disease. Cancer Res. *31*, 1723–1729 (1971).
25. Warren, R. L., Jellife, A. M., Watson, J. V., Hobbs, C. B.: Prolonged observations on variations in serum copper in Hodgkin's disease. Clin. Radiol. *20*, 247–256 (1969).

26. WERNER, M.: Serum protein changes during the acute-phase reaction. Clin. Chim. Acta *25*, 299–305 (1969).
27. WHITFIELD, J. B., POUNDER, R. E., NEALE, G., MOSS, D. W.: Serum γ-glutamyl transpeptidase activity in liver disease. Gut *13*, 702–708 (1972).

Biology of the Human Malignant Lymphomas

A. L. EPSTEIN and H. S. KAPLAN

Introduction

In the decade following the successful cultivation of African Burkitt's lymphoma cells by EPSTEIN and BARR [10], hundreds of lymphoblastoid cell lines have been established in vitro from patients with leukemias and lymphomas, as well as from individuals with infectious mononucleosis and normal subjects. Because lymphoblastoid cells mimic certain attributes of neoplastic cells, it was not appreciated for several years that they are nonneoplastic B-lymphocytes infected with the Epstein-Barr virus (EBV).

In 1973, a new research program directed at the biology, virology, and immunology of the human malignant lymphomas was inaugurated in this laboratory. It was evident that the successful continuous cultivation of a spectrum of lymphomas was an essential first step. It was recognized, moreover, that it would be necessary to prove rigorously that all such established cell lines were neoplastic (by the criteria of aneuploidy and heterotransplantation) and were not lymphoblastoid (not B cells and/or devoid of the EBV genome). Cell lines meeting these criteria were first established from malignant effusions of three patients with a biopsy diagnosis of diffuse histiocytic lymphoma, and were designated SU-DHL-1, -2, and -3 [5]. Subsequently, cell lines have been established from seven additional patients with diffuse histiocytic lymphoma, three patients with North American Burkitt's lymphoma, and one patient with acute lymphoblastic leukemia. Many of these cell lines have been characterized with respect to cell surface markers and cytochemical features [9], heterotransplantability [8], and adaptation to clonal growth on agar [6]. Two of the North American Burkitt's lymphoma cell lines have been studied for the presence of the EBV genome [7] and the chromosome 14 translocation [14], which had previously been detected in biopsies and cell cultures from patients with African Burkitt's lymphoma [13, 20, 33]. It is the purpose of this communication to summarize the culture characteristics, surface markers, morphologic and cytochemical features, cytogenetic abnormalities, and biologic behavior of the cell lines established to date in this investigative program.

Materials and Methods

Details of the methods used for in vitro establishment and cloning, morphological and cytochemical characterization, identification of cell surface markers, chromosome analysis, intracranial heterotransplantation into the *nude* mouse, and EBNA tests for the presence of the EBV genome have been presented in earlier publications [5–9, 14]. Lymphoma cells were obtained from malignant pleural or peritoneal effusions, lymph node biopsies, and spleen specimens removed at staging laparotomy. All histologic sections of biopsy and surgical staging material were reviewed and classified by DR. RONALD F. DORFMAN, co-director of the Laboratory of Surgical Pathology, according to the histopathologic classification of RAPPAPORT [27].

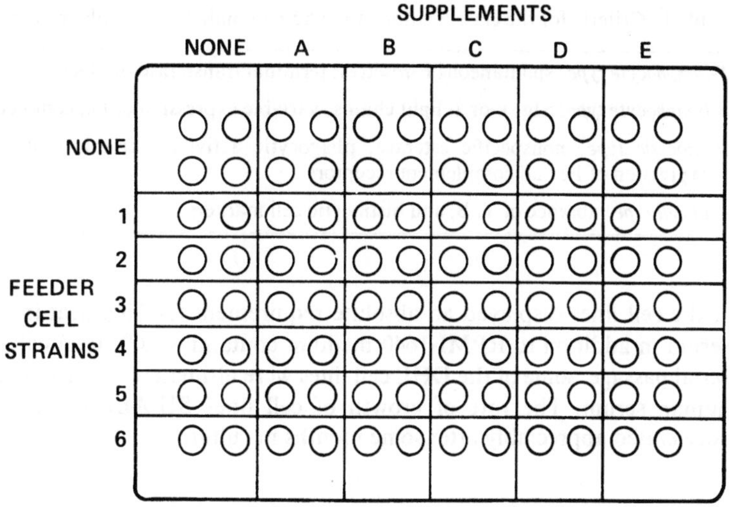

Fig. 1. Growth support system for the initial establishment of the human malignant lymphomas. Feeder cell strains 1–6 are plated in the horizontal set of wells 7 days prior to the addition of 5×10^4 lymphoma cells to each of 96 wells of a microtiter II tissue culture plate. Growth supplements A–E diluted in complete medium were then added to the vertical sets of wells. Direct observation of cell growth established the optimal nutritional requirements for each biopsy specimen

In order to identify the nutritive growth requirements of each tumor specimen, microtiter II tissue culture plates were used to screen a variety of parameters, including media, sera, effusion fluids, and feeder layers (Fig. 1). By cloning tumor cells from biopsy specimens and established cell lines on 0.5% Noble agar substrates, it was possible to quantitatively determine the optimal in vitro requirements of each lymphoma. As an important first step in the establishment of the cell lines, cell suspensions of the biopsy specimens were frozen at −1°C/min in medium containing 10% dimethylsulfoxide. When initial attempts at establishment in vitro failed, cells from thawed ampules were used to experimentally define new culture requirements. By the use of these methods, consecutive cases of malignant lymphomas were established in continuous suspension culture and frozen in liquid nitrogen for permanent storage.

Established cell lines were examined for the presence of nonspecific esterase by the α-naphthyl acetate method [32], for the capacity to form spontaneous (E) rosettes [3], IgG-EA and IgM-EAC rosettes [29], for the presence of Fc receptors [4], surface immunoglobulin (SIg) [25], κ- and λ- light chains of immunoglobulin [18], for lysozyme production by the lysoplate method of OSSERMAN and LAWLOR [23], and for phagocytic activity, using heat-killed *Candida albicans*. The criteria utilized in identifying tumor cell types are presented in Table 1.

Results

Establishment of Cell Lines

Cell lines have been successfully grown in continuous suspension culture from ten patients with a histopathologic diagnosis of diffuse histiocytic lymphoma (designated SU-DHL-1–10), three with North American Burkitt's lymphoma [designated SU-AmB-1, -2, and -3 (one of whom had ataxia telangiectasia)], and one with acute lymphoblastic leukemia (designated SU-ALL-1). All but two of these cell lines initially required a fibroblastic or epithelial cell feeder layer (Fig. 2) from which they were weaned after 1–3 weeks in culture (Fig. 3). Except for SU-ALL-

Table 1. Criteria for the classification of the human malignant lymphomas and leukemias

T-lymphocyte type: spontaneous E-rosettes; terminal transferase production
B-lymphocyte type: SIg; κ-or λ- light chains; variable expression of Fc, complement, and EBV receptors
Histiocytic type; nonspecific esterase; phagocytic activity; variable synthesis of lysozyme; variable expression of Fc and complement receptors
Null cell type: absence of T, B, and histiocytic cell markers

1, the cell lines displayed an absolute requirement for 10% heat-inactivated, pooled human serum in addition to RPMI-1640 medium containing 20% fetal calf serum. After prolonged serial passage, some of the DHL cell lines were ultimately adapted to growth in the absence of human serum. The rate of growth of cell lines SU-ALL-1, SU-DHL-6, and SU-DHL-7 accelerated appreciably after some months in culture.

Clonal Growth on Agar

Several diffuse histiocytic and Burkitt's lymphoma cell lines were successfully cloned on agar (Fig. 4). In the presence of human serum and selected feeder monolayers, cloning efficiencies increased significantly from less than 1% to 15%–25% (Table 2). In addition, the cloning efficiencies of certain cell lines showed a concentration-dependent increase with specific supplements, including dithiothreitol, L-cysteine (Fig. 5), 2-mercaptoethanol, and malignant pleural effusion fluids. A given cell line had an identical cloning efficiency when plated on the surface of the agar and in semisolid agar suspension. After a single passage on agar, cells subpassaged from visible colonies showed markedly increased cloning efficiencies, to levels as

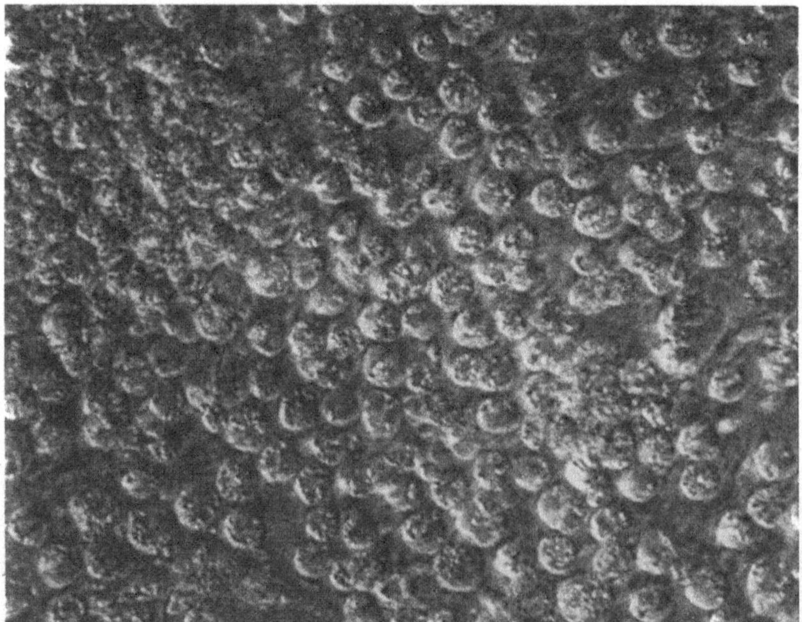

Fig. 2. SU-DHL-1 cells growing as a weakly attached sheet on the contact-inhibited epithelial monolayer after 10 days in culture (phase contrast × 500). Reproduced from Epstein and Kaplan (5)

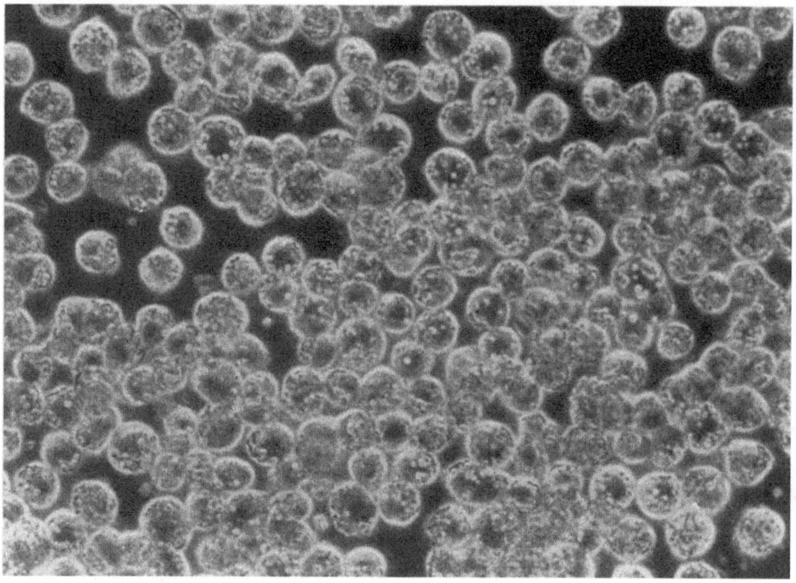

Fig. 3. Homogeneous culture of SU-DHL-1 tumor cells growing in the absence of the epithelial feeder layer after 20 days (phase contrast, × 500). Reproduced from EPSTEIN and KAPLAN (5)

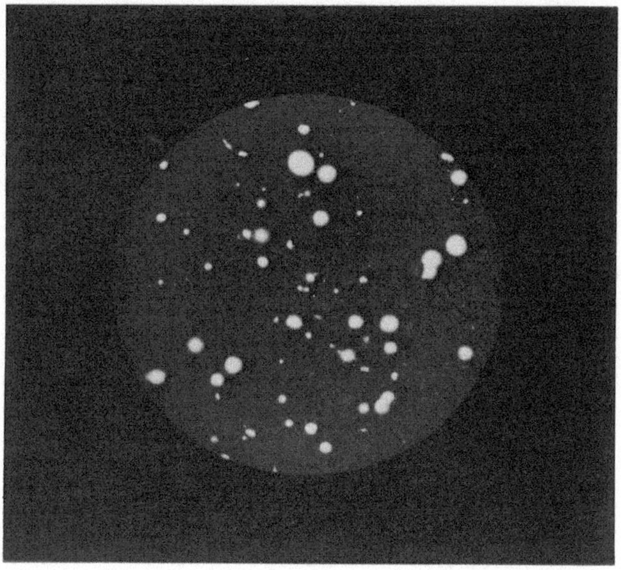

Fig. 4. Appearance of SU-DHL-4 cell colonies after 2 weeks on 0.5% Noble agar

high as 50%. Such cloning efficiencies, coupled with the use of replica plating [17], make this technique applicable to cytogenetic and quantitative radiobiologic, immunologic, and chemotherapeutic studies.

Characterization of Cell Lines

Based on the sets of criteria listed in Table 1, cell lines SU-DHL-1 and -2 were found to be of the histiocytic type, cell lines SU-DHL-3, -4, -5, -6, -7, and -10 of the B-lymphocyte type, and

Table 2. Effects of feeder layers and human serum on the cloning efficiency of human malignant lymphoma cell lines

Feeder layers (No.)	Cell lines				
	SU-DHL-1	SU-DHL-2	SU-DHL-4	SU-DHL-5	SU-AmB-1
Without human serum					
2	0[a]	<1	0	0	0
6	0	1	0	<1	0
8	0	<1	0	0	0
9	0	0	0	0	0
With human serum					
2	0	14	15	5	5
6	0	13	11	11	25
8	0	0	0	0	0
9	0	0	0	0	0
10	0	0	0	0	0

[a] Percentage cloning.

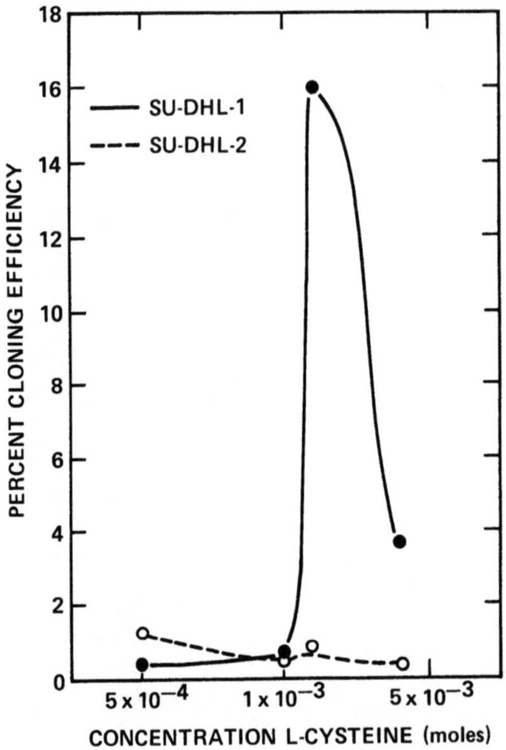

Fig. 5. The effects of various concentrations of L-cysteine on the cloning efficiences of two diffuse histiocytic lymphoma cell lines

cell lines SU-DHL-8 and -9 of the null cell type. Although nine out of the ten DHL cell lines tested were not found to synthesize lysozyme, the report by Sundström and Nilsson [30] of lysozyme production by the DHL cell line U-937 suggests that a small minority of diffuse histiocytic lymphomas, like the monocytic leukemias [23], synthesize this enzyme.

The two North American Burkitt's lymphoma cell lines studied to date displayed different marker characteristics, but were nonetheless identifiable as B-lymphocyte in origin [7]. The acute lymphoblastic leukemia cell line, SU-ALL-1, showed a high percentage of E-rosette formation, terminal transferase production, and was devoid of all B-lymphocyte and histiocytic type characteristics (A. L. EPSTEIN et al., in preparation). It was, therefore, found to resemble other previously reported T-lymphocyte type acute lymphoblastic leukemia cell lines [12, 16, 21].

Epstein-Barr Virus Studies

In collaboration with Drs. Werner and Gertrude Henle, the cell lines were studied for the presence of the EBV genome by the EBNA test. Although many of the DHL patients had positive serologies to EBV antigens, all ten DHL cell lines were EBNA-negative. Because of these findings, the DHL cell lines were clearly distinguishable from lymphoblastoid cultures [22]. In addition, the results strongly suggest that EBV plays no etiologic role in the induction of the human histiocytic lymphomas. The SU-ALL-1 cell line, like other malignant T-cell cultures [12, 16, 21], was also EBNA-negative.

The SU-AmB-1 cell line was EBNA-negative, in keeping with observations which had previously been made on several North American Burkitt's lymphoma biopsies [24]. In direct contrast, the SU-AmB-2 cell line proved to be EBNA-positive. It was also successfully superinfected with EBV and was susceptible to the induction of other EBV antigens by treatment with halogenated pyrimidine analogues [7]. A small number of other North American Burkitt's lymphomas have since been reported to be EBNA-positive or to contain EBV DNA [11, 34]. Our findings suggested the hypothesis that two different classes of morphologically indistinguishable undifferentiated B-cell lymphomas exist, one of which is positive for the presence of EBV genomes and occurs endemically in Africa and New Guinea and sporadically in other parts of the world, the other of which is EBV-negative and occurs sporadically throughout the world, including the endemic areas [7]. EBV studies of the SU-AmB-3 cell line are presently in progress.

Chromosome Studies

With the establishment of two North American Burkitt's lymphoma cell lines, one of which is EBV-negative, a karyotypic study was initiated to search for the presence of the 14q+ translocation, first detected by MANOLOV and MANOLOVA [20] in several EBV-positive African Burkitt's lymphomas. In collaboration with DRS. BARBARA KAISER-MCCAW and FREDERICK HECHT [14], Giemsa banding studies performed on the SU-AmB-1 and -2 cell lines and on three African Burkitt's lymphoma cell lines revealed the presence of a translocation from the long arm of chromosome 8 onto the long arm of chromosome 14 in all of the cell lines (Figs. 6 and 7). Since the 8q-/14q+ translocation was observed in both EBV-positive and EBV-negative North American Burkitt's lymphoma cell lines, this chromosomal abnormality appears to correlate with lymphocytic neoplasia rather than with EBV. In support of this conclusion, the 14q+ translocation has not been observed in EBV-transformed lymphocytes or in lymphoblastoid cell lines derived from peripheral lymphocytes of seropositive normal individuals or patients with infectious mononucleosis [13]. In addition, EBV infection of an EBV-negative lymphoma cell line, which reportedly did not contain the 14q+ translocation, failed to produce the translocation in the derived subline [33]. Like the Philadelphia chromosome seen in chronic myelogenous leukemia [28], the 14q+ translocation may, therefore, represent a tissue-specific, nonrandom chromosomal abnormality characteristic of lymphoid malignancies. All of the DHL cell lines exhibited aneuploidy, providing evidence of their neoplastic nature. Giemsa banding studies of the DHL and SU-ALL-1 cell lines are currently in progress.

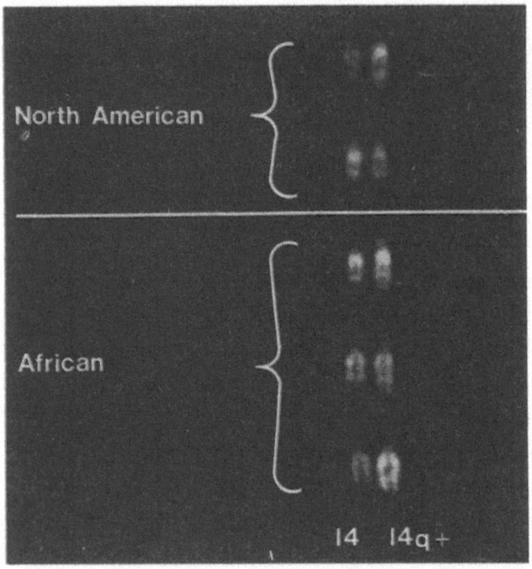

Fig. 6. The number 14 chromosomes from two North American and three African Burkitt's lymphoma cell lines. From top to bottom the cell lines are SU-AmB-1 and SU-AmB-2 (both of North American origin) and EB3, HR-1, and Raji (all of African origin). The chromosomes are quinacrine stained. The number 14 on the right in each instance (labeled 14q+) is longer than usual due to addition of material to the long arm (q). Reproduced from KAISER-McCAW et al. (14)

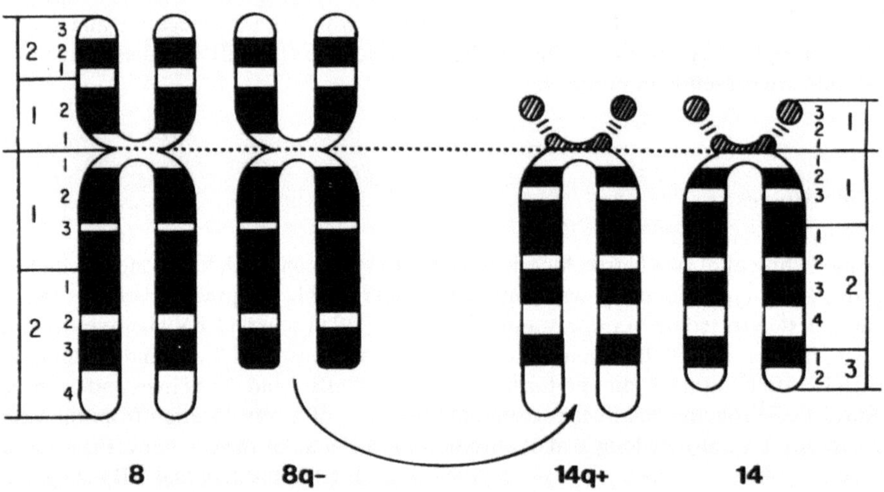

Fig. 7. Diagram of the translocation found in both North American and African Burkitt's lymphoma cell lines. The bands and their numbering are in keeping with the standard Paris Chromosome Conference nomenclature. Reproduced from KAISER-McCAW et al. (14)

Heterotransplantation

Intracranial heterotransplantation in the nude, athymic mouse proved to be a highly successful technique for the in vivo cultivation of both primary human malignant lymphomas taken directly from the patient and cell lines initially established in vitro [8]. Take rates were approximately 90% by the intracranial route of inoculation and very low by the subcutaneous

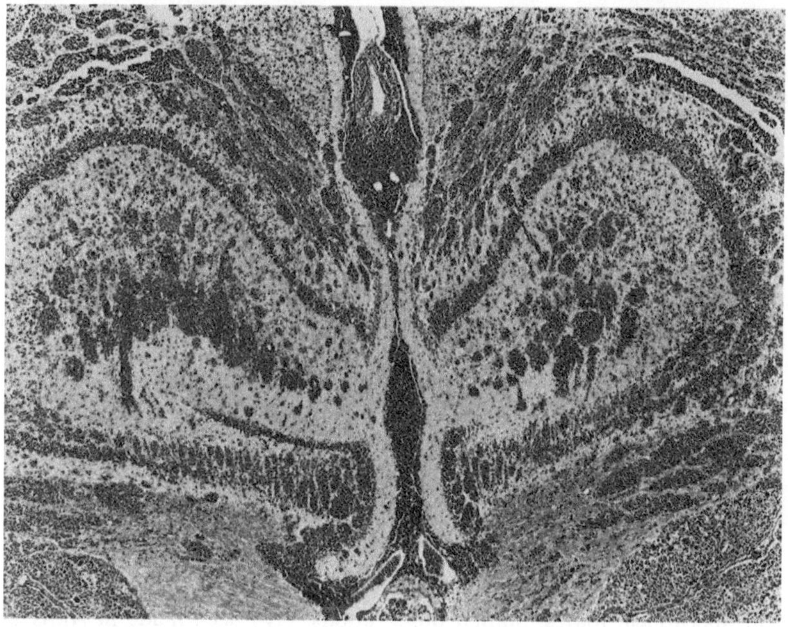

Fig. 8. Tumor infiltration blending into the normal CNS as a caricature of the preexisting architecture. SU-DHL-3 cells infiltrating the deep white matter, hippocampus, third ventricle, stria medullaris, and thalamus (hematoxylin and eosin × 30). Reproduced from EPSTEIN et al. (8)

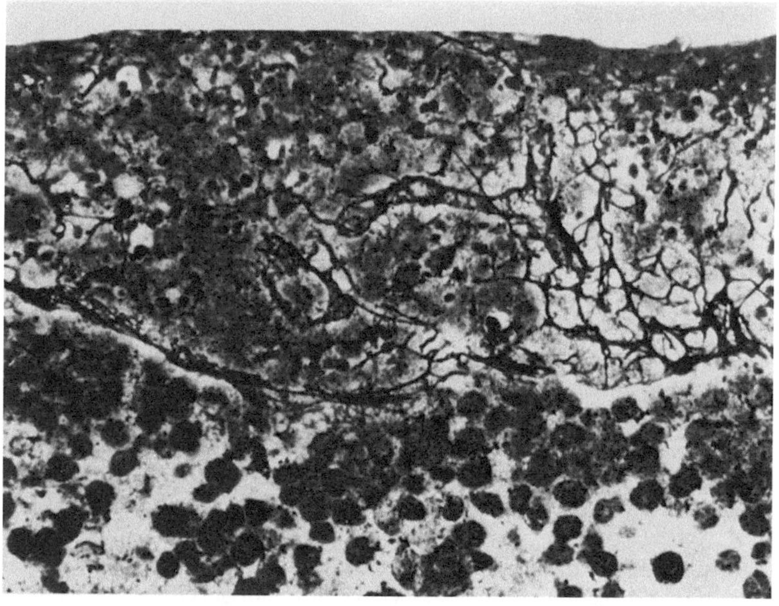

Fig. 9. Disruption of the meningeal reticulin-fiber network and subpial spread by invading SU-DHL-2 cells (silver for reticulin × 400)

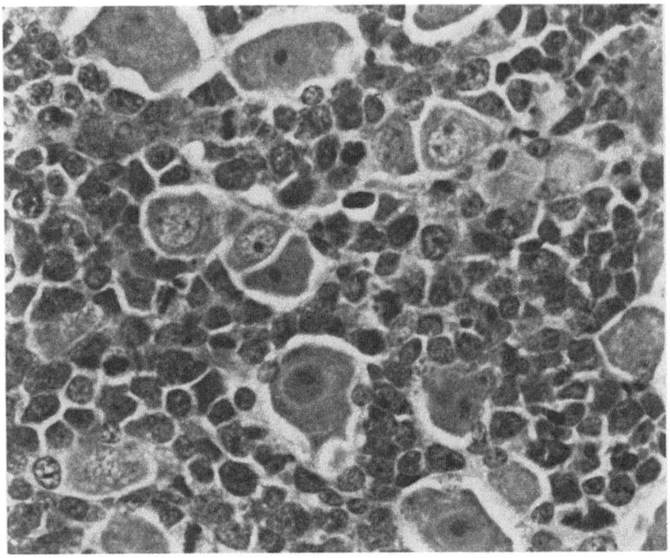

Fig. 10. Invasion of the dorsal root ganglion by SU-AmB-1 cells (hematoxylin and eosin, × 400)

or intraperitoneal routes. Similar observations have been made in ARNSTEIN et al. [1]. The autonomous, neoplastic nature of these human malignant lymphoma cell lines was further manifested by their ability to infiltrate and spread widely in the brain and meninges (Figs. 8 and 9) and occasionally in the spinal cord and dorsal root ganglia (Fig. 10). The tumor cells in the brain were convincingly demonstrated to be human in origin by their positive immunofluorescent staining reactions with heterologous antibodies prepared against human spleen cells and absorbed in mice. Vascular invasion, manifested by the presence of lymphoma cells in the lumina of small blood vessels, was readily demonstrable in several cases. Paradoxically, however, no evidence of systemic dissemination of the human lymphoma cells could be detected.

Discussion

The new techniques developed during the course of these investigations have opened the way to the successful in vitro cultivation of a widening spectrum of human malignant lymphomas, thus greatly extending the scope of human lymphoma research beyond the African Burkitt's lymphomas [10] and the handfull of T-lymphoblastic lymphomas and leukemias [12, 16, 21] previously available for study. The differential diagnosis of histiocytic, B-lymphocyte, and null cell lymphomas, which has not been possible on the basis of conventional morphology alone [19], has been convincingly achieved by the application of a battery of cytochemical, functional, and cell surface marker tests, which succeeded in identifying two of ten cell lines established from patients with a biopsy diagnosis of diffuse histiocytic lymphoma as histiocytic, six as malignant B-lymphocytes, and two as null cells. Lysozyme secretion, noted in the only other known histiocytic cell line established to date [26, 30], was absent in SU-DHL-1 and SU-DHL-2.

The availability of these pure cell cultures, devoid of contaminating stromal elements, should facilitate the detection of tumor-associated or tumor-specific antigens by immunofluorescence with appropriately absorbed heterologous antibodies prepared against the cultured cells. The development of such immunologic reagents may provide still another approach to the histopathologic differentiation of these neoplasms. Moreover, such immunologic reagents may permit the detection and ultimate indentification of viral agents other than EBV which may be present and perhaps of etiologic significance in these tumors. The cell cultures should also facilitate biochemical studies for the detection of oncornavirus "fingerprints" such as reverse transcriptase [2, 31], and some of the cell lines, as has already occurred with SU-DHL-1 [15], may initiate the production and release of candidate human lymphoma viruses during continuous in vitro cultivation. It is hoped that these methods will be widely adopted by other investigators interested in the biology, cytology, virology, and immunology of this fascinating spectrum of human neoplasms.

Acknowledgements

These studies were supported by research contract NO1-CP-43228 from the National Cancer Institute, National Institutes of Health, Department of Health, Education, and Welfare, and by gifts to the Joseph Edward Luetje Memorial Fund for Lymphoma research. Alan Epstein is a medical and graduate student in the Medical Scientist Training Program, Stanford university School of Medicine, supported by NIH grant GM-01922.

References

1. Arnstein, P., Taylor, D. O., Nelson-Rees, W. A., Huebner, R. J., Lennette, E. H.: Propagation of human tumors in antithymocyte serum-treated mice, J. Natl. Cancer Inst. *52*, 71–84 (1974).
2. Baltimore, D.: RNA-dependent DNA polymerase in virions of RNA tumor viruses. Nature *226*, 1209-1211 (1970).
3. Bentwich, Z., Douglas, S., Seigal, F., Kunkel, H.: human lymphocyte-sheep erythrocyte rosette formation: some characteristics of the interaction. Clin. Immunol. Immunopathol. *1*, 511 (1973).
4. Dickler, H., Kunkel, H.: Interaction of aggregated gamma-globulin with B lymphocytes. J. Exp. Med. *136*, 191–196 (1972).
5. Epstein, A. L., Kaplan, H. S.: Biology of the human malignant lymphomas. I. Establishment in continuous cell culture and heterotransplantation of diffuse histiocytic lymphomas. Cancer *34*, 1851–1872 (1974).
6. Epstein, A. L., Kaplan, H. S.: feeder layer and nutritional requirements for the establishment and cloning of human malignant lymphoma cell lines. Proc. Am. Soc. Clin. Oncol. *18*, 293 (abst. C-108) (1977).
7. Epstein, A. L., Henle, W., Henle, G., Hewetson, J. F., Kaplan, H. S.: Surface marker characteristics and Epstein-Barr virus studies of two established North American Burkitt's lymphoma cell lines. Proc. Natl. Acad. Sci. U.S.A. *73*, 228–232 (1976a).
8. Epstein, A. L., Herman, M. M., Kim, H., Dorfman, R. F., Kaplan, H. S.: Biology of the human malignant lymphomas. III. Intracranial heterotransplantation in the nude, athymic mouse. Cancer *37*, 2158–2176 (1976b).
9. Epstein, A. L., Kim, H., Polliack, A., Levy, R., Dorfman, R., Kaplan, H.: Morphological and functional characterization of seven diffuse histiocytic lymphoma cell lines. Proc. Am. Assoc. Cancer Res. *18*, 95 (abst. 377) (1977).
10. Epstein, M. A., Barr, Y. M.: Cultivation in vitro of human lymphoblasts from Burkitt's malignant lymphoma. Lancet 1964 *i*, 252–253.
11. Gravell, M., Levine, P. H., McIntyre, R. F., Land, V. J., Pagano, J. S.: Epstein-Barr virus in an American patient with Burkitt's lymphoma: Detection of viral genome in tumor tissue and establishment of a tumor-derived cell line (NAB). J. Natl. Cancer Inst. *56*, 701–704 (1976).
12. Itoh, U., Minowada, J., Moore, G. E., Pressman, D.: Rosette-forming human lymphoid cell lines (T-cell line Molt). II. Ability for clonal growth. J. Natl. Cancer Inst. *52*, 1403–1407 (1974).
13. Jarvis, J. E., Ball, G., Rickinson, A. B., Epstein, M.A.: Cytogenetic Studies on human lymphoblastoid cell lines from Burkitt's lymphomas and other sources. Int. J. Cancer *14*, 716–721 (1974).

14. Kaiser-McCaw, B., Epstein, A. L., Kaplan, H. S., Hecht, F.: Chromosome 14 translocation in African and North American Burkitt's lymphoma. Int. J. Cancer *19*, 482–486 (1977).
15. Kaplan, H. S., Goodenow, R. S., Epstein, A. L., Gartner, S., Decleve, A., Rosenthal, P. N.: Isolation of a C-type RNA virus from an established human histiocytic lymphoma cell line. Proc. Natl. Acad. Sci. U.S.A. *74*, 2564–2568 (1977).
16. Kaplan, J., Shope, T. C., Peterson, W. D., jr.: Epstein-Barr virus-negative human malignant T-cell lines. J. Exp. Med. *139*, 1070–1076 (1974).
17. Kuroki, T.: Colony formation of mammalian cells on agar plates and its application to Lederberg's replica plating. Exp. Cell. Res. *80*, 55–62 (1973).
18. Levy, R., Warnke, R., Dorfman, R. F., Haimovich, J.: The monoclonality of human B cell lymphomas. J. Exp. Med. *145*, 1014–1028 (1977).
19. Lukes, R., Collins, R.: Immunologic characterization of human malignant lymphomas. Cancer *34*, 1488–1503 (1974).
20. Manolov, G., Manolova, Y.: Marker band in one chromosome 14 from Burkitt lymphomas. Nature *237*, 33–34 (1972).
21. Minowada, J., Ohnuma, T., Moore, G. E.: Rosette-forming human lymphoid cell lines. I. Establishment and evidence for origin of thymus-derived lymphocytes. J. Natl. Cancer Inst. *49*, 891–894 (1973).
22. Nilsson, K., Ponten, J.: Classification and biological nature of established human hematopoietic cell lines. Int. J. Cancer *15*, 321–341 (1975).
23. Osserman, E. F., Lawlor, D. P.: Serum and urinary lysozyme (muramidase) in monocytic and monomyelocytic leukemia. J. Exp. Med. *124*, 921–951 (1966).
24. Pagano, J., Huang, C. H., Levine, P.: Absence of Epstein-Barr viral DNA in American Burkitt's lymphoma. N. Engl. J. Med. *289*, 1395–1399 (1973).
25. Rabellino, E., Colon, S., Grey, H. M., Unanue, E. R.: Immunoglobulins on the surface of lymphocytes. I. Distribution and quantitation. J. Exp. Med. *133*, 156–167 (1971).
26. Ralph, P., Moore, M., Nilsson, K.: Lysozyme synthesis by established human and murine histiocytic lymphoma cell lines. J. Exp. Med. *143*, 1528–1533 (1976).
27. Rappaport, H.: Tumors of the hematopoietic system. In: Atlas of Tumor Pathology. Washington, D.C.: Armed Forces Institute of Pathology 1966, pp. 91–123.
28. Rowley, J.: A new consistent chromosomal abnormality in chronic myelogenous leukemia identified by quinacrine fluorescence and Giemsa staining, Nature *243*, 290–293 (1973).
29. Shevach, E., Jaffe, E., Green, I.: Receptors for complement and immunoglobulin on human and animal lymphoid cells. Transplant Rev. *16*, 3–28 (1973).
30. Sundstrom, D., Nilsson, K.: Establishment and characterization of a human histiocytic lymphoma cell line (U-937). Int. J. Cancer *17*, 565–577 (1976).
31. Temin, H. M., Mizutani, S.: RNA-dependent DNA polymerases in virions of Rous sarcoma virus. Nature *226*, 1211–1213 (1970).
32. Yam, L. T., Li, C. Y., Crosby, W. H.: Cytochemical identification of monocytes and granulocytes. Am. J. Clin. Pathol. *55*, 283–290 (1971).
33. Zech, L., Haglund, U., Nilsson, K., Klein, G.: Characteristic chromosomal abnormalities in biopsies and lymphoid-cell lines from patients with Burkitt's and non-Burkitt's lymphomas. Int. J. Cancer *17*, 47–56 (1976).
34. Ziegler, J. L., Anderson, M., Klein, G., Henle, W.: Detection of Epstein-Barr virus DNA in American Burkitt's lymphoma. Int. J. Cancer *17*, 701–706 (1976).

Comparison Between Membrane Markers and Enzyme Markers in 26 Cases of Non-Hodgkin's Malignant Lymphomas

C. MICHEAU and D. BELPOMME

We performed cytoenzymic reactions and PAS stains on 26 cases of malignant lymphomas for which the results of membrane markers were available. The enzyme markers—acid phosphatases and β-glucuronidase—are generally regarded as specific markers of T-cell proliferations. These hydrolases are located in lysosomes near the Golgi apparatus and appear as a red spot in the cytoplasm close to the nuclei (Fig. 1) according to the methods of KATAMAYA and HAYASHI [1, 2] (Table 1) which we used.

Comparison between histologic diagnoses, membrane markers, and enzyme markers was made, and the results are compiled in Tables 2–4. We found complete agreement between membrane and enzyme markers for all cases of T-cell origin. The PAS stain was negative in all

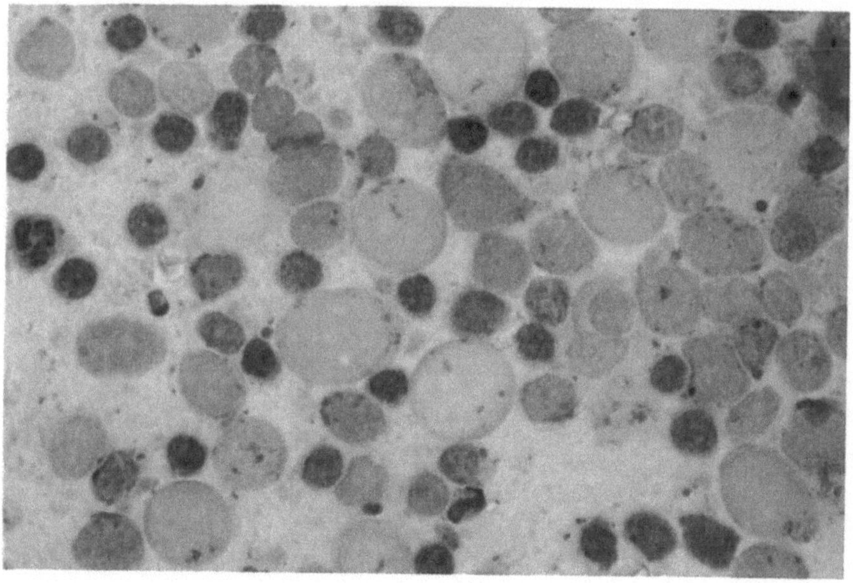

Fig. 1. T-cell malignant lymphoma (LB–D). the positive reaction for B-glucuronidase appears as red deposit in the area of the Golgi apparatus. Hayashi method. (× 800)

Table 1. Malignant lymphomas: cytoenzytic markers (methods)

Acid Phosphatase[a]	Naphthol AS-BI	Phosphoric acid (sodium salt)	Hexazoted pararosanilin	pH = 5.2 h
β-Glucuronidase[b]	Naphthol AS-BI	β-d-glucuronic acid	Hexazoted pararosanilin	pH = 5.2 h

[a] According to KATAYAMA (1972). [2].

[b] According to HAYASHI (1963–1964). [1].

Table 2. Malignant lymphomas: comparison between membrane markers and enzymic markers (26 cases)

1. T-cell markers

Membrane markers	Acid phosphatase	β-Glucuronidase	PAS	Histologic diagnosis	
T	±[a]	±	—	119/119	Lennert's lymphoma
T	±	+[b]	—	108/193	LB
T	±	±	—	LC	(D)
T	+	+	—	LB	(D)
T	+	+	—	114/146	LB

[a] Less than 70% cells.
[b] More than 70% cells.
LB = Lymphoblastic sarcoma;
LC = Lymphocytic sarcoma;
D = Diffuse.

Table 3. Malignant lymphomas: comparison between membrane markers and enzymic markers (26)

2. B-cell markers

Membrane markers	Acid phosphatase	β-Glucuronidase	PAS	Histologic diagnosis	
B.M.K.	+[a]	—	—	120/496	PLC—N
B.	—	—	—	120/174	PLC—D
B.	±[b]	+	+	131/389	PLC—N
B.M.K.	—	—	—	92/899	PLC—D
B.G.λ	—	—	—	132/189	I.D.
B.M.K.	—	—	—	125/848	I.D.
B.M.D.λ	±	+	±	125/554	PLC—D
B.M.K.	±	—	—	120/571	PLC—N
B.M.λ	—	—	+	125/805	LB
B.M.K.	+	+	—	119/348	PLC—N
B.M.λ	—	—	—	119/865	PLC—D
B.M.λ	+	+	—	132/193	ID
B.M.K.D.	—	—	—	131/980bis	LB

[a] More than 70% cells.
[b] Less than 70%cells.
PLC = Prolymphocytic lymphoma;
I = Immunoblastic sarcoma;
LB = Lymphoblastic sarcoma;
LC = Lymphocytic sarcoma;
RS = Reticulum cell sarcoma;
N = Nodular;
D = Diffuse.

Table 4. Malignant lymphomas: comparison between membrane markers and enzymic markers (26 cases)

3. Null cells[a]

Membrane markers	Acid phosphatase	β-Glucuronidase	PAS	Histologic diagnosis
N	+[b]	±[c]	—	119/945[2] LB
N	∓	—	—	120/086 LB—D
N	±	—	—	119/562 RS?
N (?)	±	+	—	120/938 RS?

[a] Four cases composed of mixed T- and B-cell populations were eliminated.
[b] More than 70% cells.
[c] Less than 70% cells.
LB = Lymphoblastic sarcoma;
RS = Reticulum cell sarcoma;
N = Nodular;
D = Diffuse.

cases (Table 2). Table 3 reveals a discrepancy between the two markers in 6 out of 13 cases and especially in three cases in which the histologic diagnosis was nodular prolymphocytic lymphoma. The PAS stain was more or less positive in three cases. Table 4 shows that three out of four cases identified as null cell lymphomas by membrane markers have T-cell enzyme markers. PAS was negative in all cases.

The interpretation of these results is quite difficult. It should be said that the correlation is very good for tumors identified as T-cell lymphomas by membrane markers, not very good for lymphomas with B-cell membrane markers and very poor for null cell lymphomas.

The questions are: what is the respective value of the membrane and enzyme markers for identifying the T- and B-cell origin of malignant lymphomas? Are the latter more precise and more reliable than the former? Can the enzyme markers detect pre-T cells which are not detected by routine membrane markers, as suggested by the results obtained for null cell lymphomas? These preliminary results have to be correlated with the clinical history and evolution of the diseases; this study is in progress. As a result, further studies have to be carried out in order to know whether enzyme markers may be considered reliable or not.

References

1. Hayashi, M., Nakajima, Y., Fishman, W. H.: The cytologic demonstration of B-glucuronidase employing Naphthol AS-BI glucuronide and hexazonium pararosanilin; a preliminary report. J. Histochem. Cytochem. *12*, 293–297 (1964).
2. Katayama, I., Li, C. Y., Yam, L. T.: Histochemical study of acid phosphatase isoenzyme in leukemic reticuloendotheliosis. Cancer, *29*, 157–164 (1972).

Hairy Cell Leukemia: B-Lymphocyte and Monocytic Properties Displayed by One Cell

E. P. Rieber, M. Hadam, R. P. Linke, J. G. Saal, G. Riethmüller, H. W. v. Heyden, and H. D. Waller

Although hairy cell leukemia (HCL; leukemic reticuloendotheliosis) is clinically and pathologically well-defined [1, 2, 3, 4, 5], the origin of the hairy cells (HC) remains controversial. In a number of reports, the B-lymphocyte origin of HC has been rendered likely by the demonstration of surface immunoglobulins (SIg) [3, 6, 17] and very recently by the biosynthesis of immunoglobulins (Ig) [7]. On the other hand, characteristic properties of monocytes such as phagocytosis [3, 6, 18] and adherence to glass and plastic surfaces [3, 10], as well as the failure of monocyte production seen in some patients [16], suggested that the HC belong to the monocytic lineage. These differences with regard to monocytic and B-lymphocyte properties, reported by several authors, prompted us to investigate whether characteristics of both cell populations could simultaneously be demonstrated on individual HC. Particular interest centered on the class distribution of SIg and their synthesis by the HC themselves.

Here we report on the HC of six patients. In most of our experiments, the HC were cytochemically identified by the demonstration of the tartrate-resistant isoenzyme 5 of the acid phosphatase (TRAP), which is reported to be a marker enzyme of HC [9]. This proved to be particularly useful in patients where the HC accounted for only a small percentage of the mononuclear blood cells. By combination of cytochemistry with radioautography for the detection of surface markers and with functional tests, e.g., phagocytosis, it was possible to evaluate three different characteristic properties on a single cell simultaneously.

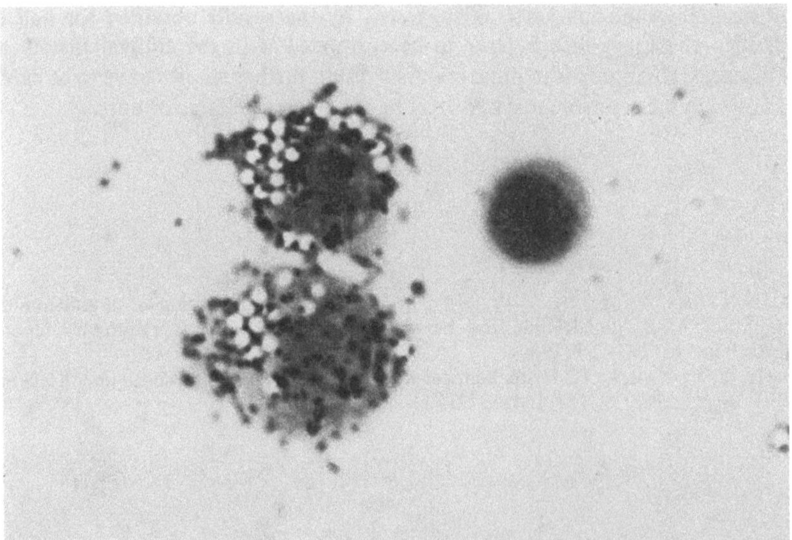

Fig. 1. Radioautograph of mononuclear blood cells in hairy cell leukemia after ingestion of latex particles and labeling with ^{125}I-Fab$_2$ anti-δ chain antibodies

As typical monocytic properties, the capacity of the HC to adhere to glass and plastic surfaces and to phagocytose particles were studied. After 2h. of incubation at 37°C, the TRAP-positive HC of all patients studied adhered to glass coverslips and, when examined by phase-contrast microscopy, showed typical spreading, thus being morphologically almost indistinguishable from normal blood monocytes. The adherence of HC was at least as strong as that of normal monocytes as judged from its resistance to treatment with EDTA-trypsin [14].
The TRAP-positive HC of all patients readily ingested latex particles of more than 1 μm diameter. Figure 1 shows HC after phagocytosis of latex particles; on the same cell surface, IgD is demonstrated by radioautography. Serial sections in electron microscopy revealed that the latex particles were indeed ingested by the HC [14]. Despite the marked phagocytosis of latex particles, HC were not found to engulf larger particles, e.g., erythrocytes, either untreated or sensitized with IgG or IgM antibodies, whereas under identical conditions, normal blood monocytes were heavily loaded with erythrocytes. Phagocytosis of latex particles, however, may not be sufficient to support the monocytic character of HC, as lymphoid cells have also been reported to ingest small particles [18, 19].
Fc Receptors (FcR) have been shown to be surface markers of both monocytes and B-lymphocytes. Determination of the uptake of ^{125}I-labeled aggregated IgG revealed that monocytes bound significantly more aggregates than normal B-lymphocytes. When HC were investigated in the same way, they were found to bind even more aggregates than normal monocytes [12]. However, when aggregate-binding was evaluated by grain count distribution analysis, a broad range of FcR density was detected on the TRAP-positive HC of each patient, which is in marked contrast to the rather homogeneous distribution observed in purified normal cell populations (RIEBER et al., in prep.).
Autochthonous SIg is taken as an exclusive marker for B-lymphocytes [8]. To obviate interactions with the FcR, only Fc-free antibody preparations were used for the detection of surface Ig. Thus, ^{125}I-labeled Fab_2 fragments were prepared from anti-Ig antibodies, which had been purified and rendered monospecific for immunoglobulin heavy and light chains by the use of affinity chromatography. To reduce the amount of serum Ig adsorbed to the cell surface, cells were cultured for at least 12h. in human serum-free medium prior to labeling with the radioactive antibodies. Table 1 shows the results abtained for the TRAP-positive HC of the six patients investigated. Only one light chain type was detected in individual patients, suggesting monoclonality of SIg in HC. In three patients μ and δ-chains were simultaneously expressed on single HC, as usually found on normal B-lymphocytes [15] and cells of chronic lymphocytic leukemia [11]. In two patients, only γ-chains were found, and in one patient the unusual combination of γ and δ-chains was observed. Similar to what has been found for the FcR, the density of SIg on HC of individual patients varied considerably.
In order to prove the synthesis of SIg by HC, we tried to remove the SIg and assess their reappearance during cell culture. Since we were not able to completely digest off the SIg with trypsin without damaging the cells, SIg was removed by capping. It has previously been shown

Table 1. Labeling of TRAP-positive mononuclear blood cells in hairy cell leukemia by ^{125}I-Fab_2 anti-heavy and light chain antibodies in radioautography

Patient	μ	δ	γ	α	κ	λ
M.D.	+	+	—	—	—	+
F.W.	—	—	+	—	+	—
K.F.	—	+	+	—	+	—
W.R.	+	+	—	—	—	+
R.R.	+	+	—	—	—	+
W.S.	—	—	+	—	—	+

that SIg on HC can very effectively be redistributed by incubation with bivalent anti-Ig antibodies at 37°C [13]. For example, in one patient, after removal by capping, both IgM and IgD were found to reappear on the HC surface during cell culture in human serum-free medium. However, it took 4 days of culture until SIg could again be detected on HC, whereas normal B-lymphocytes treated identically reexpressed their SIg already after 24h. [14]. Thus, resynthesis of SIg did take place in HC, but seemed to be much slower than in normal B-lymphocytes. However, in both HC and normal B-lymphocytes, the density of SIg reexpressed after capping was much lower when compared with noncapped control cells incubated under identical conditions. Whether this has possibly been caused by inappropriate culture conditions or by a suppressing signal induced by the capping, remains open. The synthesis of Ig by HC was also demonstrated by labeling pure HC populations obtained from patients' spleens with ^{3}H-leucine. Labeled Ig could be precipitated with heavy or light chain specific anti-Ig antibodies from both cell lysates and culture supernatants. Preliminary results from polyacrylamide gel electrophoresis indicate that most of the radioactivity precipitated from culture supernatants was associated with light chains (RIEBER et al., in prep.).

In conclusion, it is clearly demonstrated that HC can display both monocytic and B-lymphocytic properties at the same time. An explanation for the marked heterogeneity with regard to functional capacities and surface marker expression described in the literature has to be given.

Acknowledgements

This work was supported by Deutsche Forschungsgemeinschaft Bonn-Bad Godesberg.

References

1. BOURONCLE, B. A., WISEMAN, B. K., DOAN, C. A.: Leukemic reticuloendotheliosis. Blood *13*, 609–630 (1958).
2. BURKE, J. S., BYRNE, G. E., RAPPAPORT, H.: Hairy cell leukemia (Leukemic reticuloendotheliosis). I. A clinical pathological study of 21 patients. Cancer *33*, 1399–1410 (1974).
3. CATOVSKY, D., PETTIT, J. E., GALETTO, J., OKOS, A., GALTON, D. A. G: The B-lymphocyte nature of the hairy cell of leukemic reticuloendotheliosis. Br. J. Haematol. *26*, 29–37 (1974a).
4. CATOVSKY, D., PETTIT, J. E., GALTON, D. A. G., SPEIRS, A. S. D., HARRISON, C. V.: Leukemic reticuloendotheliosis ('Hairy' cell leukemia): a distinct clinico-pathological entity. Br. J. Haematol. *26*, 9–27 (1974b).
5. FLANDRIN, G., DANIEL, M. T., FOURCADE, M., CHELLOUL, N.: Leucémie à tricholeucocytes (hairy cell leukemia). Étude clinique et cytologique de 55 observations. Nouv. Rev. Fr. Haematol. *13*, 609–640 (1973).
6. FU, S. M., WINCHESTER, R. J., RAI, K. R., KUNKEL, H. G.: Hairy cell leukemia. Proliferation of a cell with phagocytic and B-lymphocytic properties. Scand. J. Immunol. *3*, 847–851 (1974).
7. GOLDE, D. W., STEVENS, R. H., QUAN, S. G., SAXON, A.: Immunoglobulin synthesis in hairy cell leukemia. Br. J. Haematol. *35*, 359–365 (1977).
8. JONDAL, M., HOLM, G., WIGZELL, H.: Surface markers on human T- and B-lymphocytes. I. A large population of lymphocytes forming non immune rosettes with sheep red blood cells. J. Exp. Med. *136*, 207–215 (1972).
9. KATAYAMA, I., LI, C. Y., YAM, L. T.: Histochemical study of acid phosphatase isoenzyme in leukemic reticuloendotheliosis. Cancer *29*, 157–164 (1972).
10. KING, G. W., HURTUBISE, P. E., SAGONE, JR., A. L., LO BUGLIO, A. F., METZ, E. N.: Leukemic reticuloendotheliosis. A study of the origin of the malignant cell. Am. J. Med. *59*, 411–416 (1975).
11. KUBO, R. T., GREY, H. M., PIROFSKY, B.: IgD: a major immunoglobulin on the surface of lymphocytes from patients with chronic lymphatic leukemia. J. Immunol. *112*, 1952–1954 (1974).
12. RIEBER, E. P., SAAL, J. G., RIETHMÜLLER, G., HEYDEN, H. W., WALLER, H. D.: Strong expression of Fc-receptors on leukemic cells in hairy cell leukemia. Z. Immunitaetsforsch. *151*, 282–288 (1976a).

13. Rieber, E. P., v. Heyden, H. W., Linke, R. P., Saal, J. G., Riethmüller, G., Waller, H. D.: Hairy cell leukemia. Characterization of the leukemic cell: surface immunoglobulins, Fc-receptors and stimulation by mitogens. Klin. Wochenschr. *54*, 1011–1019 (1976b).
14. Rieber, E. P., Linke, R. P., Hadam, M., Saal, J. G., Riethmüller, G., v. Heyden, H. W., Waller, H. D., Schwarz, H.: Hairy cell leukemia: simultaneous demonstration of autochthonous surface-Ig and monocytic functions of hairy cells. In: Immunological Diagnosis of Leukemias and Lymphomas. Thierfelder, S., Rodt, H., Thiel, E. (ed.) Berlin-Heidelberg-New York: Springer-Verlag 1977, pp. 157–161.
15. Rowe, D. S., Hug, K., Forni, L., Pernis, B.: Immunoglobulin D as a lymphocyte receptor, J. Exp. Med. *138*, 965–972 (1973).
16. Seshadri, R. S., Brown, E. J., Zipursky, A.: Leukemic reticuloendotheliosis. A failure of monocyte production. N. Engl. J. Med. *295*, 181–184 (1976).
17. Stein, H., Kaiserling, E.: Surface immunoglobulins and lymphocyte specific surface antigens on leukemic reticuloendotheliosis cells. Clin. Exp. Immunol. *18*, 63–71 (1974).
18. Utsinger, P. D., Yount, W. J., Fuller, C. R., Logue, M, J.,Orringer, E. P.: Hairy cell leukemia: B-lymphocyte and phagocytic properties. Blood *49*, 19–27 (1977).
19. Zucker-Franklin, D.: the percentage of monocytes among "mononuclear" cell fractions obtained from normal human blood. J. Immunol. *112*, 234–240 (1974).

Facultative Phagocytosis by Leukemic B-Lymphocytes: Further Proof of the B-Cell Nature of Hairy Cells

D. CATOVSKY, P. SPERANDIO, and M. O'BRIEN

Almost since the first good description of hairy cell leukemia (HCL), also known as leukemic reticuloendotheliosis (LRE), was given by BOURONCLE et al. [3], there have been conflicting arguments on the origin of the characteristic hairy cell. Possible candidates for the origin of hairy cells are shown in Table 1. A more detailed discussion of the subject is given elsewhere [4]. Most workers have argued the possibility that these cells are related to monocytes or B-lymphocytes. Evidence for B-lymphocyte origin has been provided primarily by the demonstration of surface-bound immunoglobulins (SIg), mainly IgM and IgD, and less frequently IgG, usually, but not always, shown to be monoclonal [4, 5, 9, 11, 12, 13, 18]. Furthermore, several groups have now demonstrated resynthesis of monoclonal immunoglob-

Table 1. Candidates for the origin of hairy cells

1. Monocyte—macrophage [15]
2. B-lymphocyte [4, 5, 9, 10, 12, 13, 16, 18]
3. K cells [4]
4. Human equivalent to the mouse 'dendritic' cell [8]
5. B-lymphocyte with phagocytic properties [11, 17, 19]

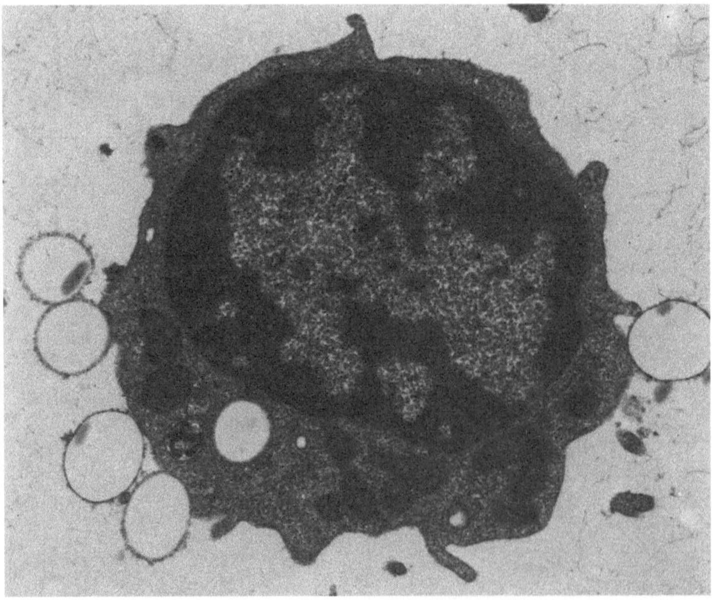

Fig 1. A peripheral blood lymphocyte from a case of chronic lymphocytic leukemia (B-cell type) showing binding of latex particles and one ingested particle. (Lead-uranyl acetate; × 15,000)

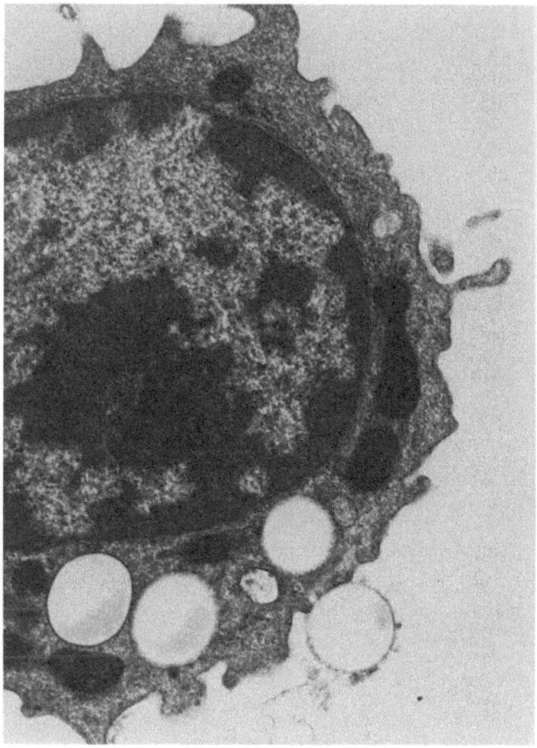

Fig. 2. A peripheral blood cell from a case of prolymphocytic leukemia (B-cell type) showing three latex particles phagocytosed. (Lead-uranyl acetate; × 13,000)

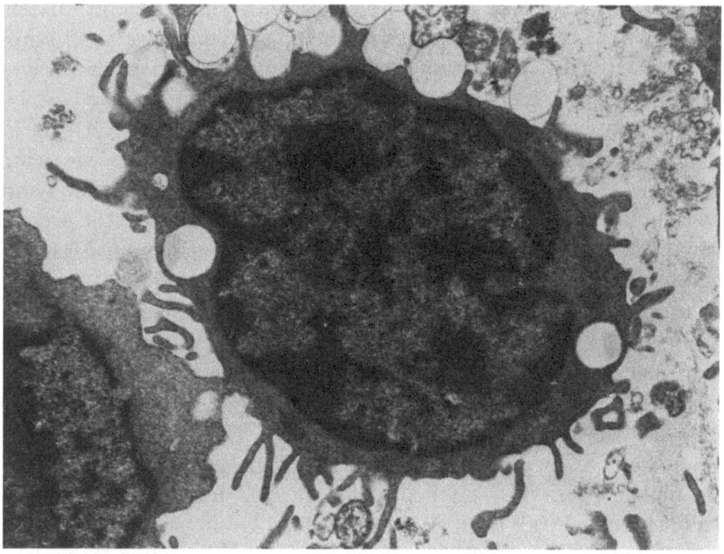

Fig. 3. A hairy cell from the spleen of a case of HCL showing phagocytosis (two particles) and surface binding (several particles) of latex. (Lead-uranyl acetate; × 11,000)

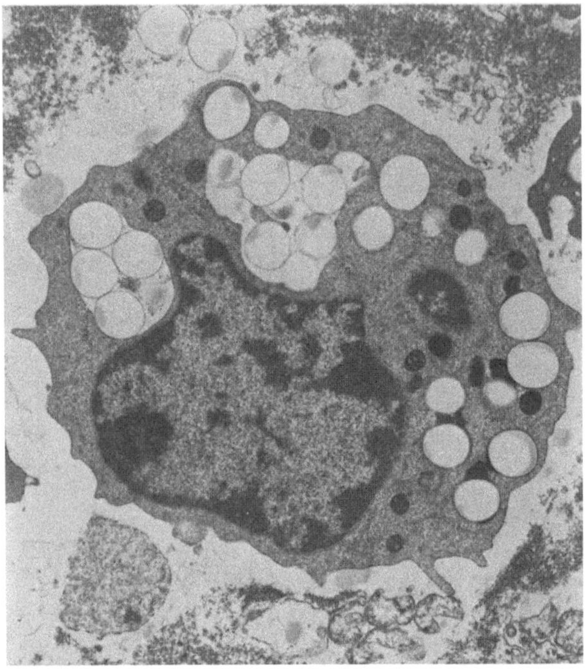

Fig. 4. A normal peripheral blood monocyte with numerous ingested latex particles. Note that several particles are contained within the same phagocytic vacuole. (Lead-uranyl acetate; ×8000)

ulins after the SIg have been removed by a variety of means (trypsinization, prolonged incubation at 37° in serum-free media, etc.) [10, 11, 12, 16, 17, 19]. The lymphocyte nature is also supported by the binding of mouse RBC [6] and in rare cases of sheep RBC [1]. On the other hand, other workers have emphasized the undoubted capacity of hairy cells to phagocytose latex particles and some microorganisms [8, 11, 15, 17, 19], a function primarily related to monocytes and not lymphocytes. The finding of both B-cell surface characteristics and phagocytic potential led to the suggestion that hairy cells may correspond to a hitherto unrecognized cell type: a B-lymphocyte with phagocytic properties [11, 19]. However, few workers have carried out studies on the phagocytic capacity of lymphocytes. Early reports [2, 14, 20, 21] suggested that some cells, morphologically identified as lymphocytes, may be able to phagocytose. We have recently studied the phagocytic capacity of lymphocytes from patients with B-lymphoproliferative disorders other than HCL [7]. Using latex particles of 0.8 μ in diameter and fresh human serum in the incubation mixture, we demonstrated phagocytosis in approximately 15% of lymphocytes from nine cases of chronic lymphocytic leukemia (CLL) and three of prolymphocytic leukemia. In all these samples the predominant cell type (ca. 90%) was a leukemic lymphocyte with SIg and/or binding of mouse RBC [6]. The observations were made both at light microscopy and at ultrastructural level.

In most cases phagocytic lymphocytes were seen predominantly with one or two ingested particles (Fig. 1). In two cases, however, 17%–30% of lymphocytes were seen ingesting three or more latex particles (Fig. 2). This was even higher than in two cases of HCL which were included in that study (Fig. 3). Monocytes usually phagocytose ten or more particles (Fig. 4). Phagocytosis was not observed in the absence of serum but occurred in the presence of serum inactivated at 56°C. Binding of latex particles to the surface of lymphocytes correlated significantly with the degree of phagocytosis. On the other hand, no phagocytosis or binding was observed in cells from two cases of T-CLL and one of Sezary's syndrome. It would appear that phagocytosis by leukemic B-lymphocytes is mediated through their Fc receptor for IgG, which is absent from T-lymphocytes, and that this activity may also be demonstrated in some tonsil lymphocytes (DC and PS, unpublished observation). This study [7] demonstrated that in the same way as hairy cells, other leukemic B-lymphocytes are also facultative phagocytes. Phagocytic capacity as such is not an exclusive property of monocytes, although these cells are, indeed, professional phagocytes. These studies should remove the last remaining argument against hairy cells being lymphocytes in the pathway of B-cell differentiation. However, it does not provide any clue as to the existence of a normal counterpart with the characteristic morphological and cytochemical features of hairy cells; thus, the possibility remains that they are only the result of the neoplastic process.

Acknowledgements

We thank Mr. William Hinkes for the microphotographs. DR. PAOLO SPERANDIO is a Research Fellow from the Division of Medical Oncology, Ospedale Civile di Padova, Italy.

References

1. ADVANI, S. H., TALWALKAR, G. V., NADKARNI, J. S., NADKARNI, J. J., SIRSAT, S. M., SRINIVASAN, U.: Hairy Cell Leukaemia: A case report and review of literature. Indian J. Cancer *13*, 283–287 (1976).
2. BERMAN, L., POLLACK, R.: Erythrophagocytosis by human lymphocytes in vitro. J. Reticuloendothel. Soc. *4*, 219–222 (1967).
3. BOURONCLE, B. A., WISEMAN, B. K., DOAN, C. A.: Leukemic reticuloendotheliosis. Blood *13*, 609–630 (1958).
4. CATOVSKY, D.: Hairy Cell leukaemia and prolymphocytic leukaemia. Clin. Haematol. *6*, 245–268 (1977).
5. CATOVSKY, D., PETTIT, J. E., GALETTO, J., OKOS, A., GALTON, D. A. G.: The B-lymphocyte nature of the "hairy" cell of leukaemic reticuloendotheliosis. Br. J. Haematol. *26*, 29–37 (1974).
6. CATOVSKY, D., CHERCHI, MARIA, OKOS, A., HEGDE, U., GALTON, D. A. G.: Mouse red-cell rosettes in B-lymphoproliferative disorders. Br. J. Haematol. *33*, 173–177 (1976).
7. CATOVSKY, D., SPERANDIO, PAOLA, O'BRIEN, MAUREEN, CHERCHI, MARIA, GALTON, D. A. G.: Phagocytic potential of leukaemic B-lymphocytes. Scand. J. Haematol. *19*, 211–216.
8. DANIEL, M. T., FLANDRIN. G.: Fine structure of abnormal cells in hairy cell (tricholeukocytic) leukemia, with special reference to their *in vitro* phagocytic capacity. Lab. Invest. *30*, 1–8 (1974).
9. DEEGAN, M. J., COSSMAN, J., CHOSNEY, B. T., SCHNITZER, B.: Hairy Cell leukemia: an immunologic and ultrastructural study. Cancer *38*, 1952–1961 (1976).
10. DEBUSSCHER, L., BERNHEIM, J. L., COLLARD-RONGE, E., GOVAERTS, A., HOOGHE, R., LEJEUNE, F. J., ZEICHER, M., STRYCKMANS, P. A.: Hairy Cell Leukemia: Functional, Immunologic, Kinetic and Ultrastructural characterization. Blood *46*, 495–507 (1975).
11. FU, S. M., WINCHESTER, R. J., RAI, K. R., KUNKEL, H. G.: Hairy Cell Leukemia: Proliferation of a Cell with Phagocytic and B-lymphocyte properties. Scand. J. Immunol. *3*, 847–851 (1974).
12. GOLDE, D. W., STEVENS, R. H., QUAN, S. G., SAXON, A.: Immunoglobulin synthesis in hairy cell leukaemia. Br. J. Haematol. *35*, 359–365 (1977).
13. HAEGERT, D. G., CAWLEY, J. C., COLLINS, R. D., FLEMANS, R. J., SMITH, J. L.: Leukaemic reticuloendotheliosis: a morphological and immunological study of four cases. J. Clin. Pathol. *27*, 967–972 (1974).
14. HUGHES, N. R.: Erythrocyte phagocytosis by human lymphocytes. Nature (Lond.) *212*, 1575–1576 (1966).
15. KING G. W., HURTUBISE, P. E., SAGONE, A. L., JR., LOBUGLIO, A. F., METZ., E. N.: Leukemic Reticuloendotheliosis: a study of the origin of the malignant cell. Am. J. Med. *59*, 411–416 (1975).
16. LEECH, J., ROY, R. M., FLEXNER, J. M., GLICK, A. D., WALDROM, J. A., COLLINS, R. D.: Evidence for synthesis of surface immunoglobulin in leukemic reticuloendotheliosis. Blood *46*, 1037 (Abst.) (1975).
17. RIEBER, E. P., LINKE, R. P., HADAM, M., SAAL, J. G., RIETHMÜLLER, H. W., v. HEYDEN, H. W., WALLER, H. D., SCHWARZ, H.: Hairy Cell leukemia: simultaneous demonstration of autochtonous surface-Ig and monocytic functions of hairy cells. In: Immunological Diagnosis of Leukemias and Lymphomas (Haematology and Blood Transfusion). THIERFELDER, S., RODT, H., THIEL, E. (eds.) Berlin: Springer-Verlag 1977, Vol. XX, 157–162.

18. Smith, W. L., Jr., Zidar, B. L., Winkelstein, A., Whiteside, T. L., Rabin, B. S., Shaddick, R. K., Zeigler, Z., Brietfeld, V., Silverberg, J. H., Rosenbach, L. M.: Hairy Cell leukaemia: a case with B-lymphocyte origin. Am. J. Clin. Pathol. *68*, 778–786 (1977).
19. Utsinger, D., Yount, W. J., Fuller, C., Logue, M. J., Orringer, P.: Hairy Cell Leukemia: B-lymphocyte and phagocytic properties. Blood *49*, 19–27 (1977).
20. Zucker-Franklin, D.: The percentage of monocytes among mononuclear cell fractions obtained from normal human blood. J. Immunol. *112*, 234–240 (1974).
21. Zucker-Franklin, D., Davidson, M., Thomas, L.: The interaction of mycoplasmas with mammalian cells. II. Monocytes and lymphocytes. J. Exp. Med. *124*, 533–542 (1966).

Hairy Cell Leukemia: Vascular Changes in Spleen and Liver

C. W. BERARD and K. NANBA

In 14 cases of hairy cell leukemia, we have observed unique vascular lesions in surgically resected spleens and in wedge biopsies of liver. All 14 spleens contained variably prominent distended spaces filled with erythrocytes. These structures resembled dilated sinuses, and they have been interpreted as such by the authors of one recent paper [1]. In routine sections of our material, however, they often appeared to be lined by hairy cells rather than sinus endothelial cells. Special histochemical and enzymic studies confirmed that these blood-filled spaces were in fact *pseudosinuses*, devoid of the ring fibers and endothelial cells of normal splenic sinuses [2]. These lesions appear to be qualitatively specific for hairy cell leukemia, since similar changes were not observed either in normal spleens or in spleens involved by other forms of chronic leukemia. Wedge biopsies of liver were available from five patients, and in three of the five there were similar hepatic *angiomatous lesions* in multifocal aggregates resembling hemangiomas [2]. These *splenic pseudosinuses* and *hepatic angiomatous lesions* may be pathogenetically related to adherence of hairy cells to stromal reticulum fibers in involved organs.

References

1. DIEBOLD, J., CHOMETTE, G., REYNES, M., TRICOT, G.: The spleen in hairy cell leukemia. Virchows Arch. A. Pathol. Anat. Histol. *372*, 325–336 (1977).
2. NANBA, K., SOBAN, E. J., BOWLING, M. C., BERARD, C. W.: Splenic pseudosinuses and hepatic angiomatous lesions. Distinctive features of hairy cell leukemia. Am. J. Clin. Pathol. *67*, 415–426 (1977).

Upon the Nature of Hodgkin's Disease and the Reed-Sternberg Cell

C. R. TAYLOR

Introduction

The pathologic diagnosis of Hodgkin's disease depends upon the observation of characteristic Reed-Sternberg cells in an appropriate histologic setting. Historically, in 1863, VIRCHOW [57] seems to have been the first to refer to these "large peculiar cells," which he termed lymphadenoma cells. In 1872, LANGHANS [18] provided a more detailed description: "grössere Zellen mit 2–4 und mehr Kernen und etwas dunkelkörniger Zellsubstanz, auch wirklich Riesenzellen von länglicher Form." Six years later, GREENFIELD [13] also observed similar giant cell forms: "large numbers of multi-nucleated cells (containing from four to eight to twelve nuclei) adherent to the trabeculae."

These characteristic cells derive their name from the more precise descriptions of STERNBERG [44, 45] and REED [39] which, though they differed in detail, served to establish the principal histologic features defining this abnormal cell type: thus REED [39]—

> Large giant cells vary from the size of two or three red blood cells to cells twenty times this size. The nucleus is always large in proportion to the size of the cell. it may be single or multiple . . . one or more large nucleoli are always present . . .

Subsequently, additional histological features, such as the common presence of a juxtanuclear "hof," were reported—"a pale area adjacent to, and often indenting, the nucleus or nuclei" [14], and several variants of the classical Reed-Sternberg cell were described. The mononuclear relative of the Reed-Sternberg cell, having similar nuclear characteristics and one or more large nucleoli, was recognized and was dubbed the "Hodgkin" cell by MOESCHLIN [30]. Similar mononuclear variants had previously been observed by others, including both REED and STERNBERG, the latter regarding it as an intermediate type in the development of the classical Reed-Sternberg cell. This concept of the evolution of the Reed-Sternberg cell was described minutely, and beautifully illustrated, by FAVRE and CROIZAT [9] (Fig. 1).

With the recognition and acceptance of the Reed-Sternberg cell as a distinctive neoplastic form, there followed a fierce controversy as to its cellular derivation. The following are but a select few of the many diverse theories propounded: from sinus endothelial cells [39], from lymphoblasts [24], from "adventitial" or "reticular" elements [17], from monocyte-like cells [26], from plasmacytic or reticuloendothelial cells [55], from hemohistioblasts [9], from megakaryocytes [27], from reticulum cells [37, 43], from myeloblasts [20], and from malignant histiocytes [3, 38]. Over this period, some sort of general consensus developed that the Reed-Sternberg cell was "reticulum cell derived," with the implication that the reticulum cell was some sort of stem cell and/or was related to the histiocyte series.

In the last decade, immunological studies have added a new dimension to our concepts of lymphocytic neoplasia in general [50]. The radical behavioral and morphologic changes occurring during the process of lymphocyte "transformation," in response to specific antigen, have been recognized. In addition, distinct functional subgroups of the lymphocytes (T and B cells) have been defined, and the origin of the immunoglobulin-secreting plasma cell from the B-lymphocyte has been established. These developments have profoundly influenced our

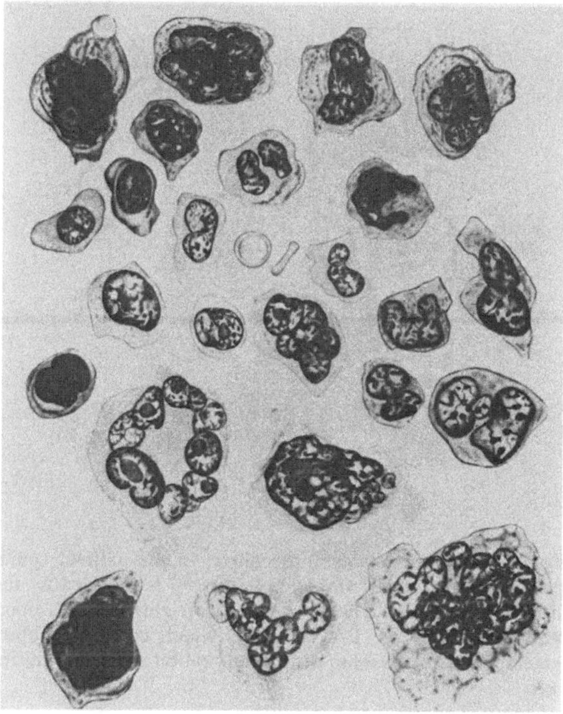

Fig. 1. "Evolution de la jeune cellule de Sternberg," according to FAVRE and CROIZAT (1931) [9]

concepts of the cellular derivation of the neoplastic cells in lymphomas other than Hodgkin's disease. Thus, in essence it is now believed that the neoplastic cell, previously regarded as a malignant reticulum cell (reticulum cell sarcoma, [40, 41]), or malignant histiocyte (malignant lymphoma, histiocytic [38]), is in fact a derivative of the transformed lymphocyte or immunoblast [47, 49]; hence the designation immunoblastic sarcoma [19, 22, 42]. In the study of Hodgkin's disease, these revelations have shed new light and cast new doubts over the controversy concerning the origin of the Reed-Sternberg cell.

This paper describes the development of immunoperoxidase procedures leading to the finding of cytoplasmic immunoglobulin within Reed-Sternberg cells [47–50, 10, 11]. The possible implications of this observation regarding the origin of the Reed-Sternberg cell and the interrelationship of Hodgkin's disease with the other lymphomas are discussed.

Materials and Methods

The Immunoperoxidase Procedure

Immunoperoxidase methods were developed for application for formalin-paraffin sections, the aim being to combine the excellent morphology of hematoxylin and eosin stained paraffin sections with the facility possessed by labeled antibody methods for specifically detecting tissue antigens. The development of the various immunoperoxidase procedures for application to the study of lymphomas has been described in detail elsewhere [47–54]. In our laboratories, two methods have been used extensively, the first involving the use of horseradish peroxidase

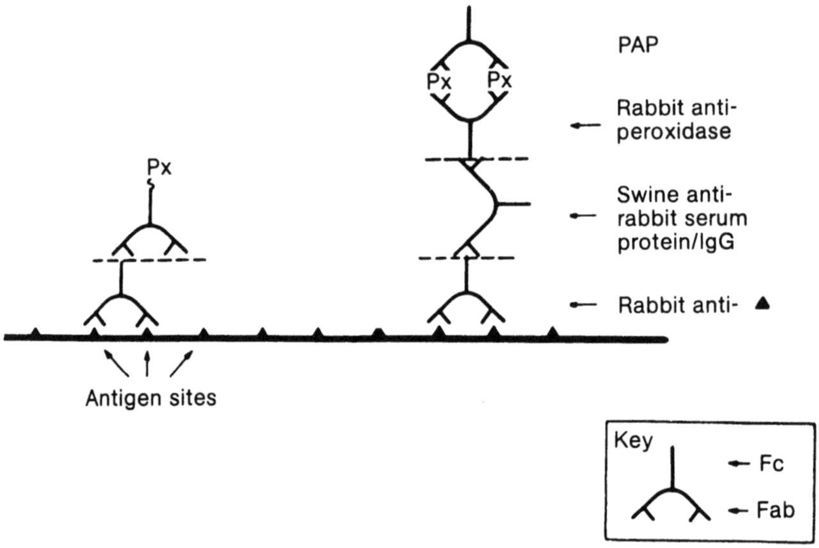

Fig. 2. Immunoperoxidase procedures. In the indirect conjugate method (left), the localization of the specific primary antiserum (rabbit anti-▲) is revealed by the addition of peroxidase-conjugated swine antirabbit antibody. The PAP method (right) depends upon an excess of unlabeled swine antirabbit antibody to link the PAP reagent (which contains rabbit antibody to horseradish peroxidase and horseradish peroxidase) to the primary rabbit antiserum (rabbit anti-▲)

(HRP) conjugated to antibody (indirect conjugate method (Fig. 2), and the second utilizing immune complexes of HRP antigen and rabbit antibody to HRP (peroxidase-antiperoxidase, PAP, method; Fig. 2). Both methods rely upon the enzymic action of HRP with a chromogenic substrate (usually diaminobenzidine—DAB) to produce a stable colored reaction product, visible by light microscopy. Following counterstaining with hematoxylin and mounting in DPX or permount, a high degree of resolution is obtainable by light microscopy, and the overall histologic detail is excellent, equivalent to orthodox hematoxylin and eosin stained sections.

The PAP method is preferred by reason of its exquisite sensitivity [100–1000 times greater than immunofluorescence according to STERNBERGER [46]] and relative freedom from problems of nonspecific staining. The principle of the method is illustrated in Figure 2, and theoretic and practical aspects have been described in detail elsewhere [46–50]. In each case, sections were screened for the presence of immunoglobulin-containing cells with anti-κ and with anti-λ antisera, with antilysozyme (muramidase) antiserum serving as control. In selected cases, staining for heavy chains was performed subsequently, and double staining procedures were employed in some cases as described in the results.

Case Population

Immunoperoxidase staining for immunoglobulin and lysozyme (muramidase) was performed on formalin-paraffin sections of lymph node biopsies from the surgical pathology files of two major teaching hospitals, the University of Oxford Medical School, Radcliffe Infirmary, Oxford and the University of Southern California Medical School (USC), Los Angeles County Medical Center, Los Angeles.

A total in excess of 400 lymphomas and lymphoid neoplasms was examined (Table 1), including 233 non-Hodgkin's lymphomas of different categories, 77 cases of Hodgkin's disease, and 62 cases of multiple myeloma and related conditions. This study of non-Hodgkin's lymphoma and

Table 1. Lymphomas and lymphocyte-derived neoplasms[c] examined by the immunoperoxidase procedure for the presence of cytoplasmic immunoglobulin and lysozyme

Classification[a] ROBB-SMITH *Oxford* (1964)		RAPPAPORT (1966)		LUKES, COLLINS *University of Southern California* (1975)
Lymphoid follicular reticulosis and lymphoblastic reticulosarcoma (follicular)	20	ML, lymphocytic, WD and PD nodular	51	Follicular center cell lymphoma
Lymphosarcoma	5	ML, lymphocytic, WD and PD diffuse		
Lymphoblastic reticulosarcoma (diffuse)	11			
Syncytial reticulosarcoma	16	ML, diffuse, mixed and histiocytic	81	Immunoblastic sarcoma
Dictyosyncytial reticulosarcoma	5			
Dictyocytic/histocytic reticulosarcoma	7			
Polymorphic reticulosarcoma	11			
Plasma cell reticulosarcoma	9			
Myeloma and related conditions	33	Myeloma	10	Plasmacytoid lymphocytic lymphoma
			29	Myeloma
Unclassified	7	—	—[b]	
Hodgkin's disease	45	Hodgkin's disease	32	Hodgkin's disease
Total	169		203	

[a] The classifications given in the Table are those in use at the designated centers over the period of this study (Oxford, 1970–75, ROBB-SMITH [40, 41]; USC, 1975–77, LUKES and COLLINS [22]). Very crude comparative groupings of these diagnostic categories are possible and are indicated by brackets. Precise correlation is not feasible, without re-examination of all of the original slides, and this was not possible for the Oxford study. An equally crude matching with the RAPPAPORT classification [38] is given for reference purposes. (ML = malignant lymphoma, WD and PD = well and poorly differentiated.)

[b] A number of cases have been omitted because of classification difficulties, principally due to the presence of variable features making it difficult to assign to a single category or because of inadequate material for evaluation.

[c] A lesser number of cases of other diagnostic categories have also been examined, including hairy cell leukemia, acute and chronic lymphocytic leukemia, convoluted lymphoma (Sternberg sarcoma, mediastinal lymphoblastic lymphoma), Burkitt's lymphoma, mycosis fungoides, "true histiocytic lymphoma," and malignant histiocytosis.

myeloma, coupled with similar studies of tissues from approximately 100 nonlymphomatous tissues (including nonspecific lymphadenitis, toxoplasmosis, sarcoidosis, infectious mononucleosis, dilantin hyperplasia, and angioimmunoblastic lymphadenopathy) provides a sound basis for the study and interpretation of the findings in Hodgkin's disease.

Antisera

The majority of antisera used in these studies were obtained from commercial sources, principally Dakopatts AS, (through Mercia Diagnostics Sandown Road, Watford, Herts, England). The specificity of these reagents under the conditions employed in this study has been established by extensive reference to control populations of reactive plasma cells and cases of myeloma of predetermined light and heavy chain type. Also by hemagglutination techniques these antisera were shown to possess a high degree of discrimination between different light chains [25]. In checkerboard titration studies, the antisera were found to give specific reactions, without evidence of cross-reactivity in control tissues, at dilutions of 1/20 (for anti-κ and anti-λ). The possibility of significant cross-reactivity occurring at dilutions of 1/3000 (i.e., more than 100 times greater), as used in this study, must be considered remote.

Results

The results of some of these studies have been published elsewhere—non-Hodgkin's lymphomas and Hodgkin's disease (Oxford cases [47–49]), multiple myeloma (Oxford cases [54]), Hodgkin's disease, nodular sclerosing category (USC cases [2]). Only the findings in Hodgkin's disease will be considered in detail here, primarily including material previously available only on a restricted basis [48] and more recent unpublished observations from USC cases.

Pattern of Immunoglobulin Staining in Hodgkin's Disease

Immunoglobulin-containing plasma cells were clearly demonstrable in all cases of Hodgkin's disease (HD), their number varying considerably, from almost none in HD-LP (lymphocyte predominant) to numerous in some cases of HD-NS (nodular sclerosing) and HD-MC (mixed cellularity) (Table 2). The staining reactions of the plasma cell populations for κ- and λ-light chains and for γ-, α-, μ-, and δ-heavy chains were consistent with a polyclonal reactive plasma cell response, comparable to that observed in reactive lymph nodes.

In most cases of Hodgkin's disease, however, the striking feature was the observation of distinct immunoglobulin staining within classical Reed-Sternberg cells and in mononuclear variants (Hodgkin's cells) (Fig. 3). Not all Reed-Sternberg or Hodgkin's cells were immunoglobulin-positive in any one case, the percentage varying from less than 5% to 80% or more (Table 3). The intensity of positive staining of Hodgkin's and Reed-Sternberg cells ranged from very faint to heavy but was usually less than that observed in adjacent plasma cells, which served as valuable intrinsic controls. These observations are in close agreement with other independent studies [11].

Table 2. Correlation of histologic subgroups[a] with immunoglobulin-positive plasma cells in Hodgkin's disease [48]

Histological subgroup	No. of immunoglobulin-positive plasma cells +	++	+++	Totals
LP	3	1	—	4
NS	10	12	8	30
MC	3	4	2	9
LD[b]	2	—	—	2
Totals	18	17	10	45

[a] Rye conference recommendations [23].
[b] Extensive necrosis was present in cases classified as HD-LD, making interpretation difficult. In addition, three cases which might by others have been classified as HD-LD were included in the polymorphic reticulosarcoma group (Table 1).
LP: lymphocyte predominant; NS: nodular sclerosing; MC: mixed cellularity; LD: lymphocyte dominant.

Table 3. Correlation of histologic subgroups[a] of Hodgkin's disease with immunoglobulin positivity of Reed-Sternberg and variants (including mononuclear Hodgkin's cells and lacunar cells) [48]

Histological subgroup	Immunoglobulin positivity—semiquantitative intensity and number –	± to +	+ to ++	+++	Totals
LP	3	1	—	—	4
NS	5	16	8	1	30
MC	—	2	4	3	9
LD[b]	2	—	—	—	2
Totals	10	19	12	4	45

[a]Rye conference recommendations [23].
[b]Extensive necrosis was present in cases classified as HD-LD, making interpretation difficult.
+ equivalent to about 20% of Hodgkin's and Reed-Sternberg cells.
LP: lymphocyte dominant; NS: nodular sclerosing; MC: mixed cellularity; LD: lymphocyte dominant.

Of the 45 Oxford cases, 10 were judged not to show definite immunoglobulin staining of Reed-Sternberg cells. Three of these cases were in the HD-LP group, in which only rare diagnostic cells were encountered for examination. Of the 35 immunoglobulin-positive cases, 23 showed definite staining for both κ- and λ-light chains, and in these cases at least some cells apparently stained with both antisera (bitypic). In five cases (two HD-MC and three HD-NS), the pattern of immunoglobulin staining was consistent with concepts of a monoclonal B-cell origin (three exclusively κ, two exclusively λ), and in seven the decision (monoclonal or bitypic staining) was uncertain.

The "bitypic" staining of individual cells with both antisera (anti-κ and anti-λ) was unexpected and without precedent but was confirmed by examining the same cell in serial sections and by

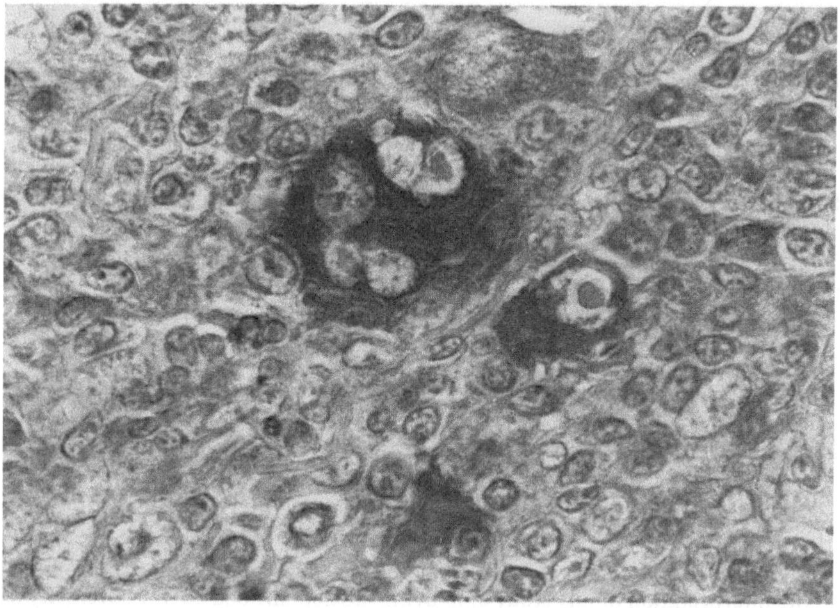

Fig. 3. Hodgkin's disease. Reed-Sternberg cell variant and Hodgkin's cell stained for immunoglobulin (shades of grey to black) with anti-λ antiserum by the immunoperoxidase (PAP) method. Formalin-paraffin section, counterstain hematoxylin. (×800)

double staining techniques, in which the immunoperoxidase procedure was performed twice, first with anti-κ antisera followed by DAB (brown coloration) and second with anti-λ antisera followed by α-naphthol pyronin (an alternative substrate giving a red color) [53]. In "double" stained preparations clear discriminatory staining of plasma cells by anti-κ and anti-λ antisera was observed, with no evidence of cross-reaction. Yet adjacent Reed-Sternberg cells clearly contained two colored reaction products, denoting specific binding with both anti-κ and anti-λ antisera. Specificity was further confirmed by serial dilutions of anti-κ and anti-λ antisera to dilutions of more than 1/3000 and by simple absorption with urinary concentrates of κ and λ Bence-jones proteins. Control preparations omitting the anti-immunoglobulin antisera, or substituting anti-lysozyme antiserum, showed no staining of plasma cells or Reed-Sternberg cells. Staining of histiocytes, sometimes multinucleate in form, was observed with antilysozyme antiserum in some cases. These multinucleate histiocytes were usually distinguishable from Reed-Sternberg cell variants by the distinct nuclear membrane and prominant nucleolus of the latter cell type.

These basic findings were confirmed in 32 additional cases at USC, including 22 HD-NS, and 10 HD-MC. In addition, a small number of cases of HD-LP and HD-LD were also examined. The pattern of heavy chain staining was determined in a small number of cases of the Oxford series and in 20 cases of the USC group. In the majority of instances, Reed-Sternberg and Hodgkin's cells staining for κ- or λ-chains, or both, stained also for γ-chain. Only two cases stained for μ-chain in the absence of γ-staining, and staining for more than one heavy chain was observed rarely.

In all instances, immunoglobulin-positive Reed-Sternberg and Hodgkin's cells were characterized by large nucleoli with distinct nuclear membranes and usually the presence of a large nucleolus. Cytoplasm was usually extensive and basophilic in H and E preparations and pyroninophilic in methyl green pyronin stains. Other Reed-Sternberg and mononuclear variants, not staining for immunoglobulin, tended to possess more irregularly folded or lobulated nuclei, with more delicate nuclear membranes and inconspicuous nucleoli. GARVIN and colleagues [11] also observed ultrastructural differences between immunoglobulin-positive and immunoglobulin-negative Reed-Sternberg cells.

Immunoglobulin-Positive Reed-Sternberg-Like Cells in Lymphomas Other than Hodgkin's disease

Also of great interest was the observation of cells closely resembling, or indistinguishable from, Reed-Sternberg cells or Hodgkin's cells in some non-Hodgkin's lymphomas (principally those classified as immunoblastic sarcoma or plasmacytic reticulosarcoma, including cases developing from preceding monoclonal myeloma cell populations). These cells also sometimes showed a bitypic staining pattern for κ and γ, even when associated with a population of morphologically similar mononuclear cells of monoclonal type (Fig. 4).

Discussion

Specificity of Staining for Immunoglobulin

In the interpretation of any study employing labeled antibodies, the specificity of the antisera is of prime importance [51]. Thus, the staining of Reed-Sternberg cells with anti-immunoglobulin antisera might be attributable to some unrealized specificity of the antisera against a cell constituent other than immunoglobulin, or it might represent nonspecific staining. The

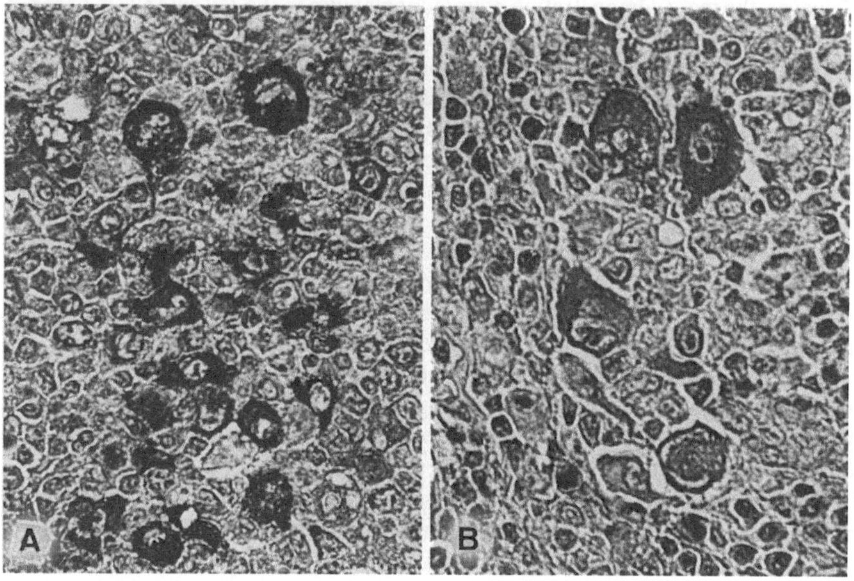

Fig. 4. Immunoblastic sarcoma.
(A) Immunoblasts and lymphoma cells showing close resemblance to Reed-Sternberg cell variants staining positively for immunoglobulin (shades of grey to black) with anti-κ antiserum;
(B) In serial sections stained with anti-λ, the mononuclear immunoblasts show absence of staining (monoclonal) while the large bizarre cells demonstrate definite staining for λ-light chain, as well as for κ-chain (bitypic staining). Formalin-paraffin section, counterstain haematoxylin. (× 300)

inclusion of control preparations, omitting each of the stages of the PAP immunoperoxidase procedure in turn, and substituting the primary anti-immunoglobulin antisera by an antiserum of irrelevant specificity (e.g., antilysozyme), demonstrates conclusively that staining of Reed-Sternberg cells is only observed with specific anti-immunoglobulin antisera (anti-κ, anti-γ, anti-μ, anti-α, anti-δ). In addition, binding of rabbit antisera to the section through Fc receptor activity [51] can be discounted, as this would occur randomly for all the different antisera used, and aggregated rabbit immunoglobulin itself shows no evidence of binding to Reed-Sternberg cells. Finally, absorption of antisera by whole immunoglobulin abolishes staining. Thus, the staining observed with anti-immunoglobulin antisera can reasonably be attributed to the presence of immunoglobulin within the cells. This conclusion has been drawn independently by Garvin et al. [10, 11] who, using an immunoperoxidase method, also observed IgG within Reed-Sternberg cells, and by Denton [7] using immunofluorescence.

Immunoglobulin in Reed-Sternberg Cells: Significance

The demonstration of immunoglobulin in Reed-Sternberg cells and in mononuclear Hodgkin variants is open to several interpretations [47–50]. Firstly, the presence of immunoglobulin within the cell cytoplasm might be indicative of in situ synthesis. Secondly, immunoglobulin might be taken into the cell actively, by pinocytosis or by phagocytosis, possibly in the form of immune complexes. Thirdly, degenerating cells fail to maintain the integrity of their plasma membranes, thus allowing immunoglobulin freely to enter the cytoplasm. Specific antibody directed against cellular antigens might, therefore, gain access to the cytoplasm, having first induced cell membrane damage.

According to present beliefs, the synthesis of immunoglobulin is limited to differentiated cells of the B-lymphocyte series which in their fully specialized form are termed plasma cells.

However, the mere demonstration of immunoglobulin in the cell cytoplasm does not necessarily construe synthesis by the cell, for immunoglobulin could enter the cell passively, or by pinocytosis, or by phagocytosis of immune complexes. Present concepts of clonal selection restrict individual B-lymphocytes and their derivatives (plasma cells) to the production of a single light chain (either κ or λ) and a single heavy chain, although sequential changes in heavy chain production (e.g., from μ to γ) do appear to occur during B-cell maturation [12, 58]. Thus, the demonstration of a single light chain and a single heavy chain within a cell can reasonably be taken as evidence of in situ synthesis, for absorbed or phagocytosed immunoglobulin would inevitably consist of both light chain classes and possibly two or more heavy chain classes.

In those cases of non-Hodgkin's lymphoma and multiple myeloma in which staining for immunoglobulin is observed, the pattern of staining usually meets the conditions for monoclonality (monotypic, i.e., exclusively one light chain and one heavy chain). This is consistent with the B-lymphocytic derivation of these neoplasms and with production of the immunoglobulin by the neoplastic cell population. In addition, in some of these cases bizarre lymphoma cells, having a very close morphological resemblance to Reed-Sternberg cells, also appear to contain immunoglobulin as a result of synthesis (Fig. 4).

In Hodgkin's disease, however, a "monotypic" or monoclonal staining pattern is the exception, rather than the rule, the majority of immunoglobulin-positive cells showing bitypic staining with both anti-κ and anti-λ antisera, and usually also with anti-γ antiserum. At first sight, this observation weighs heavily against the proposal that Reed-Sternberg cells are B-lymphocyte derived and that the cytoplasmic immunoglobulin is present as the result of synthesis. A more plausible explanation would seem to be that Reed-Sternberg cells might be histiocyte derived, containing IgG (IgG-λ and IgG-κ) by virtue of phagocytosis of free immunoglobulin or immune complexes. Such cells might also carry surface immunoglobulin due to Fc receptor adsorption of IgG (IgG-γ and IgG-κ), although this could not account for the cytoplasmic distribution of staining in sections. However, in a minority of cases, indistinguishable on morphologic grounds, the pattern of staining in Reed-Sternberg cells does appear to be monoclonal, and such a pattern cannot be explained by phagocytosis but only by synthesis [11, 47, 49].

"Bitypic" κ-λ Staining of Reed-Sternberg Cells

If the immunoperoxidase staining pattern is a result of synthesis of immunoglobulin by Hodgkin's or Reed-Sternberg cells, then an explanation must be sought for the apparent presence of κ and γ within the same cell, since this is not allowable by current theory. Obviously, the specificity of the antilight chain antisera must be suspect. However, purification of antilight chain antisera by absorption with purified κ- or γ-light chain (Bence–Jones protein) fails to abolish the bitypic staining reaction, and this has been confirmed independently in other laboratories [59]. The ultimate control of specificity in a system having the high sensitivity of the PAP method must depend upon the use of adequate biologic controls [51]. In this respect, the antilight chain antisera used in this study show no evidence of cross-reactivity in normal plasma cell populations. In addition, neoplastic cells of myeloma tissues used as controls show staining exclusively for κ or for γ, the alternate light chain being completely negative in the great majority of cases. Finally, in double staining procedures, plasma cells reacting only with anti-κ chain can be seen adjacent to plasma cells reacting only with anti-λ chain and to Reed-Sternberg cells showing reaction with both antisera. This constitutes strong evidence that antigenic determinants defining both light chains are present within individual Reed-Sternberg cells.

To date, there is little evidence that normal or neoplastic plasma cells are able to secrete both light chains. However, all the cytoplasmic components within an immunoglobulin-producing cell need not necessarily be secreted (as in cases of nonsecretory myeloma in which the neoplastic cells may contain immunoglobulin). Also, it is possible that during intracellular synthesis and assembly, antisera may detect common determinants on κ- and λ-light chain precursors that are not revealed on the secreted intact immunoglobulin molecules. There is evidence that in rare instances neoplastic plasma cells contain and may actually secrete immunoglobulins of both light chain classes [in biclonal myeloma, IgG-κ and IgG-λ of identical idiotype [5, 33, 36, 50, 56], in in vitro lymphocyte culture experiments [21], and in murine plasmacytomas [31]].

Regarding Reed-Sternberg cells, the ultimate answer perhaps awaits evidence of immunoglobulin synthesis in vitro, and a preliminary report of two cases by BOECKER et al. [4] suggest that Reed-Sternberg cells may, in fact, be capable of immunoglobulin synthesis in prolonged culture.

Non-Hodgkin's Lymphomas: Immunoblastic Sarcoma

Further information pertaining to the immunoglobulin staining of Reed-Sternberg cells may be derived from studies of other lymphomas. In non-Hodgkin's lymphomas, and in myeloma, the great majority of immunoglobulin-positive cases show monotypic (monoclonal) staining. However, a proportion of those cases with a prominent immunoblastic component (i.e., some cases of immunoblastic sarcoma and "poorly differentiated" myeloma) do show an anomalous bitypic staining pattern in that cells, which are judged to be part of the neoplastic population by orthodox morphologic criteria, show staining with both anti-κ and anti-λ light chain antisera [52]. In some of these cases, it is possible to demonstrate unequivocal staining of individual malignant cells by both antisera; in other cases, two separate populations appear to be present. Even more remarkable is the observation that the bitypic ($\kappa\lambda$) staining cells are often large and bizarre, with marked resemblance to Reed-Sternberg cell variants (Fig. 4). In some cases, such cells occur as part of an immunoblastic sarcoma, in which the neoplastic cells otherwise show a monoclonal staining pattern.

Monoclonal but Polymorphous

On the basis of immunologic and morphologic studies [6, 19, 22, 47–50], it has been postulated that many of the lymphomas, including large cell lymphomas, previously known as reticulum cell sarcomas or malignant lymphomas of histiocytic type, are B-lymphocyte derived. The B-lymphocyte undergoes distinct morphologic and behavioral changes during its cell cycle (Figs. 5 and 6), from a small circulating cell to one undergoing transformation within the follicle, to a fully transformed lymphocyte (immunoblast) leaving the follicle, and ultimately to an immunoglobulin-secreting plasma cell. The corresponding B-lymphocyte derived lymphomas show analogous patterns of morphology, surface marking, and behavior, represented by chronic lymphocytic leukemia (CLL), follicular center cell lymphoma, immunoblastic sarcoma, and Waldenström's disease and multiple myeloma (Fig. 5).

However, certain logical consequences of these proposals have largely been ignored. For example, the close relationship of multiple myeloma and immunoblastic sarcoma, in terms of the postulated cell of origin, has not been recognized in most classifications (Fig. 6). Our concepts are also vulnerable in other areas in that we think of monoclonal neoplastic cell populations as being of a single cell type with a basically uniform ("monoclonal-monomorphous") morphology. This view, which carries the implication that neoplasms proliferate by division of recognizably neoplastic cells, also leads to a further omission of our logical reasoning. Thus, just as normal plasma cells do not develop from other plasma cells, but from small lymphocytes by lymphocyte transformation, so neoplastic plasma cells would be expected

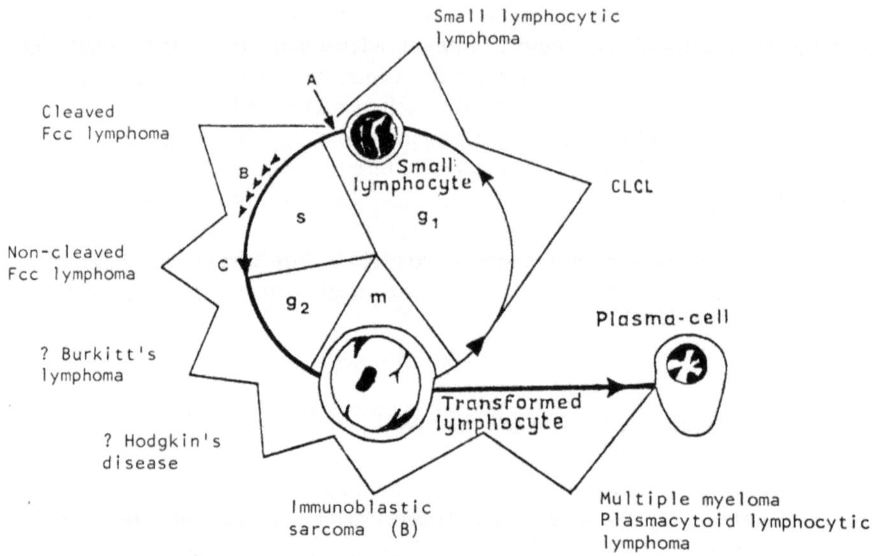

Fig. 5. Postulated relationship between B-cell lymphomas (classified according to LUKES and COLLINS, 1975) and the various morphologic forms assumed by the lymphocyte during its cell cycle (from [50]).
A: Stimulation by antigen or other mitogen;
B: Metamorphosis from small lymphocyte to transformed lymphocyte, probably involving cleaved cell forms in the B-series;
C: Thickened line represents immunoglobulin synthesis, initially expressed on the cell surface, but present in the cytoplasm and secreted during maturation to the plasma cell;
g_1, s, g_2, m: phases of cell cycle; g_1: diploid cells; s: DNA and RNA synthesis; g_2: tetraploid premitotic cells; m: mitosis

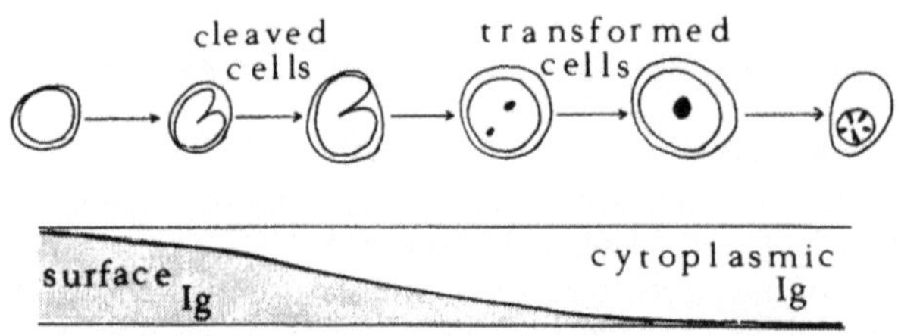

Fig. 6. Variation of surface and cytoplasmic immunoglobulin in lymphocyte transformation and maturation to the plasma cell (from [50]). There is an inverse relationship between SIg (highest on circulating and tissue small B-lymphocytes) and cytoplasmic immunoglobulin (present in the greatest amounts in the plasma cell). Transforming (cleaved) cells in follicular centers show intermediate patterns

to develop, not from division of other neoplastic plasma cells, but from neoplastic small lymphocytes by a parody of the normal process of lymphocyte transformation. Indeed, there is evidence that this occur. For example, ABDOU and ABDOU [1] and MELLSTEDT and colleagues [28, 29] have shown that in multiple myeloma a proportion of the circulating small lymphocytes, morphologically indistinguishable from other circulating small lymphocytes, carry synthesized surface immunoglobulin with the same idiotypic specificity as that secreted by the myeloma cells. Thus, these small lymphocytes appear to be an integral part of the same neoplastic clone as the recognizable myeloma cells, although they are not recognizably neoplastic by the usual criteria. Also, in bone marrow sections from cases of multiple myeloma it is possible, by immunoperoxidase methods, to detect a variable proportion of immunoblasts (transformed lymphocytes), which show a pattern of staining for light and heavy chain immunoglobulin components identical to that of the predominant neoplastic plasma cell population (i.e., the myeloma cells). These observations suggest that in multiple myeloma the neoplastic clone is composed of a wide range of different morphologic expressions of the neoplastic B-lymphocyte, corresponding to the various behavioral and morphologic expressions of the normal B-lymphocyte at different phases of the cell cycle (Fig. 7). The overall histologic appearance of the neoplasm is governed by the predominant cell type (i.e., the predominant phase of the cell cycle), which in the case of multiple myeloma is the plasma cell (Fig. 7).

Similar reasoning applied to CLCL (Fig. 8) or follicular center cell lymphoma reveals that expansion of the neoplastic clone can only occur through the process of lymphocyte transformation. Thus, by definition, the neoplastic cell population must contain a proportion of transformed cells (immunoblasts) which, when present in small numbers, are generally overlooked in histologic assessment or dismissed as part of a reactive infiltrate. Cases in which the rate of proliferation is high contain a larger proportion of cells in the dividing phase of the cell cycle (i.e., cells morphologically resembling transformed lymphocytes or immunoblasts), and if this type of cell is predominant, then the diagnosis will be one of immunoblastic sarcoma (Fig. 9). This may arise de novo, or it may evolve from established cases of CLCL, follicular center cell lymphoma, or multiple myeloma which have progressed to a more aggressive rapidly proliferating state.

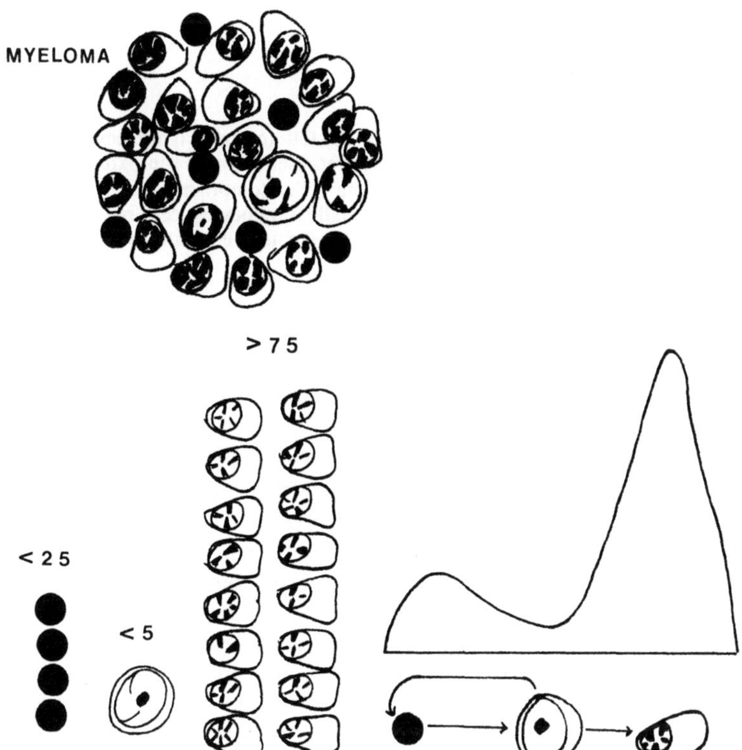

Fig. 7. Monoclonal, but polymorphous—multiple myeloma, relationship to B-lymphocyte transformation. Diagrammatic representation of approximate proportions (%) of different cell forms (lymphocytes, immunoblasts, plasma cells) comprizing a single neoplastic clone in multiple myeloma. The majority of the neoplastic cells resemble plasma cells. Cells resembling the immunoblasts are in the division phase of the cell cycle, and a proportion of circulating neoplastic small lymphocytes are present (from [52])

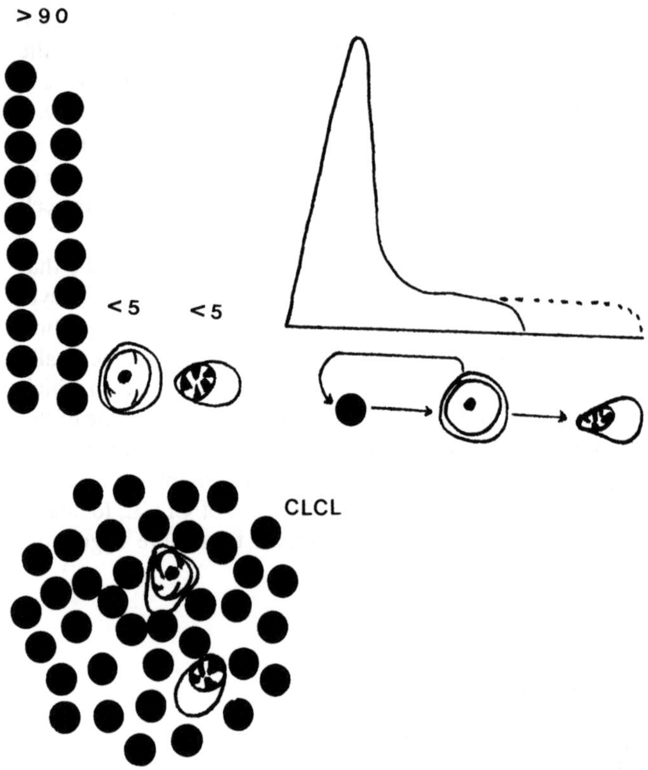

Fig. 8. Monoclonal, but polymorphous—CLCL (chronic lymphocytic leukemia)—relationship to B-lymphocyte transformation. Diagrammatic representation of approximate proportions (%) of different cell forms (lymphocytes, immunoblasts, plasma cells) comprising a single neoplastic clone in CLCL. The majority of the neoplastic cells resemble small lymphocytes; cells resembling the immunoblast are in the division phase of the cell cycle. In rare instances, some neoplastic cells differentiate through to plasma cells (from [52])

Histologic Features of Hodgkin's Disease Related to a Postulated Lymphocytic origin

All this has important implications for Hodgkin's disease, which, if derived from the B-lymphocyte as implied by the studies reported here, must also conform to the above logic. According to current concepts, Hodgkin's disease differs from all other malignant neoplasms in that in Hodgkin's disease the presumptive neoplastic cell (the mononuclear Hodgkin's cell or the Reed-Sternberg cell) may be quite rare, comprising 1% or less of the total cells in any microscopic section (Fig. 10), the remaining cells being considered to be reactive lymphocytes, reactive plasma cells, reactive histiocytes, reactive eosinophils, etc. PULLINGER [37] explained the presence of these diverse cell types quite logically, although perhaps not quite correctly according to current beliefs: "... The reticulum cell is the proliferating cell of Hodgkin's disease; ... all other cellular manifestations ... are due to subsequent differentiation of the reticulum cell ... into one or several of the possible cell progeny." However, current beliefs, while decrying the reticulum cell theory of PULLINGER, have not produced a logical alternative explanation for the presence of these cell types or the paucity of the neoplastic cells in Hodgkin's disease.

Many of these conceptual problems may be resolved if it transpires that in fact Reed-Sternberg cells do evolve from transformed lymphocytes, possibly via the sequential changes proposed by

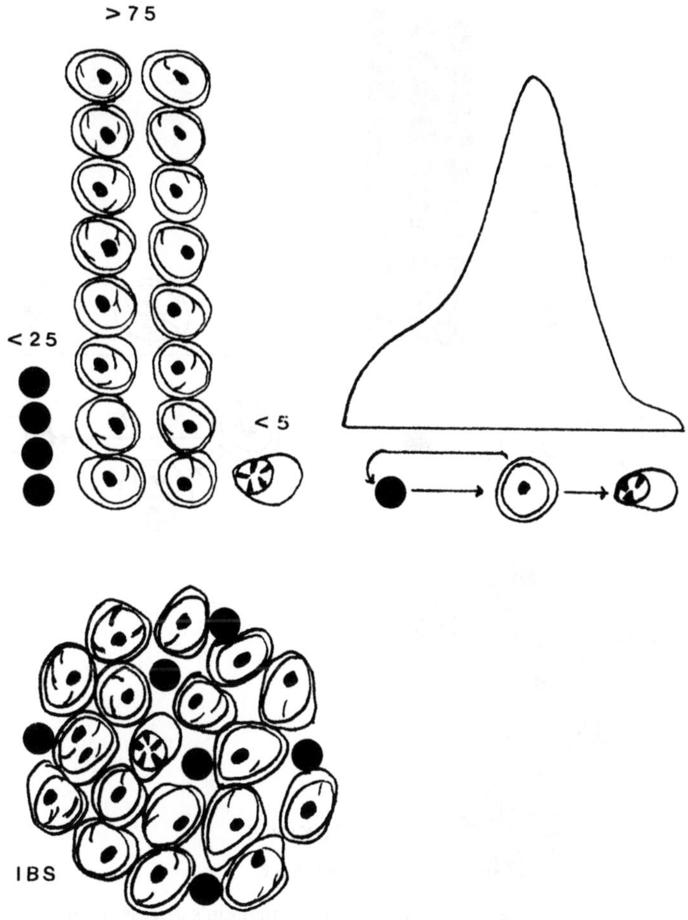

Fig. 9. Monoclonal, but polymorphous—B-cell IBS (immunoblastic sarcoma, B-cell type)—relationship to lymphocyte transformation. Diagrammatic representation of approximate proportions (%) of the different cell forms (lymphocytes, immunoblasts, plasma cells) comprizing the neoplastic clone in immunoblastic sarcoma. The majority of the neoplastic cells resemble immunoblasts and are in the division phase of the cell cycle. A small proportion of neoplastic cells differentiate to plasma cells, and some may remain as circulating small neoplastic lymphocytes (from [52])

Anagnostou [2]. For example, if the Reed-Sternberg cell and Hodgkin variant do indeed represent malignant derivatives of the transformed B-lymphocyte, then ultimately they must be derived from, and related to, neoplastic small lymphocytes. Indeed, a proportion—possibly large—of the lymphocytes present in Hodgkin's disease might in reality be part of the neoplastic process, rather than simply reactive. Olinici [32], in fact, has shown chromosomal abnormalities, resembling those present in Hodgkin's and Reed-Sternberg cells, in the lymphocytes in Hodgkin's disease, suggesting that morphologically normal lymphocytes are also involved as part of the neoplastic process.

The situation in Hodgkin's disease is complicated by three factors. Firstly, a proportion of the malignant transformed lymphocytes (equivalent to the proliferating Hodgkin's cells [34, 35]) apparently fail to complete the cell cycle, undergoing some sort of arrest in S or G_2, yielding bizarre multinucleate forms including Reed-Sternberg cells [47–49]. Secondly, the admixture of histiocytes, eosinophils, and plasma cells tends to obscure the nature of the underlying cell population. It has been proposed that the granulocytes and histiocytes might accumulate as a result of the activity of specific chemotactic factors or lymphokines released, either by

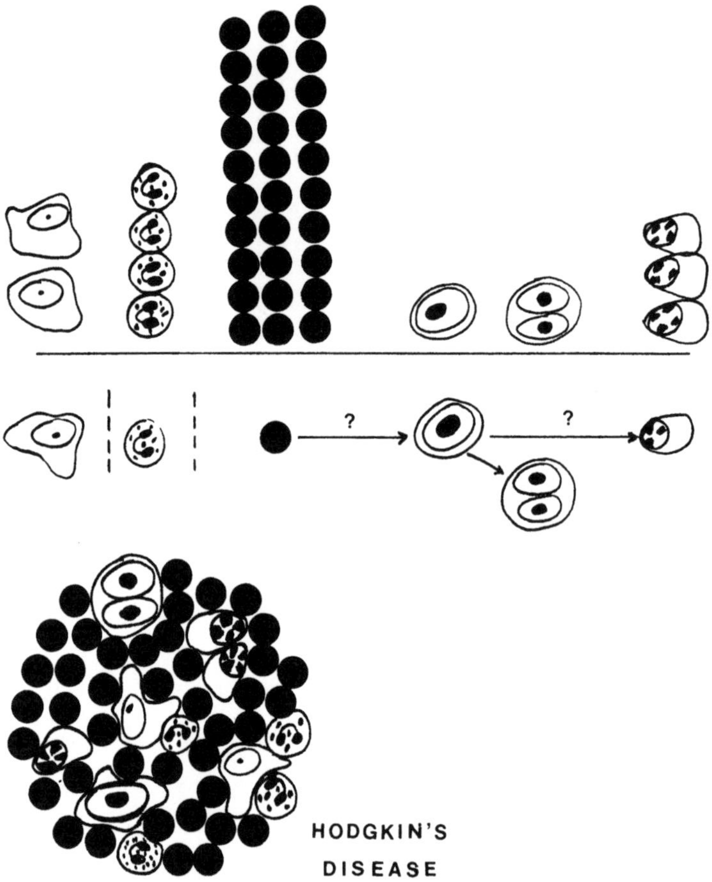

Fig. 10. ? Monoclonal, but polymorphous--Hodgkin's disease, relationship to B-lymphocyte transformation. Diagrammatic representation of approximate proportions of cell types (lymphocytes, immunoblasts, plasma cells, eosinophils, histiocytes) in section from a typical case of Hodgkin's disease. Reed-Sternberg cells, Hodgkin's cells, lymphocytes, and plasma cells may represent different morphologic expressions of a single neoplastic clone (viz. Figs. 7, 8, and 9). The Hodgkin's cells, resembling the immunoblast, correspond to that part of the clone in the division phase of the cell cycle [34, 35]. Histiocytes and eosinophils may be present in response to lymphokine release by the neoplastic lymphocytes or as part of an associated immune reaction [47–50]

malignant lymphocytes (or their derivatives, Reed-Sternberg cells [47, 49]) or by reactive lymphocytes involved in some sort of immune response against the Hodgkin's disease cells [8, 16]. Thirdly, plasma cells might be present as part of this reactive response. Alternatively, a proportion of the plasma cells might form part of the primary neoplastic process, representing that fraction of the neoplastic clone which has retained the ability to complete the differentiation pathway of the B-lymphocyte, as occurs in some cases of immunoblastic sarcoma and in multiple myeloma.

Conclusion

Clearly, the recognition of the radical morphologic and behavioral changes occurring during lymphocyte transformation and the realization that many of the non-Hodgkin's lymphomas are related to the transformed lymphocyte, of B- or T-cell origin, has far-reaching implications for our understanding of these disease processes [50, 52]. At present, we only dimly perceive the impact of these beliefs on our criteria for histologic diagnosis, classification, and staging of non-Hodgkin's lymphomas. In Hodgkin's disease, our concepts are still less clear, for we still await conclusive proof of the cellular origin of Hodgkin's disease, whether from the B-lymphocyte, the T-lymphocyte [8], or the histiocyte [15]. Nevertheless, the principles entertained above still apply, for the lymphomas are dynamic parodies of normal lymphocyte transformation and function, involving multiple cytologic forms and multiple behavioral attributes within a single clone. Current methods of diagnosis recognize only the predominant, and morphologically grossly abnormal, fraction of the total neoplastic population. The histologic assessment of just this recognizably abnormal fraction is perhaps an insufficient basis for meaningful classification of the lymphomas. That this may be so is suggested by the observation that 30 or more classifications of lymphoma have been proposed during the last half century but, having failed to pass the test of time, have been discredited or simply forgotten.

Finally, in presenting this possibility for the origin of the Reed-Sternberg cell, it should be remembered that many of the theories advanced in previous years had respectable scientific support at the time of their conception, and that in the future it is not impossible that present immunologic concepts of lymphoma might be viewed more dispassionately.

Summary

Immunoglobulin components have been demonstrated within Reed-Sternberg cells in Hodgkin's disease using immunoperoxidase techniques. The possibility that this finding is indicative of a B-lymphocytic origin for the Reed-Sternberg cell is considered, and the implications that such a conclusion might have regarding the histiopathology of Hodgkin's disease and the relationship of Hodgkin's disease to other lymphomas is discussed.

References

1. Abdou, N. I., Abdou, N. L.: The monoclonal nature of lymphocytes in multiple myeloma. Effects of therapy. Ann. Intern. Med. *83*, 42–45 (1975).
2. Anagnostou, D., Parker, J. W., Taylor, C. R., Tindle, B. H., Lukes, R. J.: Lacunar cells of nodular sclerosing Hodgkin's disease. An ultrastructural and immunohistologic study. Cancer *39*, 1032–1043 (1977).
3. Bessis, M.: Cytologie sanguine normale et pathologique, Vol. I. Paris: Masson 1948.
4. Boecker, W. R., Hossfeld, D. K., Gallmeier, W. M., Bruntsch, U., Schmidt, C. G.: Clonal growth of Hodgkin cells. Nature *258*, 235–236 (1975).
5. Bouvet, J. P., Buffe, D., Oriol, R., Liacopoulos, P.: Two myeloma globulins IgGl-κ and IgGl-λ from a single patient (Im). II. Their common cellular origin as revealed by immunfluorescence studies. Immunology *27*, 1095–1101 (1974).
6. Braylan, R. C., Jaffe, E. S., Berard, C. W.: Malignant lymphomas: Current classification and new observations. Pathology Annual. Somers, S. C. (ed.) New York: Appleton-Century-Crofts 1975.
7. Denton, P. M.: Immune responsiveness in Hodgkin's disease. Br. J. Cancer *28*, Suppl. I, 119–127 (1973).
8. De Vita, V. T., Jr.: Lymphocyte reactivity in Hodgkin's disease: a lymphocyte civil war. N. Engl. J. Med. *239*, 801–802 (1973).
9. Favre, M., Croizat, P.: Caractères généraux du granulome malin, tirés de son étude anatomoclinique. Ann. Anat. Pathol. *8*, 838–900 (1931).

10. GARVIN, A. J., SPICER. S. S., PARMLEY, R. T., MUNSTER, A. M.: Immunohistochemical demonstration of IgG in Reed-Sternberg cells and other cells in Hodgkin's disease. J. Exp. Med. *139*, 1077–1083 (1974).
11. GARVIN, A. J., SPICER, S. S., MCKEEVER, P. E.: The cytochemical demonstration of intracellular immunoglobulin. In: Neoplasms of lymphoreticular tissue. Am. J. Pathol. *82*, 457–477 (1976).
12. GEARHART, P. J., SIGAL, N. H., KLINMAN, N. R.: Production of antibodies of identical idiotype but diverse immunoglobulin classes by cells derived from a single stimulated B cell. Proc. Nat. Acad. Sci. USA *72*, 1707–1711 (1975).
13. GREENFIELD, W. S.: Specimens illustrative of the pathology of lymphadenoma and leucocythaemia. Trans. Path. Soc. London *29*, 272–304 (1878).
14. HOSTER, H. A., DRATMAN, M. B.: Hodgkin's disease—(Part I). 1832–1947. Cancer Res. *8*, 1–78 (1948).
15. KAY, M. M. B.: Hodgkin's disease: a war between T-lymphocytes and transformed macrophages? In: Recent Results in Cancer Research Vol. 56. Lymphocytes, Macrophages and Cancer. MATHE, G., FLORENTIN, I., SIMMLER, M. C. (eds.) Berlin/New York: Springer-Verlag 1976, pp. 111–121.
16. LANCET EDITORIAL: Blind alleys in the Hodgkin's maze. Lancet *1*, 556–557 (1975).
17. LANG, F. J.: In: Handbook of Hematology. DOWNEY, H. (ed.) New York: P. B. Hoeber, Inc. 1938, Vol. III, p. 2103.
18. LANGHANS, T.: Das maligne Lymphosarkom (Pseudoleukämie). Virchows Arch. (Pathol. Anat.) *54*, 509–537 (1872).
19. LENNERT, K., STEIN, H., KAISERLING, E.: Cytological and functional criteria for the classification of malignant lymphomata. Br. J. Cancer *31*, Suppl. II, 29–43 (1975).
20. LEWIS, M. R.: The behavior of Dorothy Reed cells in tissue culture. Am. J. Med. Sci. *201*, 467 (abst.) (1941).
21. LITWIN, S. D., LIN, P. K., HUTTEROTH, T. H., CLEVE, H.: Multiple heavy chain classes and light chain types on surfaces of cultured human lymphoid cells. Nature (New Biol.) *246*, 179–180 (1973).
22. LUKES, R. J., COLLINS, R. D.: New approaches to the classification of the lymphomata. Br. J. Cancer *31*, 1–28 (1975).
23. LUKES, R. J., CRAVER, L. F., HALL, T. C., RAPPAPORT, H., RUBEN, P.: Report of the nomenclature committee. Cancer Res. *26*, 1311 (1966).
24. MALLORY, F. B.: The principles of pathologic histology. Philadelphia: W. B. Saunders Co. 1914, p. 333.
25. MASON, D. Y.: Measurement of kappa: lambda light chain ratios by hemagglutination techniques. J. Immunol. Methods *6*, 273–282 (1975).
26. MCJUNKIN, F. A.: Histologic resemblance of the rous chicken sarcoma no. 1 to Hodgkin's granuloma. Cancer Res. *12*, 47–52 (1928).
27. MEDLAR, E. M.: An interpretation of the nature of Hodgkin's disease. Am. J. Pathol. *7*, 499–513 (1931).
28. MELLSTEDT, H., HAMMARSTROM, S., HOLM, G.: Monoclonal lymphocyte population in human plasma cell myeloma. Clin. Exp. Immunol. *17*, 371–384 (1974).
29. MELLSTEDT, H., PETTERSSON, D., HOLM, G.: Monoclonal B-lymphocytes in peripheral blood of patients with plasma cell myeloma. Relation to activity of the disease. Scand. J. Haematol. *16*, 112–120 (1976).
30. MOESCHLIN, S., SCHWARZ, E., WANG, H.: Die Hodgkinzellen als Tumorzellen. Schweiz. Med. Wochenschr. *80*, 1103–1104 (1950).
31. MORSE, H. C., II, PUMPHREY, J. G., POTTER, M., ASOFSKY, R.: Murine plasma cells secreting more than one class of immunoglobulin heavy chain. I. Frequency of two or more M-components in ascitic fluids from 788 primary plasmacytomas. J. Immunol. *117*, 541–547 (1976).
32. OLINICI, C. D.: Cytogenetic observations on different cell lines in Hodgkin's disease. Acta Haematol. (Basel) *48*, 283–287 (1972).
33. ORIOL, R., HUERTA, J., BOUVET, J. P., LIACOPOULOS, P.: Two myeloma globulins, IgGl-κ and IgGl-λ, from a single patient (Im). I. Purification and immunochemical characterization. Immunology *27*, 1081–1093 (1974).
34. PECKHAM, M. J., COOPER, E. H.: Proliferation characteristics of the various classes of cells in Hodgkin's disease. Cancer *24*, 135–146 (1969).
35. PECKHAM, M. J., COOPER, E. H.: Cell biology. In: Hodgkin's Disease. SMITHERS, D. (ed.) London: Churchill, Livingstone 1973, p. 64.
36. PREVAL, C. DE, FOUGEREAU, M.: Absence of preferential reassociation between heavy and light chains of two human immunoglobulins from common cellular origin. Biochem. Biophys. Res. Commun. *67*, 236–239 (1975).
37. PULLINGER, B. D.: Histology and histogenesis. Rose research in lymphadenoma. Bristol, England: John Wright 1932, p. 117.
38. RAPPAPORT, H.: Tumors of the hematopoietic system. In: Atlas of Tumor Pathology, section 3, fascicle 8. Washington, D.C.: Armed Forces Institute of Pathology 1966.

39. REED, D. M.: On the pathological changes in Hodgkin's disease, with especial reference to its relation to tuberculosis. Johns Hopkins Hosp. Rep. *10*, 133–196 (1902).
40. ROBB-SMITH, A. H. T.: The lymph node biopsy. Recent Adv. Clin. Pathol. 350, London: Churchill, Livingstone 1947.
41. ROBB-SMITH, A. H. T.: The classification and natural history of the lymphadenopathies. In: Treatment of Cancer and Allied Diseases, 2nd Edition, Vol. 9. PACK, G. T., ARIEL, I. M. (eds.) New York: Hoeberg 1964.
42. ROBB-SMITH, A. H. T., TAYLOR, C. R.: An Approach to Lymph Node Diagnosis. London: Harvey Miller Publishers, 1976 (in press).
43. ROSS, J. M.: The pathology of the reticular tissue illustrated by two cases of reticulosis with splenomegaly, and a case of lymphadenoma. J. Pathol. Bact. *37*, 311–324 (1933).
44. STERNBERG, C.: Ueber eine eigenartige unter dem Bilde der Pseudoleukämie verlaufende Tuberkulose des lymphatischen Apparates. Z. f. Heilk. *19*, 21–90 (1898).
45. STERNBERG, C.: Eigenartige unter dem Bilde der Pseudoleukämie verlaufende Tuberkulose des lymphatischen Apparates. Erg. allg. Path. Path. Anat. *9*, 502–512 (1903).
46. STERNBERGER, L. A.: Immunocytochemistry. New Jersey: Prentice-Hall 1974.
47. TAYLOR, C. R.: The nature of Reed–Sternberg cells and other malignant "reticulum" cells. Lancet *2*, 802–807 (1974).
48. TAYLOR, C. R.: An immunohistological study of human and murine lymphomata. Thesis. Oxford: 1974.
49. TAYLOR, C. R.: An immunohistological study of follicular lymphoma, reticulum cell sarcoma and Hodgkin's disease. Eur. J. Cancer *12*, 61–75 (1976).
50. TAYLOR, C. R.: Hodgkin's Disease and the Lymphomas. Annual Research Reviews. HORROBIN, D. F. (ed.) Montreal: Eden Press/London, Edinburgh: Longman, Churchill, Livingstone 1976.
51. TAYLOR, C. R.: Immunoperoxidase techniques: practical and theoretical aspects. Arch. Pathol. *102*, 113–121, 1978.
52. TAYLOR, C. R.: Hodgkin's disease and the Lymphomas Vol. II. Annual Research Reviews. HORROBIN, D. F. (ed.) Montreal: Eden Press/London, Edinburgh: Longman, Churchill, Livingstone 1977.
53. TAYLOR, C. R., BURNS, J.: The demonstration of plasma cells, and other immunoglobulin-containing cells in formalin-fixed, paraffin-embedded tissues using peroxidase-labelled antibody. J. Clin. Pathol. *27*, 14–20 (1974).
54. TAYLOR, C. R., MASON, D. Y.: Immunohistological detection of intracellular immunoglobulin in formalin-paraffin sections from multiple myeloma using the immunoperoxidase technique. Clin. Exp. Immunol. *18*, 417–429 (1974).
55. VASILIU, T., GOIA, I.: La granulomatose maligne; la lymphogranulomatose ou maladie de Hodgkin-Paltauf-Sternberg. Ann. Anat. Pathol. *4*, 33–61 (1927).
56. VILLIAUMEY, J., BOUVET, J.-P., MENZA, C. DI, BOCCARA, M.: Myélome plasmocytaire "monoclonal" à deux paraprotéines, IgG κ et IgG λ. Nouv. Presse Med. *3*, 2707–2711 (1974).
57. VIRCHOW, R.: Die krankhaften Geschwülste. Berlin: Hirschwald Verlag 1863, Vol. I, p. 728.
58. VOSSEN, J. M., HIJMANS, W.: Membrane-associated immunoglobulin determinants on bone marrow and blood lymphocytes in the pediatric age group and on fetal tissues. Ann. N.Y. Acad. Sci. *254*, 262–279 (1975).
59. WARNKE, R.: Personal communication at N.I.H. Symposium on immunoperoxidase procedures, Bethesda, Maryland, May, 1977.

Part III

Natural History of Lymphoid Neoplasias: Human and Experimental Models

Evolution of Immunoblastic Lymphoma in Angioimmunoblastic Lymphadenopathy[1]

B. N. Nathwani, H. Rappaport, E. M. Moran, G. A. Pangalis, and H. Kim

Angioimmunoblastic lymphadenopathy (AILD) [4, 5] or immunoblastic lymphadenopathy [7] is a systemic disease clinically characterized by fever, generalized lymphadenopathy, and hepatosplenomegaly. Polyclonal hypergammaglobulinemia, and Coombs' positive hemolytic anemia are frequently present. The lymph nodes in AILD reveal a polymorphic picture consisting of a proliferation of small vessels, immunoblasts, and plasma cells. Similar clinical and histologic observations have been reported under other designations [3, 10, 14].

AILD differs from malignant lymphomas by the high frequency of constitutional symptoms, generalized lymph node enlargement, hepatosplenomegaly, cutaneous manifestations, and polyclonal hypergammaglobulinemia at the time of clinical onset. Histologically, AILD is characterized by obliteration of the architecture, small vessel proliferation, proliferation of small mature lymphocytes, plasma cells and immunoblasts which are scattered throughout the involved tissue without forming cohesive clusters or masses, and the presence of an eosinophilic amorphous intercellular material which is generally PAS positive. Based on our study of 24 patients [4, 5], AILD was considered as a nonneoplastic disorder, a view also expressed for immunoblastic lymphadenopathy [7, 10]. However, progression of both AILD [2, 9, 15] and immunoblastic lymphadenopathy [1, 6, 7, 13] into immunoblastic lymphoma (IL) has been reported. For this reason, we were particularly interested in establishing histologic criteria that would allow us to recognize the occurrence of malignant lymphoma in lymph nodes exhibiting features of AILD.

Eighty-four cases of AILD with and without histologic features of IL were studied [8]; 42 of these were interpreted as AILD, 36 as AILD co-existing with immunoblastic lymphoma (AILD + IL), and six as AILD in the initial (diagnostic) biopsy and AILD + IL in follow-up biopsies. Analysis of the histologic features in the diagnostic and follow-up biopsies in some of these patients strongly suggested that the earliest phase of malignant progression can be recognized by the presence of transformed large lymphoid cells in clusters or islands (Table 1). The clusters may be of varying sizes and may be intravascular or extravascular. As the disease progresses, the clusters and islands become confluent and form monomorphic areas of large lymphoid cells with or without plasmacytoid features, and when this has taken place, the malignant lymphoma is readily diagnosable. Such progression was observed in eight of ten patients with AILD + IL in whom a second lymph node biopsy became available in the course of the patients' illness (Table 1) [18].

In order to investigate the validity of our histologic criteria for malignancy, we compared 42 patients in whom AILD was found in one or more biopsies with 36 patients in whom AILD + IL was diagnosed on the basis of the first biopsy with respect to: 1) clinical features, 2) response to therapy, 3) survival, and 4) presence and extent of malignant lymphoma at autopsy. We found no differences in the clinical presentation between AILD and AILD + IL. However, patients with AILD tended to respond better to prednisone or to chemotherapeutic agents than patients with AILD + IL. There was a significant difference in the incidence of complete

1 Supported by Grant Number R10 CA 18044 awarded by the National Cancer Institute, NIH, DHEW, and by Haematopathology Tutorial.

Table 1. Evolution of disease in 10 patients with AILD + IL who had a follow-up biopsy and at autopsy

Pt.	Findings in first LN biopsy	Interval between biopsies (months)	Findings in follow-up biopsy[a]	Interval between last biopsy and death (months)	Autopsy
R.J.	AILD + IL clusters, islands	1	IL diffuse	1	AILD
C.O.	AILD + IL clusters[b]	2	IL diffuse	4	AILD + IL (LN, spleen) islands
E.L.	AILD + IL clusters, islands, clear cells	2	IL diffuse (splenectomy)	6	Not done
G.P.	AILD + IL clusters	3½	IL diffuse	1	IL (LN) diffuse
M.L.	AILD + IL clusters, clear cells	5	IL diffuse	4	IL (LN) diffuse
A.C.	AILD + IL clusters, diffuse	9½	IL diffuse (splenectomy)	½	IL (LN) diffuse
F.B.	AILD + IL clusters, islands	16	IL diffuse	2	AILD + IL (LN, BM) islands
A.Y.	AILD + IL clusters	2½	IL clusters, islands, diffuse	2	Not done
J.D.	AILD + IL clusters, diffuse	9	AILD + IL clusters, diffuse	2	IL (LN) diffuse
L.G.	AILD + IL clusters	2½	AILD	1	IL (LN) diffuse

[a] Of lymph nodes, except in patients A.C. and E.L.
[b] A lymph node biopsy obtained 214 months earlier had shown AILD only (Table 2).
LN: lymph node; BM: bone marrow.

remission following prednisone or chemotherapy between patients with AILD (63%) and those with AILD + IL (26%) ($p = 0.01$).The median survival was 35 months in patients with AILD versus 6 months in patients with AILD + IL ($p = 0.0004$). Malignant lymphoma was evident at autopsy in two of ten patients (20%) in the AILD group in contrast to 18 of 22 patients (82%) in the AILD + IL group ($p < 0.005$). Extranodal involvement by malignant lymphoma at autopsy was observed in only one patient (10%) with AILD, whereas it was seen in 14 patients (64%) with AILD + IL ($p < 0.025$) [8].

Spontaneous clinical remissions lasting longer than 6 months and consisting of disappearance of clinical symptoms and regression of lymphadenopathy occurred in four patients with AILD and in three patients with AILD + IL. Of the four patients with AILD, two are alive and well 50 and 56 months, respectively, after onset of the disease. One patient died from pneumonia 45 months after onset of the disease, and at autopsy no evidence of AILD or IL was found. The fourth patient had a repeat biopsy after 60 months, revealing AILD + IL, and he died 10 months thereafter. Of three patients with AILD + IL who had spontaneous remissions, two are alive without treatment 12 and 28 months after diagnosis and one had a relapse after 9 months and died 2 months later.

Thirteen patients with AILD had a second lymph node biopsy after intervals of 2–214 months; evidence of malignant lymphoma was found in six of them (Table 2). This tends to indicate that malignant lymphoma may develop in patients with AILD after latent periods of unpredictable duration. The four long-term spontaneous remissions in AILD would be consistent with the histologically benign appearance of the disease. The two relatively short spontaneous remissions in AILD + IL without relapse are not readily explained but could be attributed either to the fact that the removed tissue may have contained the only focus of tumor in the host or that the total tumor cell mass outside the removed tissues may have been still small enough to be controlled by the immunologic defenses of the host.

Table 2. Evolution of AILD to malignant lymphoma, as seen in follow-up biopsies and at autopsy

Pt.	Findings in 1st biopsy	Interval between biopsies months	Findings in 2nd biopsy	Interval between 2nd biopsy and death (months)	Autopsy
V.R.	AILD	2	AILD + IL islands, diffuse	8	IL (LN, BM, spleen, liver, kidney, lung, thyroid) diffuse
H.F.	AILD	4½	IL diffuse	3	IL (LN, liver, kidney) diffuse
O.S.	AILD	5	AILD + IL islands, clear cells	14	Not done
R.J.	AILD	48	IL diffuse	3	AILD + IL (Skin) diffuse
R.L.	AILD	60	IL diffuse	10	Not done
C.O.	AILD	214	AILD + IL clusters	6	AILD + IL (LN, spleen) islands

LN: lymph node; BM: bone marrow.

Table 3. Results of immunoperoxidase reaction in 32 patients with AILD + IL

	Immunoglobulin chains demonstrated by monospecific antisera		
	Plasma cells	Immunoblasts in AILD areas	Immunoblasts in IL areas
Light chains (LC)	32 κ, λ	18 κ, λ 14 no LC	5 κ, λ 27 no LC
Heavy chains (HC)	18 α, γ, μ	6 α, γ, μ 7 α, γ 5 no HC	2 α, γ, μ 16 no HC
	9 α, λ	4 α, λ 1 λ 4 no HC	2 α, λ 7 no HC
	2 α, μ 1 α	2 no HC 1 no HC	2 no HC 1 no HC
	2 no HC	2 no HC	2 no HC

We were also interested in correlating the functional activity of the plasma cells and of the large lymphoid cells (immunoblasts) by demonstrating the presense of intracytoplasmic immunoglobulins in tissue sections by using the peroxidase-anti-peroxidase (PAP) method [11, 12]. We found that in all cases tested, the plasma cell population was polyclonal. In approximately half of them, scattered immunoblasts in the AILD areas showed both light chains as well as the heavy chains corresponding to those observed in the plasma cells, in the same sections. In the remaining cases, only the plasma cells, but not the immunoblasts, contained immunoglobulin (Table 3). The ultrastructural findings in some of these cases showed that many of the large lymphoid cells had abundant polyribosomes but no rough endoplasmic reticulum. This is in keeping with the absence of demonstrable immunoglobulin in most of the neoplastic cells by the PAP method (Table 4). Whether this indicates neoplastic differentiation or lack of plasmacytic differentiation is not clear at this time. It is of great interest, however, that in those cases in which clusters or islands were a prominent feature, all or most of the component cells of these clusters or islands were negative for immunoglobulins, although the immunoblasts in the rest of the lymph node contained them. This suggests a functional difference between the immunoblasts inside and outside the clusters or islands. However, in five instances in which immunoglobulin could be detected in areas of IL, the immunoblastic proliferation proved to be polyclonal.

Table 4. Correlation of ultrastructural findings with light microscopic and immunoperoxidase findings

Patient	Light microscopy	Immunoperoxidase for immunoglobulin chains in large lymphoid cells	Ultrastructure
R.J.	Monomorphic IL (large lymphoid cells with plasmacytoid features)	Negative	Rare rough endoplasmic reticulum, not dilated. Abundant polysomes
A.C.	Polymorphic IL (large lymphoid cells with plasmacytoid features and plasma cells)	Negative	Rare rough endoplasmic reticulum, not dilated. Abundant polysomes
G.P.	Monomorphic IL (large lymphoid cells with plasmacytoid features)	Positive for κ, λ, α, γ	Occasional rough endoplasmic reticulum, rarely dilated with immunoglobulin. Abundant polysomes

It would have been of interest to study in a larger series of cases whether evolution of immunoblastic lymphoma could in any way be related to changes in the serum immunoelectrophoretic pattern. We were unable to establish a definite correlation between changes in serum immunoglobulin levels and the evolution of immunoblastic lymphoma. However, in 7 of 14 patients with AILD + IL, in whom follow-up serum immunoglobulin determinations were available, the immunoglobulin levels decreased in the course of the disease and in six of them hypogammaglobulinemia developed (Table 5). This would suggest that as the functioning plasma cells and large lymphoid cells of AILD are replaced by a neoplastic immunoblastic population, the capacity for forming immunoglobulin diminishes and hypogammaglobulinemia may ensue. In two patients, the serum immunoglobulin levels increased suggesting an increase in the immunoglobulin-producing cell mass.

In summary [8], our findings indicate that: 1. A differentiation between AILD and AILD + IL can be made only histologically, and there are no distinguishing clinical or laboratory features between them. 2. The evolution of malignant lymphoma in AILD can have several morphologic expressions. The accuracy of our criteria for the diagnosis of malignant lymphoma has been

Table 5. Follow-up serum immunoglobulin (Ig) levels in 14 patients with AILD + IL

Initial Ig	No. of patients	Follow-up Ig	No. of patients
Polyclonal hypergammaglobulinemia	11	Essentially no change	3[a]
		Increase of polyclonal hypergammaglobulinemia	2
		Decrease of lg to normal	1
		Hypogammaglobulinemia	5
Normal	3	Normal Ig	2
		Hypogammaglobulinemia	1

[a] In one patient, IgG decreased from 3980 mg% to 2420 MG%. IgA remained about the same (610 vs, 565 mg%), and IgM increased from 350 mg% to 740 mg%.

tested by observations in sequential biopsies, response to therapy, length of survival, and incidence and extent of malignant lymphoma at autopsy. The data thus obtained indicate that the evolution of AILD into IL can be recognized in tissue sections. 3. Sixty-three percent of patients with AILD had a complete remission following prednisone or chemotherapy. In contrast, only 62% of patients with AILD + IL had a complete response to prednisone or chemotherapy ($p = 0.01$). 4. In the AILD group, median survival of patients who had complete remission after prednisone was significantly longer than that of patients who had partial or no remissions ($p = 0.02$), and the same is true for patients who were given chemotherapy ($p < 0.003$). In patients with AILD + IL, the same difference was observed for patients initially treated with chemotherapy ($p < 0.007$) but not for those initially treated with prednisone only ($p = 0.31$). 5. The median survival of all patients with AILD without IL is significantly longer than that of patients with AILD = IL ($p = 0.0004$), regardless of the type of therapy. 6. Comparison of the autopsy findings of patients with an antemortem diagnosis of AILD with those of patients with an antemortem diagnosis of AILD + IL revealed that 20% of the AILD group and 82% of the AILD + IL group had malignant lymphoma at necropsy ($p < 0.005$), and that in the AILD group extranodal involvement by malignant lymphoma was observed in only 10% of autopsies while in the AILD + IL group it was found in 64% ($p < 0.025$). 7. Studies of lymph nodes and organs from various sites, both during life and at autopsy, revealed that malignant lymphoma occuring in AILD is not necessarily present in all sites sampled nor in every section from available tissue specimens. In some instances, evidence of malignancy was limited to one lymph node or extranodal site. Thus, unavoidable sampling errors can be reduced by taking as many sections from a surgical specimen as possible or by obtaining biopsies from additional lymph nodes. 8. Preliminary immunologic studies using the immunoperoxidase method confirmed the polyclonal nature of both the plasmacytic and immunoblastic cellular proliferations. They also revealed that formation of light and heavy chains, a conspicuous feature in the plasma cells, is both quantitatively and qualitatively reduced in the large lymphoid cells in the AILD areas and absent in the majority of the IL areas. However, in five instances in which immunoglobins could be detected in IL areas, the proliferations were polyclonal [8].

References

1. FISHER R.I., JAFFE, E. S., BRAYLAN, R. C., ANDERSEN, J. C., TAN, H. K.: Immunoblastic lymphadenopathy. Evolution into a malignant lymphoma with plasmacytoid features. Amer. J. Med. *61*, 553 (1976).

2. FLANDRIN, G.: Adénopathies angio-immunoblastiques avec anémie auto-immune et hyperimmunoglobulinémie polyclonale. Nouv. Presse Med. *5*, 1521 (1976).
3. FLANDRIN, G., DANIEL, M. T., EL YAFI, G., CHELLOUL, N.: Sarcomatoses ganglionnaires diffuses a différenciation plasmocytaire avec anémie hemolytique auto-immune. Actual. Haematol. (Paris) *6*, 25 (1972).
4. FRIZZERA, G., MORAN, E. M., RAPPAPORT, H.: Angio-immunoblastic lymphadenopathy with dysproteinaemia. Lancet *1*, 1070 (1974).
5. FRIZZERA, G., MORAN, E. M., RAPPAPORT, H.: Angio-immunoblastic lymphadenopathy. Diagnosis and clinical course. Amer. J. Med. *59*, 803 (1975).
6. HOWARTH, C. B., BIRD, C. C.: Immunoblastic sarcoma arising in child with immunoblastic lymphadenopathy. Lancet *11*, 747 (1976).
7. LUKES, R. J., TINDLE, B. H.: Immunoblastic lymphadenopathy. A hyperimmune entity resembling Hodgkin's disease. New Engl. J. Med. *292*, 1 (1975).
8. NATHWANI, B. N., RAPPAPORT, H., MORAN, E. M., PANGALIS, G, A., KIM, H.:Malignant lymphoma arising in angio-immunoblastic lymphadenopathy. Cancer *41*, 578 (1978).
9. PRUZANSKI, W., SUTTON, D. M. C., PANTALONY, D.: Angio-immunoblastic lymphadenopathy: An immunochemical study. Clin. Immunol. Immunopath. *6*, 62 (1976).
10. RADASZKIEWICZ, T., LENNERT, K.: Lymphogranulomatosis X. Dtsch. med. Wschr. *100*, 1157 (1975).
11. STERNBERGER, L. A., HARDY, P. H., JR., CUCULIS, J. J., MEYER, H. G.: The unlabeled antibody enzyme method of immunohistochemistry. J. Histochem. Cytochem. *18*, 315 (1970).
12. TAYLOR, C. R.: An immunohistological study of follicular lymphoma, reticulum cell sarcoma and Hodgkin's disease. Europ. J. Cancer *12*, 61 (1976).
13. TOTH, J., GARAM, T.: Immunoblastic lymphadenopathy proceeding to sarcoma. Lancet *1*, 102 (1977).
14. WESTERHAUSEN, M., OEHLERT, W.: Chronisches pluripotentielles immunoproliferatives Syndrom. Dtsch. med Wschr. *97*, 1407 (1972).
15. YATAGANAS, X., PAPADIMITRIOU, N., PANGALIS, G. A., LOUKOPOULOS, D., FESSAS, PH., PAPACHARALAMPOUS, N.: Angio-immunoblastic lymphadenopathy terminating as Hodgkin's disease. Cancer *39*, 2183 (1977).

Immunoblastic Lymphadenopathy: A Prelymphomatous State of Immunoblastic Sarcoma

R. J. LUKES and B. H. TINDLE

Introduction

We became aware of the disorder, immunoblastic lymphadenopathy (IBL), during the course of our study of Hodgkin's disease cases from World War II at the Armed Forces Institute of Pathology [6] when we were concerned with its resemblance to Hodgkin's disease. A number of years were required to accumulate a sufficient number of acceptable cases of IBL with follow-up information to determine its clinical expressions and prognostic significance. The findings were presented finally at several meetings in 1973 [9, 10] and subsequently published as a series of 32 cases in early 1975 [11]. These cases collected from hospitals throughout the United States had been investigated clinically in a variable fashion, but nevertheless permitted the presentation of a rather distinctive clinical morphologic entity as a benign appearing hyperimmune proliferation of the B-cell system with distinctive morphologic features. It frequently was initially manifested by hypersensitivity reactions to therapeutic agents (35%), with a dramatic onset of fever, rash and pruritus, and later by generalized lymphadenopathy, and less frequently hepatosplenomegaly. Anemia was common and there was a consistent polyclonal hyperglobulinemia. A lymphoma of transformed lymphocytes, immunoblastic sarcoma (IBS), developed in the subsequent course of disease in three cases and justified consideration of IBL as a prelymphomatous disorder. We have now collected histologic material in over 250 cases of IBL and related disorders, approximately 100 of which fulfill the criteria we originally proposed for IBL; 25 of the latter cases have exhibited features of both IBL and IBS, either in subsequent specimens or in different areas of the initial biopsy. From this experience, it appears that there is a broad spectrum of as yet undefined abnormal immune reactions of which IBL represents the most extreme and abnormal component. The degree of abnormality of IBL and its morphologic expressions seems to account for its prelymphomatous nature with a tendency to evolve to IBS, while the less abnormal components of the spectrum frequently subside. The disorder, angioimmunoblastic lymphadenopathy, presented subsequently by FRIZZERA et al. [1], judging from their published criteria, is not equivalent morphologically to IBL and seems to be more representative of the broad spectrum of abnormal reactions rather than the extreme component of the spectrum that we have reserved for IBL. This view is supported by the realization that none of their original cases were reported to develop immunoblastic sarcoma. In this presentation, I will review briefly: 1) the morphologic criteria of IBL for comparison with the lesion reported by FRIZZERA et al., 2) the clinical findings in the 250 cases we have accumulated for study, and 3) the basic concept of the disease of IBL.

Morphologic Criteria

The diagnostic criteria for IBL are described in detail in our original publication [11], and their clinical relevance has been supported in our large case series accumulated in the interim. There

Table 1. Morphologic criteria for diagnosis of IBL

1. Arborizing vascular proliferation with PAS + thickened vessel walls	(3–4+)	100%
2. Immunoblastic and plasma cell proliferation	(3–4+)	100%
3. Deposit of acidophilic interstitial material	(3–4+)	100%

Complete involvement of lymph node essentially *without* any residential reactive follicles. The lymph node is hypocellular and *lymphocyte depleted.*

are three essential diagnostic features that combine to involve the entire lymph node (Table 1): 1) the proliferation of arborizing small vessels with PAS-positive thickened walls, 2) an immunoblast and plasma cell proliferation, and 3) a deposit of acidophilic interstitial material associated with decrease in lymphocytes. All of these features are present to a prominent degree (3–4+). The decrease in lymphocytes is of considerable significance and relates to the general hypocellularity of the node and an appearance of lymphocyte depletion. Lymphatic follicles with reaction centers are essentially absent. Benign histiocytes with prominent acidophilic cytoplasm occurring individually and in clusters are a prominent feature in approximately 25% of the cases. Eosinophils in small numbers are commonly found but are frequently absent. In a few cases, large cells with lobated nuclei are encountered and raise concern for the possibility of Hodgkin's disease, but none fulfill the criteria for diagnostic Sternberg-Reed cells [5, 6]. Moreover, the general character of the process and the frequency of immunoblasts make Hodgkin's disease unlikely since immunoblasts in our experience are an uncommon component of Hodgkin's disease. The vessels involved in IBL are small, twisting, curling, and branching, and not the increase in the prominence of vessels resulting from endothelial hyperplasia that are typical of normal reactive lymphoid processes.

The relationship of IBL to other immunoblastic proliferations of lymph nodes is illustrated schematically in Figure 1. IBL in our opinion is a homogeneous morphologic entity that represents the extreme portion of the spectrum of immunoblastic proliferations and of abnormal immune reactions. Within this spectrum, there seems to be a gradation in the degree and abnormality of immunoblastic proliferations from that observed in normal immune reactions at one end of the spectrum to IBL at the other extreme. The severe immunoblastic reaction typical of infectious mononucleosis falls within the normal region. Even though it may contain polyploid cells indistinguishable from diagnostic Sternberg-Reed cells [5, 12], infectious mononucleosis lacks the arborizing vascular proliferation and the deposit of amorphous interstitial material. In the broad group of abnormal immune reactions, immunoblastic

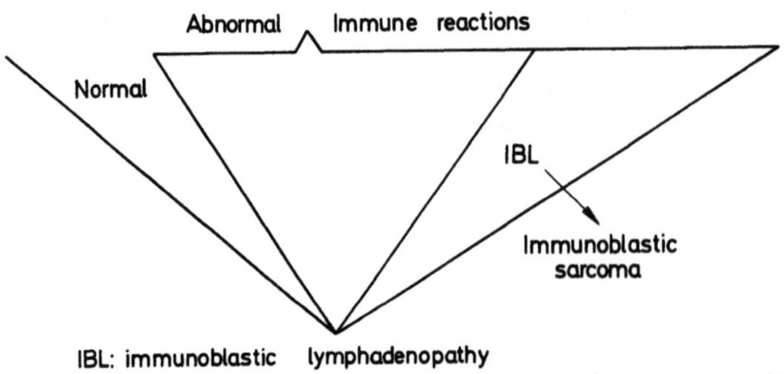

Fig. 1. A spectrum of immunoblastic proliferation is shown with normal at one extreme and the most abnormal IBL at the extreme of abnormal immune reactions. Intermediate between these extremes is a group of as yet undefined abnormal reactions some of which resemble IBL

proliferations associated with plasma cells, vascular proliferation, and deposit of interstitial material may be found, but only when all three occur in typical character and prominent degree (3–4+) does the process fulfill the criteria for IBL. At times, other features of chronic reaction are present such as chronic reactive follicles containing prominent deposits of acidophilic globular material within reaction centers. This finding is not part of IBL, although it was emphasized by FRIZZERA et al. [1, 2]. Of our accumulated 250 cases of abnormal immune reactions now under review, approximately 100 fulfill the above criteria. Those regarded as unacceptable usually fail to fulfill one or two of the above criteria, or all three features are found, but in less than prominent degree. In several cases, the typical features are limited to a small portion of a lymph node that otherwise exhibits features of reactive hyperplasia. The significance of partial lymph node involvement, however, is uncertain at the present time. Finally, the most common reason for unacceptability of cases is the hypercellularity of the process or the lack of lymphocyte depletion, even though all three other features are prominent. It might be argued, correctly, that there are two additional criteria, i.e., diffuse lymph node involvement essentially without any residual follicles and the lymphocyte depletion character of the process. We have rigidly required the above diagnostic criteria for acceptance of cases as IBL in order to determine the clinical and prognostic significance of IBL as a homogeneous morphologic process. At the same time, we believe this approach will permit the establishment of the significance of the processes included in the remainder of the spectrum of abnormal immune reactions. It is acknowledged that a number of the cases excluded may represent an earlier phase or a milder expression of IBL. Only detailed follow-up studies will clarify the meaning of these morphologic distinctions. Our experience so far indicates that when our morphologic criteria for IBL are fulfilled, the patients almost without exception have generalized symptomatic progressive disease; whereas, if the morphologic criteria are not fulfilled, the patients may be asymptomatic and have limited disease.

Comparison with the morphologic criteria published by FRIZZERA et al. [1, 2] for angioimmunoblastic lymphadenopathy (AILD) reveals several important and fundamental differences that are not generally appreciated. The deposit of acidophilic interstitial material was not an essential feature, lymphocyte depletion was not considered, and chronic reactive follicles often were a common and even a prominent finding. We can only conclude that many of the cases included by these authors would not be acceptable in our series and that immunoblastic lymphadenopathy (IBL) and AILD are not equivalent processes. The lesion reported by FRIZZERA et al. [1, 2], judging from their published criteria, appears to be representative of the broad spectrum of abnormal immune reactions and differs from the homogeneous extreme component of the spectrum we have attempted to reserve for IBL and which seems to be prelymphomatous. This observation possibly accounts for the lack of immunoblastic sarcoma in the original case series of FRIZZERA et al. [1, 2]. It will also account for the wide variation in clinical expressions and the more benign course of the disease of their case series [1, 2].

The morphologic criteria for immunoblastic sarcoma (IBS) are those of a monomorphous proliferation of transformed lymphocytes. The process may involve a part or the entire lymph node or tissue and the cytologic features vary widely from essentially normal appearing transformed lymphocytes to pleomorphic lobated or multinucleolated, cells. At times, binucleated cells are found with large nucleoli, and as a result they resemble diagnostic Sternberg-Reed cells. IBS developing in abnormal immune proliferations may be limited in extent and occur as focal or multifocal processes with foci as small as a microscopic field. Obviously, the diagnosis is established with great caution when found in minor degree. We believe the diagnosis can be accurately established if it is monomorphous in character, and particularly if the transformed lymphocytes are pleomorphic.

The detailed criteria for recognizing IBS of T or B-cell types will be the subject of a subsequent detailed report by our investigative group. In general, IBS of B-cell type exhibits plasmacytoid features to varying degrees, while IBS of T-cell type has lightly amphophilic cytoplasm that may appear almost water-clear in hematoxylin- and eosin- stained sections. The cells have nuclei of medium to large size with finely dispersed nuclear chromatin giving the nucleus a vesicular appearance. There are one to three medium size nucleoli often situated near the thick nuclear membrane. Immunoblasts must be distinguished from the large noncleaved or transformed follicular center cell (FCC) that we described [7, 8].

Clinical findings

The clinical findings in our accumulated cases of IBL and related abnormal immune reactions are the subject of a current study and will be reported in detail subsequently. The clinical expressions encountered in the 100 cases fulfilling the morphologic criteria for IBL are even more consistent than reported in our original study [11]. Many cases have had dramatic presentations and have been readily recognized clinically. The initial manifestation of hypersensitivity has continued at approximately the same frequency (35%), and we suspect that it may prove even more common with more sensitive immunologic techniques in prospective studies. Generalized lymphadenopathy often with splenomegaly in a symptomatic febrile patient, often with a rash, anemia, and usually polyclonal hyperglobulinemia provide a readily recognizable clinical entity. The development of IBS in a patient with IBL is often heralded by a dramatic change in the enlargement of lymph nodes, the intensity of systemic symptoms, and the rate of progression of the disease. In a number of cases, the morphologic features of both IBL and IBS were found in different portions of the initial lymph node biopsy. This observation suggests that IBL may have existed for varying periods in these patients without clinical recognition.

Basic Concept of Disease

IBL presents the morphologic features of a benign hyperplastic process. The diffuse involvement of lymph nodes without residual follicles, together with the prominent immunoblasts and plasma cell proliferation, the arborizing vascular proliferation, and the deposit of interstitial acidophilic material associated with lymphocyte depletion combine to from a distinct proliferative process that is distinguishable from both a normal benign reactive self-limited lymphoid proliferation and malignant lymphoma. The disease has a malignant progressive clinical course, but morphologic evidence of malignant neoplasm as IBS was found in only three of our original series of 32 cases, two in subsequent biopsies, and one in the follow-up autopsy material. Chromosomal abnormalities have been reported in two cases and presented as potential evidence of neoplasia although no detailed morphologic description of the biopsy or information regarding the subsequent course of the disease have been provided [3]. We have concluded that the morphologic features of IBL although not indicative of malignant lymphoma, are evidence of a persistent and progressive abnormal immune process that represents a "switch on" of the lymphocyte transformation mechanism that seems uncontrolled and possibly accounts for the tendency to evolve to IBS.

The obvious questions that immediately arise relate to the significance of the morphologic features of the abnormal immune process and how they might explain the development of IBS. The prominent proliferations of transformed lymphocytes (immunoblasts) in IBL are individually similar morphologically to normal immunoblasts found in both mild and severe reactive processes of the interfollicular tissue. In IBL, they are prominent in number and often plasmacytoid, as evidence of their B-cell nature, and apparently relate to the commonly observed polyclonal hyperglobulinemia. The latter is also evidence of the nonneoplastic character of the process. This finding is supported by the results of the immunoperoxidase studies of cytoplasmic immunoglobulin performed by DR. CLIVE TAYLOR in our laboratory which demonstrate polyclonal cytoplasmic immunoglobulin in all the cases of IBL investigated with this technique. Thus, the immunoblasts not only morphologically appear benign in character, but the proliferating population of immunoblasts is not monomorphous, as evidenced by the polyclonal character of the cytoplasmic immunoglobulin and the associated polyclonal character of the hyperglobulinemia. The character and severity of the vascular proliferation, however, confers a morphologic indication of an abnormal immune process. The involvement of small arborizing vessels of lymph nodes, spleen, and bone marrow in association with an initial hypersensitivity reaction suggests that a fundamental hypersensitivity phenomenon selects certain small vessels as part of the basic process in IBL. The prominent deposit of acidophilic interstitial material that is associated with lymphocyte depletion suggests the possible existence of a lymphocytoxin in the IBL process. If a lymphocytoxic factor plays a role in the typical IBL process, there may be loss of effective lymphocyte function, i.e., decrease in suppressor or helper factors. The loss of suppressor cells or factors could be hypothesized to relate to the loss of control of lymphocyte transformation and result in the persistence of immunoblast proliferation and even play a role in the development of IBS. A parallel process is observed in the immunosuppressed graft rejection state in which IBS develops when the suppression of lymphocyte function apparently permits immunoblasts to proliferate (derepression). Under similar conditions lymphomas have also been produced experimentally by KRUEGER et al. [4]. Finally, the diffuse involvement of lymph nodes without residual reactive follicles indicates the severity of the process and also the apparent postfollicular nature of the process in which the proliferation essentially involves the B-immunoblast to the plasma cell portion of the B-cell system rather than the follicular component according to our FCC concept [7, 8]. The occurrence of malignant lymphoma, IBS type in IBL, parallels the developments of IBS in a variety of abnormal immune states, such as SJÖGREN's syndrome, systemic lupus erythematosis (SLE), α-chain disease, Hashimoto's disease, the immune suppressed graft rejection patient, and finally, the most common abnormal immune state, senescence. It also occurs in the low-grade malignant lymphomas, the plasmacytoid lymphocyte type associated with macroglobulinemia, and the small B-lymphocyte, the tissue expression of chronic lymphocytic leukemia. The occurrence of IBS in these conditions as well as IBL, suggests that chronic lymphoid proliferations in defective immune states are prone to a switch on (derepression) of lymphocyte transformation and that the control mechanism possibly related to suppressor cells or factors may be defective and permit the transformation to persist.

Conclusions

1. IBL appears established as a distinctive clinical morphologic entity with a progressive and commonly fatal termination. Morphologically, IBL is a benign hyperproliferation of the B-cell system and represents the extreme component of the spectrum of abnormal immune proliferations with a predilection for evolving into IBS, a lymphoma of transformed lymphocytes.

2. IBL is characterized morphologically by 1) immunoblast and plasma cell proliferation, 2) a proliferation of arborizing small vessels with PAS-positive thickened walls, and 3) an interstitial deposit of acidophilic amorphous material. All of these features occur in prominent degree, involve lymph modes diffusely, lack a follicular component, and are associated with a decrease in lymphoctes (lymphocyte depletion). The remaining proliferations of the spectrum may have one or more of these features in minor degree and appear to represent possibly a number of, as yet, undefined abnormal immune reactions. The findings described for AILD by FRIZZERA et

al., [1, 2] lack the lymphocyte depletion and often the amorphous interstitial material as well, and frequently possess a follicular component. We can only conclude that the lesion, AILD, is representative of the entire spectrum of abnormal immune reactions and is not equivalent to IBL. Unquestionably, these differences in criteria account for their lack of cases evolving to IBS in their original cases series. IBL, as the extreme component of the spectrum, is a more homogeneous and abnormal morphologic entity, which is associated with the development of IBS and is, therefore, a prelymphomatous state.

3. The basic process in IBL appears to involve an alteration in the control mechanism of lymphocyte transformation in the B-cell system; if the control mechanism is severely and persistently limited, the hyperproliferation of the B-cell system may evolve into IBS. The benign morphologic appearance of IBL is supported by the findings of polyclonal cytoplasmic and serum immunoglobulins. The distinctive arborizing vascular proliferation in association with the initial hypersensitivity reaction suggests a hypersensitivity vascular component in the process that selects specific vessels. The lymphocyte depletion component of IBL is possibly an expression of an existent lymphocytoxin and could lead to reduction of suppressor cells or factors that normally play a role in regulating B-lymphocyte transformation and immunoglobulin synthesis. Limitation of the control of B-lymphocyte transformation when severe and persistent permits severe hyperproliferation and represents the prelymphomatous state of IBS.

Acknowledgements

This investigation has been supported in part by National Institutes of Health training grant No. CA 19449–02 and the Beaumont Foundation.

References

1. FRIZZERA, G., MORAN, E. M., RAPPAPORT, H.: Angio-immunoblastic lymphadenopathy with dysproteinaemia. Lancet *1*, 1070–1073 (1974).
2. FRIZZERA, G., MORAN, E. M., RAPPAPORT, H.: Angio-immunoblastic lymphadenopathy. Diagnosis and clinical course. Am. J. Med. *59*, 803–818 (1975).
3. HOSSFELD, D. K., HOFFKEN, K., SCHMIDT, C. G., DIEDRICHS, H.: Chromosome abnormalities in angioimmunoblastic lymphadenopathy. Lancet *1*, 198 (1976).
4. KRUEGER, G., MALMGREN, R. A., BERARD, C. W.: Malignant lymphomas and plasmacytosis in mice under chronic immunosuppression and persistent antigenic stimulation. Transplantation *11*, 138–144 (1971).
5. LUKES, R. J.: Criteria for involvement of lymph node, bone marrow, spleen, and liver in Hodgkin's disease. Cancer Res. *31*, 1755–1767 (1971).
6. LUKES, R. J., BUTLER, J. J., HICKS, E. B.: Natural history of Hodgkin's disease as related to its pathologic picture. Cancer *19*, 317–344 (1966).
7. LUKES, R. J., COLLINS, R. D.: Immunologic characterization of human malignant lymphomas. Cancer *34*, 1488–1503 (1974).
8. LUKES, R. J., COLLINS, R. D.: New approaches to the classification of the lymphomata. Br. J. Cancer *31*, suppl. II, 1–28 (1975).
9. LUKES, R. J., TINDLE, B. H.: Immunoblastic lymphadenopathy. Presented at meeting of Pathology Panel and Repository Center for Lymphoma Clinical Trials, National Cancer Institute, Bethesda, Maryland, January 26–28, 1973.
10. LUKES, R. J., TINDLE, B. H.: Immunoblastic lymphadenopathy: a new hyperimmune entity resembling Hodgkin's disease. Presented at the Workshop on Classification of Non-Hodgkin's Lymphomas, University of Chicago, Chicago, Illinois, June 25–29, 1973.
11. LUKES, R., TINDLE, B. H.: Immunoblastic lymphadenopathy. A hyperimmune entity resembling Hodgkin's disease. New Engl. J. Med. *292*, 1–8 (1975).
12. TINDLE, B. H., PARKER, J. W., LUKES, R. J.: "Reed-Sternberg Cells" in infectious mononucleosis? Am. J. Clin. Pathol. *58*, 607–617 (1972).

Angioimmunoblastic Lymphadenopathy: Clinical, Biologic, and Follow-up Study of 14 Cases

G. Flandrin

Angioimmunoblastic lymphadenopathy (AILD) is a recently invidualized atypical lymphoid disease [5, 9, 14]. It is characterized by the presence of peripheral lymph node enlargement, hepatosplenomegaly, cutaneous rash, and constitutional symptoms. The diagnosis of this disorder is based on examination of lymph nodes, the anatomic alterations of which meet the following histologic criteria [26, 9]:

1. Diffuse effacement of nodal architecture;
2. Abundance of small vessels;
3. Marked proliferation of pleomorphic lymphoid cells: lymphocytes, plasma cells, and immunoblasts.

All these criteria must be present to enable the diagnosis of this disease to be made.

Despite this apparently coherent histologic definition, the confines of the disorder appear to be somewhat nebulous in the light of the already numerous reports published. The clinical picture, biologic aspects, and course are not absolutely superimposable from one report to the next. There is also discussion as to the seriousness of the disorder and its treatment [6, 15]. Our purpose in this paper is to make a contribution to this dossier by reporting the detailed clinical and biologic data obtained during the follow-up of 14 patients.

Materials and Methods

This work is not a retrospective study but is based on the clinical follow-up of 14 patients admitted in the same clinical hematology department (Hematologic Disease Research Institute, Hôpital Saint-Louis, Paris; Director, Professor Jean Bernard) between 1968 and 1976. The first six patients included in this study were previously reported in 1972 under the name of "Diffuse Plasma Cell Differentiated Lymph Node Sarcomatosis with Autoimmune Hemolytic Anemia" [3]. These 14 patients all exhibited characteristic histologic alterations in their lymph nodes. At least one or two lymph node biopsy specimens were available for each patient.

Transcutaneous lymph node aspirates and/or imprints of biopsy specimens were available in every case for cytologic examination after staining with Giemsa's stain. Serial blood counts and at least one, and in most cases several, bone marrow aspirates were obtained. At least one bone marrow biopsy specimen was obtained in 12 patients. Other routinely performed laboratory tests included electrophoretic and immunoelectrophoretic study of serum proteins and Coombs' test. In all 14 patients, these investigations were performed before therapy and particularly before therapy with prednisone (except for patient 6 who had been on low-dose prednisone for several years because of chronic rheumatic disease). These biologic tests were routinely performed before and after therapy as well as during the course of the disease. Other routine investigations performed included tests for antitissue antibodies (stomach, thyroid, smooth muscle), antinuclear antibodies, antimitochondrial antibodies, rheumatoid factor, and serologic tests for toxoplasmosis, infectious mononucleosis, and syphilis. Immunofluorescence studies were performed on fixed cells from lymph nodes, blood, or bone marrow in five patients.

Surface membrane Ig of viable cells were investigated in three patients. These studies were done by the immunofluorescence technique using five monospecific antisera: anti-μ, γ, α, κ, and λ [12]. Roentgenographic investigations included a standard chest film in 14 patients, a pedal lymphangiogram in seven patients, and a complete bone series in four patients.

Results

Clinical Observations

Age and Sex (Table 1)

This series includes five female and nine male patients. Their ages ranged from 31–80 years with a mean age of 60 years.

Onset of Disease and Clinical Picture

Symptoms were generally rapidly progressive, the interval between the first examination and initiation of therapy being 1–6 months (mean 2.5 months) (Table 7). Superficial lymph node enlargement was the most consistent clinical finding. These enlarged lymph nodes were initially restricted to a limited region in six patients (axillary in one case and cervical in five cases) (Table 7), while in five patients generalized lymphadenopathy was present at the time of initial examination. Spontaneously, the lymph nodes increased in size and spread, so that after variable periods of time all patients had superficial generalized lymphadenopathy (Tables 1 and 7). In most instances, this intumescence of lymphoid organs was attended from the onset by constitutional symptoms including fever, sweats, asthenia, and weight loss (Table 9).
Most patients exhibited highly variable cutaneous manifestations at some time during their clinical course (11 patients). These manifestations were either confined to pruritus (two cases) or characterized by an often pruritic maculopapular rash sometimes with signs of purpuric vasculitis. Joint pain was commonly encountered. The spontaneous course in all our patients was one of aggravation, sometimes interspersed with phases of relative improvement, but ultimately leading to a severely febrile disease with generalized superficial lymphadenopathy, involvement of deep lumbar nodes (7/7 abnormal lymphangiograms), splenomegaly in the majority of cases (11 patients), and constant hepatomegaly. In all cases, standard chest films ruled out the presence of mediastinal lymph nodes (Table 1). As a rule, cutaneous manifestations tended to get worse as the disease progressed or to appear secondarily if they were absent when the first enlarged lymph nodes were diagnosed. In three cases, they appeared to follow treatment with penicillin. In a fourth case, prescription of penicillin led to worsening of a preexisting rash. In two cases, skin nodules containing specific histologic infiltrates were documented.

Laboratory Investigations

Severe anemia (hemoglobin < 9 g/100 ml) was virtually a regular finding (13 cases) (Table 2) but was absent in approximately one case out of two at the time of the initial workup (Table 12). Anemia was aplastic with a low reticulocyte count and erythroblastopenia in five cases,

Table 1. Signs and symptoms

Case No.	Age (years)	Sex	Lymphadenopathies			Splenomegaly	Hepatomegaly	Skin manifestations	Hypersensitivity reaction
			Peripheral generalized	Positive lymphangiogram	Mediastinal adenopathy				
1	53	M	+ +		0	+	+ +	Maculopapular rash	0
2	60	F	+ +	+ +	0	+ +	+ +	Maculopapular rash	0
3	59	M	+ +	+ +	0	+	0	Purpuric vasculitis	0
4	57	M	+ +		0	0	+	Pruritus	0
5	57	M	+ +		0	+	+ +	Rash + purpuric vasculitis	0
6	72	M	+ +	+ +	0	0	+	Purpuric vasculitis	0
7	49	F	+ +		0	+	+ +	0	Penicillin
8	72	F	+ +	+ +	0	+	+	Rash + specific infiltrates	0
9	71	F	+ +		0	0	+	Rash + specific infiltrates	Penicillin
10	57	M	+ +	+ +	0	+	+ +	Maculopapular rash	0
11	80	F	+ +		0	+ +	+	0	0
12	47	M	+ +	+ +	0	+	+	0	0
13	71	M	+ +		0	+	+	Rash + purpuric vasculitis	Penicillin
14	31	M	+	+ +	0	+	+	Pruritus	0

Table 2. Laboratory findings (1) anemia

Case No.	Peripheral blood			Bone marrow aspiration erythroblasts (%)	Unconjugated bilirubin (mg/liter)	Plasma iron (γ/100 ml)	Direct Coombs' test	Cold agglutinins
	Hemoglobin[a] (g/100 ml)	RBC[a] (10^6/cmm)	Reticulocytes (%)					
1	5	2.2	0.2	1	15	140	+ IgG IgMC′	
2	6.5	1.5	10	35	25.5	145	+ IgG IgMC′	+
3	8.5	2.9	10	32	8.5	75	+ IgM C′	
4	5.5	1.7	0.1	3	10	125	+ C′	+1/64
5	9	2.5	6	53	10	140	+ IgG IgMC′	
6[b]	16	4.8	0.5	21	7	55	−	
7	8.5	2.5	10	62	10	100	+ IgG	
8	7.1	2.5	0.1	0–4	12	145	+ IgG	
9	6.8	2.1	0.1	12	10	80	−	+1/32
10	8.2	2.7	0.1	0–3	10	155	+ IgG	
11	7.7	2.8	0.1	15	8	55	+ C′	
12	3.6	1.2	6	49	16	65	+ IgG IgMC′	
13	6	1.6	11	49	76	155	+ IgG C′	
14	8.8	2.6	1.5	16	8	35	+ IgG C′	+1/256

[a] Lowest values before chemotherapy.
[b] Patient on prednisone therapy before first examination.

Table 3. Laboratory findings (2) WBC and platelets

Case No.	Peripheral blood		Bone marrow		Platelets (10^3/cmm)		Bone marrow aspiration megacaryocytes
	WBC/cmm	Plasma cell and/or immunoblasts (%)	Aspiration: plasma cells and/or immunoblasts (%)	Lymphoid cell aggregates on bone marrow biopsy	First examination	Lowest level before any treatment	
1	4000–10,000	2–7	3	+	150	100	Normal
2	4000–17,000	1–10	6–18	+	200	120	Normal
3	8000–20,000	3–10	7–10	+	200	55	Normal
4	7000–12,000	5–30	29	+	180	80	Decreased
5	2500–3,000	3–7	4–10	+	140	20	Normal
6	4000–5,000	2–10	2–4	+	240	40	Normal
7	5200–8,800	1–35	0	+	230	80	Normal
8	3400–10,300	0–12	3	0	300	70	Sparse
9	5500	13	1			80	Normal
10	6900–10,000	0	0		250	40	Nil
11	9800–15,000	5–13	22	+	240	45	Normal
12	9300–11,400	2–11	0	+	260	120	Normal
13	5000–10,800	0–2	2	+	350	25	Decreased
14	3300–9,400	4–11	13	0(?)	180	90	Decreased

Table 4. Laboratory findings (3) immunologic study

Case No.	Serum electrophoresis			Cryoglobulin	Antibodies			
	Total protein (g/l)	Serum albumin (g/l)	Gammaglobulin (g/l)		Anti-IgG	Antinuclear	Antimitochondria	Antismooth muscle
1	93	27.5	47.5	⊖	⊖	⊖	⊖	⊕
2	102	28	62.5	⊖	⊖	⊖	⊖	⊕
3	71	21.5	38.5	⊖	⊖	⊖	⊖	⊕
4	86	19	59	⊖	⊖	⊖	⊖	⊕
5	85	21	52	⊕	⊕	⊖	⊖	⊕
6	81	41.5	24	⊖	⊖	⊖	⊖	⊕
7	84	31.5	38[a]	⊖				⊕
8	84	24.5	55	⊖	⊖	⊖	⊖	
9	87	42	23	⊖	⊖	⊖	⊖	⊖
10	70	34	41[a]	⊖	⊖	⊖	⊖	⊕
11	83	16.5	61	⊖	⊖	⊖	⊖	⊕
12	70	28	40	⊖	⊖	⊖	⊖	⊕
13	70	27	30	⊖	⊖	⊖	⊖	⊕
14	60	29	16	⊖	⊖	⊖	⊖	⊕

[a] Monoclonal Ig appearing during clinical course (one case Bence Jones and one case IgG spike).

successively erythroblastopenic and hemolytic in one case, and hemolytic with a high reticulocyte count and bone marrow erythroblastosis in six cases.

Coombs' test, which was always performed at least once, was found to be positive in 12 patients. In two cases, the test was initially negative but became positive at the time of clinical aggravation prior to initiation of therapy (Table 12). Owing to the fact that Coombs' test was not done at the time of the initial workup in five patients, the test was initially positive in only five patients and negative in four. The platelet count was normal initially but always dropped in patients with advance disease prior to treatment (11 patients out of 14 with advanced disease had a platelet count of less than 100,000/mm^3) (Table 3).

The white blood cell count was highly variable from one patient to the next and even in a given patient at different times during the course of the disease (Table 3). The WBC count was often normal during the early phases, and sometimes there was mild hyperleukocytosis due to increased numbers of granulocytes with a few sparse atypical hyperbasophilic lymphoid cells (immunoblasts) and/or plasma cells (11 cases out of 14). These pleomorphic cells increased in number during the course of the disease to reach quite high levels in some patients (10%–30% in six cases), giving a WBC picture reminiscent of that seen in infectious mononucleosis. In addition to the previously mentioned alterations of the erythroblast and megacaryocyte series (Tables 2 and 3), bone marrow aspirates and biopsies showed variable but small numbers of hyperbasophilic lymphoid cells (immunoblasts) and/or plasma cells (10 cases).

The study of serum proteins (Table 5) by electrophoresis revealed hypergammaglobulinemia exceeding 20 g/l in 13 cases. Immunoelectrophoresis confirmed the polyclonal nature of this hyperglobulinemia, which was accompanied by hypoalbuminemia. These changes were sometimes absent at the time of the initial examination, often progressed rapidly in the space of a few weeks (Table 8), and were usually concomitant with clinical aggravation. All three classes of immunoglobulins were elevated, but the most marked rise was observed for IgG, peak levels of which ranged from 16–62.5 g/l with a mean peak level of 42 g/l (11 patients had an IgG level exceeding 30 g/l). The diffuse nature of hyperimmunoglobulinemia is suggestive of the polyclonal character of the plasma cell infiltration seen in lymph nodes, bone marrow,

Table 5. Survival and therapy

Case No.	Therapy	Survival from the first lymph node biopsy	Maintenance therapy	Follow-up		
				Remission	Relapse	Cause of death
1	MOPP (6 months)	78 months	Oncovin chlorambucil	Remission		Still alive
2	MOPP (3 months)	3 months		Improvement		Septicemia
3	MOPP (1 month)	1 month				Unknown
4	MOPP (6 months)	9 months		Remission	Relapse	Occlusion
5	MOPP (3 months)	4 months		Improvement		Unknown
6	MOPP (6 months)	58 months	Oncovin	Remission		Still alive
7	Velbe, thiotepa, Rufochromomycin bleomycin	29 months		Remission		Still alive
8	MOPP (1 month)	6 months		Improvement	Relapse after 1 month	Pulmonary infection
9	MOPP (4 months)	12 months	Chlorambucil	Remission	Relapse after 10 months	Severe herpes zoster
10	MOPP (1 month)	3 months		Improvement		Septicemia
11	MOPP (2 months)	3 months		Improvement		Renal failure
12	MOPP (6 months)	12 months	Chlorambucil	Improvement		Still alive
13	MOPP (15 days)	1 month				Septicemia
14	MOPP (8 months)	30 months	Chlorambucil	Remission	Relapse after 24 months	Infection

Table 6. Immunocytologic studies

Case No.	Tissues studied	Intracytoplasmic Ig (% nucleated cells)						Surface Ig %[a]						Aggregated IgG (%)[a]	E-rosettes (%)[a]
		δ	μ	γ	α	κ	λ	δ	μ	γ	α	κ	λ		
2	Bone marrow		4.4	13	7.7	14.6	9.5								
5	Bone marrow		<1	9	2	7	4								
9	Lymph node		<1	3	3	4	5		23	20	10	18	33	50	7
9	Blood[b]		10	40	17	38	27		[c]	[c]	[c]	[c]	[c]	72	3–6
11	Lymph node	0		20	3.5	15	8								50
12	Lymph node	0	7	19	4	18	9	1	12	12	2	14	11	25	29
Mean normal values	Blood[b]	Few positive cells (≤1% for all Ig classes)						8	11	4	2	12.5	4.5	18	70

[a] % on mononucleated cell.
[b] On mononuclear cell after Ficoll–Triosil separation.
[c] About 75% positive cells with all anti-Ig.

and peripheral blood. This polyclonal nature of the cell proliferation, or at least of part of the cell proliferation, was shown (Table 6) by an intracytoplasmic immunofluorescence study on fixed cells in five patients and by investigation of surface membrane Ig of viable cells in three of these. Tests for autoantibodies (Table 4) other than antierythrocyte antibodies (Table 2) were performed. Tests for rheumatoid factor proved to be negative, as did those for antinuclear, antimitochondrial, and antiorgan (stomach, thyroid) antibodies. In contrast, antismooth muscle antibodies were very often detected (11 cases).

Lymph Node Pathology and Cytology

Nodal architecture was diffusely obliterated by a pleomorphic cell proliferation (Fig. 1). The capsule and pericapsular region sometimes, but not consistently, showed infiltration. In most cases, the peripheral and medullary sinuses remained uninvolved and were visible. An abundance of neoformed small vessels of the caliber of postcapillary venules was consistently observed (Fig. 2) and these exhibited markedly hypertrophic endothelial cells. Cytologic examination on sections and particularly on imprints showed the highly pleomorphic nature of the cellular infiltrates, which contained a variable mixture of lymphocytes, mature plasma

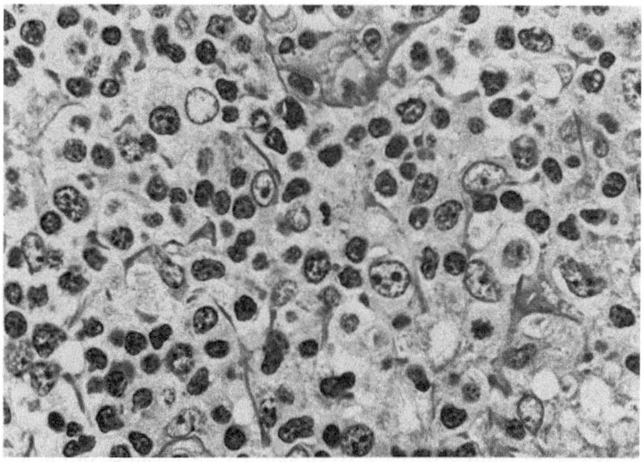

Fig. 1. Lymph node histology. Hematoxylin and eosin stain (× 63). Cellular pleomorphism of the infiltrate in which lymphocytes, immunoblasts, and mature plasma cells are evident

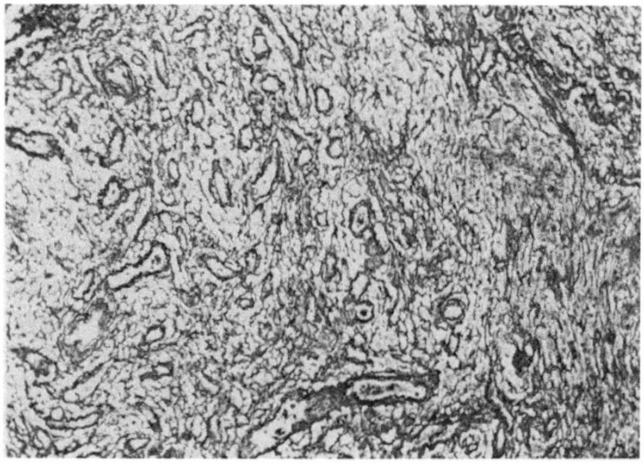

Fig. 2. Lymph node histology. Gomori's stain (× 25). Reticulin staining showing the marked degree of vascular proliferation

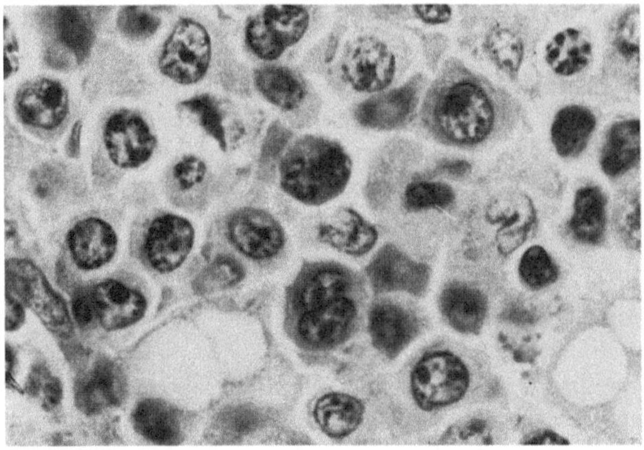

Fig. 3. Lymph node histology. Hematoxylin and eosin stain (× 100). High-power view of the pleomorphic cellular infiltrate: binucleated plasma cells and immunoblasts

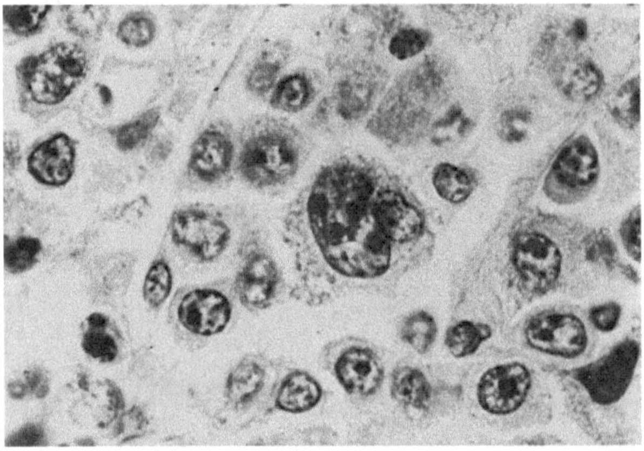

Fig. 4. Lymph node histology. Hematoxylin and eosin stain (× 100). Presence of large immunoblastic cells which differ from Sternberg-Reed cells by the absence of nucleolar abnormalities

cells, large, sometimes bi- or multinucleated plasma-like cells (Fig. 3), and immunoblasts. These immunoblasts were characterized by their large size, their young nucleus, and abundant and intensely basophilic cytoplasm. The intensity of this basophilia was absolutely remarkable in this disorder. The impression of a lack of clear-cut separation between these various cell types added to the characteristic pleomorphism of the lymph nodes. These distinctive features are particularly evident on imprints stained with Giemsa's stain and often go unnoticed on examination of sections if the appropriate staining techniques are not used.

Occasional large, sometimes multinucleated cells, may be seen. These are similar in size to Sternberg-Reed cells, but they differ from the latter by their intensely basophilic cytoplasm and by the absence of major nucleolar abnormalities (Fig. 4). Eosinophils may be seen in the infiltrates, but in our experience this was an inconsistent and minor finding.

In all our patients the lymphoid follicles virtually disappeared, the general appearance of the lymph node being mistakable for other types of malignant lymphomas on low-power views. In one case (patient 8), two successive biopsy specimens were taken. The first specimen showed a picture of nonspecific adenitis. Two months later, when immunoglobulin levels increased and Coombs' test became positive, the second biopsy specimen revealed the above-described abnormalities.

Table 7. Evolution before treatment

Case No.	Date	First symptoms	News signs and symptoms before treatment	Duration of disease before chemotherapy
1	Dec. 68	Localized ly. node (axillary)	Generalized ly. nodes, skin rash, fever	3 months
2	Jan. 69	Generalized ly. nodes	Fever, weight loss, increasing size of ly. node	6 months
3	Jun. 69	Generalized ly. nodes, weight loss, fever	Jaundice	1 month
4	Nov. 70	Asthenia, fever, joint pain, pruritus	Generalized ly. nodes	1 month
5	Jan. 71	Asthenia, weight loss	Generalized ly. nodes, hemolytic anemia	4 months
6	Dec. 71	Localized ly. node (submaxillary)	Generalized ly. nodes, fever, weight loss, skin rash	3 months
7	Feb. 73	Localized ly. node (cervical tonsillar)	Generalized ly. nodes	3 months
8	Jan. 73	Localized ly. node (cervical)	Generalized ly. nodes, specific skin infiltrates	5 months
9	Aug. 72	Localized ly. node, weight loss, fever, pruritus	Generalized ly. nodes, specific skin infiltrates	5 months
10	Feb. 73	Generalized ly. nodes, fever, hemolytic anemia		1 month
11	Aug. 74	Generalized ly. nodes, fever, weight loss		2 months
12	Feb. 75	Generalized ly. nodes, fever		1 month
13	Sept. 75	Generalized ly. nodes, fever, hemolytic anemia		1 month
14	Aug. 74	Joint pain, skin rash	Generalized ly. nodes	3 months

Course

Within the space of several months, or more often several weeks, all the symptoms gradually became more pronounced and the patients' condition regularly declined, sometimes with transient periods of minor improvement. Tables 7, 8, and 12 give a general idea of the clinical and biologic changes occurring before therapy and the rapidity of these changes.

Progressing anemia was usually the most striking manifestation of a declining clinical course and was accompanied by severe weight loss, the onset or accentuation of cutaneous manifestations, joint pain, oliguria, edema, and sometimes pleural and peritoneal effusion. Obnubilation, disturbances of consciousness, and a drop in blood pressure often added to the severity and alarming character of the clinical picture which raised fears of a fatal outcome. Owing to this rapid clinical course, all these patients had to be treated despite the uncertainty of the pathologic diagnosis in many cases. This diagnostic uncertainty accounted for the often long interval between the onset of symptoms and initiation of treatment (Table 7).

In a few cases, treatment with prednisone led to the disappearance of hemolysis, conversion of Coombs' test to negative, and an initial drop in elevated serum immunoglobulin levels (Table 8). However, prednisone alone never produced lasting clinical improvement and did not prevent renewed aggravation. All patients were treated with combined chemotherapy (MOPP—nitrogen mustard, vincristine, procarbazine, and prednisone in 13 cases out of 14) (Table 5). In all cases but one (a patient who died after 2 weeks), this regimen produced rapid clinical improvement with reduction in lymph node size, disappearance of fever, resumption of normal urinary output, and regression of edema. This clinical improvement was paralleled

Table 8. Evolution of biologic symptoms before treatment
Coombs' test

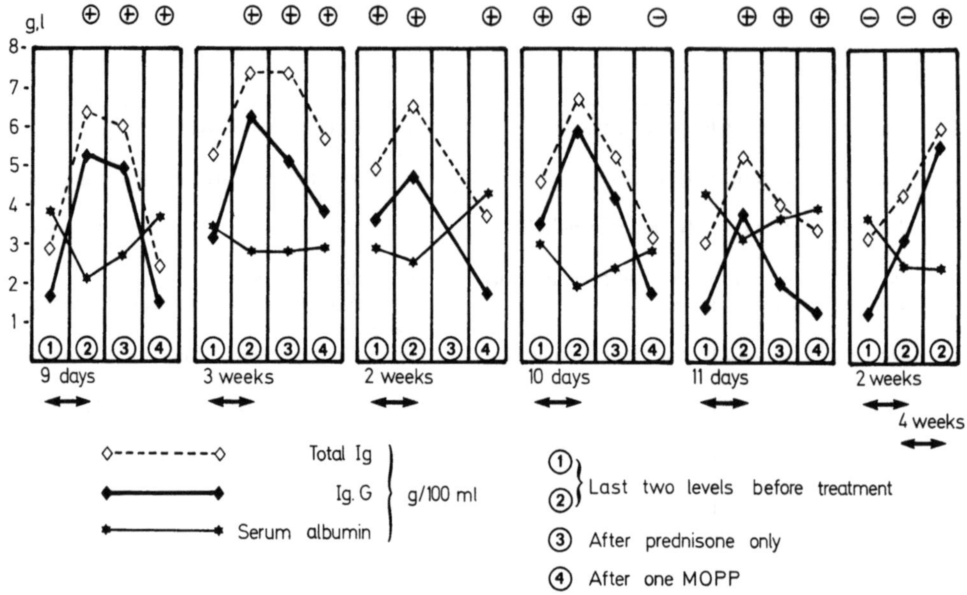

by the correction of biologic abnormalities with a very rapid return of serum protein levels to normal (Table 8), disappearance of hemolysis, and conversion of Coombs' test to negative. Leukocyte alterations disappeared very rapidly in all cases, whereas the increase in the platelet count often took longer, as did complete correction of anemia.

Four patients are still alive with a follow-up of 78, 58, 29, and 12 months (Table 5). Two patients died during a relapse after 12 and 9 months. One patient achieved a second remission after clinical and biologic relapse (hemolytic anemia and hyperimmunoglobulinemia) during the 24th month. This patient died at 30 months. The other patients showed only partial and transient improvement, survival being less than 4 months in four cases. Necropsy was performed in three patients and in one revealed multiple visceral involvement consistent with the diagnosis of sarcomatosis. In the other two cases, only the lymph nodes contained pleomorphic cellular infiltrates comparable to those observed on biopsy specimens. In one of these patients, the bone marrow was hypoplastic while in the other there was extensive myelofibrosis without abnormal cell infiltration.

Discussion

AILD represents a type of immunoproliferative syndrome remarkable because of its association with a distinctive clinical and biologic picture suggesting the presence of an immunologic reaction [9]. The 14 patients whose clinical course we followed from beginning to end clearly illustrate this since hypergammaglobulinemia exceeding 2 g/100 ml was present in 13 cases out of 14, Coombs-positive anemia in 12 cases, apparently immunologically related thrombocytopenia in 14 cases, and peripheral hyperbasophilic lymphoid cells in 13 cases. The incidence of this highly distinctive biologic syndrome appears to be considerably lower in the other major series published [6, 9, 11, 14] (Table 10). Our cases also differ from previously published series in other respects (Table 9), chiefly with regard to mediastinal lymph nodes, which we found to

Table 9. Signs and symptoms

	FRIZZERA et al. (1975) 24 cases	LUKES et al. (1975) 32 cases	MOORE et al. (1976) 14 cases	RADASZKIEWICZ et al. (1975) 50 cases	FLANDRIN (1976) 14 cases
Pruritus	9/24	6/19	2/14	25/38	11/14
Maculopapular rash	9/24	8/20	4/14	16/42	9/14
Sweats	17/24	9/12	6/14		14/14
Fever		13/22	8/14	33/45	14/14
Hypersensitivity reactions	8/24	2/22	3/14	10	3/14
Lymphadenopathy					
Generalized	24/14	21/29	9/14	47/50	14/14
Localized		8/29	5/14	3/50	
Abnormal lymphangiogram	3/3				7/7
Mediastinal adenopathy	9/24		1/14		0/14
Splenomegaly	17/24	11/16	8/14	26/44	11/14
Hepatomegaly	20/24	11/16	7/14	26/44	13/14
Dermal infiltrate	5				2
Bone marrow involvement	8	4/10	0/8	5/27	10/12

Table 10. Laboratory findings

	FRIZZERA et al. (1975) 24 cases	LUKES et al. (1975) 32 cases	MOORE et al. (1976) 14 cases	RADASZKIEWICZ et al. (1975) 50 cases	FLANDRIN (1975) 14 cases
● Anemia	13/24	7/19	8/14	29/40	13/14
● Severe anemia <30% HT	7/24				13/14
● Thrombopenia <100,000	2/22			8/33 (<125,000)	11/14
● Atypical lymphoid cells in the peripheral blood					13/14
● Positive Coombs' test	8/14	3/7	8/14	1/3	12/14
● Polyclonal hyperglobulinemia	17/22	13/14	4/10	18/38	13/14
● Monoclonal Ig	1/15	0	2/14		2/14

be absent but which have been reported to be common [6, 10, 11, 16, 18], as high as 9/24 in the series of FRIZZERA et al. [6].

An attempt to account for these differences is perhaps not devoid of interest. One of the factors underlying the different incidents of biologic alterations observed is possibly the moment at which the investigations were performed, as is suggested by our study on the changes in biologic abnormalities during the pretherapeutic course (Table 12). The rather long period of observation prior to initiation of therapy (2.5 months on the average in our cases; Table 7) may have allowed more time for the distinctive biologic picture to appear in these patients. This may also account for our impression of a more severe clinical picture when treatment is initiated. Differences in the clinical picture, and particularly the presence of mediastinal lymph nodes in certain series and their absence in others, can only be accounted for by differences in patient recruitment. The explanation undoubtedly lies in the histologic criteria considered for the diagnosis of AILD. The diffuse obliteration of nodal architecture, which we considered a fundamental diagnostic feature in our patients and which is stated as a requirement in the

Table 11. Age, sex, therapy, and survival

	Frizzera et al. (1975) 24 cases	Lukes et al. (1975) 32 cases	Moore et al. (1975) 14 cases	Radaszkiewicz et al. (1975) 50 cases	Flandrin (1975) 14 cases
● Age (years)					
Range	44–80	28–92	45–81	21–84	31–80
Mean	68	57	64	59	60
● Sex					
M	10	19	7	23	9
F	14	13	7	27	5
● Survival, dead patients (months)	16 cases	18 cases	10 cases	18 cases	10 cases
Range	1–45	6–192	2–60	1–42	1–30
Mean		15	19		7
● Survival, living patients (months)	8 cases	10 cases	3 cases	23 cases	4 cases
Range	24–67	6–72	15–84	2–60	12–78
Mean	37	13	53		44
● Therapy (No. of cases)					
With chemotherapy	16	"Usually treated"	14	20	14
Without chemotherapy	8		0		0

Table 12. Comparison of signs and symptoms between first examination and last examination before treatment

Flandrin (14 patients)	Signs and symptoms	
	At first examination	At last examination before chemotherapy
● Lymphadenopathies		
Generalized	5	14
Localized	6	0
● Splenomegaly	7	11
● Skin manifestations	7	9
● Severe anemia (<30% HT)	7	13
● Thrombocytopenia (<100,000/cmm)	0	11
● Positive Coombs' test	5[a]	12
● Polyclonal hyperglobulinemia (IgG>20 g/liter)	9	13

[a] Coombs' test not done at first examination in 5 patients.

definition of this disease [4, 5, 6, 14], does not appear to be complete in certain series. In the series reported by Frizzera et al. [6], the persistence of altered "burnt out" lymphoid follicles is common (11 cases out of 24), as is the apparent presence of an epithelioid granuloma [6, 14]. It is very likely that these differences in recruitment account for the different opinions as to the severity of the spontaneous course of this disorder and the indications for chemotherapy. No sufficiently clear-cut correlation between prognosis and any distinctive histologic feature has emerged from the detailed histologic study performed by Frizzera et al. [6] to indicate a well-defined choice of management.

In our experience, active treatment appeared to be the only way of influencing an unrelenting course. Despite the reservations expressed about cytotoxic chemotherapy, it appears to have been used frequently in all the series published in the literature (Table 11). Although steroids do exert a certain degree of efficacy, used alone they have not enabled us to achieve complete eradication of symptoms and lymphadenopathy, whereas this has been possible in most cases with combined chemotherapy.

The theoretic discussion as to the "malignant" character of AILD should not be confused with the study of its clinical activity. From a histologic standpoint, as has been pointed out by FRIZZERA et al. [6], despite the loss of normal lymph node morphology, neither marked cellular pleomorphism nor abundant vasculature is a usual finding in malignant lymphomas. The same may be said for the polyclonal nature of the B-lymphoid cells found in lymph nodes, peripheral blood, and bone marrow which has been demonstrated in this study. Indeed, all known malignant B-lymphoid cell proliferations are monoclonal. This is the case for example for the majority of malignant lymphomas and for macroglobulinemia, despite the marked cytologic pleomorphism of the latter. As further evidence against the malignant nature of this disease, FRIZZERA et al. [6] drew attention to the absence of tumor masses in extralymphatic organs at autopsy. During the course of the disease, however, these classic features of nonmalignancy may change. In two of our cases, a monoclonal protein appeared secondarily, a finding also reported by other authors [1, 6, 8, 11, 13, 17, 19], and in three cases reported by LUKES and TINDLE [9] as well as in one of our cases, malignant lymphoma-like tumor masses were found at autopsy. The chromosomal abnormalities observed in two cases by HOSSFELD et al. [7] may provide an argument in favor of malignancy.

In view of the fact that there is still considerable uncertainty as to the histologic diagnostic criteria of AILD, it is more than likely that somewhat disparate cases will be grouped under this new heading. It is for this reason that once the histologic diagnosis has been established, management should be based solely on the clinical and biologic course.

References

1. ABU-ZAHRA, H. T., MCDONALD, D. B., HORNE, W. I. Angio-Immunoblastic Lymphadenopathy with dysproteinemia. Lancet, 1975, *1*, 114.
2. DORFMAN, R. F., WARNKE, R. Lymphadenopathy simulating the malignant lymphomas. Human Pathol. 1974, *5*, 519–550.
3. FLANDRIN, G., DANIEL, M. Y., EL YAFI, G., CHELLOUL, N. Sarcomatoses ganglionnaires diffuses à différenciation plasmocytaires, avec anémie hémolytique auto-immune—I—. Actual. Hematol. 1972, *6*, 25–41.
4. FLANDRIN, G. Adénopathies angio-immunoblastiques avec anémie auto-immune et hyperimmunoglobulinémie polyclonale. Nouv. Pres. Med. 1976, *5*, 1521–1524.
5. FRIZZERA, G., MORAN, E. M., RAPPAPORT, H. Angio-Immunoblastic Lymphadenopathy with dysproteinemia. Lancet, 1974, *1*, 1070–1073.
6. FRIZZERA, G., MORAN, E. M., RAPPAPORT, H. Angio-Immunoblastic Lymphadenopathy—Diagnosis and clinical course. Am. J. Med., 1975, *59*, 803.
7. HOSSFELD, D. K., HOFFKEN, K., SCHMIDT, C. G., DIEDRICHS, H. Chromosome abnormalities in Angio-Immunoblastic Lymphadenopathy. Lancet, 1976, *1*, 198.
8. LAPES, M. J., VIVACQUA, R. J., ANTONIADES, K. Immunoblastic Lymphadenopathy associated with Phenytoin (Diphenylhydantoin). Lancet, 1976, *1*, 198.
9. LUKES, R. J., TINDLE, B. H. Immunoblastic Lymphadenopathy—A hyperimmune entity resembling Hodgkin's disease. New. Engl. J. Med. 1975, *292*, 1–8.
10. MATHÉ, G., AMIEL, J. L., GERARD-MARCHANT, R., CAILLOU, B., PICO, J. L., MACHOVER, D. Les adénopathies angio-immunoblastiques. Nouv. Press. Med., 1976, *5*, 1515–1519.
11. MOORE, S. B., HARRISON, E. G., WEILAND, L. H. Angio-Immunoblastic Lymphadenopathy. Mayo Clin. Proc., 1976, *51*, 273–280.
12. PREUD'HOMME, J. L. Sarcomatose ganglionnaire diffuse à différenciation plasmocytaire II—Etude immunologique. Actual. Hematol., 1972, *6*, 42–48.
13. PRUZANSKI, W., SUTTON, D. M. C., PANTALONY, D. Angio-Immunoblastic Lymphadenopathy: an immunochemical study. Clin. Immun. Immunoathol., 1976, *6*, 62–76.

14. RADASZKIEWICZ, T., LENNERT, K. Lymphogranulomatosis X. Klinischer Bild therapic und prognose. Deutsch Med. Wocheuschr., 1975, *100* (*21*), 1157–1163.
15. RAPPAPORT, H., MORAN, E. M. Angio-Immunoblastic Lymphadenopathy. New. Engl. J. Med., 1975, *292*, 42–43.
16. SCHOENGEN, O., FEYEN, H., HAFERKAMP, O., HEIMPEL, H., KUBANE, K. B. Immunoblastische lymphadenopathy—maligne neoplasie oder hyperimmunisatorische reaction? Klin. Wschr, 1977, *55*, 265–273.
17. TANGUN, Y., SARACBASI, Z., PECKCELEN, Y., INCEMAN, S. Angio-Immunoblastic Lymphadenopathy with dysproteinemia. Lancet, 1974, *1*, 1345.
18. THOMAS, M., MANDARD, J. C., TANGUY, A., LEMENAGER, J. F. Lymphadenopathie angio-immunoblastique avec dysprotéinemie. Nouv. Press. Med., 1976, *5*, 864–865.
19. TWOMEY, J. J. Angio-Immunoblastic Lymphadenopathy with dysproteinemia. Lancet, 1974, *1*, 1345.

Hydantoin-Induced Lymphadenopathies and Lymphomas

A. RAUSING

Hydantoin derivatives have been used as anticonvulsants since about 1940. Many reports of lymph node enlargement in patients taking hydantoin drugs have been reported. SALTZSTEIN and ACKERMAN reviewed about 80 cases in 1959 [4]. The lymph node enlargement generally appears in conjunction with other side-effects. The histologic lymph node picture has been described as follicular hyperplasia, so-called atypical hyperplasia (pseudolymphoma), or in recent years, as immunoblastic lymphadenopathy. The earlier reports generally stated that the lymph node enlargement disappeared soon after drug withdrawal, but more recently, many reports have appeared on malignant lymphomas of various types in patients taking hydantoins. Some attempts at assessing the frequency of malignant lymphomas in such patients have been made, e.g., by ANTHONY, who found ten times the normal frequency [1]. LI et al. reported a frequency of 1.6% after diphenylhydantoin therapy and suggested that a small excess risk exists [3]. Both series included both Hodgkin's and non-Hodgkin's lymphomas. CLEMMESEN et al. failed to confirm an increased frequency among epileptics examined retrospectively in the Danish Cancer Registry [2].

A speculative cause of lymphoma development in these patients is the immunosuppressive effect of hydantoins found by, e.g., SORRELL et al., who reported depression of various parameters of cellular and/or humoral immune responses in a high frequency in patients taking diphenylhydantoin [5]. Carbamazepine, a nonhydantoin anticonvulsant, was found to have a similar effect.

In order to assess the frequency of lymph node complications with anticonvulsant therapy, an inquiry was performed at the Swedish Adverse Drug Reaction Committee. From 1967 to the middle of 1977, nine cases had been notified, three on diphenylhydantoin, three on mephenetoin, and three on carbamazepine (courtesy of Dr. G. BOMAN). Sweden had about 8,000,000 inhabitants during this period, and the frequency of epilepsy in the general population is about 0.5%. It thus appears as if lymph node enlargement in patients taking

Table 1. Number of patients with some types of malignant lymphomas treated with anticonvulsant drugs

Diagnosis	No. of patients with adequate clinical records	No. of patients treated	Drug	
Well-differentiated lymphocytic	115	1 (lymphoplasmacytic)	Diphenyl-hydantoin	
Histiocytic (immunoblastic)	191	3 (1.6%)	Diphenyl-hydantoin	1
			Mephenetoin	1
			Carbamazepine	1
1+2	306	4 (1.3%)		
Hodgkin's disease, all types	145	0 (one of the cases in group 2 also had lesions similar to Hodgkin's disease)		
1+2+3	451	4 (0.9%)		

anticonvulsants is rare. Çarbamazepine has not previously been reported as a cause of lymph node enlargement, but in view of its immunosuppressive effect similar to that of hydantoins such a reaction may well exist.

To study the frequency of malignant lymphomas in patients taking anticonvulsants of different kinds, an examination of the clinical records of patients histologically diagnosed as having Hodgkin's disease, malignant lymphoma of well-differentiated lymphocytic type (including chronic lymphatic leukemia), and malignant lymphoma of histiocytic (immunoblastic) type was undertaken in the Institute of Pathology, Malmö, Sweden. The results are shown in Table 1. The frequencies observed are not high, still there is a suggestion of a true increased risk, especially in the histiocytic (immunoblastic) group. It is suggested that carbamazepine may be associated with a small risk of lymph node lesions similar to those induced by hydantoin drugs, and patients treated with these drugs should be examined for such complications, benign or malignant.

References

1. ANTHONY, J. J.: Malignant lymphoma associated with hydantoin drugs. Arch. Neurol. *22*, 450–454 (1970).
2. CLEMMESEN, J., FUGLSANG-FREDERIKSEN, V., PLUM, C. M.: Are anticonvulsants oncogenic? Lancet *i*, 705–707 (1974).
3. LI, F. P., WILLARD, D. R., GOODMAN, R., VAWTER, G.: Malignant lymphoma after diphenylhydantoin (Dilantin) therapy. Cancer *36*, 1359–1362 (1975).
4. SALTZSTEIN, S. L., ACKERMAN, L. V.: Lymphadenopathy induced by anticonvulsant drugs and mimicking clinically and pathologically malignant lymphomas. Cancer *12*, 164–182 (1959).
5. SORRELL, T. C., FORBES, I. J.: Depression of immune competence by phenytoin and carbamazepine. Clin. Exp. Immunol. *20*, 273–285 (1975).

Hydantoin-Induced Lymphadenopathies and Lymphomas: Experimental Studies in Mice

G. R. F. KRUEGER and V. A. BEDOYA

As summarized by RAUSING in this volume [12], diphenylhydantoin (DPH) induces various kinds and degrees of lymphadenopathy in man and animals. Some of these changes were interpreted as hypersensitivity reactions [9] since they were accompanied by marked eosinophilia, dermatitis, and focal necroses in lymphatic tissues and bone marrow. Others were thought to be of true neoplastic nature representing in part Hodgkin's lymphoma [1, 2, 5, 12]. Searching for a model to induce Hodgkin's disease in animals we undertook a number of experiments in which we administered DPH to mice. We did not obtain Hodgkin's lymphomas in any of the experiments, yet we observed an enhanced incidence of other types of lymphomas [6, 7, 8]. The present paper reviews our results from these studies.

Materials and Methods

Female 2-months-old mice of three different strains were used: C3Hf, which are essentially resistant to lymphoma development, C57Bl, which are not resistant but show a low spontaneous incidence of lymphomas and leukemias, and SJL/J, which exhibit a high spontaneous incidence of malignant lymphomas. C3Hf and C57Bl mice were obtained from the animal production facilities of the National Institutes of Health, United States, and SJL/J mice were purchased from the Jackson Laboratory, Bar Harbor, Maine. All animals were caged in groups of six and kept on the liquid diet Metrecal, Dutch chocolate flavor, as available for humans. It had to be supplemented with folic acid (Lederle, Folvite, 0.75 mg/100 ml Metrecal) to avoid folic acid deficiency in mice. DPH (Dilantin Steri-Vials, Parke & Davis, 100 mg/2 ml) was administered at 6 mg/100 g mouse with a daily liquid consumption of 12 ml per mouse (maximum tolerated dose: 4.4 mg/10 mg mouse). The actual DPH intake being measured was between 3.84 and 4.88 mg/100 g mouse, the total uptake per mouse varied between 162.24 and 415.7 mg and largely depended upon the survival time of the animal. Control mice received Metrecal with folic acid only or were kept on the usual Purina lab chow pellets. Tap water was given to all mice ad libitum.

Complete autopsies were done at regular 8-week intervals starting 6 weeks after initiation of the experiment. Routine histology techniques were applied, including fixation in Zenker's or Carnoy's solution and staining with hematoxylin and eosin, PAS, Giemsa, methyl green pyronine Y, Masson's trichrome, and Wilder's reticulin reaction. Selected specimens were fixed in 3% glutaraldehyde solution in Sorensen's buffer, postfixed with osmium tetroxide, and embedded in Epon. Ultrathin sectioning was done on a LKB Ultrotome and microscopy with a ZEISS EM 9S-2 with 60 kv accelerating voltage.

For cytochemical characterization of tumor cells, the following reactions were carried out: PAS, Sudan black B, nonspecific esterase, peroxidase, alkaline, and acid phosphatase. T- and B-cell characteristics of lymphoma cells were determined by immunofluorescence, using monospecific antisera to mouse IgG1, IgG2, IgM, IgA, and θ (for methods see 10). From tissues grossly suggestive of tumor, 1 mm^3 particles were transplanted subcutaneously into isogeneic young mice. Tumor tissue was also explanted in medium 1640 with 15% fetal calf serum, 20 mM Hepes buffer, penicillin, and streptomycin for tissue culture (media from Flow Laboratories, Rockville, United States and Bonn, Germany).

Results

The results are summarized in Table 1. The histologic tumor type of the C57BI lymphomas and of the 25% early SJL/J lymphomas was consistent with a typical thymic lymphoma of the mouse, i.e., a malignant lymphoma, lymphoblastic cell type. Tumor cells were occasionally slightly positive for acid phosphatase but negative for all other enzymes tested. No T- or B-cell markers were demonstrated. The lymphomas of SJL/J mice occurring at 6–8 months and later, both in experimental and in control mice, were reticulum cell sarcomas type B of Dunn [3]. Immunocytologically, these tumors were B-cell lynphomas with numerous plasma cells (type immunocytoma-immunoblastoma). The lymphoblastic lymphoma originated in the thymus with subsequent spread to other tissues (Fig. 1), while the type-B reticulum cell sarcoma appeared to develop in the spleen (Fig. 2). The histologic tumor diagnosis was confirmed by isotransplantation. Lymphoblastic lymphomas grew on transplantation in 80% of the cases with a latent period of 1–4 months, while type-B reticulum cell sarcomas grew in only 10% of cases with latent periods of 6–8 months. Thymic lymphomas were readily carried on in tissue culture, but type-B reticulum cell sarcomas were not.

It is of interest to mention that none of the lymphomas observed started in salivary or

Table 1. Hyperplastic and neoplastic changes in lymphoid tissues of mice with DPH treatment

Mice	No.	Treatment	Neoplasia	Latent period	Reactive changes	Latent period
C3Hf	60	DPH—Metrecal	0%		Thymic atrophy Paracortical atrophy Diffuse reticulo-histiocytosis	Begin 4–6 weeks
	60	Metrecal—control	0%		Sinus histiocytosis	
	60	Purina—control	0%		Follic hyperplasia and secondary atrophy	
C57BI	60	DPH—Metrecal	Thymic lymphoma 12%	8 months	Same as for C3Hf mice In addition: thymic hyperplastic cortical nodules	2–3 months
	60	Metrecal—control	Thymic lymphoma 4%	18 months		
	60	Purina—control				
SJL/J	60	DPH—Metrecal	Thymic lymphoma 25% Type-B RCS 75%	4–8 months 6–8 months	Same as for C3Hf mice with thymic hyperplastic cortical nodules	2–3 months
	60	Metrecal—control	Type-B RCS 85%	8–12 months		
	60	Purina—control	Type-B RCS 85%	8–12 months		

DPH: diphenylhydantoin; RCS: reticulum cell sarcoma.

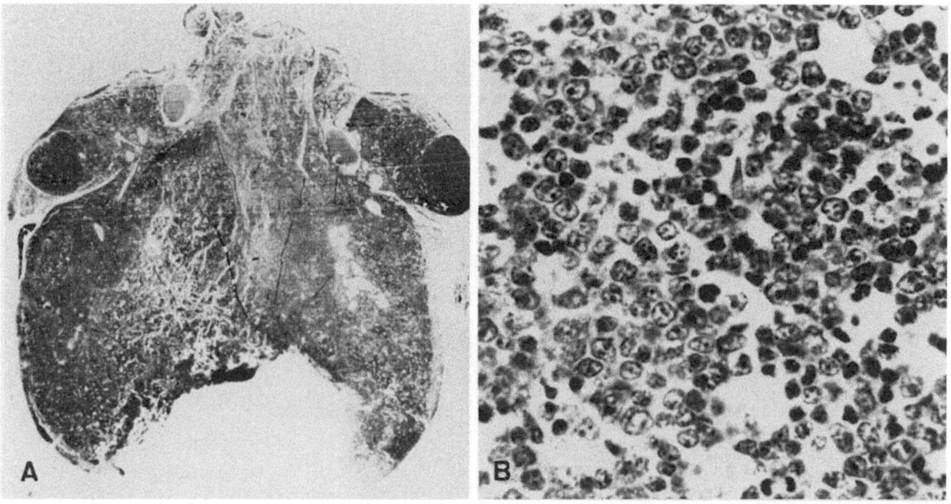

Fig. 1. Thymic lymphoma in SJL/J mouse after 4 months of DPH feeding. A: Cytology showing diffuse lymphoblastic population. Hematoxylin and eosin stains. (× 8). B: Hematoxylin and eosin stains. (× 600)

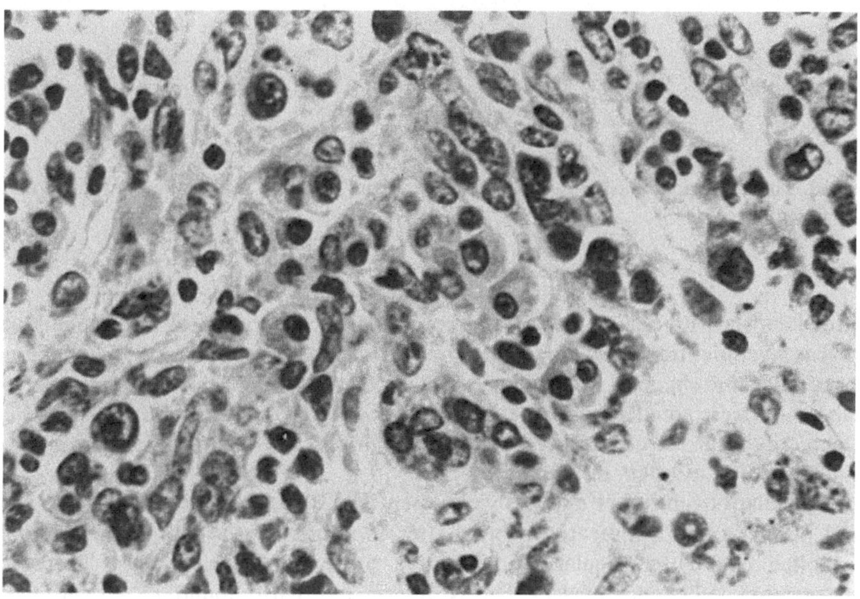

Fig. 2. Splenic type-B reticulum cell sarcoma in a SJL/J control mouse. Hematoxylin and eosin stains. (× 600)

mesenteric lymph nodes, i.e., in the lymphatic tissues which showed the most extensive nonmalignant lesions after DPH administration (the drug is probably more concentrated in these regions secondary to a secretion-reabsorption process).

By electron microscopy, thymic lymphomas were seen to be composed of lymphoblasts and small lymphocytes, dark elongated reticular cells, histiocytes, and occasional plasma cells. Predominating, however, was the lymphoblast. These cells exhibited several abnormalities such as widening of the perinuclear cisterna, dilatation of endoplasmic reticulum, and

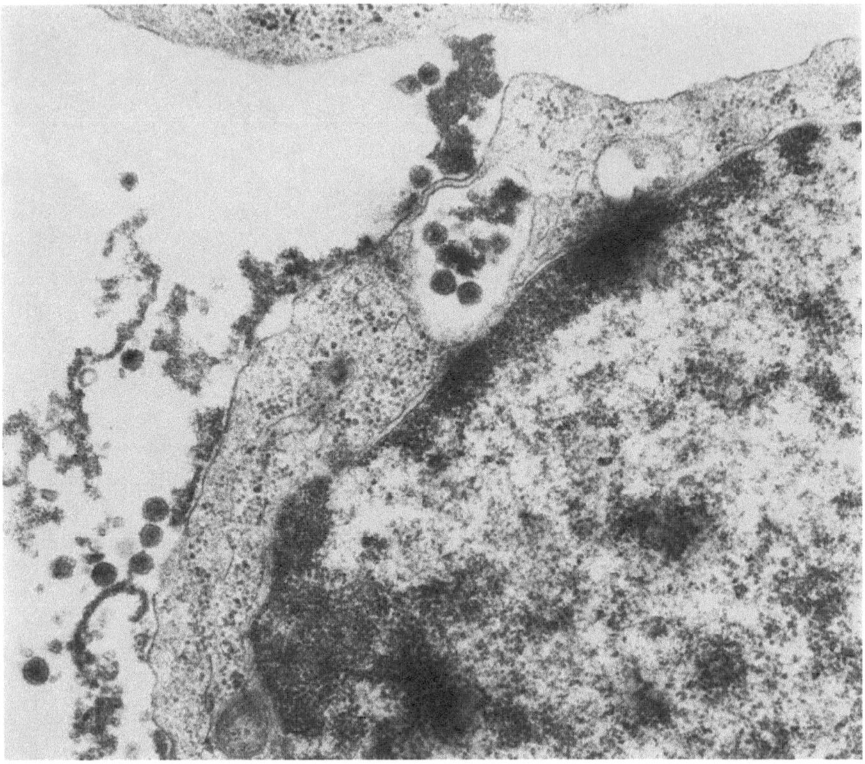

Fig. 3. Thymic lymphoblast with type-C particles from a thymic lymphoma of a C57BI mouse on DPH treatment. (× 21,000)

mitochondria with loss of cristae and occasional incorporation of ribosome-like material as well as myelinic structures. No C-type viral particles were seen intracellularly nor virus-related cytopathogenic changes. In addition, small vesicles and closely arranged granular cytoplasmic substances were noted which sometimes have been interpreted as viral in nature (Figs 3 and 4). Details of the ultrastructural investigations will be described in a separate paper (V. A. BEDOYA and G. R. F. KRUEGER, in preparation).

Cell populations in tumor cultures were essentially the same except that dense reticular cells and plasma cells disappeared shortly after initiation of the culture. Lymphoblasts often exhibited convoluted nuclei representative of thymus-derived cells. There were many degenerated cells and nuclear debris intermixed with abundant C-type particles. No intracytoplasmic C-type particles were observed.

Discussion

From our experimental results briefly outlined in this paper, we are tempted to draw the following conclusions: DPH is an effective drug for producing atrophic and reactive changes in immunocompetent tissues such as atrophy of the thymus and of thymus-dependent areas with coincident reticulohistiocytic hyperplasia. These lesions probably correspond to

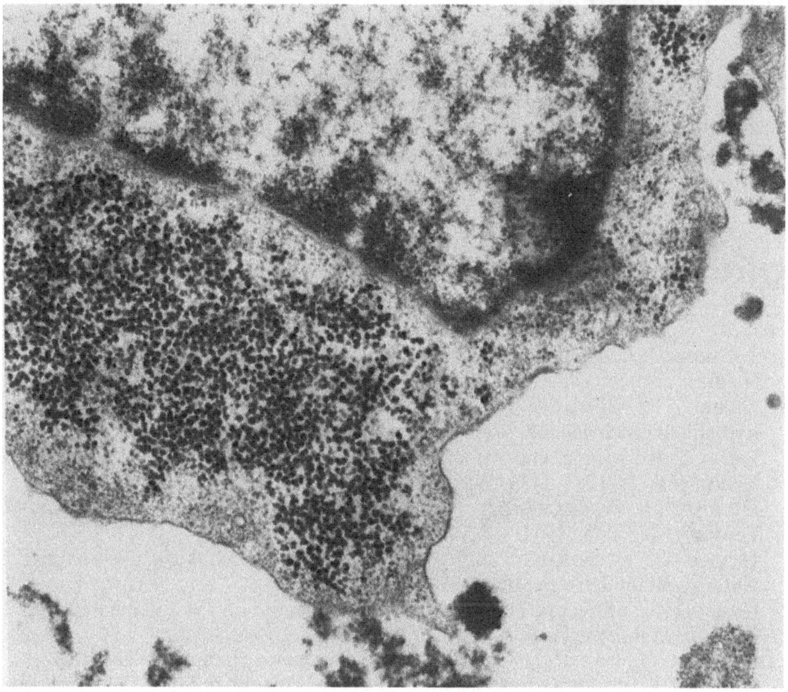

Fig. 4. Thymic lymphoblast with intracytoplasmic (virus-related?) inclusions from a thymic lymphoma of a C57Bl mouse on DPH treatment. (× 21,000)

disturbances in immune reactivity causing both a T-cell depression [8] and hypersensitivity reactions. The latter may be due to the hapteinic nature of DPH. Accordingly, in man, DPH allergies are reported [4, 13] as well as elevated serum γ-globulin and tissue histamine concentrations in patients on DPH therapy.

Reactive histologic changes after DPH administration are consequently observed quite regularly. Apart from this, there is some indication of an enhanced lymphoma development following prolonged DPH treatment in animals which are susceptible to such neoplasms. Susceptibility may be genetically determined, such as in SJL/J mice, as well as due to the presence of oncogenic viruses. All of our mice which did develop lymphomas after DPH therapy also harbored C-type particles. It thus appears to us that DPH acts rather as a kind of cocarcinogen rather than being carcinogenic per se.

It is of considerable interest that SJL/J mice, which are apparently genetically predetermined to develop type-B reticulum cell sarcomas, also developed typical thymic lymphomas at an early age when subjected to DPH treatment. The thymic lymphoma in mice is frequently observed in virus lymphoma induction [14]; it also differs immunocytologically from the common type-B reticulum cell sarcoma in SJL/J mice. We think the experiments in this mouse strain show two things: DPH, probably by turning on the action of oncogenic viruses, may lead to early thymic lymphomas in SJL/J mice; and secondly, by supporting or adding to the genetic predetermination, DPH also shortens the latent period of developing type-B reticulum cell sarcomas. The mechanism of DPH common to both pathogeneses is probably the disturbance of immune reactivity. More detailed investigations are necessary, however, to further elucidate such activities.

Acknowledgements

Part of the experiments reported in this study were done at the Laboratory of Pathology, National Cancer Institute, United States; current studies are supported by the German Science Foundation and by the Volkswagen Foundation.

References

1. ANTHONY, J. J.: Malignant Lymphoma Associated with Hydantoin Drugs. Arch. Neurol. *22*, 450–454 (1970).
2. CHAIRI, H.: Über das feingewebliche Bild der bei Mesantoinbehandlung zu beobachtende Lymphknotenschwellung. Wein. Klin. Wochenschr. *63*, 77–81 (1951).
3. DUNN, T. B.: Normal and Pathologic Anatomy of the Reticular Tissue in Laboratory Mice. J. Natl. Cancer Inst. *14*, 1281–1433 (1954).
4. GOODMAN, L. S., GILMAN, A.: The Pharmacological Basis of Therapeutics; 4th edition. London-Toronto: Macmillan 1971.
5. HYMAN, G. A., SOMMERS, S. C.: Development of Hodgkin's Disease and Lymphoma During Anticonvulsant Therapy. Blood *28*, 416–427 (1966).
6. KRUEGER, G.: Effect of Dilantin in Mice. I. Changes in the Lymphoreticular Tissues After Acute Exposure. Virchows Arch. A. Pathol. Anat. *349*, 297–311 (1970).
7. KRUEGER, G., HARRIS, D.: Is Phenytoin Carcinogenic? Lancet *I*, 323 (1972).
8. KRUEGER, G., HARRIS, D., SUSSMAN, E.: Effect of Dilantin in Mice. II. Lymphoreticular Tissue Atypia and Neoplasia After Chronic Exposure. Z. Krebsforsch. *78*, 290–302 (1972).
9. LENNERT, K.: Lymphknoten; Diagnostik in Schnitt und Ausstrich pp. 340–343. In: Handbuch der Speziellen Pathologischen Anatomie und Histologie. HENKE, F., LUBARSCH, O., RÖSSLE, R., UEHLINGER, E. (eds.), I/3A. Berlin-Göttingen-Heidelberg: Springer Verlag 1961, Vol. 1, 3A.
10. MERTENS, H., KRUEGER, G.: Percent Distribution of T- and B-Lymphoid Cells in Spleen and Lymph Nodes of Moloney Virus Infected Mice. Z. Krebsforsch. *85*, 169–175 (1976).
11. RAUSING, A.: Hydantoin-Induced Lymphadenopathies and Lymphomas. pp. 263–264 in this volume.
12. SALTZSTEIN, S. L., ACKERMAN, L. V.: Lymphadenopathy Induced by Anticonvulsant Drugs and Mimicking Clinically and Pathologically Malignant Lymphomas. Cancer *12*, 164–182 (1959).
13. VAN DER KWAST, W. A. M.: Speculations Regarding the Nature of Gingival Hyperplasia Due to Diphenyhydantoin-Sodium. Acta Med. Scand. *153*, 399–405 (1956).
14. KRUEGER, G.: Comparative Pathologic Classification of Malignant Lymphomas. Z. Krebsforsch. (in press).

Natural History of α-Chain Disease and the So-called Mediterranean Lymphoma

J. C. Rambaud, A. Galian, C. Matuchansky, F. Danon,
J. L. Preud'Homme, J. C. Brouet, and M. Seligmann

α-Chain disease (α-CD) is defined as a B-lymphoid cell proliferation involving first and foremost the IgA secretory system and producing a presumably homogeneous population of immunoglobulin molecules consisting of incomplete α-chains and devoid of light chains. It is the most frequent of the heavy chain diseases and, since its initial description in 1968 [15, 26], more than 120 cases have been recognized to our knowledge. All these patients, except three who showed an involvement of the respiratory tract, were affected with the digestive form of α-CD which is mainly located in the small intestine and the mesenteric lymph nodes.

In all cases of α-CD so far recognized, the abnormal IgA (α-CP) was present in the serum, often at a low concentration [28]. However, immunofluorescence and in vitro biosynthetic studies of the proliferating cells may lead in the future to the discovery of a "nonsecreting" form of the disease [28] among the so-called Mediterranean lymphomas with a clinicopathologic pattern identical to that of α-CD [23] but without detectable α-CP in the serum and jejunal juice [11]. The definite demonstration of the presumed monoclonal character of α-CP is still needed. The fact that all α-CP so far studied belonged to one IgA subclass only, i.e., IgA_1 [28], the finding of a single aminoacid substitution in position 12 of the protein of patient DEF [30], as well as the results of structural studies of several γ-CD proteins, strongly suggest that α-CP are in fact monoclonal. However, an essential criterion of monoclonality, i.e., the structural homogeneity of the variable region of these proteins, has not yet been demonstrated [27]. This heterogeneity of the N-terminal sequence could be due to a secondary limited proteolysis obscuring a primary internal deletion of the α-chain [27]. The usual failure of light chain synthesis in α-CD could be due to a defective translation and not to an absence of transcription. This hypothesis is supported by the finding of membrane-bound κ-light chains in a case of a α-CD (unpublished data) and of an inactive light chain messenger RNA in the cells of a nonsecretory variant of a mouse myeloma which contained an abnormally short heavy chain and failed to synthesize light chains [4]. The search for the presence of such a messenger in α-CD proliferating cells is needed and the determination of its structure could help in the demonstration of the monoclonal character of α-CP.

The clinical pattern of α-CD in its digestive form is remarkably uniform [19]. It mainly consists of a severe malabsorption syndrome which is usually associated with abdominal pains and often proceeds as exacerbations separated by more or less complete improvements. Chronic small bowel obstruction or abdominal surgical emergencies may sometimes reveal the disease, and abdominal masses may be present. But these "tumoral" signs are more often observed in the late stages of the evolution.

Pathological lesions may be classified in three stages [7]. At stage A there is a diffuse infiltration by plasma cells of the whole length of the small intestinal (or at least duodenojejunal) lamina propria. Plasma cells also infiltrate peripancreatic and mesenteric lymph nodes. At stage B the small intestinal proliferation extends in some areas to deep submucosa, or even to muscularis propria, and encompasses numerous atypical plasma cells and some large cells with cytologic and ultrastructural features of immunoblasts. The same pleiomorphic infiltrate obliterates the mesenteric lymph node architecture. At stage C an overt immunoblastic sarcoma is found in the gut and/or mesenteric lymph nodes. Pathologic involvement of extra enteromesenteric lymphoid tissue and bone marrow is a rare event, especially in the absence of intestinal or mesenteric lymph node sarcoma.

In some patients who have been repeatedly studied, the lesions progressed in a given site from the A to B, and/or from the B to C stages. The reverse evolution has never been observed [7]. However, it must be emphasized that lesions belonging to different stages may be present at the same time in different organs or even in different sites in the same organ. Moreover, a purely plasmacytic infiltration of peripheral lymph nodes may appear while entero mesenteric lesions have already reached the stage of immunoblastic sarcoma [3]. Thus, the accurate pathologic staging of α-CD requires a laparatomy with multiple samplings.

Patients with such an initial staging and with adequate long-term follow-up are still scarce. However, available data shed some light on the evolution of the disease [7]. Complete and prolonged clinical, histologic, and immunologic remissions have been obtained only in cases with stage-A lesions. Some of these patients were treated with antimitotic drugs, such as chlorambucil [10] and cyclophosphamide associated with prednisone and tetracycline [12], but at least four of them received exclusively oral antibiotics [13, 18, 20, 24]. In some other patients who underwent similar treatments, lesions apparently belonging to stage A at peroral biopsy progressed to stage B or C [7]. Since no laparotomy was performed in these patients, it is possible that lesions of stage B or C were already present at the onset of treatment. Among patients with known stage-B or -C lesions, only a few, treated by total abdominal irradiation and/or combination chemotherapy, showed clinical and sometimes immunologic and histologic remissions or improvements. Most died either from cachexia and infections or from acute surgical complications [7].

Morphologic and immunologic studies provide strongly suggestive evidence that the immunoblastic lymphomatous cells which may arise in the late course of α-CD are derived from the same clone as the initial plasma cell proliferation. Morphologically, both types of proliferation are sometimes intimately intermingled in the lymph nodes and in the gut [1]. Even when they form circumscribed tumors, immunoblastic cells are often also scattered in the persisting diffuse small intestinal or lymph node plasmacytic infiltration [7]. All transitional forms between the large immunoblastic cells and the mature plasma cells are usually found by optical and electron microscopy [7].

Immunofluorescence studies have regularly failed to show intracytoplasmic α-CP in the most undifferentiated and sometimes monstrous cells [1, 7], and α-CP can no longer be detected in the serum as the sarcoma develops [29]. However, α-chains have been identified by immunoelectron microscopy in the perinuclear cisternae of immunoblastic cells present in the bone marrow of one patient (F. Reyes, unpublished data). Membranes of immunoblastic cells forming intestinal circumscribed tumors have been found to bear α-chains and no light chains in three other patients [2, 21, and unpublished data]. In two of these, in vitro biosynthetic studies showed that these cells actually synthesized the α-CP [21, unpublished data].

Provided α-CP are definitely shown to be monoclonal, these recent data support the single clonal origin of the immunoblastic lymphomas and the preceding plasmacytic proliferations. In contrast, the benign or malignant nature of the latter is still open to question. The hypothesis of a benign process seems unlikely in those patients with very high and sometimes rising levels of the pathologic protein if its monoclonal nature is confirmed. Likewise, malignancy cannot be doubted when the plasma cell proliferation shows numerous atypical forms, destroys the mucosal crypts, penetrates deeply into the mucosa and sometimes muscularis propria, completely disorganizes the mesenteric lymph node architecture, and invades the pericapsular fat. However, in our and others' experience [with the possible exception of the patient of Guardia et al. [8]], this invasive cellular proliferation is no longer purely plasmacytic but encompasses more or less numerous and atypical immunoblasts and thus belongs to stage B, which is probably the early phase of the immunoblastic sarcoma development [7]. The possibility of an early benign stage of α-CD may be advocated when the cellular proliferation consists mainly of mature plasma cells, is limited to small intestinal lamina propria and to mesenteric lymph nodes and, overall, when complete and prolonged remissions are achieved with oral antibiotic treatment alone. It is noteworthy that in the three published cases with such remissions [13, 18, 24], the initial serum level of the α-CP was relatively low. Each of these features arguing in favor of a possible benign process deserves discussion.

The cytologic characteristics of the plasmacytic proliferation have been usually poorly described. In the cases we have studied [7], including a patient who responded to oral antibiotics [18], some plasma cells showed a central nucleus with a large nucleolus, contrasting with a well-developed rough endoplasmic reticulum. This asynchronism between nucleus and cytoplasmic maturation is usually considered as a dystrophic feature but does not constitute a sufficient criterion of malignancy. Karyotyping of plasma cells of the intestinal or lymph node infiltrate could provide useful information [23], but it is a difficult task owing to the scarcity of mitoses in fresh or cultured material.

In small intestinal lamina propria and mesenteric nodes, the plasmacytic proliferation nearly always disorganizes the normal architecture, although to a variable degree [7]. This is not observed in usual diffuse hyperplastic lymphoplasmacytic infiltrations of the lamina propria or in merely reactive lymph nodes. Even in a patient who responded to antibiotics alone [18], a limited extension of the cellular infiltration to the superficial part of the submucosa was present. Conversely, a remote spread of the plasmacytic proliferation out of the small intestinal and mesenteric lymph node areas does not necessarily militate for malignancy in view of the normal traffic of gut-associated lymphoid cells [14]. This particularly applies to the involvement of other sites of the IgA secretory system such as postnasal space, stomach, colon, and rectum, and probably also to their satellite lymph nodes. Indeed, in two patients, a gastric lamina propria [18] and a postnasal plasmacytic infiltration [25] disappeared during oral antibiotic therapy. Even an abnormal pattern of retroperitoneal lymph nodes at lymphangiography does not preclude an antibiotic-induced remission [18].

The initial serum level of α-CP is of limited significance. Indeed, there appears to be no clear relationship between the serum level of α-CP and the extension and density of the plasmacytic proliferation in the small intestinal lamina propria. This could be explained by variations in the rate of secretion of α-CP by the proliferating cells and by their belonging to the mucosal secretory system. A better correlation could be observed between the cellular mass of the abnormal clone and the level of α-CP in the intestinal fluid.

Finally, complete clinical, histologic, and immunologic remissions induced by oral antibiotics alone and lasting for several years (up to 7 years in one patient) after antibiotic withdrawal provide the strongest suggestive evidence of the benign nature of α-CD in its early stage. However, the four patients with well-documented remissions received tetracyline, either alone or in combination with other antibiotics, and a possible "nonantibiotic" effect of this drug on the plasmacytic proliferation cannot be completely ruled out. Moreover, even a "true antibiotic" mechanism of action may not completely exclude the possibility of a low-grade malignancy, the persistence of which would necessitate a continous local bacterial antigenic stimulation.

Besides these antibiotic-induced remissions, the geographic origin of the patients strongly suggests the role of such a protracted antigenic stimulation in the pathogenesis of α-CD. Although early reports on the digestive form of the disease mainly concerned patients of Mediterranean and Middle East origins, cases have now been observed in many parts of the world [28]. One factor common to these patients of various racial or ethnic origins is their exposure to an environment of poor hygiene in areas with a high degree of infections by intestinal pathogenes [28]. Studies conducted on some populations at risk have shown that chronic gastrointestinal infections and diarrheas are frequent, and serial intestinal biopsies have shown an increased lymphoid infiltration of the small bowel lamina propria [6]. Since orally ingested microorganisms are known to be a powerful proliferation stimulus to the secretory IgA-producing cells [14], the early phase of α-CD could represent an aberrant humoral immune response to such a sustained local stimulation. It is remarkable that this antigenic challenge leads preferentially to heavy chain disease rather than to plasmacytoma producing complete monoclonal IgA molecules. Whether this is due to the nature of the triggered cells or to that of the triggering agent remains a matter for speculation.

Intraluminal bacterial overgrowth and diverse parasitic infestations of the small intestine have been documented in α-CD [19], but up to now, no specific agent has been found by the limited number of bacteriologic, parasitic, and virologic studies which have been performed. However, the postulated specific agent may have initiated the disease many years before its clinical onset and may be absent in an identifiable form at the time of diagnosis. Indeed, the first symptoms of α-CD appeared in some patients more than 10 years after withdrawal from the environmental factors mentioned above [17], and the usual clinical onset of the disease during the 2nd or 3rd decade of life [27] suggests that the clonal proliferation may have begun in early childhood. The absence of the Fab fragment in α-CP precludes the identification of the putative antigenic stimulus through the demonstration of a specific binding activity of this immunoglobulin. Establishment of long-term cultures of the proliferating cells could greatly help to solve this and other problems raised by α-CD.

Bacterial lipopolysaccharides may constitute nonspecific stimuli of the humoral immune response in the gut [9]. Thus, small intestinal bacterial overgrowth could merely trigger a preexisting cell clone synthesizing α-CP, or alternatively promote the oncogenic effect of a virus intefering with genes controllong IgA synthesis [16]. In either case, the abnormal clone could have a selective advantage for proliferation because of the lack of antibody activity of its immunoglubulin product, resulting in the suppression of a feedback mechanism [16]. The clonal expansion could also be favored by an underlying immunodeficiency, possibly due to malnutrition, especially in early infancy, or to genetic factors.

In fact, the role of environmental factors does not exclude the possibility of a genetic predisposition. However, there appears to be no predilection for α-CD to cluster in families [28], and no clear immunoglobulin abnormalities have been found in a limited number of sera from close relatives of the patients. A search for genetic markers could help to identify predisposed subjects. Raised serum levels of the intestinal isoenzyme of alkaline phosphatase have been reported in some (but not all) patients with α-CD [11] and Mediterranean lymphoma [22] as well as in their healthy relatives. The histocompatibility antigens of the patients and of their relatives should be determined in view of their implication in the immune response and susceptibility to some diseases.

In conclusion, α-chain disease represents a remarkable model of an immunoproliferative disorder, characterized by a continous sequence of events ranging from a possibly benign (or low-grade malignancy) plasmacytic proliferation, induced and/or maintained by a protracted antigenic stimulation of the IgA secretory system, to an immunoblastic lymphoma. A complete understanding of its natural history may offer revealing insights into the pathogenesis of human lymphomas.

References

1. Bognel, J. C., Rambaud, J. C., Modigliani, R., Matuchansky, C., Bognel, C., Bernier, J. J., Scotto, J., Hautefeuille, P., Mihaesco, E., Hurez, D., Preud'Homme, J. J., Seligmann, M.: Etude clinique, anatomo-pathologique et immunochimique d'un nouveau cas de maladie des chaînes alpha suivi pendant cinq ans. Rev. Eur. Et. Clin. Biol. *17*, 362–374 (1972).

2. Brouet, J. C., Mason, D. Y., Danon, F., Preud'Homme, J. L., Seligmann, M., Reyes, F., Navab, F., Galian, A., Rene, E., Rambaud, J. C.: Alpha-chain disease: Evidence for common clonal origin of intestinal immunoblastic lymphoma and plasmacytic proliferation. Lancet. *1*, 861 (1977).

3. Chadli, A., Hafsia, M., Maamouri, M. T., Haddad, N., Ayed, K.: Lymphome méditerranéen avec maladie des chaînes alpha. Etude anatomo-pathologique à propos du premier cas tunisien. Arch. Anat. Pathol. (Paris) *21*, 199–210 (1973).

4. COWAN, N. J., SECHER, D. S., MILSTEIN, C.: Intracellular immunoglobulin chain synthesis in non-secreting variants of a mouse myeloma: detection of inactive light-chain messenger RNA. J. Mol. Biol. *90*, 691–701 (1974).
5. DOE, W. F.: Alpha chain disease. Clinicopathological features and relationship to so-called Mediterranean lymphoma. Br. J. Cancer, *31*, suppl. II, 350–355 (1975).
6. DUTZ, W., ASVADI, S., SADRI, S., KOHOUT, E.: Intestinal lymphoma and sprue: a systematic approach. Gut *12*, 804–810 (1971).
7. GALIAN, A., LECESTRE, M. J., SCOTTO, J., BOGNEL, C., MATUCHANSKY, C., RAMBAUD, J. C.: Pathological study of alpha chain disease, with special emphasis on evolution. Cancer *39*, 2081–2101 (1977).
8. GUARDIA, J., MORAGAS, A., PEDREIRA, J. D., FERRAGUT, A., GOMEZ-PEREZ, J., MARTINEZ-VASQUEZ, J. M., LLORENS, V.: Enfermedad de lad cadenas pesadas alfa (Enfermedad de Seligmann). Rev. Clin. Esp. *127*, 923–926 (1972).
9. JONES, P. P., CRAIG, S. W., CEBRA, J. J., HERZENBERG, L. A.: Restriction of gene expression in B lymphocytes and their progeny. II. Commitment to immunoglobulin heavy chain isotype. J. Ex. Med. *140*, 452–469 (1974).
10. LAROCHE, C., SELIGMANN, M., MERILLON, H., TURPIN, G., MARCHE, C., CERF, M., LEMAIGRE, G., FOREST, M., HUREZ, D.: Nouvelle observation d'une maladie des chaînes lourdes alpha au cours d'un lymphome abdominal de type méditerranéen avec tuberculose isolée des ganglions mésentériques et pelvi-spondylite. Presse Med. *78*, 55–59 (1970).
11. LEWIN, K. J., KAHN, L. B., NOVIS, B. H.: Primary intestinal lymphoma of "western" and "mediterranean" type, alpha chain disease and massive plasma cell infiltration. A comparative study of 37 cases. Cancer *38*, 2511–2528 (1976).
12. MANOUSOS, O. N., ECONOMIDOU, J. C., GEORGIADOU, D. E., PRATSIKA-OUGOURLOGLOU, K. G., HADZIYANNIS, S. J., MERIKAS, G. E., HENRY, K., DOE, W. F.: Alpha-chain disease with clinical, immunological and histological recovery. Br. Med. J. *2*, 409–412 (1974).
13. MONGES, H., AUBERT, L., CHAMLIAN, A., REMACLE, J. P., MATHIEU, B., COUGARD, A., ARROYO, H.: Maladie des chaînes alpha à forme intestinale. Présentation d'un cas traité par antibiothérapie avec rémission clinique, histologique et immunologique. Arch. Fr. Mal. App. Dig. *64*, 223–231 (1975).
14. PARROTT, D. M. V.: The gut as a lymphoid organ. Clin. Gastroenterol. *5*, 211–228 (1976).
15. RAMBAUD, J. C., BOGNEL, C., PROST, A., BERNIER, J. J., LE QUINTREC, Y., LAMBLING, A., DANON, F., HUREZ, D., SELIGMANN, M.: Clinico-pathological study of a patient with "Mediterranean" type of abdominal lymphoma and a new type of IgA abnormality ("alpha chain disease"). Digestion *1*, 321–336 (1968).
16. RAMBAUD, J. C., MATUCHANSKY, C.: Alpha-chain disease. Pathogenesis and relation to Mediterranean lymphoma. Lancet *1*, 1430–1432 (1973).
17. RAMBAUD, J. C., MATUCHANSKY, C., BOGNEL, J. C., BOGNEL, C., BERNIER, J. J., SCOTTO, J., PEROL, C., FERRIER, J. P., MIHAESCO, E., HUREZ, D., SELIGMANN, M.: Nouveau cas de maladie des chaînes alpha chez un eurasien. Ann. Med. Interne (Paris) *121*, 135–148 (1970).
18. RAMBAUD, J. C., MODIGLIANI, R., GALIAN, A., LECLERC, J. P., HAUTEFEUILLE, P., DANON, F., BERNIER, J. J.: Rémission complète clinique, histologique et immunologique d'un cas de maladie des chaînes alpha traité pendant deux mois par antibiothérapie orale. Gastroenterol. Clin. Biol. (Paris) *2*, 49–61 (1978).
19. RAMBAUD, J. C., SELIGMANN, M.: Alpha-chain disease. Clin. Gastroenterol. *5*, 341–358 (1976).
20. RAMOT, B.: Alpha chain disease and related small intestinal lymphoma. Report of a WHO meeting of investigators. Arch. Fr. Mal. App. Dig. *65*, 591–607 (1976).
21. RAMOT, B., LEVANON, M., HAHN, Y., LAHAT, N., MOROZ, C.: The mutual clonal origin of the lymphoplasmocytic and lymphoma cell in alpha-heavy chain disease. Clin. Exp. Immunol. *27*, 440–445 (1977).
22. RAMOT, B., STREIFLER, C.: Raised serum-alkaline phosphatase. Lancet *2*, 587 (1966).
23. RAPPAPORT, H., RAMOT, B., HULU, N., PARK, J. K.: The pathology of so-called Mediterranean abdominal lymphoma with malabsorption. Cancer *29*, 1502–1511 (1972).
24. ROGE, J., DRUET, P., MARCHE, C.: Lymphome méditerranéen avec maladie des chaînes alpha. Triple rémission clinique, anatomique et immunologique. Pathol. Biol. (Paris) *18*, 851–858 (1970).
25. ROSS, I. N., JEFFERIS, R., JOHNS, P., THOMPSON, R. A., ASQUITH, P.: Alpha heavy chain disease complicated by a post nasal lymphoma, responding to antibiotics. Gut *17*, 820 (1976).
26. SELIGMANN, M., DANON, F., HUREZ, D., MIHAESCO, E., PREUD'HOMME, J. L.: Alpha-chain disease: a new immunoglobulin abnormality. Science *162*, 1396–1397 (1968).
27. SELIGMANN, M., MIHAESCO, E., FRANCIONE, B.: Studies on alpha-chain disease. Ann. N.Y. Acad. Sci. *190*, 487–500 (1971).
28. SELIGMANN, M., RAMBAUD, J. C.: Alpha-chain disease, a possible model of pathogenesis of human lymphomas. In: The Immunopathology of Lymphoreticular Neoplasms. GOOD, R. A., TWOMEY, J. J. (eds). New York: Plenum Press, 1978, p. 425–447.

29. TEULIERES, J. P.: La maladie des chaînes lourdes alpha. M.D. Thesis (1975). Claude Bernard University, Lyon, France.
30. WOLFELSTEIN-TODEL, C., MIHAESCO. E., FRANCIONE, B.: "Alpha-chain disease" protein Def: Internal deletion of a human immunoglobulin A_1 heavy chain. Proc. Natl. Acad. Sci. USA *71*, 974–978 (1974).

Neoplastic Proliferation and Natural History of B-Cell Neoplasia

S. E. SALMON

Introduction

Advances in immunology and laboratory and clinical oncology have provided a basis for a unifying view of various human neoplastic disorders arising from cells of the B-cell series of immunocytes. Over the past decade, our clinical research group has applied a variety of immunologic, cytokinetic, marker-kinetic, and cell culture techniques to the study of these malignancies. In this paper, I will attempt to summarize observations obtained in clinical investigations of the human disorders and hypotheses which we have derived from this work. I will also attempt to focus on those features which distinguish the more indolent from the more aggressive B-cell neoplasms and potential mechanisms for transformation over time to more aggressive states. The techniques which we have found most useful have been (1) quantitative studies of immunoglobulin synthesis and tumor cell number, (2) measurement of the tritiated thymidine labeling index, (3) Gompertzian kinetic analysis of tumor growth and regression, and (4) bioassay of tumor stem cells in soft agar. Observations obtained from these various independent approaches have helped to frame a pattern of pathophysiology of these disorders; however, many details remain yet to be filled in.

Immunoglobulin Synthesis and Total Body Tumor Mass

One of our first approaches to characterizing these disorders was to attempt to quantitate the total body tumor burden [14] in patients with the secretory (plasmacytic) B-cell disorders: multiple myeloma (MM), benign monoclonal gammopathy (BMG), and macroglobulinemia (MG). These studies took advantage of the secreted monoclonal Ig protein, as precise quantitation of this marker (in vitro and in vivo) could be used to calculate total tumor cell number from the following relationship:

$$\text{total body tumor cell number} = \frac{\text{rate of M-component synthesis (total body/24 h in vivo)}}{\text{rate of M-component synthesis (per tumor cell/24 h in vitro)}}$$

Using in vivo metabolic turnover studies (and more recently, calculations based on such studies), the total body mass turnover of M-component can be measured or predicted with reasonable accuracy [19]. Measurement of in vitro synthesis of M-component by relatively small numbers of tumor cells required development and application of sensitive immunoassay techniques. By application of this approach, we were able to determine that patients with MM, MG, and BMG all have a relatively large tumor burden present at the time of diagnosis [15]. At diagnosis, in excess of 3×10^{11} tumor cells are present in the body, as measured immunologically. Patients with BMG generally have less than 1×10^{12} tumor cells/m^2 of body surface area (BSA), whereas typical cases of MM and MG have greater than 1×10^{12} tumor cells/m^2, although there are marked differences in the distribution of tumor cells in different organs in these latter two disorders. Myeloma cases with bone destruction usually have greater than 1.5×10^{12} tumor cells/m^2 present and may have as many as 4×10^{12} cells/m^2 at the termination of their clinical course.

Tritiated Thymidine Labeling Index (LI)

This relatively simple kinetic technique is applied to fresh aspirated bone marrow (collected in heparin). Autoradiographs are prepared by our high-speed technique which can provide useful results within hours [3]. The LI measures the percentage of tumor cells in the S-phase of the cell cycle and can thereby serve as a marker of the "growth fraction," which is likely to be no greater than twice that of LI. In general, patients with MM and MG have LIs in the range of 1%–3%, with BMG patients having substantially lower LIs, generally far less than 1%. My colleague, Dr. Durie, has recently shown that LI is inversely related to tumor mass in myeloma, with the patients with low tumor mass (less than 0.6×10^{12} tumor cells/m^2) more frequently having LIs of greater than 3% [4]. Thus, as tumor mass increases in myeloma, the growth fraction appears to decrease, with fewer of the tumor cells entering the proliferative cycle. The very low LI in BMG corresponds with the clinical findings of negligible growth in the tumor burden over many years of observation.

Gompertzian Kinetic Analysis of Tumor Growth and Regression

The above-mentioned studies provide static images of a disseminated neoplasm at a given point in time. The availability of electrophoretic measurement of the M-component marker facilitates serial study of tumor mass behavior in both the untreated state and following the perturbations that are induced with chemotherapy [10, 19].

In order to use the M-component marker most accurately, we have primarily studied cases with serum M-components and have measured plasma volumes (routinely in MG and often in MM cases with a high concentration of an IgG or IgA M-component). We have also developed computer programs to carry out relatively complex metabolic equations [11]. More recently, we have used the increasingly sophisticated programmable pocket calculators for these calculations [16]. When such techniques were applied to myeloma growth, we were able to establish that myeloma grew in accord with Gompertzian kinetics. Thus, a curving-off and plateauing phenomenon was apparent, with a progressive decrease in the growth rate as the total tumor burden increased. Although an eventual plateau tumor mass could be predicted (beyond which further tumor growth would not occur), this was generally projected in the range of 10^{13} cells (a supralethal level) (Fig. 1). The typical "doubling time" in myeloma in the clinical phase of disease is in the range of 3–6 months. By back calculation by computer (using those constants derived from the clinical phase of greater than 10^{11} tumor cells), we could estimate that the initial doubling of the first monoclonal tumor stem cell (from one cell to two), took about 3 days. Thus, it appeared that despite the 3–6 month doubling time in the clinical phase of disease, the total duration of myeloma from its initiation from a single malignant monoclone is in the range of 1–3 years [19]. Until recently, we did not have techniques to directly assess the proliferative rates of human tumor stem cells, but as will be apparent from our stem cell work discussed later, our back extrapolations from total tumor mass growth curves appear to predict reasonably well the proliferative potential of low dilutions of myeloma stem cells. In contrasting the growth kinetics of BMG and MM, several points appear to be clear: 1) BMG can develop

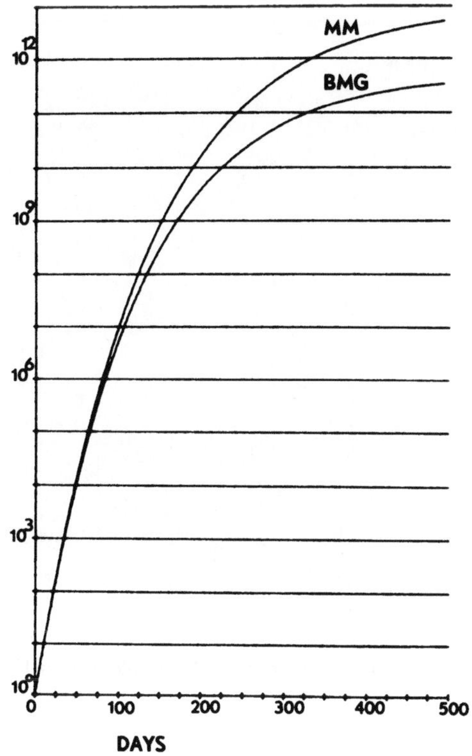

Fig. 1. Gompertzian kinetic growth curves for multiple myeloma (MM) and benign monoclonal gammopathy (BMG). The standard Gompertz relationship developed for monoclonal neoplasms has been applied (SULLIVAN and SALMON). A 3-day initial doubling time has been assumed (one cell to two). Values selected for the retardation constant α were 0.007718 for MM and 0.00857 for BMG. Thus, in the MM case, plateau tumor mass would be reached at a supralethal 10^{13} cells, whereas in BMG, the plateau is at about 5×10^{11} cells and similar in tumor burden to a stage I myeloma case

relatively quickly as in the circumstance of development of a benign monoclone after pneumonia, hepatitis, or bone marrow transplantation, and 2) BMG reaches a plateau at a lower total tumor mass, which is often in the mass range of a stage I myeloma case. Furthermore, the tumor mass usually remains in plateau for many years in BMG (Fig. 1).

Bioassay of Human Tumor Stem Cells in B-Cell Neoplasia

The most important cells in a cancer are the tumor stem cells, as they are responsible for population renewal and for the colonization which occurs in a neoplasm that is capable of metastasis. Starting over a decade ago, a series of workers at the Ontario Cancer Institute [1, 7, 8] showed that tumor stem cells from murine lymphoma and myeloma could be bioassayed in vivo or in vitro with tumor colony-forming assays. The studies of mouse myeloma stem cells also showed that differential sensitivity was present with respect to anticancer drugs and that the in vitro assay was predictive of in vivo results. Within the past 1½ years, my associate, Dr. Hamburger, and I have developed similar in vitro soft agar colony-forming assays for human myeloma and lymphoma stem cells (and other neoplasms as well) [5]. We have thus far studied

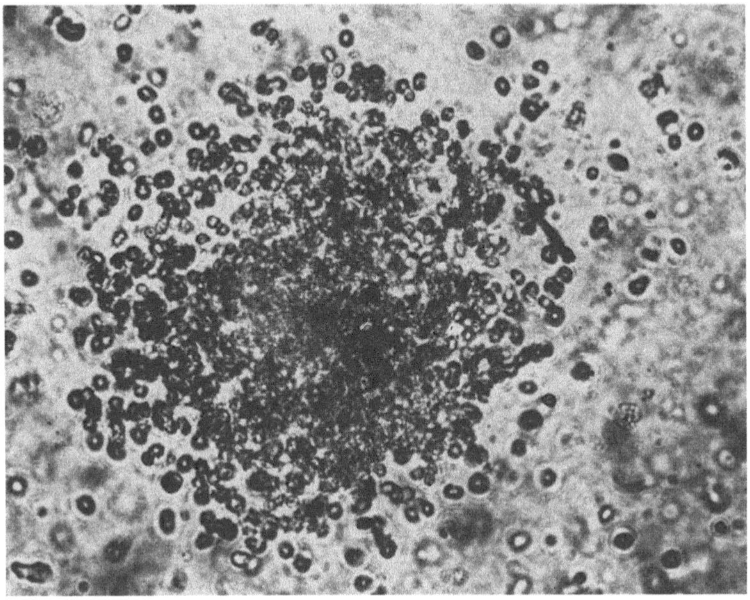

Fig. 2. A typical human myeloma colony after 17 days of culture. (× 200)

more than 65 myeloma and 41 lymphoma cases, as well as several patients with BMG or MG [12]. A typical myeloma colony is depicted in Fig. 2. We have observed tumor colony formation to occur in vitro within 2–3 weeks, with colonies growing more rapidly in lymphoma than myeloma. Plating efficiencies are low (in the range of 0.1%) but quite similar to those for normal human marrow granulocyte or erythroid colony formation. However, in myeloma and lymphoma, the colonies grown with our system have the morphologic, histochemical, and immunofluorescent characteristics of the specific neoplasm present in the patients studied [12, 6]. In vitro doubling times of cells in individual colonies are in the range of 2–3 days [and in accord with our earlier predictions from Gompertzian kinetics [19]]. Our success rate for colony formation has been in the range of 80% in myeloma cases who were untreated or in relapse. A similar percentage positivity was observed in patients with lymphoma who had histopathologically proven marrow involvement [12].

It is interesting that lymphoma colonies grew from two of ten cases whose marrows were histopathologically negative for tumor. Both of these patients had nodular lymphoma (NL), indicating that tumor stem cells for this B-cell neoplasm may be present in the marrow even when it is clinically free of involvement. Such occult marrow disease supports the concept that nodular lymphoma is frequently disseminated even though it may clinically appear to be localized. Thus, nodular lymphomas appear to be B-cell neoplasms which share significant biologic as well as immunologic features with MM, MG, and BMG. Much as BMG occasionally terminates in MM, NL occasionally transforms into a diffuse neoplasm of B-cell type. Although we have studied relatively few cases of MG or BMG with this colony-forming system, such patients' marrows have also formed plasma cell colonies in vitro with growth rates quite similar to those observed in myeloma cases. This suggests that the different in vivo behavior of these disorders may relate to a similarity in growth modulation in the host. We have not been able to grow lymphoid or plasmacytic colonies from normal marrows, nor were they observed in a single healthy individual studied who had a reactive plasmacytosis some weeks after a viral infection.

Significance of Feedback Inhibition in B-Cell Neoplasms

It is clear that growth kinetics of different B-cell neoplasms show many features in common. Perhaps the major difference observed to date between MM and BMG is the susceptibility to plateauing, presumably in relation to tumor mass-related feedback inhibition (Fig. 1). While our kinetic studies provide functional and theoretic evidence for such an inhibitor [10], biochemical evidence for the existence of an inhibitor of normal B-cell proliferation has been obtained in murine myeloma [20] and more recently in human myeloma [2]. While this inhibitor has yet to be characterized, its effects may be mediated by a suppressor T-cell or a macrophage, and it is, therefore, uncertain whether this effect is due to a chalone or not. The acquired antibody deficiency syndrome observed in BMG cases can be every bit as severe as that observed in myelomas, even though tumor growth in BMG appears far more indolent. It is, therefore, reasonable to propose that a central feature which may make BMG "more benign" than MM is the retention of a greater degree of sensitivity by the tumor cells themselves to feedback inhibition of their proliferation by an inhibitor of B-cell proliferation which they themselves produce. Occasional cases of BMG do eventually transform into myeloma, even after many years of observation. Such transformations may be "subcloning" events, in which the new mutant is less sensitive to feedback inhibition than its progenitors.

"Two-Hit Phenomenon" for Myeloma Development

About 4 years ago, Professor SELIGMANN and I formulated several hypotheses with respect to B-cell neoplasia and proposed that a two-hit phenomenon might be responsible for myeloma induction [13]. That concept, which still seems sound, is summarized in Fig. 3. It is based on some of the kinetic studies discussed above, plus clinical observations in patients with M-components with antibody activity [17, 18], and studies of myeloma induction in BALB/c mice [9]. The same hypothesis could conceivably apply to certain lymphomas. In this construct, the

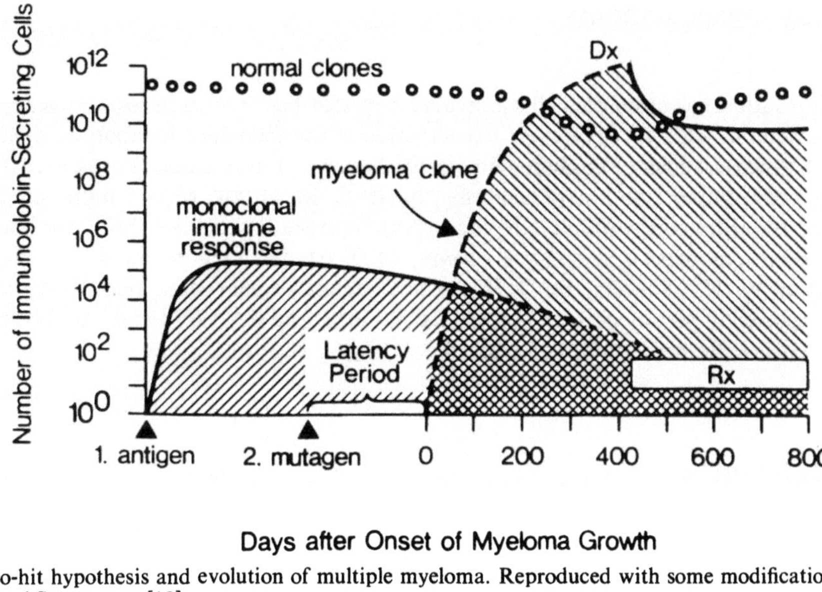

Fig. 3. The two-hit hypothesis and evolution of multiple myeloma. Reproduced with some modification from SALMON and SELIGMANN [13]

first hit is due to antigen and results in monoclonal B-cell proliferation. This could be a preneoplastic state. If the clone is 10^{11} cells in size, it may be a detectable benign gammopathy. Such clones may involute or may subsequently be transformed into myeloma.
The second hit (which may occur months or years later) is the oncogenic or mutagenic event (e.g., oncornavirus) which transforms a susceptible subclone in the population. Thus, with this view, BMG itself can be thought of as heterogeneous. In some instances, it may be an exuberant monoclonal immune response (with persistent antigen present) and in others a "minimal deviation" malignancy after the second hit.

Summary

In this analysis, I have concentrated on advances in immunology, kinetics, and clinical oncology which have provided a substantial basis for identifying major common features in the natural history and pathophysiology of B-cell neoplasia as diverse as MM, MG, BMG, and NL. Observations on the natural history of both experimental and clinical myeloma as well as studies of kinetics of proliferation of MM and BMG in man provide the basis for reasonable hypotheses. Firstly, malignant variants of B-cell neoplasms may result from a two-hit evolution. In this scheme, the first hit is a triggering by specific antigen which leads to a required monoclonal expansion, while the second hit is the oncogenic event. Some cases of BMG seem to be examples of an unusually prolific response to the first hit, while others appear to be minimal deviation malignancies after the second hit. In this latter circumstance, the neoplastic clone in BMG usually retains a significant degree of sensitivity to tumor mass-related feedback inhibition. This may occasionally be lost during subsequent subcloning. Significant future testing of these hypotheses may prove feasible through the application of the in vitro tumor colony-forming assay system as it lends itself to study of a number of the salient features of these disorders.

Acknowledgements

The author has attempted to summarize a related but diverse series of investigations he has carried out with the invaluable participation of the following collaborators: Beth A. Smith, B.S. (measurement of immunoglobulin synthesis and tumor mass); Peter W. Sullivan, M.D. (use of Gompertzian kinetic analysis), Brian G. M. Durie, M.D. (studies of clinical staging and the tritiated thymidine labeling index), Maxime Seligmann, M.D. (development of the two-hit hypothesis), Stephen E. Jones, M.D. (studies of non-Hodgkin's lymphomas), and Anne W. Hamburger, Ph.D. (bioassay of human tumor stem cells). This work has been supported in part by grants CA-14102, CA-13612, and CA-17094 from the National Institutes of Health, Bethesda, Maryland 20014.

References

1. Bruce, W. R., Meeker, B. E., Valeriote, F. A.: Comparison of the sensitivity of normal hematopoietic and transplanted lymphoma colony-forming cells to chemotherapeutic agents administered in vivo. J. Natl. Cancer Inst. *37*, 233 (1966).

2. BRODER, S., HUMPHREY, R., DURM, M., BLACKMAN, M., MEADE, B., GOLDMAN, C., STROBER, W., WALDMANN, T.: Impaired synthesis of polyclonal (non-paraprotein) immunoglobulins by circulating lymphocytes from patients with multiple myeloma. New Engl. J. Med. *293*, 887 (1975).
3. DURIE, B. G. M., SALMON, S. E.: High speed scintillation autoradiography. Science *190*, 1093 (1975).
4. DURIE, B. G. M., VAUGHT, L., SALMON, S. E.: Prognostic significance of tritiated thymidine labeling index (LI) in multiple myeloma and acute myeloid leukemia. Proc. of 68th Meeting of the American Association of Cancer Research, p. 80, Denver, May, 1977.
5. HAMBURGER, A. W., SALMON, S. E.: Primary bioassay of human tumor stem cells. Science *197*, 461 (1977).
6. HAMBURGER, A. W., SALMON, S. E.: Primary bioassay of human myeloma stem cells. J. Clin. Invest. *60*, 846 (1977).
7. OGAWA, M., BERGSAGEL, D. E., MCCULLOCH, E. A.: Chemotherapy of mouse myeloma: quantitative cell culture predictive of reponse in vivo. Blood *41*, 7 (1973).
8. PARK, C. H., BERGSAGEL, D. E., MCCULLOCH, E. A.: Mouse myeloma stem cells: a primary cell culture assay. J. Natl. Cancer Inst. *46*, 411 (1971).
9. POTTER, M.: The developmental history of the neoplastic plasma cell in mice: a brief review of recent developments. Semin. Hematol. *10*, 19 (1973).
10. SALMON, S. E.: Immunoglobulin synthesis and tumor kinetics of multiple myeloma. Semin. Hematol. *10*, 135 (1973).
11. SALMON, S. E., DURIE, B. G. M.: Cellular kinetics in multiple myeloma. Arch. Intern. Med. *135*, 131 (1975).
12. SALMON, S. E., HAMBURGER, A. W., JONES, S. E.: Primary bioassay of human tumor stem cells in myeloma and lymphoma. Proc. of 68th Meeting of the American Association of Cancer Research, p. 88, Denver, May, 1977.
13. SALMON, S. E., SELIGMANN, M.: B-cell neoplasia in man. Lancet II, 1230 (1974).
14. SALMON, S. E., SMITH, B. A.: Immunoglobulin synthesis and total body tumor cell number in IgG multiple myeloma. J. Clin. Invest. *49*, 1114 (1970).
15. SALMON, S. E., SMITH, B. A.: Paraprotein synthesis and tumor cell number in myeloma and macroglobulinemia. Proc. of the 13th International Congress of Hematology, p. 353, 1970, J. F. Lehmanns, Pub.
16. SALMON, S. E., WAMPLER, S. B.: Multiple myeloma: quantitative staging and assessment of response with a programmable pocket calculator. Blood *49*, 379 (1977).
17. SELIGMANN, M., DANON, F., BASCH, A., BERNARD, J.: IgG myeloma cryoglobulin with antistreptolysin activity. Nature *220*, 711 (1968).
18. SELIGMANN, M., SASSY, C., CHEVALIER, A.: A human IgG myeloma protein with anti-2 macroglobulin antibody activity. J. Immunol. *110*, 85 (1973).
19. SULLIVAN, P. W., SALMON, S. E.: Kinetics of tumor growth and regression in IgG myeloma. J. Clin. Invest. *51*, 1697 (1972).
20. TANAPATCHAIYAPONG, P., ZOLLA, S.: Humoral immunosuppressive substance in mice bearing plasmacytomas. Science *186*, 748 (1974).

Castleman's Disease

R. F. DORFMAN and M. CIBULL

In 1956, CASTLEMAN studied a group of patients with "asymptomatic, large, benign hyperplastic mediastinal lymph nodes that resembled thymomas" [3]. Although a similar lesion was subsequently described by others under various designations including lymph nodal hamartoma [1], angiofollicular mediastinal lymph node hyperplasia [7], and benign lymphoid mass of probable hamartomatous nature [10], this disorder is referred to in many countries as "Castleman's disease." The lesion has a predilection for the mediastinum, but has been described at other sites, usually involving lymph nodes, although on occasion in extranodal locations [4]. The latter observation has provided support for the theory that the lesion represents a lymphoid hamartoma [10].

In 1972, KELLER et al. [9] analyzed 81 cases and introduced the term "giant lymph node hyperplasia." The cases were subdivided into two histologic types: "hyaline-vascular" form, conforming with the previous designation, angiofollicular lymph node hyperplasia, and the "plasma cell" lesion, characterized by large follicles with intervening sheets of plasma cells. KELLER et al. [9] reported that systemic manifestations such as fever, anemia, and hyperglobulinemia were frequently associated with the plasma cell lesion. The literature is now replete with reports describing additional unusual manifestations, including anemia associated with an antierythropoietic factor [2], peripheral neuropathy [11, 14], growth failure [13], the nephrotic syndrome [8], and even myasthenia gravis [6] (Table 1). Of particular interest is the observation that excision of isolated tumors has often resulted in the disappearance of all symptoms and a return to normality [5, 12].

Review of the files in the Laboratory of Surgical Pathology at Stanford University Hospital disclosed 33 cases during the years 1969–1977. Only two of the patients had been admitted to Stanford Hospital. The remaining cases comprised consultations to one of us (RFD) and were derived from institutions throughout the United States and other countries. It is thus impossible to comment on the incidence of this disorder, which nevertheless is rarely encountered in any one institution.

Histopathologic Findings

Using the criteria of KELLER et al. [9], we observed the characteristics of the hyaline-vascular type in 24 cases and those of the plasma cell type in nine.

Hyaline–Vascular Type (Fig. 1)

The most conspicuous features include lymphoid follicles with a tight concentric layering of small lymphocytes in the mantle zone surrounding small follicular centers containing arborizing vessels with thickened, hyalinized walls. Some thick-walled vessels enter these follicles in an

Table 1. Giant lymph node hyperplasia (Castleman's disease)

Unusual manifestations
Anemia (refractory)
Abnormal iron metabolism
Hypoferremia (antierythropoietic factor)
Peripheral neuropathy
Growth failure
Hyperglobulinemia
Hypoalbuminemia
Nephrotic syndrome
Raised erythrocyte sedimentation rate
Fever
Leukocytosis
Disturbed liver function

unusual radial fashion. In some cases, rounded masses of hyaline material, deposited in a concentric fashion, often associated with hyalinized vessels, are presumed to represent progressive hyalinization of lymphoid follicles. We have observed extensive hyalinization associated with focal ossification. Arborizing vessels are also prominent in the interfollicular stroma, which consists predominantly of small lymphocytes, occasional plasma cells, eosinophils, and often large lymphoid cells (so-called immunoblasts). Focal involvement of lymph nodes may occur with a thin, compressed rim of normal lymphoid tissue containing either lymphoid follicles with secondary centers devoid of the hyaline-vascular component or in other cases, patent sinuses. In some lesions the hyaline-vascular structures are lobulated or dumbbell-shaped. Variable numbers of plasma cells may be noted in the interfollicular stroma but never to the extent seen in the plasma cell type.

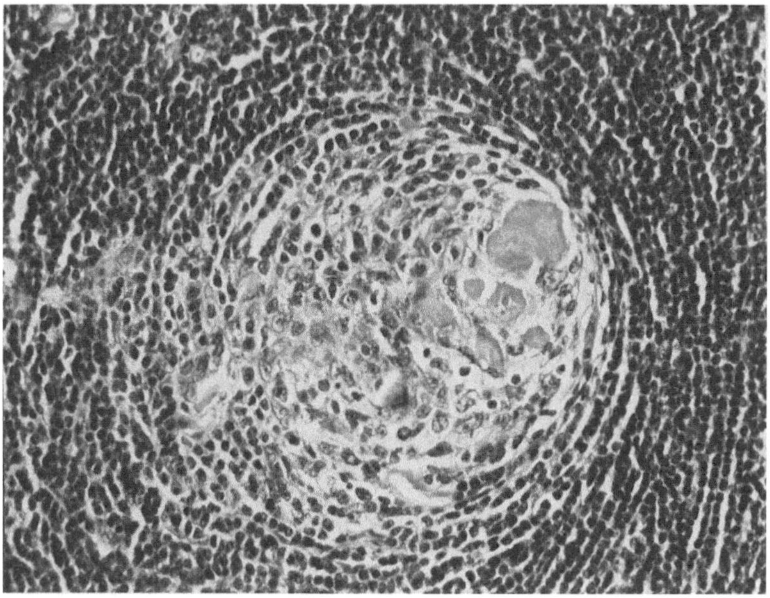

Fig. 1. Giant lymph node hyperplasia, hyaline-vascular type. Small follicle with hyalinized vessels. Note tight concentric layering of lymphocytes in mantle zone (onion-skin appearance). Hematoxylin and eosin stains. (× 250)

Plasma Cell Type

Lymphoid follicles with secondary centers are prominent and for the most part lack the hyaline-vascular component. Occasional cases are encountered in which both large reactive follicles and occasional small hyaline-vascular structures are present. The most conspicuous feature in the plasma cell type comprises an extensive plasma cell infiltrate in the interfollicular stroma, often associated with Russell bodies. The interfollicular stroma is also well-vascularized. Partial involvement of lymph nodes may also occur, with remnants of normal lymph node architecture containing patent sinuses.

Clinical Manifestations

Although most of the reports in the literature have described solitary masses, most often in the mediastinum or involving mesenteric lymph nodes, we have encountered a number of patients with multiple sites of involvement. In most instances, these have involved lymph nodes, but we have observed both the hyaline-vascular and plasma cell lesions in the spleen and two patients have had concomitant hepatomegaly. Table 1 indicates the remarkable variety of clinical manifestations reported in the literature. Several of our patients were found to have anemia and hypergammaglobulinemia of the polyclonal type. While these manifestations are more often associated with the plasma cell lesions, we have observed anemia and hypergammaglobulinemia in rare instances of the hyaline-vascular type.

Conclusions

The etiology of these lesions is not known. The histologic features in the plasma cell type bear a strong resemblance to those observed in lymph nodes from patients with rheumatoid arthritis (Felty's syndrome) [9]. The concept that these lesions are lymphoid hamartomas [10] is controversial and yet intriguing. Although most lesions appear to involve lymph nodes, we have observed others in unusual sites, including the broad ligament of the uterus and soft tissues of the shoulder in an infant, and such lesions have been devoid of identifiable subcapsular and trabecular sinuses.

Giant lymph node hyperplasia is presumed to represent a benign disorder and removal of the lesion is usually curative, with resolution of symptomatology and abnormal laboratory findings. Nevertheless, in three cases that we have encountered, all of the hyaline–vascular type, recurrence of the lesion occurred, once in the mediastinum and once involving axillary lymph nodes. In one patient with a cervical mass, the lesion recurred twice.

Acknowledgements

We are grateful to Ms. PATRICIA SCHOLL who typed the manuscript and Mr. PHILLIP HORNE who prepared the illustration.

References

1. Abel, M. R.: Lymphnodal hamartoma versus chronic choristoma of pulmonary hilum. Arch. Pathol. *64*, 584–588 (1957).
2. Burgert, E. O., Jr., Gilchrist, G. S., Fairbanks, V. F., Lynn, H. B., Dukes, P. P., Harrison, E. G., Jr.: Intra-abdominal angiofollicular lymph node hyperplasia (plasma cell variant) with an anti-erythropoietic factor. Mayo Clin. Proc. *50*, 542–546 (1975).
3. Castleman, B., Iverson, L., Menendex, V.: Localized mediastinal lymph-node hyperplasia resembling thymoma. Cancer *9*, 822–830 (1956).
4. Cohen, H.: Tumor-like proliferations of lymphoid tissue. Occurrence in deltoid muscle and mediastinum. J. Mt. Sinai Hosp. *24*, 750–760 (1957).
5. Dorfman, R. F., Warnke, R.: Lymphadenopathy simulating the malignant lymphomas. Hum. Pathol. *5*, 519–550 (1974).
6. Emson, H. E.: Extrathoracic angiofollicular lymphoid hyperplasia with coincidental myasthenia gravis. Cancer *31*, 241–245 (1973).
7. Harrison, E. G., Bernatz, P. E.: Angiofollicular mediastinal lymph node hyperplasia resembling thymoma. Arch. Pathol. *75*, 284–292 (1963).
8. Humphreys, S. R., Holley, K. E., Smith, L. H., McIlrat, D. C.: Mesenteric angiofollicular lymph node hyperplasia (lymphoid hamartoma) with nephrotic syndrome. Mayo Clin. Proc. *50*, 317–321 (1975).
9. Keller, A. R., Hochholzer, L., Castleman, B.: Hyaline-vascular and plasma cell types of giant lymph node hyperplasia of the mediastinum and other locations. Cancer *29*, 670–683 (1972).
10. Lattes, R., Pachter, M. R.: Benign lymphoid masses of probable hamartomatous nature. Cancer *15*, 197–214 (1962).
11. Mallory, A., Spink, W. W.: Angiomatous lymphoid hamartoma in the retroperitoneum presenting with neurologic signs in the legs. Ann. Int. Med. *69*, 305 (1968).
12. Miller, J. S., Miller, J. J.: Benign giant lymph node hyperplasia presenting as fever of unknown origin. J. Pediatr. *87*, 237–245 (1973).
13. Neerhout, R. C., Larson, W., Mansur, P.: Mesenteric lymphoid hamartoma associated with chronic hypoferremia, anemia, growth failure, and hypergobulinemia. New Engl. J. Med. *280*, 922 (1969).
14. Yu, G. S. M., Carson, J. W.: Giant lymph node hyperplasia, plasma cell type of the mediastinum with peripheral neuropathy. Am. J. Clin. Pathol. *66*, 46–53 (1976).

Benign and Malignant Lymphoid Proliferation in Autoimmunity

N. Talal

In autoimmune disorders, the organism's ability to discriminate self from foreign antigens is disturbed, leading to autorecognition and autodestruction due to a variety of immunopathologic mechanisms. Autoantibodies and immune complexes may be present in the serum, and target organs may undergo vasculitic destruction or become infiltrated with lymphocytes and plasma cells. Quite recently, immunologists have come to appreciate that autorecognition of histocompatibility antigens on lymphocyte membranes is an important regulatory mechanism allowing the immune system to react against viral and other foreign antigens [17]. Either by an alteration of these self-antigens or by a dual recognition mechanism, immune reactions against these foreign antigens are facilitated through recognition of the self-antigenic component.

The immune system is exquisitely regulated. In part, this regulation is dependent upon specific immune response genes which are located within the major histocompatibility complex. Genetic factors influence specialized subpopulations of T-lymphocytes, which function either to suppress or enhance immune responses. Recognition of idiotypic receptors on lymphocyte membranes by antibody or by other lymphocytes can also result in either suppression or priming of an immune response. Since these regulatory mechanisms play an important role in immunologic control, one must look to some derangement in their function to explain the existence of autoimmunity and autoimmune disorders [13].

Genetic factors play an important role in autoimmunity [1]. Certain autoimmune disorders occur more frequently in individuals with particular histocompatibility antigens. For example, several autoimmune diseases are associated with the histocompatibility antigen, HLA-B8. Sjögren's syndrome, an autoimmune disorder characterized by lymphocytic destruction of salivary and lacrimal glands, is one such disease that shows a statistically significant association with HLA-B8 [2, 4]. Another is celiac disease in which patients suffer from malabsorption and have atrophy of intestinal villi.

Patients with Sjögren's syndrome complain of dryness of the eyes and mouth and may have an associated connective tissue disorder (most often rheumatoid arthritis). The diagnosis can be made on the basis of characteristic findings of salivary and lacrimal gland insufficiency and can be confirmed by biopsy of the minor salivary glands of the lower lip which show the charactersitic lymphocytic and plasma cell infiltrates [3]. Rheumatoid factor, antinuclear factor, antisalivary duct antibody, and certain tissue precipitating antibodies are frequently present in the serum [12]. Many patients have evidence of decreased T-cell number and function [16].

Thirteen years ago we reported an increased incidence of malignant lymphoma in patients with Sjögren's syndrome [15]. There are now over 50 examples of this association in the medical literature. The autoimmune disorder may precede the development of lymphoma by intervals as long as 20 years. The lymphomas are of two major types: either composed of highly undifferentiated cells and termed reticulum cell sarcoma or histocytic lymphoma, or highly pleomorphic and sometimes associated with monoclonal macroglobulinemia. In the first type, antibodies tend to disappear and hypogammaglobulinemia may develop when the malignancy appears. The lymphoma may involve salivary glands or major parenchymal organs such as lungs, kidney, and gastrointestinal tract. One patient in our series died from generalized reticulum cell sarcoma 13 years after the resection of a localized process of the same histologic type which involved only inguinal lymph nodes.

Some patients with Sjögren's syndrome develop a clinical picture suggestive of a malignant lymphoma which cannot be clearly classified as malignant after tissue biopsy. Features of autoimmunity are present. The term "pseudolymphoma" has been applied to such cases. The course of these patients is quite variable, and many of them respond to corticosteroids or immunosuppressive drugs. Some, however, develop a frankly malignant histiocytic lymphoma.

Two patients will serve to illustrate the relationship between autoimmunity and lymphoid proliferation:

Patient 1 (L.B.R.)

This patient was 49 years old when she first developed dry mouth, dry eyes, and bilateral parotid gland swelling. Right parotid gland biopsy revealed a benign lymphoepithelial lesion. She developed generalized lymphadenopathy, hepatosplenomegaly, various serum autoantibodies, and a pulmonary lymphoid infiltrate which responded to prednisone therapy. When the prednisone dosage was tapered, more extensive pulmonary infiltrates appeared accompanied by a rise in serum IgM concentration and a small monoclonal spike seen on electrophoresis. The increase was due entirely to a rise in λ-type IgM molecules. Although the total level of serum IgM never exceeded 7 mg/ml, the response appeared monoclonal. Increasing the prednisone brought about a decrease in lymphocytic infiltration and IgM concentration. This patient ultimately died of vasculitic and renal complications of Sjögren's syndrome. There was no evidence of lymphoid malignancy at postmortem examination. She represents an example of a benign monoclonal gammopathy (IgM type) that may develop in Sjögren's syndrome.

Patient 2 (S.M.)

This patient developed dry mouth, dry eyes, and parotid gland swelling at the age of 41. A parotid biopsy early in her course revealed a benign lymphoepithelial lesion with many epimyoepithelial islets. Parotid swelling only partially subsided on prednisone therapy. She consistently demonstrated a decrease in T-rosette-forming cells (48% compared to 65% in normal subjects) and a decreased proliferative response to suboptimal concentrations of phytohemagglutinin. She underwent a mastectomy for a carcinoma of the breast, and shortly thereafter developed marked bilateral parotid gland swelling. Parotid biopsy revealed a diffuse histiocytic lymphoma. She developed aplastic anemia and died from infectious complications. This patient demonstrates the transition from a benign to a malignant lymphoproliferative process occurring in the parotid glands.

Immunologic mechanisms may contribute to the gastrointestinal lesions that occur in celiac disease, another HLA-B8 associated disorder that shows a significantly increased risk of malignancy [5] (particularly reticulum cell sarcoma). As in Sjögren's syndrome, T-cell number and function are decreased in celiac disease [8,10].

Malignant lymphomas also develop in New Zealand black/white (NZB/NZW) mice who are genetically predisposed to an autoimmune disorder resembling systemic lupus erythematosis. They spontaneously develop antinuclear factors, antibodies to DNA and RNA, immune complex glomerulonephritis, and generalized lymphoid proliferation. The disorder occurs earlier and with greater severity in females than in males. We have recently shown that sex hormones greatly modify autoimmunity, nephritis, and survival, with estrogens accelerating and androgens suppressing disease [9].

There is a significant incidence of lymphoid tumors and monoclonal macroglobulinemia in these NZB/NZW F_1 mice [11]. The monoclonal nature of these macroglobulins was confirmed by light chain analysis and demonstration of idiotypic characteristics. There was less evidence of autoimmunity in mice that had monoclonal proteins, suggesting a possible inverse relationship between autoimmunity and monoclonal lymphoid proliferation.

Discussion

Current hypotheses implicate genetic, immunologic, and possibly viral factors in the pathogenesis of autoimmunity [14]. Much evidence suggests that autoimmunity can arise from a defect in the regulation of immune responses mediated by helper and suppressor T cells. Either a deficiency in the function of suppressor cells or an inappropriate augmentation of helper function could trigger potentially autoreactive B cells to proliferate and synthesize autoantibodies. There is now extensive evidence that such potentially autoreactive B-lymphocytes with immunoglobulin receptors for autoantigens exist in normal healthy individuals [14]. Either immunologic or viral mechanisms (or a combination of the two) could create a regulatory imbalance and activate these autoreactive cells.

Current theories also put great emphasis on the role of T-lymphocytes in immunologic defense against malignancy (although there are other important immunologic mechanisms that kill cancer cells). The increased incidence of lymphoid malignancies in Sjögren's syndrome and celiac disease is associated with a particular histologic type (reticulum cell or histiocytic lymphoma). This suggests a mechanism more specific than one based on generalized immune defense against neoplasia. In exploring possible mechanisms to explain malignant lymphoid proliferation, one might examine those put forth to explain the benign lymphoproliferation associated with autoimmunity. Foremost among these theories would be mechanisms involving the activity of regulatory T cells.

Recent studies by Drs. Joseph Michalski and Candace McCombs in my laboratory have investigated the decreased response to phytomitogens seen in Sjögren's syndrome. Leventhal et al. [6] originally reported a decreased response to phytohemagglutinin (PHA) and an impaired ability to develop hypersensitivity to dinitrochlorobenzine in this disease. The recent studies have shown an impaired lymphocyte activation in response to suboptimal concentrations of PHA in a majority of patients with Sjögren's syndrome [7]. This defect is particularly pronounced in patients who express the HLA-B8 antigen.

Fortunately, the development of malignant lymphoid proliferation in a patient with autoimmune disease is a rare event. The factors that predispose to autoimmunity and benign lymphoid proliferation may also, at least in part, predispose to malignant lymphoid proliferation. We have found a genetic factor (the presence of HLA-B8) and an immunologic factor (decreased lymphocyte activation in response to a suboptimal concentration of PHA) associated with autoimmune and benign lymphoproliferative features of Sjögren's syndrome. These factors, no doubt combined with additional new factors promoting neoplasia, may create an environment of augmented susceptibility to the development of malignant lymphomas. Evidence based on animal models such as the NZB mouse and a recently described mouse strain called MRL/1, which develops autoimmunity and extensive lymphoproliferation, suggest that these clinical observations may have a broader biologic and medical significance.

Acknowledgements

This work was supported by an Arthritis Foundation Clinical Center Grant and research support from the U.S. Veterans Administration.

References

1. Bach, F. H.: The Major Histocompatibility Complex and its Relationship to Autoimmune Disease. In: Autoimmunity: Genetic, Immunologic, Virologic and Clinical Aspects. Talal, N. (ed.) New York–London: Academic Press, p. 4–32 (1977).

2. Chused, T. M., Kassan, S. S., Opelz, G., Moutsopoulus, H. M., Terasaki, P. I.: Sjögren's syndrome associated with HLA-DW. New Engl. J. Med. *296*, 895–897 (1977).
3. Daniels, T. E., Silverman, S., Michalski, J. P., Greenspan, J. S., Sylvester, R. A., Talal, N.: The oral component of Sjögren's syndrome. Oral Surg. *39*, 875–885 (1975).
4. Fye, K. H., Terasaki, P. I., Moutsopoulos, H., Daniels, T. E., Michalski, J. P., Talal, N.: Association of Sjögren's syndrome with HLA-B8. Arthritis Rheum. *19*, 883–886 (1976).
5. Holmes, G. K. T., Stokes, P. L., Sorahan, T. M., Prior, P., Waterhouse, J. A. H., Cooke, W. T.: Coeliac disease, gluten-free diet, and malignancy. Gut *17*, 612–619 (1976).
6. Leventhal, B. G., Waldorf, D., Talal, N.: Impaired lymphocyte transformation and delayed hypersensitivity in Sjögren's syndrome. J. Clin. Invest. *46*, 1338–1345 (1967).
7. Michalski, J. P., McCombs, C.: Decreased lymphocyte reactivity to a suboptimal concentration of phytohemagglutinin in Sjögren's syndrome. Arthritis Rheum. *20*, 851–858 (1977).
8. O'Donoghue, D. P. O., Lancaster-Smith, M., Laviniere, P., Kumar, P. J.: T cell depletion in untreated adult coeliac disease. Gut *17*, 328–331 (1976).
9. Roubinian, J. R., Papoian, R., Talal, N.: Androgenic hormones modulate autoantibody responses and improve survival in murine lupus. J. Clin. Invest. (in press).
10. Scott, B. B., Losowsky, M. S.: Depressed cell-mediated immunity in coeliac disease. Gut *17*, 900–905 (1976).
11. Sugai, S., Pillarisetty, R. J., Talal, N.: Monoclonal macroglobulinemia in NZB/NZW F_1 mice. J. Exp. Med. *138*, 989–1002 (1973).
12. Talal, N.: Recent clinical and experimental developments in Sjögren's syndrome—Medical Staff Conference, University of California, San Francisco. West. J. Med. *122*, 50–58 (1975).
13. Talal, N.: Disordered immunologic regulation and autoimmunity. Transplant. Rev. *31*, 240–263 (1976).
14. Talal, N.: Immunologic and viral factors in autoimmune diseases. Med. Clin. North Am. *61*, 205–215 (1977).
15. Talal, N., Bunim, J. J.: The development of malignant lymphoma in the course of Sjögren's syndrome. Am. J. Med. *36*, 529–540 (1964).
16. Talal, N., Sylvester, R. A., Daniels, T. E., Greenspan, J. S., Williams, R. C.: T and B lymphocytes in peripheral blood and tissue lesions in Sjögren's syndrome. J. Clin. Invest. *53*, 180–189 (1974).
17. Zinkernagel, R. M., Doherty, P. C.: Hz compatibility requirement for T cell-mediated lysis of target cells infected with lymphocytic choriomeningitis virus. J. Exp. Med. *141*, 1427–1436 (1975).

Lymphomagenesis and Autoimmunization Caused by Reactions of T-Lymphocytes to Incompatible Structures of the Major Histocompatibility Complex: A Concept of Pathogenesis

E. GLEICHMANN, C. J. M. MELIEF, and H. GLEICHMANN

The classic animal model for induction of graft-versus-host reactions (GVHRs) [1] is the parent → F_1 hybrid system (Fig. 1). A variety of different pathologic lesions can be induced in this system, as has recently been reviewed in great detail [28, 54]. In the present article, we shall focus on a pathogenetic concept of lymphomagenesis and autoimmunization which was prompted on the one hand by experiments performed with GVH model and on the other hand by important recent discoveries concerning the physiologic reactions of T-lymphocytes to structures of the major histocompatibility complex (MHC). Since T-cell anti-MHC reactions that are comparable to those seen during the GVHR may also occur in an autologous system (i.e., between the cells of the same individual), it has been postulated that they may lead to the same diseases as in the semiallogeneic parent → F_1 hybrid system [49, 54]. This hypothesis will be reexamined in the light of recent findings obtained by several groups of investigators.

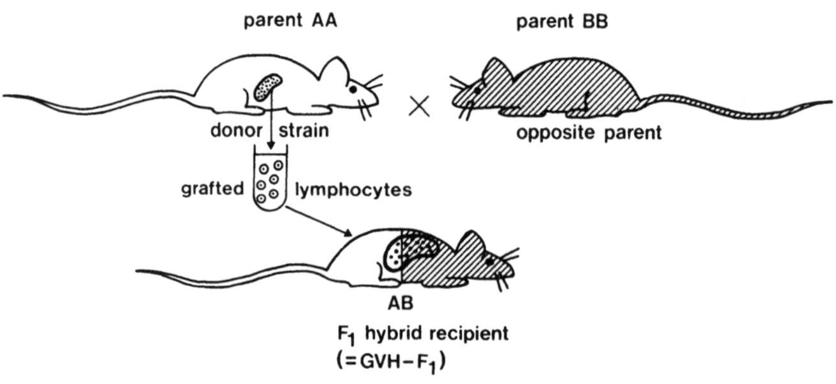

Fig. 1. Scheme of induction of graft-versus-host reactions using a parent → F_1 hybrid combination. The histocompatibility antigens of both parental strains are expressed in the heterozygous F_1 hybrid. For this reason, it fails to recognize parental strain tissues, e.g., spleen cells, grafted to it as foreign. In contrast, T-lymphocytes of the parental donor strain AA injected into the F_1 host AB recognize the histocompatibility antigens inherited from the opposite parental strain BB as foreign and react against them. The critical incompatibility in the F_1 hybrid, against which parental T cells must react for induction of pathologic lesions, is provided by its H-2 complex [3]; other histoincompatibilities are incapable of doing so

Lymphadenopathy in the Semiallogeneic GVH Model

Histopathology of GHV Lymphomagenesis

When groups of GHV F_1 mice were serially killed at various times after injection of parental strain spleen cells and their lymphoid tissues histologically examined, it appeared that there was a gradual transition with time from lymphoreticular hyperplasia to overt malignancy [6,

10]. Four different phases of alterations in spleens and lymph nodes were distinguished during this course [6]: 1) follicular hyperplasia, 2) plasmacytosis accompanied by the appearance of larger cells having a vesicular nucleus and one or more prominent nucleoli, 3) prelymphoma, and 4) malignant lymphoma.

The most common tumor developing during this sequence of events has been termed "reticulum cell sarcoma, type B" according to the nomenclature of DUNN and DERINGER [33]. Within the past 5 years, however, detailed immunologic and cytologic investigations of reticulum cell sarcomas in man have shown that this terminology is not correct, since the majority of cells in such tumors consists not of reticulum cells but of cells with the morphology of stimulated lymphocytes [94, 158]. Moreover, STEIN and co-workers [149], who analyzed tissue extracts from lymphoma specimens for their immunoglobulin content, were the first to relate some reticulum cell sarcomas to the B-lymphocyte series, a conclusion that was subsequently confirmed by studying the cells of such tumors with additional immunologic methods [158].

These findings raised the question of whether the reticulum cell sarcomas of GVH F_1 mice would also predominantly consist of B-lymphoblasts. The following lines of indirect evidence were compatible with this possibility:

1. The development of GVH lymphomas in the B-cell-dependent area of the lymphoid tissue and their association with plasmacytosis [6, 10, 52, 139];
2. The fact that the majority of lymphoma cells from GVH F_1 mice were Thy 1.1 (θ)-negative when tested in a complement-dependent cytotoxicity test [55 and unpublished results of E.G.];
3. The well-known stimulatory effect of parental strain T cells on B cells during the GVHR (see p. 299);
4. The frequent occurrence in GVH F_1 animals of phenomena such as hypergammaglobulinemia [153] and formation of autoantibodies to erythrocytes [50, 92, 154] and nuclear antigens [39, E.G. and H.G., unpublished results].

Recently, TAYLOR [157], using an immunoperoxidase technique, was able to directly demonstrate intracytoplasmatic immunoglobulin in a considerable portion of lymphoma cells obtained from (BALB/c × A)F_1 (CAF_1) hybrids that had been injected with BALB/c spleen cells. He concluded that the reticulum cell sarcomas of GVH CAF_1 mice are B-lymphocyte-derived and resemble the *immunoblastic sarcoma* group in man. The latter conclusion was also drawn by K. LENNERT and two of us when recently examining a number of GVH lymphomas by light microscopy (K. LENNERT, E.G. and H.G., unpublished observations).

It is generally agreed that the histopathologic distinction between abnormal hyperplastic alterations and malignant changes of the lymphoreticular tissue is difficult. This is particularly so in the case of GVH lymphomas [6, 52, 157]. That at least some of these tumors were truly malignant was demonstrated by their growth in other mice following transplantation [54] and the detection of tumor cells with chromosomal translocations or hyperdiploid sets of chromosomes [53, 138]. Furthermore, in many instances, malignancy was indicated by the metastatic behavior of lymphomas in the original GVH F_1 mouse [54].

Immunosuppression and GVH Lymphomagenesis

The possible relationship of GVHR-induced immunosuppression and lymphomagenesis was investigated in two independent studies [131, 146] using a battery of different test antigens and parent → F_1 combinations with high, medium, and low lymphoma incidence. The results indicated that immunosuppression during the chronic GVHR was either absent or, if present, completely failed to correlate with the lymphoma incidences observed in the different parent → F_1 combinations. SOLNIK and her colleagues [146] also investigated the effect of deliberate immunosuppression on the development of lymphomas in the same F_1 hybrid lines they used for analysis of the GVHR. They administered antithymocyte serum for this purpose. Although the degree of immunosuppression in the serum-treated animals far exceeded that detected in syngeneic F_1 hybrids undergoing the GVHR, only the latter animals developed a notable incidence of malignant lymphomas. The results of this experiment supported the conclusion that a lack of immune surveillance cannot explain the induction of lymphomas during the GVHR. Moreover, it is relevant to this argument that in the numerous experiments on GVHR-induced neoplasms, an increased incidence of *non*-lymphoreticular malignancies was never observed. This indicates that the oncogenic stimulans operating in GVH F_1 mice leads exclusively to *lymphomas* and cannot be explained by a decreased immune surveillance of neoplastic cells in general.

Are Endogenous C-Type RNA Viruses Involved in the Development of Lymphadenopathy During GVHR?

C-type RNA viruses naturally cause lymphoid tumors in a variety of species, including mice [62, 159]. All wild and laboratory mice that have been tested carry in their genome the DNA copy (provirus) of at least one of the murine classes of C-type RNA virus [1]. At any moment during the lifetime of a mouse, the proviral information can spontaneously be transcribed and translated, resulting in the production of complete infectious virus particles [1]. Because of the ubiquity of these viruses either as latent proviruses or as infectious particles, their involvement in the induction of lymphomas during chronic GVHRs deserves serious consideration.

Based on spread and replication in tissue culture, three classes of infectious murine C-type viruses can be distinguished: ecotropic, xenotropic, and amphotropic viruses. The in vitro host range behavior of these classes of virus is shown in Table 1. Xenotropic viruses have never been found to cause tumors under natural or laboratory conditions [86]. Amphotropic viruses were only recently detected [66] and might turn out to be important, naturally-occurring mediators of viral oncogenesis. Ecotropic viruses are naturally involved in tumor causation in strains that have been selected for high leukemia or lymphoma incidence, such as AKR [91, 127], as well as in strains that were not so selected [99, 111, 112] and in wild mice [45]. An important feature of oncogenesis by ecotropic viruses is that a correlation exists between the titer of infectious virus in mouse tissues and the chance of developing lymphoma or leukemia [45, 91, 99]: the higher the virus titer, the higher the chance of tumor development.

Of utmost importance for the current discussion is the natural pattern of expression of infectious, ecotropic viruses in the inbred mouse strains that have been used in the induction

Table 1. In vitro host range of endogenous C-type RNA virus of mice

Class	Host range	Types
Ecotropic virus	Spreads and replicates well in mouse cells but poorly if at all in cells of other species	*N-tropic virus*: replicates 10–1000 times better in Fv-$^{n/n}$ than in Fv-$1^{b/b}$ cells *B-tropic virus*: replicates 10–1000 times better in Fv-$1^{b/b}$ than in Fv-$1^{n/n}$ cells *NB-tropic virus*: replicates equally well in Fv-$1^{n/n}$ and Fv-$1^{b/b}$ cells
Xenotropic virus	Spreads and replicates in cells of other species but poorly if at all in mouse cells	
Amphotropic virus	Spreads and replicates well in both mouse cells and cells of other species	

of chronic GVHR. In high leukemia strains such as AKR, every single animal harbors large amounts of infectious virus within 3 weeks of birth [129]. In contrast, the low leukemia incidence strains such as BALB/c, C57BL/10 and its congenic strains employed in lymphoma induction by GVHR display a peculiar nonhomogeneous pattern of expression of C-type viruses. The majority of young animals of such strains do not harbor infectious ecotropic viruses [1, 9, 101, 109, 110, 127, 128]. Upon aging, the proportion of animals displaying expression of infectious virus increases, as is evident from both tests for infectious virus and from radioimmunossay for antibody to viral envelope antigens (VEA) [9, 44, 74, 75, 101, 109, 128]. The latter assay was found to be a reliable indicator of the presence of infectious virus [140].

In BALB/c (Fv-$1^{b/b}$] mice, N-tropic virus was the only ecotropic virus recovered from some young mice, whereas either N- or B- tropic viruses were recovered from a proportion of mice over 6 months of age [109, 128]. Hence, despite the fact that BALB/c mice are inbred, the phenotypic expression of C-type viruses in this strain is nonhomogeneous at any given age. Most of the ecotropic viruses and all of the xenotropic viruses observed in individual mice presumably represent derepression of endogenous RNA provirus [1].

In the GVHR, activation of latent C-type RNA virus was first described by HIRSCH et al. [71]. Ecotropic virus was recovered from the spleens of CAF_1 (BALB/c × A/J) mice that had been injected with BALB/c parental lymphocytes but not from the spleens of BALB/c mice of the same age as those whose cells were used for injection nor from the spleens of uninjected CAF_1 mice. Since then, the findings in the BALB/c → CAF_1 combination have been confirmed and extended [5, 7, 8, 9, 72]. Thus, it was postulated that such viruses were the etiologic agents responsible for the development of neoplasias during GVHR [7, 9, 71], and this view was thought to be strengthened by the observation that cell-free extracts prepared from the spleens of animals with GVHR upon injection into newborn hosts caused lymphoid tumors of the same histologic type as the GVHR-induced tumors [5, 7, 8, 9]. The oncogenic cell-free extracts from CAF_1 mice with GVHR uniformly contained B-tropic virus, and the view that B-tropic virus was responsible for tumorigenesis was supported by the finding that tumors arose in Fv-$1^{b/b}$ but not Fv-$1^{n/n}$ recipients of extract [7, 9].

Even though at face value these findings strongly argue in favor of a viral etiology for GVHR-associated neoplasms, with activation of endogenous DNA proviruses as the underlying mechanism, several objections against this attractive hypothesis can be raised. Firstly, SHERR et al. [143] failed to observe activation of ecotropic viruses during GVHR in the BALB/c → CAF_1 combination. They noted, in contrast, expression of endogenous xenotropic virus during GVHR, but not in CAF_1 mice injected with CAF_1 cells. Levy et al. [87] were likewise unable to confirm the activation of ecotropic viruses in CAF_1 mice injected with BALB/c spleen cells. Again, expression of endogenous xenotropic C-type viruses was seen in all animals with GVHR. The specificity of this finding for GVHR may be questioned, however: three out of nine uninjected CAF_1 mice and one out of seven control BALB/c mice injected with BALB/c spleen cells also expressed xenotropic virus. In fact, in a second study by the same investigators, GVHR and control mice all expressed xenotropic virus [29].

A similar lack of agreement exists with regard to activation of C-type viruses in mixed lymphocyte culture (MLC), the in vitro counterpart of the GVHR. Whereas HIRSCH et al. [72] reported the activation of ecotropic viruses in mixed lymphocyte culture, this could not be confirmed by SHERR et al. [143], DATTA et al. [27], and one of us (C.J.M., unpublished observations). The MLC studies of HIRSCH et al. [72] are inconclusive since their method of assay for ecotropic virus was much less sensitive than a technique developed later [100] and since they only tested for virus replicating in Fv-$1^{n/n}$ but not Fv-$1^{b/b}$ cells. Consequently, they may have overlooked the presence of infectious ecotropic virus in either BALB/c or CAF_1 spleen cell suspensions before they were mixed in culture. In our experience [27 and C.J.M., unpublished observations], ecotropic virus was only detected in MLC when it was already present in one of the two cell suspensions *before* MLC. Furthermore, HIRSCH et al. [72]

performed no titrations with carefully counted known numbers of cultured lymphocytes. They were, therefore, more likely to detect infectious virus in mixed (parent → F_1) cultures, since cell counts in MLC are higher than in control cultures.

Xenotropic virus was recovered by SHERR et al. [143] from mixed lymphocyte culture of BALB/c and NIH Swiss spleen cells but not from cultures containing either BALB/c or NIH Swiss spleen cells alone. This preliminary observation needs to be confirmed. It appears established beyond doubt that nonspecific B-lymphocyte mitogens such as lipopolysaccharide can induce the release of xenotropic virus from cultured lymphocytes [61, 103, 104, 113, 114, 136]. We will return later to the possible implications of this finding.

A major flaw in experimental designs to test the specific activation of C-type viruses in GVHR has been the regular omission of one essential control: injection of cells from the same pool of donor (usually BALB/c) spleen cells as used for the induction of GVHR into syngeneic (BALB/c) mice. In order to induce GVHR in an appreciable number of recipients, each recipient is injected with pooled inocula from a large number of donor mice. Any donor containing eco- or xenotropic viruses will contaminate the pool. As pointed out before, young BALB/c mice occasionally harbor ecotropic viruses [109,128]. Hence, contamination of the donor cell pool with virus is a real hazard. Next to virus assay of uninjected CAF_1 mice, it is necessary to test for virus in the spleens of BALB/c mice injected with the same pools of BALB/c spleen cells as inoculated into CAF_1 recipients. Assays for virus on the pooled BALB/c spleen cells at the time of injection [9] do not obviate the need for injection into syngeneic recipients; at the time of injection, the amount of spontaneously expressed infectious virus may still be below detectable levels. The injection of BALB/c spleen cells into syngeneic animals also serves the purpose of checking for age-dependent spontaneous expression of C-type RNA viruses which in this strain is known to increase with age [9, 109, 128]. Since BALB/c cells injected into CAF_1 recipients survive in these hosts [6, 51, 53], upon aging they may express C-type RNA viruses in the same way as BALB/c cells injected into syngeneic recipients. It is not unlikely that age-dependent expression of C-type viruses in BALB/c mice injected with large numbers of syngeneic spleen cells occurs earlier than in nonmanipulated BALB/c mice. Indeed, ARMSTRONG et al. [8, 9] detected N-tropic viruses early in the course of GVHR induced by infection of BALB/c spleen cells into CAF_1 recipients, but late in the course of GVHR they found B-tropic viruses in this combination. This corresponds precisely with the age-dependent expression of C-type viruses in natural BALB/c mice. In young BALB/c animals, only N-tropic virus was seen, and B-tropic virus appeared in mice over 6 months of age [9, 109, 128]. Furthermore, the oncogenic potency of cell free extracts from the spleens of GVHR mice in the studies of ARMSTRONG et al. [7, 8] was low. Not all newborn recipients of extract developed tumors, and the latent period before the appearance of lymphoreticular tumors was longer (mean 16 months) than the average latent period of lymphoma appearance after GVHR induction [6]. This corresponds again with the findings in normal BALB/c mice. B-tropic viruses isolated from such mice were similarly oncogenic upon injection into newborn syngeneic recipients after a comparably long latent period (about 15 months) [111, 112].

On the basis of these considerations, it appears likely that the enhanced expression of ecotropic viruses in the spleens of CAF_1 mice injected with BALB/c spleen cells represents age-related expression of ecotropic viruses in the BALB/c donor cells. This might have been detected by performing the syngeneic control experiment of injecting the same BALB/c donor spleen cells into BALB/c recipients. This important control experiment is notably absent in the studies claiming specific activation of ecotropic viruses in GVHR [5, 7, 8, 9, 71, 72]. When this control experiment was recently carried out by DATTA and SCHWARTZ [29], BALB/c recipients injected with BALB/c spleen cells were all positive for ecotropic viruses (B-tropic virus or a mixture of N- and B-tropic virus) and xenotropic virus, just like the CAF_1 recipients injected with the same pools of BALB/c spleen cells. This outcome raises serious doubts about the specificity of activation of ecotropic and xenotropic viruses during GVHR.

In several other parent → F_1 combinations, similar observations were made [29]. Despite the presence of eco- and xenotropic viruses in both GVHR animals and syngeneic control mice, lymphomas only developed in mice with GVHR. In one combination (SWR spleen cells injected into (SWR × NZB)F_1 recipients), lymphomas developed in the absence of expression of ecotropic viruses. Xenotropic virus was expressed in both experimental and syngeneic control animals. These findings indicate that GVHR-induced lymphomas can develop in the absence of detectable infectious ecotropic viruses.

In summary, ecotropic viruses do not appear to be specifically activated by GVHR nor in mixed lymphocyte reactions (MLR), the in vitro counterpart of GVHR. Furthermore, GVHR-associated lymphomas can develop in the absence of detectable ecotropic viruses. These considerations do not rule out a tumor-enhancing role of ecotropic viruses when present in GVHR-activated tissues. Specific activation of xenotropic viruses in GVHR is questionable since in one report such viruses were isolated more frequently from GVHR tissues than from the tissues of syngeneic control mice [87], whereas in a second study comparable titers of xenotropic virus were seen in both experimental and control animals [29]. An earlier report of specific activation of xenotropic virus during GVHR is hard to evaluate since the authors did not inject the same pool of donor (BALB/c) spleen cells into syngeneic recipients [143]. The same group of investigators [143] has reported the only instance of activation of xenotropic virus in mixed lymphocyte reaction in a well-controlled study, a result which needs confirmation. Extensive studies have shown that xenotropic viruses can be activated by nonspecific B-cell mitogens such as lipopolysaccharide, but not T-cell mitogens such as phytohemagglutinin and concanavalin A. Hence, activation of xenotropic viruses in MLR and GVHR, which are specific T-cell reactions, cannot be expected at first sight. It has been shown, however, that polyclonal B-cell activation is one of the sequelae of a protracted GVHR (cf. p. 293 and 299). Therefore, one of the several consequences of polyclonal B-cell activation might be the enhanced release of xenotropic viruses.

Xenotropic viruses were found in chronic GVHR whenever an assay was performed [29, 87, 143]. It is, therefore, impossible to decide at this moment whether lymphomas can develop during GVHR in the absence of detectable xenotropic virus. An oncogenic influence of xenotropic virus in this situation would be unique, however, since all assays for oncogenicity of xenotropic mouse viruses so far have been negative [86].

It remains to be elucidated whether GVHR-associated lymphomas develop independently of C-type virus expression or whether lymphoid tissues activated by chronic GVHR across H-2[1] differences provide a greatly favored microenvironment for the induction of lymphomas by C-type RNA viruses of otherwise low oncogenic potential. A possibility to be kept in mind is that lymphomas arising during chronic GVHR could be mediated by a class of oncogenic virus for which an assay has not yet been performed, such as the recently described recombinant virus of aging AKR mice [67]. Such a virus cannot be involved, however, in the causation of lymphomas seen after injection of SWR spleen cells into (SWR × NZB) F_1 recipients, since in this combination the virus recovered from animals with GVHR did not grow in mouse cells [29] and, therefore, could not have been like recombinant virus of AKR mice, which grows both in mouse cells and non-mouse cells.

Need for Donor T-Lymphocytes Reacting Toward an I-Region Incompatibility in the F_1 Recipient

In the F_1 hybrid recipients of parental strain spleen cells, a genetic disparity within the I-region of the H-2 complex was found to be necessary for lymphomagenesis [54]. Which one(s) of the

1 H-2 is the MHC of mice corresponding to HLA in man.

I-subregions is (are) responsible for this process remains to be determined. H-2 incompatibilities at the right hand side of the I-region, i.e., the D-, X(G)-, and S-regions, were found to be irrelevant; a possible participation of the K-region, however, cannot yet be excluded on the basis of the parent → F_1 hybrid combinations studied so far. *Non*-H-2 loci, including the minor lymphocyte stimulation (MLS) locus, were completely ineffective in triggering lymphomagenesis under the experimental conditions applied [52, 54]. On the grounds of these genetic histoincompatibility requirements and by analogy with acute GVH assays such as the popliteal lymph node assay, Simonsen splenomegaly assay, and MLR, which all require a T-cell anti-I-region reaction for maximal lymphocyte stimulation, it was postulated that T-lymphocytes among the donor spleen cells also represented the critical cell population for the induction of lymphadenopathy in the chronic GVHR [for references, see 54].

Preliminary experimental results obtained recently corroborate this concept. Thus, administration of C57Bl/10 cortisone-resistant thymocytes of (C57BL/10 × DBA/2) F_1 recipients proved to be capable of inducing not only autoantibodies to erythrocytes [50] and nuclear antigens but, in some of the 6-month survivors of these experiments, also immunoblastic sarcoma (E.G. and H.G., unpublished observations). In contrast, when the same numbers of C57BL/10 bone marrow cells were administered to F_1 hybrids, neither autoantibody production [50] nor malignant lymphomas (unpublished data) were induced. The morphology of the lymphomas induced by cortisone-resistant parental thymocytes showed no differences from that of tumors induced by parental spleen cells. When these lymphomas were typed in a complement-mediated cytotoxicity test using antisera against Thy 1.1 and the H-2 antigens of C57BL/10 and DBA/2, more than 95% of the tumor cells were found to be of F_1 origin while the percentage of Thy 1.1-positive lymphocytes was not increased (E.G., unpublished results). Apparently the injected donor T cells had triggered a persistent proliferation of non-T cells of the F_1 recipient. A possible mechanism for this persistent lymphoproliferation will be discussed below (p. 299).

Determination of Host and Donor Type Lymphomas

The initiation of lymphomas during the GVHR is a consequence of an immune reaction of the donor against the recipient [6, 52]. Since immune responses involve proliferation of lymphocytes, the theoretic expectation has always been that GVHR-induced lymphomas should consist of donor cells that were persistently stimulated by F_1 antigens [138, 161]. However, the majority of neoplasms induced by the chronic GVHR actually consists predominantly of host cells [53, 54]. In this respect, lymphoproliferation during the chronic GVHR again essentially parallels the one observed during acute GVHRs [36, 54, 82]. According to our pathogenetic concept of GVH-induced lymphomas (see p. 299), both donor type and host type lymphomas depend on a common primary event, a persistent anti-F_1 reaction of parental T cells, which *non*specifically recruits all other cells in the tumor whether they be donor or host-derived. This concept is consistent with the results of Hilgard [70], who studied the contribution of bone marrow cells to the development of splenomegaly in irradiated F_1 mice injected with various mixtures of nonirradiated parental and F_1 cells. While the immunologic specificity required for initiation of splenomegaly was found to rest in parental thymus cells, bone marrow cells acted synergistically in that they increased splenomegaly. It is relevant to our argument that no differences were found whether bone marrow cells of F_1 hybrids or the donor strain were added to the parental thymus cells.

Pathogenetic Concept of the Development of GVH-Induced Immunoblastic Sarcoma

Previous investigations on the pathogenesis of malignant lymphomas in GVH F_1 mice can best be summarized by the following statement: for the development of immunoblastic sarcoma (reticulum cell sarcoma) during the GVHR, *immunocompetent parental T-lymphocytes must react towards incompatible I-region structures* of the F_1 hybrid. As we have already mentioned, these immunogenetic requirements for triggering of long-term lymphocyte proliferation in vivo, i.e., lymphomagenesis, are identical with those needed for maximal lymphocyte stimulation in short-term assays such as Simonsen's splenomegaly assay, the popliteal lymph node assay, and the in vitro mixed lymphocyte reaction [54]. In view of this stringent parallelism, we feel encouraged to apply the principles derived from investigations of maximal lymphoproliferation during the short-term GVH assays to explain lymphocyte proliferation during the chronic GVHR. The reader should be aware, however, that this approach is based on analogy and is therefore speculative.

A major assumption in this approach, which has been discussed in detail elsewhere [54], holds that the anti-H-2 reaction of parental T-lymphocytes in GVH F_1 mice persists during the entire period of progressive lymphoreticular hyperplasia, i.e., for at least several months. If existent, this persistent anti-F_1 reaction of parental T cells could readily explain the progressive proliferation of other lymphoreticular cells such as F_1 B cells on the basis of a persistent lymphokine release by the ongoing immune response. Studies using short-term assays, including the MLR, have provided solid evidence for the release of mitogenic lymphokines during GVHR. With respect to the pathogenesis of GVH lymphomas consisting mostly of F_1 B cells, the phenomenon of *backstimulation* [162] seems to be particularly relevant. It denotes the fact that parental T-lymphocytes, when co-cultivated in vitro with H-2-different F_1 lymphoreticular cells, release mitogenic factor(s) into the culture medium which can induce a marked proliferation of various F_1 cells, in particular F_1 B cells [65, 115, 162].

Recently, Romano and co-workers [125] demonstrated that this backstimulation of F_1 B cells under the influence of a parental T-cell signal also occurs in vivo. The assay used was measurement of ^{3}H-thymidine uptake by nonirradiated F_1 B cells that were injected together with mitomycin-treated parental T cells into irradiated H-2 heterozygous F_1 hybrids. If B cells of the parental donor, instead of the F_1 hybrid, were injected along with the parental T cells, they could likewise be recruited into proliferation by the parental T-signal. However, parental B cells alone were unable to respond to the F_1 antigens. Earlier studies on the development of GVH splenomegaly induced by parental lymphocytes in H-2-incompatible irradiated F_1 recipients had already demonstrated a synergism between parental T cells and parental bone marrow cells [12, 70] as well as between parental T cells and F_1 bone marrow cells [70]. As we have already mentioned, both the initiation and the specificity of the immune responses were found to rest completely in the parental T cell population.

Rolstad [123] and Rolstad and Fossum [124] also found that when *non*-irradiated MHC-heterozygous F_1 hybrids were used as recipients of parental T cells, the overwhelming majority of cells in the enlarged popliteal lymph nodes were host cells. While the majority of the proliferating cells were B cells, macrophages did not proliferate. These authors argued that mitogenic signals *selective* for B cells need not be postulated to account for the preferential proliferation of host B cells as compared to host T cells, since these two lymphocyte populations normally have different migration pathways and transit times through lymphatic tissues [73] and might thus be unequally exposed to nonselective mitogenic signals.

Together with the mitotic stimulation of F_1 B cells, Romano et al. [125] also noted a typical allogeneic effect [77] in their system, i.e., an enhanced anti-hapten response of primed F_1 B cells stimulated by parental T cells and hapten on a noncross-reacting carrier. Their findings seem to be closely related to the rapid formation of Fc receptor-bearing host cells [24], host plasma cells [92, 156], and autoantibodies [92] in F_1 hybrids undergoing short-term GVHR.

Since in the *chronic* GVH model the injection of parental strain T cells into MHC-incompatible F_1 hybrids likewise leads to polyclonal autoantibody responses [39, 50, 154] and host cell proliferation in the B cell-dependent areas [50, 54], it is very likely that the same mechanisms of nonspecific B cell stimulation as in the acute GVHR and the MLR are involved. If this argument is correct, the main difference between the two systems would lie in the different observation periods: while in the MLR and the acute GVHR the observation times range from 3 days to maximally 2–3 weeks, they range from about 3 weeks up to 2 years in the chronic GVHR, with a minimum of 4 months required for the formation of malignant lymphoma [54]. Several other investigations may be quoted which all lend further support to the concept that proliferation of F_1 lymphoid cells during the GVHR is procured by nonspecific mitotic factors released by those parental T cells which specifically react towards the incompatible H-2 structures on F_1 cells. Using their in vitro system of GVHR, AUERBACH and GLOBERSON [11] showed that parental spleen cells released a factor into the culture medium which was able to pass through a cell-impermeable millipore membrane and cause considerable cell proliferation and enlargement of F_1 hybrid spleen fragments cultured in the same medium. This in vitro splenomegaly was accompanied by many of the histologic changes of the in vivo GVHR. WARD and VOLKMAN [164] demonstrated that mixtures of allogeneic lymphoid cells in vitro produced a monocyte-chemotactic factor and were able to isolate a similar factor from ongoing local GVHRs in the kidneys of F_1 rats which had been injected with parental thoracic duct cells 1 week before. Interesting results were also obtained by KORČÁKOVÁ and HAŠKOVÁ [81] who measured RNA synthesis in the popliteal lymph nodes of mice 24 h after injection of soluble products into the hind feet. The products were obtained from the supernatants of in vitro MLRs. Supernatants from cells differing only at non-H-2 loci had no activating effect, whereas a significant degree of lymph node activation occurred after injection of the supernatants from mixed cultures derived from H-2 congeneic-resistant strains. The active products reacted with lymph nodes of *both* the parental donor strain and the F_1 hybrid, a finding which corrobrated the authors' conclusion that the factor was lymphokine and not an immunogen. ROEHM [122], who assayed the mitogenic effect of cell-free medium from murine MLRs upon spleen fragments cultured in vitro, essentially reached the same conclusions. Recently, however, DATTA and SCHWARTZ [28] offered an explanation for the proliferation of F_1 hybrid cells during chronic GVHR which differs from the explanation given above. They propose that the progressive hyperplasia of F_1 lymphoid cells results from a specific immune response toward the parent's idiotypic recognition structures that are complementary to the MHC components of the F_1 hybrid [14]. The present authors consider this to be an unlikely explanation for the following reasons:

1. Idiotypes are weak immunogens, which require extensive immunization before anti-idiotypic antibodies appear. With parental anti-F_1 idiotypes of mice in particular, antibodies often fail to develop even after prolonged immunization (E. P. RIEBER and G. RIETHMÜLLER, personal communication).
2. If a specific anti-idiotype response of the F_1 hybrid were to account for the tremendous host cell proliferation during the GVHR, one would have to assume the presence of a single clone whose proliferative capacity by far exceeds that of other clones reacting to much stronger immunogens. In contrast to this assumption, however, the stimulatory effect of the GVHR can nonspecifically enhance proliferation of several clones, e.g., those reacting to xenogeneic erythrocytes [79, 93, 108]. Observations of KORČÁKOVÁ et al. [82] obtained with the popliteal lymph node assay in MHC-different rats are also relevant here. While histologic changes in the node were very similar in both the GVHR (parent → F_1) and the host-versus-graft reaction (HVGR) (F_1 → parent), the extent of lymphoreticular proliferation and trapping was two to three times higher in the GVHR than the HVGR. Thus, under otherwise identical experimental conditions, lymph node enlargement in the GVHR exceeded that seen during an immune response to highly immunogenic antigens. Furthermore, the kinetics of the popliteal lymph node assay using presensitized donor cells also fail to favor the anti-idiotype response as a cause of host cell proliferation. Using as their donor inoculum parental spleen cells that were presensitized to F_1 antigens, EMESON and THURSH [37] and one of us (E.G., unpublished data) found that not only the magnitude but also the speed of popliteal lymph node enlargement was significantly enhanced. The accelerated F_1 response in this experimental setting can only be

attributed to preimmunization of donor cells, but not to an accelerated specific reaction of the recipient.
3. Since anti-F_1 idiotypes were found to be present on both parental T and B cells [14], these cells should exert a comparable stimulatory effect on F_1-lymphocytes according to the anti-idiotype concept. However, only parental T cells, but not B cells, can induce the proliferation of F_1 cells seen during the MLR (65, 115, 162), popliteal lymph node assay [13], and SIMONSEN'S splenomegaly assay [19, 58] as well as the chronic GVHR [50, 54, and p. 298).
4. The anti-idiotype concept fails to account for why under identical experimental conditions one GVHR F_1 mouse may develop a lymphoma consisting predominantly of F_1 cells, while the lymphoma of another animal consists of donor cells (mostly non-T cells) [53, 55]. By contrast, according to the findings of ROMANO et al. [125] and HILGARD [70], mentioned above, both host and donor type lymphomas can readily be explained by a persistent release of nonspecific mitogenic signals from F_1-reactive parental T cells; this is followed by proliferation of adjacent cells irrespective of whether these are donor or host derived.
5. Finally, in view of the results obtained by BINZ [13], it is much easier to visualize how an anti-idiotype response by the recipient could mitigate the donor's anti-F_1 response and, as a consequence, depress the proliferation of host cells rather than stimulate it. BINZ showed that preincubation of parental spleen cells with certain anti-idiotype sera and complement eliminated the F_1-reactive parental T cells able to initiate popliteal lymph node enlargement.
We shall conclude this section on the pathogenesis of GVH lymphomas with a more general remark. While the facts allowed us to discuss the mechanism responsible for initiation of lymphoreticular hyperplasia and, possibly, also for its progression, the final step responsible for transition from hyperplasia to malignancy is completely unknown. Unfortunately, in this respect, neoplasia in the chronic GVHR is no exception from other models of tumor development.

T-Cell Reactions Toward Self-MHC Structures

Apart from bone marrow transplantation, the possible relevance of animal GVHRs as models for the pathogenesis of human diseases is two-fold. First, the possibility exists that maternal T cells occasionally pass across the placenta to the fetus and induce GVHRs [137]. Secondly and more importantly, there is now evidence that T cells can react toward self-MHC structures in an essentially similar way as they react toward allogeneic MHC structures. This opens up the possibility that T-cell anti-MHC reactions, which take place between the cells of *one* individual, may lead to the same pathologic symptoms as seen in F_1 hybrids infected with parental strain T cells. That T-lymphocytes also recognize MHC structures that are genetically identical was discovered by ZINKERNAGEL and DOHERTY [167] and SHEARER [141] and subsequently confirmed and extended by many investigators [15, 17, 30, 40, 59, 83, 88, 116, 121, 134, 160]. Cells whose surfaces were altered by either an infection with one of a variety of different viruses or coupling of a hapten to their membrane could all elicit a strong immune response by MHC identical *killer* (T^K) T cells. In each case so far analyzed, both the foreign antigen introduced by infectious agent or hapten *and* self-MHC structures had to be present on target cells for effective cytotoxicity by killer T cells (32, 38, 41, 42, 47, 60, 69, 133, 135). More exactly, the H-2 structures involved were specified by the D- and/or K-regions of H-2 [15, 40, 121, 142, 168], the same structures which also elicit maximal cytotoxicity in allogeneic T-cell killing [107, 132]. In the case of hapten-modified cells, this H-2 restriction of T cell recognition exists even though the hapten was also shown to be attached to membrane structures other than H-2 [42].
Recent findings of MILLER and co-workers [102] indicate that for the expression of *delayed-type hypersensitivity* to heterologous proteins or dinitrofluorobenzene, primed T cells must also

match the cells in their environment with respect to H-2 structures. In the case of hypersensitivity to fowl γ-globulin, identity at the I-A-subregion was shown to be critical. Comparable results were recently obtained by ZINKERNAGEL and colleagues [166] who investigated the histocompatibility requirements for expression of delayed-type hypersensitivity to *Listeria monocytogenes*. It is probably significant in this context that a typical delayed cutaneous hypersensitivity reaction can also be elicited by the parent → F_1 hybrid GVHR and that here again the only antigens capable of eliciting this reaction were specified by the F_1 hybrid's H-2 complex [150].

Finally coming to *T-B cell cooperation* in antibody production, it has been shown that identity at the I-A and I-B-subregions of H-2 is required for effective cooperation between hapten-specific precursor B cells and carrier-specific T^H cells (a subclass of T-lymphocytes which help B-lymphocytes to produce antibody) primed in a self-environment [78]. In the presence of allogeneic I-region structures [54] on hapten-primed B cells or macrophages, unprimed T cells may cooperate with B cells via the allogeneic effect, i.e., in the absence of a carrier molecule for hapten [77, 84, 97]. Whether alterations of autologous cell membranes by viruses or chemicals are likewise capable of eliciting help from unprimed T^H cells is a matter of speculation at present. By analogy to T^K cells reacting to the foreign antigen plus self-D/K-region structures, T^H cells in this situation would have to react to the foreign antigen *and* self-I-region structure. That such effects may occur is tentatively suggested by a recent observation of WAGNER and colleagues [163]. When they cultured hapten-modified spleen cells together with syngeneic T cells, they noted the generation not only of specific T^K cells reacting toward hapten and self-D/K-region structures, but also of "allogeneic effect factor", which was able to bypass the need for T^H cells in the in vitro antibody response of B cells to sheep red blood cells.

These and other findings lead to the conclusion that MHC structures, whether they are allogeneic or self, play a unique role in T cell triggering and effector function. T^K cells preferentially react toward structures coded by the D- and K-region, while T^H cells and T^D cells (a hypothetic subclass of T cells concerned specifically with delayed hypersensitivity [16]) preferentially react toward certain I-region structures [16, 20, 105, 120]. What is still unknown is the nature of T cell receptors and their precise mode of recognition of self-MHC structures plus antigen on the one hand and allogeneic MHC structures on the other. These controversial issues were discussed in recent review articles [16, 26, 31, 76, 105, 120].

If our concept that T cell reactions toward allogeneic MHC structures are essentially similar to T cell reactions toward antigen in an autologous system is valid, then the diseases induced by T cell anti-MHC reactions during GVHR can be considered to be prototypes for the pathogenesis of the same diseases developing after infections and exposure to sensitizing chemicals such as drugs. Thus, a unifying pathogenetic concept is offered for a variety of diseases which may be caused by multiple etiologic agents (Table 2). What all these different etiologic agents are postulated to have in common is a nonselective alteration of cell surfaces of lymphoid cells which, from the point of view of T cells, is indistinguishable from specific binding of antigen to the cell surface.

Possible Relationship Between Reactions of T Cells Toward Self-MHC Structures and Lymphomagenesis Caused by Viral Infections or Sensitizing Drugs

One candidate lesion in man, where a T cell anti-MHC reaction might be involved, is postvaccination lymphadenopathy, which in some individuals develops locally after inoculation of vaccinia virus. In most cases, this is a benign transient lesion, but occasionally it is

Table 2. Pathologic symptoms shared by GVHR chimeras and nonchimeric human beings suffering from viral infections or drug allergy[a]

Pathologic symptoms	Conditions for which a common pathogenesis is postulated				
	Systemic GVHR		Representative conditions in nonchimeric human patients		
	Hamster or mouse (parent → F_1)	Man	Allergy to hydantoin	Infectious mononucleosis	Smallpox vaccination
Dermatitis (especially maculopapular or erythematous rash)	+	+	+	+	
Toxic epidermal necrolysis[b]	+	+	+		+
Hepatitis	+	+	+	+	
Hyper- or dysgammaglobulinemia	+	+	+	+	
Nephrotic syndrome and/or immune complex glomerulonephritis	+		+	+	+
Autoantibodies to:					
Erythrocytes	+		+	+	
Lymphocytes	+		+	+	
Nuclear antigens	+		+	+	
Lymphoreticular hyperplasia due to proliferation of reticulum cells and histiocytes	+	+	+	+	+
Malignant lymphomas (reticulum cell sarcoma, lymphosarcoma, or Hodgkin's disease)	+		+		+[c]

[a] For detailed bibliography, see reference [49].
[b] Toxic epidermal necrolysis (Lyell's disease) is probably but an extreme variant of multiform erythema and Stevens-Johnson syndrome [49].
[c] Validity of diagnosis not certain.

indistinguishable from Hodgkin's disease or reticulum cell sarcoma [18, 68]. Today, the latter lesion is diagnosed as immunoblastic sarcoma (see contributions by K. Lennert and R. J. Lukes, this volume). In mice, a generalized lymphadenopathy termed "reticulosis with transition to hemocytoblastosis" was observed after injection of live vaccinia virus at the age of 2 weeks [96]. It is probably significant here that this virus will also lead, by an unknown mechanism, to the appearance of strongly immunogenic *allogeneic* H-2 specificities on the membrane of infected cells [46] and elicit a T^K cell reaction toward virus-induced antigen plus self-H-2 [83]. Conceivably, the failure of young immature mice to react with a vigorous cytotoxic T cell response and, instead, react preferentially by T^H and T^D cells toward the MHC structures of vaccinia-infected cells led to the development of GVH-like lymphadenopathy after infection with this virus. It is of interest in this context that other nononcogenic viruses of man such as the rubella virus may also mimic immunoblastic sarcoma in certain individuals (see discussion remark of K. Lennert after contribution of R. J. Lukes).

Another malignant lymphoma to be discussed in this context is the spontaneously developing reticulum cell sarcoma of SJL mice [34, 106]. Like the lymphomas developing in the NZB strain and in GVH F_1 mice, the tumor of SJL is a B cell lymphoma [21, 145, 157]. In a series of elegant studies, Thorbecke and her colleagues demonstrated that Ia antigens, or unknown antigens closely associated with them, on normal B cells as well as lymphoma cells from SJL mice induced an extremely strong in vitro proliferation in the T cells from normal syngeneic mice [117] without any accompanying development of cytotoxic cells [118]. At the present, it is not known whether the strong T cell response in SJL mice contributes to lymphomagenesis by the mechanism of backstimulation as discussed above or whether it is an epiphenomenon and B cell lymphomagenesis progresses independently of T cells. The latter possibility is favored by the observation that neonatal thymectomy does not decrease the incidence of reticulum cell sarcomas in the SJL strain [64, 98]. Possibly leukemogenic viruses, which appear to be present in this strain [23, 25], stimulate B cells directly.

The distinction between these two possibilities, which are not mutually exclusive, is of general importance. It also arises in the context of Epstein-Barr virus (EBV) infections in man. While on the one hand this virus is a polyclonal B cell stimulator [126] and may thus directly lead to the lymphadenopathy and autoantibody formation of infectious mononucleosis (Table 2), on the other hand it also elicits a strong response to the infected B cells by autologous T cells [130]. The latter finding is, of course, reminiscent of the GVHR. Future experiments will have to determine if only T^K cells are generated in response to the EBV-infected B cells or if T^K and T^D cells respond as well, which by analogy with the GVHR, might aggravate the autoantibody formation and lymphadenopathy of infectious mononucleosis.

An example of in vivo MLR between congeneic lymphocytes which emphasizes the pathogenetic potential of T cell anti-MHC reactions will now be discussed. KOBOW and WEILER [80] recently showed that the onset of wasting syndrome characteristic of aging athymic BALB/c nu/nu mice can be markedly enhanced by the administration of small numbers of thymus cells from congeneic BALB/c +/nu mice. Furthermore, spleen cells from wasting nudes, but not from healthy ones, caused popliteal lymph node enlargement when injected into adult BALB/c +/nudes and a typical runt disease (including lymphoreticular alterations) after injection into newborn BALB/c +/nudes. Preliminary findings suggested that donor and host had to be identical at H-2 in order to elicit runt disease in their system (U. KOBOW and E. WEILER, personal communication). These observations may be explained by the following assumption: the H-2 structures of BALB/c nu/nu mice were rendered "foreign" by undefined viral infections from which nu/nu mice suffer because of their lack of T cells. These "altered" MHC structures were capable of eliciting strong GVH- and HVG-like responses, respectively, by congeneic T cells. An observation that may be explained in a corresponding fashion was recently made when spleen cells obtained from 15-month-old inbred mice, which had been depleted of T cells at 2 months (B mice), were used in a syngeneic transfer system. Such cells, when injected into the hind feet of intact syngeneic animals, often caused an enormous degree of popliteal lymph node enlargement after 4-7 days. The magnitude of this response was sometimes even greater than that regularly detectable after injection of H-2-incompatible allogeneic spleen cells from normal mice (E.G., unpublished finding).

Immunoblastic lymphadenopathy, which occasionally appears to progress into immunoblastic sarcoma (cf. contributions by H. RAPPAPORT, R. J. LUKES, and G. FLANDRIN, in this volume), also deserves consideration here. Although this disease has been given different names such as "immunoblastic lymphadenopathy" [95], "angioimmunoblastic lymphadenopathy with dysproteinemia" [43], and "lymphogranulomatosis X" [119], it nevertheless may represent a nosologic entity. FRIZZERA et al. [43] pointed out that not only the histopathology of these lymphomas but also the accompanying constitutional symptoms and autoantibodies (cf. 63) are highly reminiscent of the GVHR in laboratory animals. We might add that this provocative view is further supported by two other observations made in these patients, i.e., dysgammaglobulinemia and angiogenesis in the T cell region of the affected lymph nodes. Both dysgammaglobulinemia [49, 153] and local angiogenesis [144] can be specific products of GVHR. Moreover, immunoblastic lymphadenopathy resembles not only the lymphoreticular alterations seen during GVHR but also those of infectious mononucleosis, hypersensitivity to hydantoin, and post vaccinal lymphadenopathy [18, 95, 119], which are discussed elsewhere in this article. Another symptom noted in several of the patients with immunoblastic lymphadenopathy was hypersensitivity to one of a variety of different drugs [95, 119]. A rational explanation for the development of this complex immunologic disorder would be a GVH-like reaction that was triggered by either viruses or fixation of a drug to the surface of lymphocytes (including B cells) and the subsequent reaction of T cells to their MHC structures and the drug [49, 54].

The lymphadenopathy and generalized autoimmunization induced by the antiepileptic drug *hydantoin* (for references, see 49] are of special interest in this context. Benign as well as malignant lymphomas have been described after hydantoin intake, and some of these tumors were diagnosed as immunoblastic sarcoma [4, 90, and the contribution by G. Rausing, this volume). Although this small hapten is *not* a B cell mitogen, and thus differs from EBV, it can nevertheless mimic all the symptoms of infectious mononucleosis including those of lymphadenopathy (Table 2). According to our hypothesis, this amazing effect may be explained by the single assumption that the drug attaches to the surface of lymphocytes and then elicits T cell anti-MHC reactions comparable to the GVHR [49].

Autoimmunity in the Semiallogeneic GVH Model

Like virtually all other pathologic lesions developing during the GVHR, autoantibody formation can only be induced by a reaction of parental T cells toward incompatible MHC structures of the F_1 recipient [54]. According to Weigle [165] and Allison and colleagues [2, 3,], B cells with the capacity to form antibodies toward those self-antigens which circulate in soluble form and at low concentration normally exist in all healthy individuals but fail to produce autoantibodies due to low zone tolerance on the part of autologous T cells. In F_1 hybrid animals, the lack of T cell cooperation can be overcome by the injection of parental T cells, which provide "help" by reacting toward incompatible MHC stuctures of the autoreactive B cells or nearby macrophages, i.e., via the allogeneic effect [77, 84, 97].

Autoimmune Hemolytic Anemia of GVH F_1 Animals

The development of antibodies to erythrocytes is the best studied example of GVHR-induced autoantibody formation. By means of immunoglobulin allotype analysis, it was demonstrated [50, 92] that the anti-RBC antibodies arising in H-2-incompatible F_1 recipients of parental thymocytes or lymph node cells were indeed autoantibodies, i.e., of F_1 hybrid origin. An analysis of the serologic specificities of anti-RBC antibodies induced in MHC-incompatible F_1 hamsters, which had received parental thymocytes and lymph node cells, showed that these antibodies failed to possess the narrow specificity expected from donor anti-host alloantibodies but reacted with multiple antigens. At least some of these antigens were also present on red blood cells obtained from the parental donor and from other strains and species [154], a finding that was recently confirmed in mice [50]. Hence, at the level of autoantibodies produced by F_1 B cells, the response failed to be specific for MHC specificities. In sharp contrast, however, an anti-MHC response was shown to be essential at the level of parental T cells [50], as shown schematically in Figure 2.

Antinuclear Autoantibodies of GVH F_1 mice

The induction of antinuclear autoantibodies in GVH F_1 mice was first reported by Fialkow et al. [39]. It has recently been shown that an H-2 incompatibility in the recipients was an absolute requirement for induction of such antibodies, since they were found in 100% of the H-2 heterozygous backcross recipients of parental spleen cells, but in none of the H-2 homozygous recipients of such cells. The animals used in that experiment were [(C57BL/10 × DBA/2)F_1

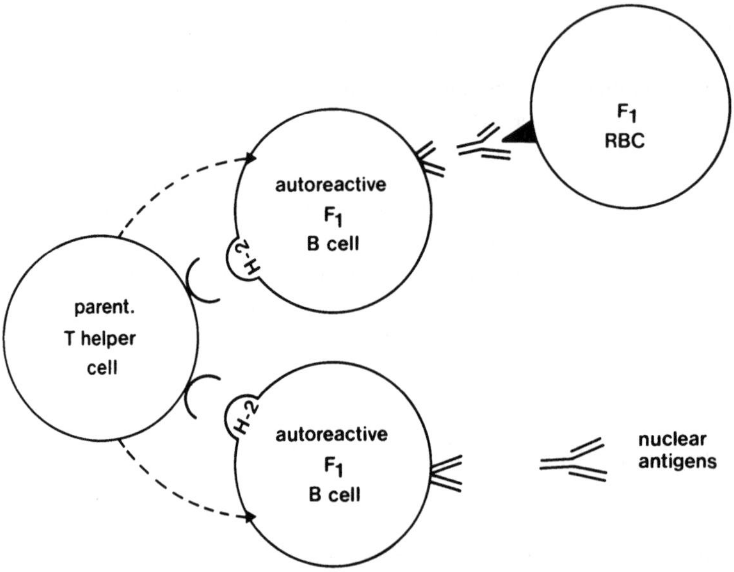

Fig. 2. Hypothetic scheme of autoimmunization through the allogeneic effect of GVHR. Parental T-lymphocytes, which were injected into an F_1 hybrid, react toward the genetically foreign H-2 structures on normally present autoreactive B cells and/or nearby macrophages (not shown). Thereafter, T cells release soluble factor(s) (see arrows), which enable B cells to differentiate into 7S antibody-secreting plasma cells. While the specificity of T cell reactivity is restricted to H-2, that of autoantibodies is not. It is proposed that essentially the same sequence of events will take place if T cells, instead of reacting to allogeneic MHC structures, react to autologous ones that were rendered foreign by viruses or drugs

× C57BL/10] backcrosses that were injected with C57 BL/10 cells (E.G., unpublished results). They were the same animals that also served to demonstrate the H-2 dependency of autoantibody formation to erythrocytes [50]

Immune Complex Glomerulonephritis of GVH F_1 Mice

In a number of murine parent → F_1 hybrid combinations, a typical nephrotic syndrome due to immune complex glomerulonephritis may result from the injection of parental strain spleen cells [56, 89]. It may or may not be associated with lymphomagenesis [52, 56] and, as far as tested, always seems to be accompanied by the formation of anti-erythrocyte and antinuclear autoantibodies (H.G., unpublished data). Once again, T-lymphocytes were demonstrated to be the critical cell population for induction of the disease by the parental donor strain [54, 57], while an incompatibility at H-2 was required of the F_1 recipient [54, 56]. Upon closer genetic analysis, an incompatibility somewhere within the K-end of H-2 (K-region plus I-region) was shown to be necessary [48, 54].

Using a fluorescein-labeled antiserum specific for the Ig^b allotype of strain C57BL/10, which was a gift from M. Bosma, it has recently been shown that at least a substantial portion of the glomerular antibodies were of host origin (H.G., unpublished). The nephritic kidneys used in this experiment were obtained from the combination DBA/2 → (C57BL/10 × DBA)2F_1. When antibodies were eluted from these kidneys and tested in the indirect Coombs' test, they were found to lack the narrow specificity of donor anti-host alloantibodies but to react also with erythrocytes and lymphocytes from the T cell donor DBA/2 [54]. A limitation of these experiments is that no quantitative absorption studies have been performed so far. Therefore, it is not known *how many* of the glomerular immune complexes contained soluble cell surface antigens. Since the GVHR induces a generalized autoantibody formation, it is conceivable that other antigens, for instance nuclear antigens, may also be involved in the glomerular immune complexes of GVH F_1 mice.

Other Pathologic Symptoms of GVH F_1 Animals

It is important to realize that the possible pathologic consequences of T cell anti-MHC reactions encompass more than merely the direct killing of target cells, the induction of autoreactive B cells via the allogeneic effect, or the triggering of lymphoproliferation. Thus, in GVH F_1 hamsters, a generalized dissolution of the dermal-epidermal junction diagnosed as *toxic epidermal necrolysis*, was observed and was often a lethal disease. The mechanism triggering this disease was shown to be a reaction of parental T-lymphocytes toward MHC-disparate F_1 lymphoid cells, epidermolysis being only a bystander effect [151, 152].

SIDKY and AUERBACH [144] noted a striking *formation of new blood vessels* at the site of T cell administration into the dermis of mice. They provided solid experimental evidence that full-blown angiogenesis was initiated solely by a T cell anti-MHC reaction. Interestingly, angiogenesis may also be a conspicuous feature of another lesion elicited by T-lymphocytes, the tuberculin reaction (K. LENNERT, personal communication). Finally, a *serum sickness syndrome* involving vasculitis, polyarthritis, carditis, dermatitis, and alterations of the lymphoreticular tissue has been reported in rats undergoing a chronic GVHR [147, 148]. Unfortunately, the cellular and histoincompatibility requirements of this interesting model have not been analyzed so that, in this case, it is unknown whether a T cell anti-MHC reaction was indeed needed for triggering the syndrome.

Possible Relationships Between Reactions of T Cells Toward Self-MHC Structures and Autoimmune Diseases Caused by Viral Infections or Sensitizing Drugs

Our hypothesis postulates that the combined recognition of self-MHC structures and antigens such as viruses and drugs may elicit T cell reactions comparable to the GVHR and consequently, lymphadenopathy and/or a generalized autoimmunization as in the GVHR (Table 2). The following pieces of indirect evidence are compatible with this concept:

1. As already mentioned (p. 303), an "allogenic effect factor" was produced by T^H cells cocultured with hapten-modified syngeneic stimulator cells [163], a system that is already known to generate T^K cell reactions toward hapten *and* D/K-region structures [40, 142].
2. Cells infected by Friend leukemia virus will elicit a cytotoxic reaction toward self-MHC structures *and* virus-induced antigen by syngeneic or autologous T^K cells [17]. In rats injected with low doses of Friend lymphatic leukemia virus at birth, several observations were made that are highly reminiscent of a GVHR across a MHC barrier. These animals developed the typical signs of an acute GVHR, and by lymphocyte transfer experiments, it was shown that their symptoms were procured by a specific reaction of spleen and lymph node cells to virus-induced antigens on infected cells [155]. Particularly relevant to the discussion of autoimmunity is the fact some of these animals developed Coombs-positive hemolytic anemia and membranous glomerulonephritis with elevated proteinuria [85], diseases that can be specific products of T-cell anti-MHC reactions [50, 54]. In this context, it is noteworthy that Friend virus appears to infect and alter splenic B cells but not T cells [22].
3. In the congeneic donor → recipient system involving BALB/c +/nu mice as T-cell donors for athymic BALB/c nu/nu recipients which was described above (p. 304), not only symptoms of

acute GVHR can be induced [80] but also a significantly enhanced formation of autoantibodies against erythrocytes (E. GLEICHMANN, H. GLEICHMANN, W. DE RIESE, C. DE RIESE, Autoantibody Formation in Athymic Nude Mice Procured and Inhibited by Congeneic T-lymphocytes, in preparation). The assumed pathogenetic mechanism in this system is a reaction of normal T^H cells toward syngeneic H-2 structures of recipient which were rendered foreign by infectious agents from which athymic nude mice are known to suffer. It was formally demonstrated in the parent → F_1 hybrid model that incompatible H-2 structures of the recipient were the only antigens capable of triggering formation of autoantibodies to red blood cells [50].

Concluding Remarks and Summary

In F_1 hybrid animals undergoing chronic GVHR, autoantibody formation is triggered by the abnormal help provided to normally present but inactive autoreactive B cells of the F_1 recipient by donor T cells reacting to their incompatible H-2 structures (allogeneic effect). The present authors favor the view that a related immunologic mechanism termed *backstimulation* is responsible for the proliferation of H-2-incompatible F_1 B cells in the presence of donor T cells. The persistent proliferation, mainly of F_1 B cells, eventually leads to the development of immunoblastic sarcoma in GVH F_1 mice. Immunosuppression fails to play a role in lymphomagenesis of the GVHR.

The evidence for the claim that GVH-associated lymphomas are caused by latent leukemia viruses that are specifically activated by the GVHR has been critically reviewed. At present, it is unresolved whether GVH-induced lymphomas develop independently of C-type RNA virus expression or whether lymphoid tissues stimulated by chronic GVHR provide a greatly favored microenvironment for a virus of otherwise low oncogenic potential. The possibility cannot be excluded that GVH lymphomagenesis is caused by C-type RNA viruses for which an assay has not yet been developed.

The hypothesis has been discussed that the spontaneously developing (angio-) immunoblastic lymphadenopathy of man as well as the various autoantibodies and constitutional symptoms, which often accompany this disease, may also be mediated by reactions of T-lymphocytes toward incompatible MHC structures on adjacent lymphoid cells. This concept is based on two different lines of experimental evidence:

1. Results obtained with animal GVH models, in which immunoblastic sarcoma, angiogenesis, and autoantibody formation are known to be induced by reactions of parental T-lymphocytes toward genetically incompatible MHC structures.
2. Recent discoveries pointing to an essential similarity in T cell reactions toward genetically foreign MHC structures on the one hand and self-MHC structures on cells that were rendered foreign by chemicals or infectious agents on the other hand. Hence, it is conceivable that infections with various viruses as well as sensitization to various drugs may lead to (angio-) immunoblastic lymphadenopathy via a common pathogenetic pathway that is comparable to the one operating in GVHR. This concept implies that small numbers of T-lymphocytes are crucial for the pathogenesis of certain lymphomas which, according to current nomenclature and thinking, are thought to be exclusively disorders of B-lymphocytes.

Acknowledgements

Partially supported by a grant from the Foundation Queen Wilhelmina Fund/Netherlands Organization against Cancer, Amsterdam.

References

1. Aaronson, S. A., Stephenson, J. R.: Endogenous type-C RNA virus of mammalian cells. Biochim. Biophys. Acta *458*, 323–354 (1976).
2. Allison, A. C., Denman, A. M.: Self-tolerance and autoimmunity. Brit. Med. Bull. *32*, 124–129 (1976).
3. Allison, A. C., Denman, A. M., Barnes, R. D.: Cooperation and controlling functions of thymus-derived lymphocytes in relation to autoimmunity. Lancet *II*, 135–140 (1971).
4. Anthony, J. J.: Malignant lymphoma associated with hydantoin drugs. Arch. Neurol. *22*, 450–454 (1970).
5. Armstrong, M. Y. K., Black, F. L., Richards F. F.: Tumor induction by cell-free extracts derived from mice with graft versus host disease. Nature (New Biol.) *235*, 153–154 (1972).
6. Armstrong, M. Y. K., Gleichmann, E., Gleichmann, H., Beldotti, L., André-Schwartz, J., Schwartz, R. S.: Chronic allogeneic desease. II. Development of lymphomas. J. Exp. Med. *132*, 417–439 (1970).
7. Armstrong, M. Y. K., Ruddle, N. H., Lipman, M. B., Pierce, S. K., Richards, F. F.: Role of endogenous murine leukemia virus in immunologically triggered lymphoreticular tumors. I. Development and use of oncogenic cell-free preparations serially passaged in vivo. J. Natl. Cancer Inst. *58*, 67–72 (1977).
8. Armstrong, M. Y. K., Ruddle, N. H., Lipman, M. B., Richards, F. F.: Tumor induction by immunologically activated murine leukemia virus. J. Exp. Med. *137*, 1163–1179 (1973).
9. Armstrong, M. Y. K., Ruddle, N. H., Richards, F. F.: Expression of endogenous murine leukemia viruses during the course of a protracted immunological disorder. J. Exp. Med. *145*, 1060–1065 (1977).
10. Armstrong, M. Y. K., Schwartz, R. S., Beldotti, L.: Neoplastic sequelae of allogeneic disease. III. Histological events following transplantation of allogeneic spleen cells. Transplantation *5*, 1380–1392 (1967).
11. Auerbach, R., Globerson, A.: In vitro induction of the graft-versus-host reaction. Exp. Cell. Res. *42*, 31–41 (1966).
12. Barchilon, J., Gershon, R. K.: Synergism between thymocytes and bone marrow cells in a graft versus host reaction. Nature *227*, 71–72 (1970).
13. Binz, H.: Local graft-versus-host reaction in mice specifically inhibited by anti-receptor antibodies. Scand. J. Immunol. *4*, 79–87 (1975).
14. Binz, H., Wigzell, H.: Shared idiotypic determinants on T and B lymphocytes reactive against the same antigenic determinants. II. Determination of frequency and characteristics of idiotypic T and B lymphocytes in normal rats using direct visualization. J. Exp. Med. *142*, 1218–1230 (1975).
15. Blanden, R. V., Doherty, P. C., Dunlop, M. B., Gardner, I. D., Zinkernagel, R. M., David, C. S.: Genes required for cytotoxicity against virus-infected target cells in K and D regions of H-2 complex. Nature *254*, 269–270 (1975).
16. Blanden, R. V., Hapel, A. J., Jackson, D. C.: Speculation. Mode of action of Ir genes and the nature of T cell receptors for antigen. Immunochemistry *13*, 179–191 (1976).
17. Blank, K. J., Freedman, H. A., Lilly, F.: T-lymphocyte response to Friend virus-induced tumor cell lines in mice of strains congenic at H-2. Nature *260*, 250–252 (1976).
18. Butler, J. J.: Non-neoplastic lesions of lymph nodes of man to be differentiated from lymphomas. Natl. Cancer Inst. Monogr. *32*, 233–255 (1969).
19. Cantor, H.: The effects of anti-theta antiserum upon graft-versus-host activity of spleen and lymph node cells. Cell. Immunol. *3*, 461–469 (1972).
20. Cantor, H., Boyse, E. A.: Functional subclasses of T lymphocytes bearing different Ly antigens. I. The generation of functionally distinct T-cell subclasses is a differentiation process independent of antigen. J. Exp. Med. *141*, 1376–1389 (1975).
21. Carswell, E. A., Lerman, S. P., Thorbecke, G. J.: Properties of reticulum cell sarcomas in SJL/J mice. II. Fate of labeled tumor cells in normal and irradiated SJL/J mice. Cell. Immunol. *23*, 39–52 (1976).
22. Cerny, J., Essex, M., Thomas, D. B.: Interactions of murine leukemia virus (MuLV) with isolated lymphocytes. III. Alterations of splenic B and T cells in Friend virus-infected mice. Int. J. Cancer *18*, 197–204 (1976).
23. Chang, K. S. S., Aoki, T., Law, L. W.: Isolation of a B-tropic type-C virus from reticulum cell neoplasma induced in BALB/c mice by SJL/J type-C virus. J. Natl. Cancer Inst. *54*, 83–87 (1975).
24. Clancy, J., Jr., Tønder, O., Boettcher, C. E.: Effect of neonatal rat graft-vs-host disease (GVHD) on Fc receptor lymphocytes, J. Immunol. *116*, 210–217 (1976).

25. CORNELIUS, E. A.: Rapid viral induction of murine lymphomas in the graft-versus-host reaction. J. Exp. Med. *136*, 1533–1544 (1972).
26. CUNNINGHAM, A. J., LAFFERTY, K. J.: Editorial discussion. A simple, conservative explanation of the H-2 restriction of interactions between lymphocytes. Scand. J. Immunol. *6*, 1–6 (1977).
27. DATTA, S. K., MELIEF, C. J. M., SCHWARTZ, R. S.: Lymphocytes and leukemia viruses: tropism and transtropism of murine leukemia virus. J. Natl. Cancer Inst. *55*. 423–430 (1975).
28. DATTA, S. K., SCHWARTZ, R. S.: Autoimmunization and graft-versus-host reactions. Transplant. Rev. *31*, 44–78 (1976).
29. DATTA, S. K., SCHWARTZ, R. S.: Susceptibility to lymphomas and expression of C-type RNA viruses during the graft-versus-host reaction. Eur. J. Cancer *12*, 977–988 (1976).
30. DENNERT, G.: Cell mediated immunity to hapten modified self and non-self antigens. Nature *255*, 712–713 (1975).
31. DOHERTY, P. C., GÖTZE, D., TRINCHIERI, G., ZINKERNAGEL, R.: Models for recognition of virally modified cells by immune thymus-derived lymphocytes. Immunogenetics *3*, 517–524 (1976).
32. DOHERTY, P. C., SOLTER, D., KNOWLES, B. B.: H-2 gene expression is required for T cell-mediated lysis of virus-infected target cells. Nature *266*, 361–362 (1977).
33. DUNN, T. B., DERINGER, M. K.: Reticulum cell neoplasm type B, or the "Hodgkin's-like lesion" of the mouse. J. Natl. Cancer Inst. *40*, 771–821 (1968).
34. EAST, J.: Immunopathology and neoplasms in New Zealand Black (NZB) and SJL/J mice. Progr. Exp. Tumor Res. *13*, 85–134, (1970).
35. EKPAHA-MENSAH, A., KENNEDY, J. C.: New indicator of histocompatibility differences in vitro. Nature (New Biol.) *233*, 174–176 (1971).
36. ELKINS, W. L.: Cellular immunology and the pathogenesis of graft versus host reactions. Progr. Allergy *15*, 78–187 (1971).
37. EMESON, E. E., THURSH, D. R.: The popliteal lymph node graft-versus-host (GVH) assay in mice (Abstr.). Fed. Proc. *32*, 972 (1973).
38. ERTL, H. C. J., KOSZINOWSKI, U. H.: Modification of H-2 antigenic sites by enzymatic treatment influences virus-specific target cell lysis. J. Immunol. *117*, 2112–2118 (1976).
39. FIALKOW, P. J., GILCHRIST, C., ALLISON, A. C.: Autoimmunity in chronic graft-versus-host disease. Clin. Exp. Immunol. *13*, 479–486 (1973).
40. FORMAN, J.: On the role of the H-2 histocompatibility complex in determining the specificity of cytotoxic effector cells sensitized against syngeneic trinitrophenyl-modified targets. J. Exp. Med. *142*, 403–417 (1975).
41. FORMAN, J., VITETTA, E. S.: Absence of H-2 antigens capable of reacting with cytotoxic T cells on a teratoma line expressing a T/t locus antigen. Proc. Natl. Acad. Sci. USA *72*, 3661–3665 (1975).
42. FORMAN, J., VITETTA, E. S., HART, D. A., KLEIN, J.: Relationship between trinitrophenyl and H-2 antigens on trinitrophenyl-modified spleen cells. I. H-2 antigens on cells treated with trinitrobenzene sulfonic acid are derivatized. J. Immunol. *118*, 797–802 (1977).
43. FRIZZERA, G., MORAN, E. M., RAPPAPORT, H.: Angio-immunoblastic lymphadenopathy with dysproteinaemia. Lancet *1*, 1070–1073 (1974).
44. GARDNER, M. B., HENDERSON, B. E., RONGEY, R. W., ESTES, J. D., HUEBNER, R. J.: Spontaneous tumors of aging wild house mice. Incidence, pathology and C-type virus expression. J. Natl. Cancer Inst. *50*: 719–734 (1973).
45. GARDNER, M. B., KLEMENT, V., HENDERSON, B. E., MEIER, H., ESTES, J. D., HUEBNER, R. J.: Genetic control of type C virus of wild mice. Nature *259*, 143–145 (1976).
46. GARRIDO, F., SCHIRRMACHER, V., FESTENSTEIN, H.: H-2-like specificities of foreign haplotypes appearing on a mouse sarcoma after vaccinia virus infection. Nature *259*, 228–230 (1976).
47. GERMAIN, R. N., DORF, M. E., BENACERRAF, B.: Inhibition of T-lymphocyte mediated tumor-specific lysis by alloantisera directed against the H-2 serological specificities of the tumor. J. Exp. Med. *142*, 1023–1028 (1975).
48. GLEICHMANN, E., GLEICHMANN, H.: Differential immunogenicity of D- and K-end antigens and its possible significance for HL-A. Transplantation *13*, 180–183 (1972).
49. GLEICHMANN, E., GLEICHMANN, H.: Graft-versus-host reaction: a pathogenetic principle for the development of drug allergy autoimmunity, and malignant lymphoma in non-chimeric individuals. Hypothesis. Z. Krebsforsch. *85*, 91–109 (1976).
50. GLEICHMANN, E., GLEICHMANN, H.: Diseases caused by reactions of T lymphocytes to incompatible structures of the major histocompatibility complex. I. Autoimmune hemolytic anemia. Eur. J. Immunol. *6*, 899–906 (1976).
51. GLEICHMANN, E., GLEICHMANN, H., SCHIEDEWITZ, A., SCHEELE, R.: Reactivation of radioresistant F_1-specific parental cells by F_1 T cells: preliminary evidence for a semiallogeneic T-T cell interaction. Transplantation *21*, 77–81 (1976).
52. GLEICHMANN, E., GLEICHMANN, H., SCHWARTZ, R. S.: Immunologic induction of malignant lymphoma: genetic factors in the graft-versus-host model. J. Natl. Cancer Inst. *49*, 793–801 (1972).

53. GLEICHMANN, E., GLEICHMANN, H., SCHWARTZ, R. S., WEINBLATT, A., ARMSTRONG, M. Y. K.: Immunologic induction of malignant lymphoma: identification of donor and host tumors in the graft-versus-host model. J. Natl. Cancer Inst. *54*, 107–116 (1975).
54. GLEICHMANN, E., GLEICHMANN, H., WILKE, W.: Autoimmunization and lymphomagenesis in parent → F_1 combinations differing at the major histocompatibility complex: model for spontaneous disease caused by altered self-antigens? Transplant. Rev. *31*, 156–224 (1976).
55. GLEICHMANN, E., PETERS, K., LATTMANN, E., GLEICHMANN, H.: Immunologic induction of reticulum cell sarcoma: donor-type lymphomas in the graft-versus-host model. Eur. J. Immunol. *5*, 406–412 (1975).
56. GLEICHMANN, H., GLEICHMANN, E., ANDRÉ-SCHWARTZ, J., SCHWARTZ, R. S.: Chronic allogeneic disease. III. Genetic requirements for the induction of glomerulonephritis. J. Exp. Med. *135*, 516–532 (1972).
57. GLEICHMANN, H., GLEICHMANN, E., PETERS, K.: Induction of immune complex glomerulonephritis in F_1 hybrid mice: superiority of cortisone-resistant parental thymocytes over spleen cells. Cell. Immunol. *14*, 123–127 (1974).
58. GOLUB, E. S.: Brain-associated θ antigen: reactivity of rabbit anti-mouse brain with mouse lymphoid cells. Cell. Immunol. *2*, 353–361 (1971).
59. GOMARD, E., DUPREZ, V., HENIN, Y., LEVY, J. P.: H-2 region product as determinant in immune cytolysis of syngeneic tumor cells by anti-MSV T lymphocytes. Nature *260*, 707–709 (1976).
60. GOMARD, E., DUPREZ, V., HENIN, Y., LEVY, J. P.: Relationships between H-2 and viral antigens in murine oncornavirus-induced tumours. J. Immunogenet. *4*, 35–45 (1977).
61. GREENBERGER, J. S., PHILLIPS, S. M., STEPHENSON, J. R., AARONSON, S. A.: Induction of mouse type C RNA virus by lipopolysaccharide. J. Immunol. *115*, 317–320 (1975).
62. GROSS, L.: Oncogenic Viruses. New York: Pergamon Press 1970 (Second Edn).
63. HAFERKAMP, O., SCHACHENMAYR, W., KLEEBERG, U.R., WILDFEUER, A., BOROWSKI, K., MEISTER, H., KONIETZKO, N., ENGELS, J., SCHREWE, K. H.: Schnell verlaufende Auszehrungskrankheit mit generalisierter Lymphadenopathie, Hauptbeteiligung und interstitieller Lungeninfiltration. Dtsch. Med. Wochenschr. *100*, 335–342 (1975).
64. HARAN-GHERA, N., KOTLER, M., MESHORER, A.: Studies on leukemia development in the SJL/J strain of mice, J. Natl. Cancer Inst. *39*, 653–661 (1967).
65. HARRISON, M. R., PAUL, W. E.: Stimulus-response in the mixed lymphocyte reaction. J. Exp. Med. *138*, 1602–1607 (1973).
66. HARTLEY, J. W., ROWE, W. P.: Naturally occurring murine leukemia viruses in wild mice: characterization of a new amphotropic class. J. Virol. *19*, 19–25 (1976).
67. HARTLEY, J. W., WOLFORD, N. K., OLD, L. J., ROWE, W. P.: A new class of murine leukemia virus associated with development of spontaneous lymphomas. Proc. Natl. Acad. Sci. USA *74*, 789–792 (1977).
68. Helman, J.: Vaccinia as a possible carcinogen. Lancet *1*, 50–51 (1957).
69. HENNING, R., SCHRADER, J. W., EDELMAN, G. M.: Antiviral antibodies inhibit the lysis of tumour cells by anti-H-2 sera. Nature *263*, 689–691 (1976).
70. HILGARD, H. R.: Synergism of thymus and bone marrow in the production of graft-versus-host splenomegaly in X-irradiated hosts. J. Exp. Med. *132*, 317–328 (1970).
71. HIRSCH, M. S., BLACK, P. H., TRACY, G. S., LEIBOWITZ, S., SCHWARTZ, R. S.: Leukemia virus activation in chronic allogeneic disease. Proc. Natl. Acad. Sci. USA *67*, 1914–1917 (1970).
72. HIRSCH, M. S., PHILLIPS, S. M., SOLNIK, C., BLACK, P. H., SCHWARTZ, R. S., CARPENTER, C. B.: Activation of leukemia viruses by graft versus host and mixed lymphocyte reactions in vitro. Proc. Natl. Acad. Sci. USA *69*, 1069–1072 (1972).
73. HOWARD, J. C., HUNT, S. V., GOWANS, J. L.: Identification of marrow-derived and thymus derived small lymphocytes in the lymphoid tissue and thoracic duct lymph of normal rats. J. Exp. Med. *135*, 200–219 (1972).
74. IHLE, J. N., COLLINS, J. J., LEE, J. C., FISCHINGER, P. J., MOENNIG, V., SCHÄFER, W., HANNA, M. G., Jr., BOLOGNESI, D. P.: Characterization of the immune response to the major glycoprotein (gp71) of Friend Leukemia Virus. I. Response in BALB/c mice. Virology *75*, 74–87 (1976).
75. IHLE, J. N., MCEWAN, R., BENGALI, K.: Radiation leukemia in C57BL/6 mice. I. Lack of serological evidence for the role of endogenous ecotropic viruses in pathogenesis. J. Exp. Med. *144*. 1391–1405 (1976).
76. JANEWAY, C. A., Jr., WIGZELL, H., BINZ, H.: Hypothesis. Two different V_H gene products make up the T-cell receptors. Scand. J. Immunol. *5*, 993–1001 (1976).
77. KATZ, D. H.: The allogeneic effect of immune responses: model for regulatory influences of T lymphocytes on the immune system. Transplant. Rev. *12*, 141–179 (1972).
78. KATZ, D. H., GRAVES, M., DORF, M. E., DIMUZIO, H., BENACERRAF, B.: Cell interactions between histoincompatible T and B lymphocytes. VII. Cooperative responses between lymphocytes are controlled by genes in the *I* region of the H-2 complex. J. Exp. Med. *141*, 263–268 (1975).

79. Kennedy, J. C., Ekphaha-Mensah, J. A.: Histoincompatibility recognition reaction by irradiated or mitomycin-treated parental cells against hybrid spleen cells produces hybrid cell proliferation and illusion of reaction of hybrid against parent. J. Immunol. *111*, 1639–1652 (1973).
80. Kobow, U., Weiler, E.: Wasting disease induced in athymic BALB/c-"nude" mice by congenic thymus cells. (Abstr.). Z. Immunitaetsforsch. *152*, 95 (1976).
81. Korčáková, L., Hašková, V.: Regional lymph node activation in mice by a soluble product released during contact of normal and allogeneic lymph node cells. Transplantation *18*, 347–349 (1974).
82. Korčáková, L., Holub, M., Hašková, V.: Regional graft-versus-host and host-versus-graft reactions: histology of the popliteal lymph nodes. Folia Biol. (Praha) *20*, 309–313 (1974).
83. Koszinowski, U., Ertl, H.: Lysis mediated by T cells and restricted by H-2 antigen of target cells infected with vaccinia virus. Nature (New Biol.) *255*, 552–554 (1975).
84. Kreth, H. W., Williamson, A. R.: Cell surveillance model for lymphocyte cooperation. Nature (New Biol.) *234*, 454–456 (1971).
85. Kuzumaki, N., Kodama, T., Takeichi, N., Kobayashi, H.: Friend lymphatic leukemia virus-induced autoimmune hemolytic anemia with glomerulonephritis in the rat. Int. J. Cancer *14*, 483–492 (1974).
86. Levy, J. A.: Endogenous C-type viruses: double agents in natural life processes. Biomedicine *24*, 84–93 (1976).
87. Levy, J. A., Datta, S. K., Schwartz, R. S.: Recovery of xenotropic virus but not ecotropic virus during graft versus host reaction in mice. Clin. Immunol. Immunopathol. *7*, 262–268 (1977).
88. Lewandowski, L. J., Gerhard, U., Palmer, J. C.: Cell-mediated cytotoxicity against murine cells infected with 6/94 virus, a parainfluenza type 1 isolate from multiple sclerosis brain tissue. Infect. Immun. *13*, 712–721 (1976).
89. Lewis, R. M., Armstrong, M. Y. K., André-Schwartz, J., Muftuoglu, A., Beldotti, L., Schwartz, R. S.: Chronic allogeneic disease. I. Development of glomerulonephritis J. Exp. Med. *128*, 653–679 (1968).
90. Li, F. P., Willard, D. R., Goodman, R., Vawter, G.: Malignant lymphoma after diphenylhydantoin (Dilantin) treatment. Cancer *36*, 1359–1362 (1975).
91. Lilly, F., Duran-Reynals, M. L., Rowe, W. P.: Correlation of early murine leukemia virus titer and H-2 type with spontaneous leukemia in mice of the BALB/c × AKR cross: a genetic analysis. J. Exp. Med. *141*, 882–889 (1975).
92. Lindholm, L., Rydberg, L., Strannegård, Ö.: Development of host plasma cells during graft-versus-host reactions in mice. Eur. J. Immunol. *3*, 511–515 (1973).
93. Lindholm, L., Strannegård, Ö.: Influence of parental lymphoid cells on the production of 19S and 7S antibodies in F_1 hybrid mice. Int. Arch. Allergy Appl. Immunol. *47*, 508–519 (1974).
94. Lukes, R. J., Collins, R. D.: Immunologic characterization of human malignant lymphomas. Cancer *34*, 1488–1503 (1974).
95. Lukes, R. J., Tindle, B. H.: Immunoblastic lymphadenopathy: a hyperimmune entity resembling Hodgkin's disease. New Engl. J. Med. *292*, 1–8 (1975).
96. Mazurenko, N. P.: Induction of leucoses in mice with infectious viruses and the significance of the latter in the aetiology of disease. Probl. Oncol. *6*, 873–882 (1960).
97. McCullagh, P.: The abrogation of immunological tolerance by means of allogeneic confrontation. Transplant. Rev. *12*, 180–197 (1972).
98. McIntire, K. R., Law, L. W.: Abnormal serum immunoglobulins occurring with reticular neoplasms in an inbred strain of mouse. J. Natl. Cancer Inst. *39*, 1197–1203 (1967).
99. Meier, H., Taylor, B. A., Cherry, M., Huebner, R. J.: Host gene control of type-C RNA tumor virus expression and tumorigenesis in inbred mice. Proc. Natl. Acad. Sci. USA *70*, 1450–1455 (1973).
100. Melief, C. J. M., Datta, S. K., Louie, S., Johnson, S., Melief, M. L., Schwartz, R. S.: Splenocyte plaque assay for the detection of murine leukemia virus. Proc. Soc Exp. Biol. Med. *149*, 1015–1018 (1975).
101. Melief, C. J. M., Louie, S., Schwartz, R. S.: Ecotropic leukemia viruses in congenic C57BL mice: natural dessemination by milk-borne infection. J. Natl. Cancer Inst. *55*, 691–698 (1975).
102. Miller, J. A. F. P., Vadas, M. A., Whitelaw, A., Gamble, J.: *H-2* linked *Ir* gene regulation of delayed-type hypersensitivity in mice. In: The Role of Products of the Histoincompatibility Gene Complex in Immune Responses. Katz, D. H., Benacerraf, B. (eds.) New York: Academic Press 1976, pp. 403–415.
103. Moroni, C., Schumann, G.: Mitogen induction of murine C-type viruses. II. Effect of B lymphocyte mitogens. Virology *73*, 17–22 (1976).
104. Moroni, C., Schumann, G., Robert-Guroff, M., Suter, E., Martin, D.: Induction of endogenous murine C-type virus in spleen cell cultures treated with mitogens and 5-bromo-2-deoxyuridine. Proc. Natl. Acad. Sci. USA *72*, 535-538 (1975).
105. Munro, A., Bright, S.: Products of the mg histocompatibility complex and their relationship to the immune response. Nature *264*, 145–152 (1976).

106. MURPHY, E. D.: SJL/J, a new inbred strain of mouse with a high, early incidence of reticulum cell neoplasms. Proc. Am. Assoc. Cancer Res. *4*, 46 (1963).

107. NABHOLZ, M., VIVES, J., YOUNG, H. M., MEO, T., MIGGIANO, V., RIJNBECK, A., SHREFFLER, D. C.: Genetic control of killer cell production and target specificities in the mouse. Eur. J. Immunol. *4*, 378–387 (1974).

108. PERREN, B., SCHUMANN, G., GISLER, R. H., DUKOR, P.: Dissociation of cytotoxicity and helper activity of irradiated thymus cells. Transplantation *17*, 393–399 (1974).

109. PETERS, R. L., HARTLEY, J. W., SPAHN, G. J., RABSTEIN, L. S., WHITMIRE, C. E., TURNER, H. C., HUEBNER, R. J.: Prevalence of the group specific (gs) antigen and infectious virus expressions of the murine C-type RNA viruses during the life span of BALB/c Cr mice. Int. J. Cancer *10*, 283–289 (1972).

110. PETERS, R. L., SPAHN, G. J., RABSTEIN, L. S.: Incidence of group specific (gs) antigen of type C tumor viruses in spontaneous neoplasms of BALB/c Cr mice. Int. J. Cancer *10*, 290–295 (1973).

111. PETERS, R. L., SPAHN, G. J., RABSTEIN, L. S., KELLOFF, G. J., HUEBNER, R. J.: Murine C-type RNA viruses from spontaneous neoplasms: in vitro host range and oncogenic potentiae. Science *181*, 665–667 (1973).

112. PETERS, R. L., SPAHN, G. J., RABSTEIN, L. S., KELLOFF, G. J., HUEBNER, R. J.: Neoplasm induction by murine type-C viruses passaged directly from spontaneous non-lymphoreticular tumors. Nature (New Biol.) *244*, 103–105 (1973).

113. PHILLIPS, S. M., STEPHENSON, J. R., AARONSON, S. A.: Genetic factors influencing mouse type-C RNA virus induction by naturally occurring B cell mitogens. J. Immunol. *118*, 662–666 (1977).

114. PHILLIPS, S. M., STEPHENSON, J. R., GREENBERGER, J. S., LANE, P. E., AARONSON, S. A.: Release of xenotropic type C RNA virus in response to lipopolysaccharide: activity of lipid-A portion upon B lymphocytes. J. Immunol. *116*, 1123–1126 (1976).

115. PIGUET, P.-F., DEWEY, H. K., VASALLI, P.: Study of the cells proliferating in parent versus F_1 hybrid mixed lymphocyte culture. J. Exp. Med. *141*, 775–787 (1975).

116. PLATA, F., JONGENEEL, V., CEROTTINI, J.-C., BRUNNER, K. T.: Antigenic specificity of the cytolytic T lymphocyte (CTL) response to murine sarcoma virus-induced tumors. I. Preferential reactivity of in vitro generated secondary CTL with syngeneic tumor cells. Eur. J. Immunol. *6*, 823–829 (1976).

117. PONZIO, N. M., DAVID, C. S., SHREFFLER, D. C., THORBECKE, G. J.: Properties of RCS cells in SJL/J mice. V. Nature of RCS surface antigen which induces proliferation of normal SJL/J T cells. J. Exp. Med. (in press).

118. PONZIO, N. M., LERMAN, S. P., THORBECKE, G. J.: Properties of RCS cells in SJL/J mice. IV. Minimal development of cytotoxic cells despite marked proliferation to syngeneic RCS in vivo and in vitro. Cell. Immunol. (in press).

119. RADASZKIEWICZ, T., LENNERT, K.: Lymphogranulomatosis X. Dtsch. Med. Wochenschr. *100*, 1157–1163 (1975).

120. RAFF, M. C.: T cell recognition at Cold Spring Harbor. Nature *263*, 10–12 (1976).

121. REHN, T. G., SHEARER, G. M., KOREN, H. S., INMAN, J. K.: Cell-mediated lympholysis of N-(3-nitro-4-hydroxy-5-phenyl-acetyl)-β-alanylglycylglyclyl-modified autologous lymphocytes. Effector cell specificity to modified cell surface components controlled by the *H-2 K* and *H-2 D* regions of the murine major histocompatibility complex. J. Exp. Med. *143*, 127-142 (1976).

122. ROEHM, N.: Induction of splenomegaly with stimulated leukocyte culture supernatants. Transplantation *23*, 49–52 (1977).

123. ROLSTAD, B.: The host component of the graft-versus-host reaction. Transplantation *21*, 117–123 (1976).

124. ROLSTAD, B., FOSSUM, S.: The host component of the popliteal lymph node graft-versus-host (GHV) reaction. Tissue Antigens *9*, 96–104 (1977).

125. ROMANO, T. J., PONZIO, N. M., THORBECKE, G. J.: Graft-vs-host reactions in F_1 mice induced by parental lymphoid cells: nature of recruited F_1 cells. J. Immunol. *116*, 1618–1623 (1976).

126. ROSEN, A., GERGELY, P., JONDAL, M., KLEIN, G., BRITTON, S.: Polyclonal Ig production after Epstein-Barr virus infection of human lymphocytes in vitro. Nature *267*, 52–54 (1977).

127. ROWE, W. P.: Studies of genetic transmission of murine leukemia virus by AKR mice. I. Crosses with Fv-1^n strains of mice. J. Exp. Med. *136*, 1272–1285 (1972).

128. ROWE, W. P., HARTLEY, J. W.: Studies of genetic transmission of murine leukemia virus by AKR mice. II. Crosses with Fv-1^b strains of mice. J. Exp. Med. *136*, 1286–1301 (1972).

129. ROWE, W. P., PINCUS, T.: Quantitative studies of naturally occurring murine leukemia virus infection of AKR mice. J. Exp. Med. *136*, 175–184 (1972).

130. ROYSTON, I., SULLIVAN, J. L., PERIMAN, P. O., PERLIN, E.: Cell-mediated immunity to Epstein-Barr-virus-transformed lymphoblastoid cells in acute infectious mononucleosis. New Engl. J. Med. *293*, 1159–1163 (1975).

131. Ruddle, N. H., Armstrong, M. Y. K., Richards, F. F.: Tumor induction by immunologically activated murine leukemia virus: cellular immunity early in the graft-versus-host reaction. J. Immunol. *112*, 706–715 (1974).
132. Schendel, D. J., Alter, B. J., Bach, F. J.: The involvement of LD- and SD-region differences in MLC and CML: a three-cell experiment. Transplant. Proc. *5*, 1651–1655 (1973).
133. Schmitt-Verhulst, A.-M., Sachs, D. H., Shearer, G. M.: Cell-mediated lympholysis of trinitrophenyl-modified autologous lymphocytes. Confirmation of genetic control of response to trinitrophenyl-modified H-2 antigens by the use of anti-H-2 and anti-Ia antibodies. J. Exp. Med. *143*, 211–217 (1976).
134. Schmitt-Verhulst, A.-M., Shearer, G. M.: Effects of sodium periodate modification of lymphocytes on the sensitization and lytic phases of T cell-mediated lympholysis. J. Immunol. *116*, 947–958 (1976).
135. Schrader, J. W., Edelman, G. M.: Participation of H-2 antigens of tumor cells in their lysis by syngeneic T cells. J. Exp. Med. *143*, 601–614 (1976).
136. Schumann, G., Moroni, C.: Mitogen induction of murine C-type viruses. I. Analysis of lymphoid cell subpopulations. J. Immunol. *116*, 1145–1150 (1976).
137. Schwartz, R. S.: Trojan-horse lymphocytes. New Engl. J. Med. *290*, 397–398 (1974).
138. Schwartz, R. S., André-Schwartz, J., Armstrong, M. Y. K., Beldotti, L.: Neoplastic sequelae of allogenic disease. I. Theoretical considerations and experimental design. Ann. N.Y. Acad. Sci. *129*, 804–821 (1966).
139. Schwartz, R. S., Beldotti, L.: Malignant lymphomas following allogenic disease: transition from an immunological to a neoplastic disorder. Science *149*, 1511–1514 (1965).
140. Schwartz, R. S., Donelly, J., Melief, C. J. M., Louie, S.: Immunity to C-type RNA viruses: antibody formation after natural or deliberate infection. J. Immunol. *116*, 657–660 (1976).
141. Shearer, G. M.: Cell-mediated cytotoxicity to trinitrophenyl-modified syngeneic lymphocytes. Eur. J. Immunol. *4*, 527–533 (1974).
142. Shearer, G. M., Rehn, T. G., Garbarino, C. A.: Cell-mediated lympholysis of trinitrophenyl-modified autologous lymphocytes: effector cell specificity to modified cell surface components controlled by *H-2K* and *H-20* serological regions of the murine major histocompatibility complex. J. Exp. Med. *141*, 1348–1364 (1975).
143. Sherr, C. J., Lieber, M. M., Todaro, G. J.: Mixed splenocyte cultures and graft versus host reactions selectively induce an "S-tropic" murine type C virus. Cell *1*, 55–58 (1974).
144. Sidky, Y. A., Auerbach, R.: Lymphocyte-induced angiogenesis: a quantitative and sensitive assay of the graft-vs.-host reaction. J. Exp. Med. *141*, 1084–1100 (1975).
145. Siegler, R., Rich, M. A.: Pathogenesis of reticulum cell sarcoma in mice. J. Natl. Cancer Inst. *41*, 125–143 (1968).
146. Solnik, C., Gleichmann, H., Kavanah, M., Schwartz, R. S.: Immunosuppression and malignant lymphomas in graft-*versus*-host reactions. Cancer Res. *33*, 2068–2077 (1973).
147. Stastny, P., Stembridge, V. A., Vischer, T., Ziff, M.: Homologous disease in the adult rat, a model for autoimmune disease. II. Findings in the joints, heart, and other tissues. J. Exp. Med. *122*, 681–692 (1965).
148. Stastny, P., Stembridge, V. A., Ziff, M.: Homologous disease in the adult rat, a model for autoimmune disease. I. General features and cutaneous lesions. J. Exp. Med. *118*, 635–648 (1963).
149. Stein, H., Lennert, K., Parwaresch, M. R.: Malignant lymphomas of B-cell type. Lancet *11*, 855–857 (1972).
150. Streilein, J. W., Billingham, R. E.: An analysis of the genetic requirements for delayed cutaneous hypersensitivity reactions to transplantation antigens in mice. J. Exp. Med. *131*, 409–427 (1970).
151. Streilein, J. W., Billingham, R. E.: An analysis of graft-versus-host disease in Syrian hamsters. I. The epidermolytic syndrome: description and studies on its procurement. J. Exp. Med. *132*, 163–180 (1970).
152. Streilein, J. W., Billingham, R. E.: An analysis of graft-versus-host disease in Syrian hamsters. II. The epidermolytic syndrome: studies on its pathogenesis. J. Exp. Med. *132*, 181–197 (1970).
153. Streilein, J. W., Stone, M. J.: GVH disease: unmasking of forbidden clones. Transplant. Proc. *5*, 861–864 (1963).
154. Streilein, J. W., Stone, M. J., Duncan, W. R.: Studies of the specificity of autoantibodies produced in systemic graft-vs-host disease. J. Immunol. *114*, 255–260 (1975).
155. Takeichi, N., Kuzumaki, N., Kobayashi, H.: Immunological studies of runting syndrome in rats inoculated with Friend virus. Cancer Res. *33*, 3096–3102 (1973).
156. Tatum, S. M., Lindquist, R. R.: Graft-versus-host reactions in isohistogenic rats. Frequency and donor-host origin of IgG-containing cells in local intrarenal graft-versus-host reactions. Transplantation *17*, 239–248 (1974).
157. Taylor, C. R.: Immuno-histological observations upon the development of reticulum cell sarcoma in the mouse. J. Pathol. *118*, 201–219 (1976).

158. TAYLOR, C. R.: Hodgkin's disease and the lymphomas. Ann. Res. Rev. Horrobin, D. F. (ed.) Montreal: Eden Press 1976.
159. TEMIN, H.: RNA viruses and cancer. Cancer *39*, 422–428 (1977).
160. TRINCHIERI, G., ADEN, D. P., KNOWLES, B. B.: Cell-mediated cytotoxicity to SV 40-specific tumour-associated antigens. Nature *261*, 312–314 (1976).
161. TYLER, A.: Clues to the etiology, pathology, and therapy of cancer provided by analogies with transplantation disease. J. Natl. Cancer Inst. *25*, 1197–1229 (1960).
162. VON BOEHMER, H.: Separation of T of B lymphocytes and their role in the mixed lymphocyte reaction. J. Immunol. *112*, 70–78 (1974).
163. WAGNER, H., STARZINSKY-POWITZ, A., PFIZENMAIER, K., RÖLLINGHOFF, M.: T cells sensitized in vivo towards hapten modified syngeneic MHC-structures generate in vivo an "allogeneic effect". (Abstr.) Z. Immunitaetsforsch. *152*, 121 (1976).
164. WARD, P. A., VOLKMAN, A.: The elaboration of leukotactic mediators during the interaction between parental-type lymphocytes and F_1 hybrid cells. J. Immunol. *115*, 1394–1399 (1975).
165. WEIGLE, W. O.: Immunological unresponsiveness and autoimmunity. Clin. Exp. Immunol. *9*, 437–447 (1971).
166. ZINKERNAGEL, R. M., ALTHAGE, A., ADLER, B., BLANDEN, R. V., DAVIDSON, W. F., KEES, U., DUNLOP, M. B., SHREFFLER, D.C.: H-2 restriction of cell-mediated immunity to an intracellular bacterium. Effector T cells are specific for *Listeria* antigen in association with H-2I region-coded self-markers. J. Exp. Med. *145*, 1353–1367 (1977).
167. ZINKERNAGEL, R. M., DOHERTY, P. C.: Restriction of in vitro cell mediated cytotoxicity in lymphocytic choriomeningitis within a syngeneic or semiallogeneic system. Nature *248*, 701–702 (1974).
168. ZINKERNAGEL, R. M., DOHERTY, P. C.: *H-2* compatibility requirement for T-cell-mediated lysis of target cells infected with lymphocytic choriomeningitis virus. Different cytotoxic T-cell specificities are associated with structures coded for in *H-2K* or *H-2D*. J. Exp. Med. *141*, 1427–1436 (1975).

Neoplasms of Immunoglobulin-Producing Cells in Mice

N. L. WARNER

Introduction

Although murine lymphoid tumors have been extensively used in experimental tumor research for many decades, their use has principally been related to virologic aspects and to studies of tumor immunity. In recent years, however, considerable interest has developed in their possible application as models of discrete lymphoid subpopulations. The underlying concept, based in part on studies of human lymphoid neoplasia, is that each lymphoid tumor represents the monoclonal neoplastic proliferation of a cell that belongs to a specific T- or B-cell subpopulation and is arrested in its differentiation at a particular stage.

Current research in this area is attempting to evaluate this concept principally through an analysis of the cell surface markers of these tumors with the view to determining whether the phenotypic characterization of each tumor is that of a known normal T- or B-cell subpopulation and does not include any additional markers that would be indicative of a partial or general derepression in the cell type.

The eventual aims and further goals of this research involve both basic immunologic aspects and considerations relevant to further analysis of human lymphomas, including:

1. The establishment of homogeneous cell populations of a single subpopulation for more extensive biochemical definition of specific cell surface components.
2. The provision of model systems for studies of the biochemical basis of differentiation in the lymphoid system.
3. The provision of a rational scientific basis for the classification of neoplasia of the immune system according to specific lymphoid cell subpopulations at particular stages of differentiation arrest.

For this latter aspect, studies of murine tumors have several particular advantages over those in man, since a wider range of genetically and immunochemically defined cell surface markers are currently available that can be used to define a cell's stage in differentiation. Such studies may be of considerable advantage in eventually defining those surface markers that may be most appropriate for specific characterization of lymphoid tumors and which should then be sought for in the human situation.

One of the major problems in this latter aspect of lymphoma classification is that cellular immunologists have yet to precisely define all the stages in normal T- and B-cell differentiation, which must be the basis for comparison with the neoplastic state. To illustrate this problem, Figure 1 depicts one of the many currently proposed schemes of B-cell differentiation. The emphasis in the scheme is to relate specific stages of differentiation with specific inducers of differentiation, which include both undefined early induction factors, a potential bursalpoietin type hormone [6], environmental factors of ill-defined nature [28], specific antigen, and helper T-cell-derived factors. This scheme of differentiation progresses from a hematopoietic stem cell to commitment into the B-cell lineage (pro-B cell) to a cell induced by bursalpoietin but still lacking detectable membrane-bound Ig, although probably synthesizing intracellular Ig [7, 16]

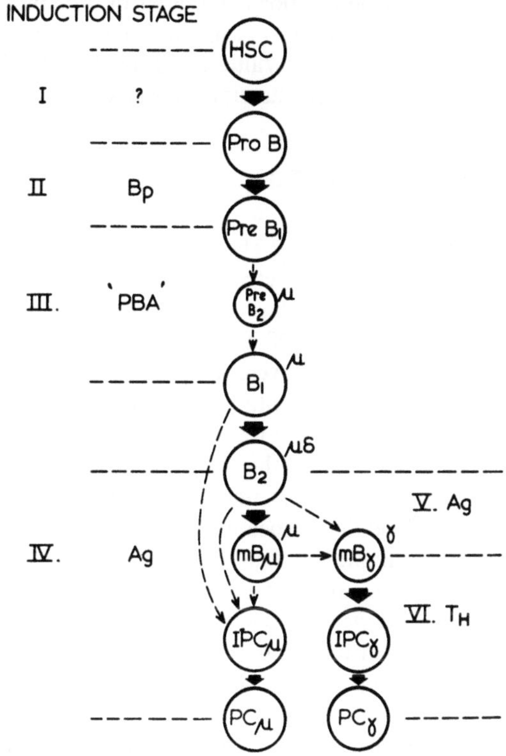

Fig. 1. Provisional scheme of B-cell maturation. Pluripotential stem cells (HSC) are induced by undefined factors into B-cell commitment (pro-B). This cell is the target for "bursalpoietin" (Bp) (6) type induction into a pre-B_1 cell that is synthesizing immunoglobulin but does not yet express membrane-bound Ig. This cell then matures into the pre-B_2 stage—a small lymphocyte with detectable cell surface IgM. This cell is then subjected to "environmental stimulation" [28], possibly of a polyclonal B-cell activation ("PBA") type which results in activation to a larger cell (B_1) still bearing only IgM (μ). Differentiation then involves expression of IgD (δ) (B_2 cell), with possibly both B_1 and B_2 cells being capable of direct antigenic (Ag) stimulation. Further maturation to immature (IPC) and mature plasma cells (PC) involves helper T-cell factors (T_H)—particularly in the case of IgG-secreting cells [17]. Memory cells (MB) arise at various stages, with currently some uncertainty as to the precise sequence of events or alternative pathways that may exist

and bearing other B-cell markers such as MBLA [27], then via "environmental stimulation" [28] into cells of varying sizes and expressing initially IgM and then IgM and IgD [9, 21, 22, 38]. The complete differentiation into antibody-secreting plasma cells requires the involvement of helper T-cell factors [13, 17, 31], and memory cells are derived at various stages. Although much of the information concerning the characterization of murine lymphoid tumors is relatively recent, several general conclusions might be provisionally advanced.

1. The majority of lymphoid tumors appear to express a phenotypic pattern of cell surface markers that are those expressed by a particular normal subpopulation of T or B cells.
2. A minority of tumors have been found that appear to express certain phenotypic combinations of cell surface markers that have not been found together on normal lymphoid cells.
3. Several lymphoid tumors have been described that express not only cell surface phenotypes of normal lymphoid cells but also certain functional properties.

Much of this information was recently considered at a National Cancer Institute workshop and will be described elsewhere in the meeting report and abstracts [24].

The following descriptions of a series of immunoglobulin-producing tumors illustrate some of the markers and patterns of marker expression that have been observed in a series of tumors recently studied at the Walter and Eliza Hall Institute [33, 35, N. L. WARNER, A. W. HARRIS, G. GUTMAN et al., manuscripts in preparation].

T-Cell Lymphomas

Examples of situation 2 above have particularly involved T-cell tumors, where a variety of surface markers were detected on T-cell lymphomas at a time when such markers were not unequivocally accepted as being expressed on any normal T-cell population.

For example, 3 out of 28 T-cell lymphomas were found to express Fc receptors [35] at a time when such receptors were considered to be expressed on B-lymphocytes but not on T-lymphocytes. Subsequently, it became clear that a distinct subpopulation of normal T cells exists that expresses Fc receptors [2, 3, 39] and thus Fc receptor-positive T-cell tumors may represent neoplasms of this subpopulation. In this regard, studies with human lymphomas will be of particular interest since two different Fc receptor-positive T-cell subpopulations have been described that respectively bind IgM (Tμ) or IgG (Tγ) [17].

A second example concerns the possible expression of I-region gene products by T cells. In vivo transplantation studies with tumors induced in congeneic recombinant mice unequivocally demonstrated the expression of I-region gene products on these tumors, whereas considerable controversy existed on the expression of such products on normal T cells. It is now quite evident that at least some subpopulations of normal T-cells express I-region gene products [20, 31].

Another possible explanation of the apparent expression of "inappropriate" surface markers is that the typing reagents are not as specific as may have been thought. Thus, for example, many anti-I-region sera may also contain anti-Qa-1 or Qa-2 antibodies [8], and these could be responsible for detection of surface markers on T cells rather than the anti-I-region antibodies in the same sera.

Possibly one of the major controversies concerning so-called "aberrant" surface marker expression is the production of immunoglobulin by T-cell lymphomas. Several T-cell lymphomas have been unequivocally shown to both synthesize [10, 11] and bear cell surface immunoglobulin [5, 11]. Since many of the tumors so studied were cultured cloned lines, the potential problem with in vivo derived cells of cytophilic-bound immunoglobulin is not relevant. The essential question, therefore, is whether this immunoglobulin parallels normal expression by at least some nonmalignant T cells or whether these tumors are in reality tumors of the B-cell lineage that are aberrant in expressing some T-cell markers. Our present concept supports the former explanation, since the latter alternative finds no experimental support. Not only do these cultured T-cell tumors express several different markers of T-cell populations, but they do not express any of the known *specific* surface markers of B-cell populations. Direct experimental support for the former explanation will depend upon identification of the nature of this T-cell immunoglobulin. Recent studies with indirect immunofluorescence using antimouse immunoglobulin antisera prepared in chickens have shown that both normal and neoplastic T cells bear a cell surface immunoglobulin whose light chain is at least cross-reactive with a B-cell-derived κ-chain, if not identical [14]. Molecular analysis of the heavy chain suggests that it is not, however, identical with any known B-cell-derived heavy chain [19], and if further studies demonstrate that T-cell immunoglobulin does have a distinct H-chain gene, then this will again demonstrate that this surface component of neoplastic T cells is representative of normal *T-cell* differentiation. A recent advantage in such studies of murine heavy chains is the description of allotypic antigens of mouse δ- [9] and μ-chains [34], and it will be of interest to determine whether or not T-cell immunoglobulin possess any of these allotypic determinants.

B-Cell Lymphomas

The analysis of immunoglobulin biosynthesis by murine B-cell tumors can be approached by a variety of methods. These include direct detection and analysis of membrane immunoglobulins, analysis of intracellular biosynthesis, and degree of secretion by the cell. Immunofluorescent reactions (either direct or indirect) can be detected either visually or quantitatively by the use of flow microfluorometry systems as described by HERZENBERG et al. [12]. Using these latter systems, it has been observed that a wide diversity exists for normal B-cell surface immunoglobulin in terms of degree of fluorescence intensity. Preliminary analysis of B-cell tumors suggests that considerably greater restriction exists in this diversity, and the possible relation of quantitation of cell surface immunoglobulin to stages in differentiation requires further elaboration.

Cell surface immunoglobulin can also be directly labeled with radioactive iodine and analyzed for chain composition by polyacrylamide gel electrophoresis. A more quantitative approach has recently been described by GUTMAN et al. (manuscript in preparation) in which iodinated cell surface immunoglobulin is specifically isolated by binding to sepharose conjugated anti-κ chain antibodies and then eluted by sodium thiocyanate. This preparation can then be used as the labeled antigen in competitive radioimmunoassays as shown in Figure 2, in which the labeled immunoglobulin from B-lymphoma WEHI-231 is precipitated by anti-μ antiserum or by an antiserum containing anti-κ and anti-γ_2 antibodies. Antisera specific for γ_1, γ_2, or γ_3 classes do not precipitate this immunoglobulin, verifying its IgM nature. Using competitive inhibition with purified myeloma proteins (only IgM proteins showing inhibition), one can determine the amount of labeled cell surface immunoglobulin from a given number of cells, which in the case of WEHI-231 yields an average of 6×10^6 molecules of IgM per cell. This tumor thus clearly represents a B-cell subpopulation of extremely high-density membrane immunoglobulin.

Biosynthesis of immunoglobulins by murine B-cell lymphomas is also currently being evaluated by the incorporation of labeled amino acids into intracellular or secreted immunoglobulin. This approach also permits quantitative radioimmunoassay analysis or polyacrylamide gel analysis

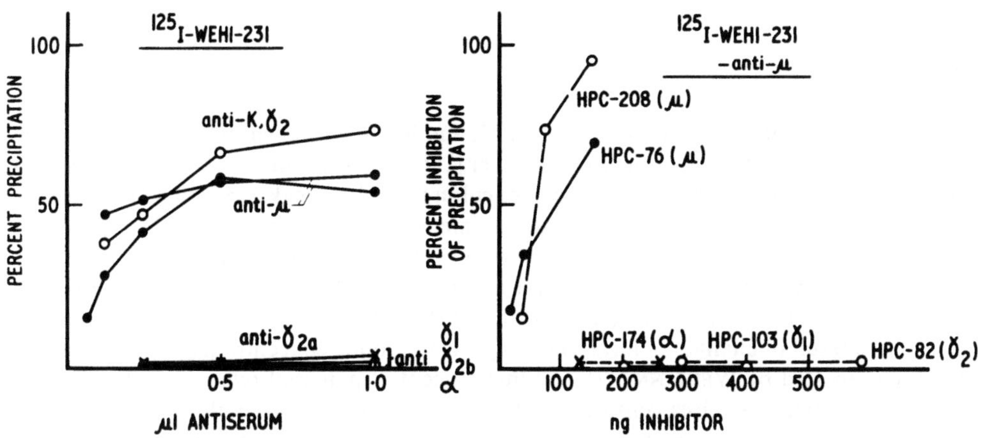

Fig. 2. Radioimmunoassay of cell surface iodinated B-lymphoma (WEHI-231) immunoglobulin (from G. GUTMAN, N. L. WARNER, and A. W. HARRIS, manuscript in preparation). Iodinated WEHI-231 cell surface immunoglobulin was isolated from an anti-κ-chain sepharose conjugate and was assayed for precipitability with various anti-immunoglobulin antisera (left graph). Two different monospecific anti-μ sera precipitate as did an antiserum containing anti-κ. The right graph shows a competitive inhibition assay with the anti-μ antibody and shows inhibition by two different IgM macroglobulins (HPC-76 and HPC-208) but not by myeloma proteins of other classes (whose H-chain type is indicated in parentheses)

Table 1. Membrane immunoglobulin and biosynthesis in murine B-cell lymphomas

Tumor line	Membrane immunoglobulins CSI page[a]	Immunofluorescence[b]					Immunoglobulin biosynthesis[c]	
		κ	μ	α	γ_1	γ_2	Intracellular	Secreted
ABE-8	κ/H	±	−	−	−	−	None detected	None detected
WEHI-231	κ/μ	++	++	−	−	−	Trace IgM	None detected
WEHI-259	NT	++	++	−	−	−	NT	NT
WEHI-279	κ/μ	++	++	−	−	−	Trace IgM	None detected
WEHI-301	NT	++	++	−	−	+	IgM	IgM (+)
WEHI-267	κ/α	+	−	±	−	−	IgA	IgA (++)
2PK3	κ/γ	+	−	−	−	+	IgG_2	IgG_2 (++)
P3K[d]	NT	+	−	−	−	−	IgG_1	IgG_1 (++++)
MPC-11[d]	NT	−	−	−	−	−	IgG_2	IgG_2 (++++)

[a] Tumor cell surfaces labeled with ^{125}I and solubilized components analyzed on polyacrylamide gels for component immunoglobulin chains. (H indicates heavy chain of unknown type).
[b] Direct immunofluorescence with fluorescein conjugated chain-specific antisera.
[c] Cultured cell lines grown with ^{75}Se methionine and intracellular immunoglobulin or secreted (into extracellular medium) immunoglobulin analyzed by PAGE or radioimmunoassay. Relative estimation of amounts of secreted immunoglobulin indicated in parentheses.
[d] Tumors P3K and MPC-11 are plasmacytomas, both actively secreting myeloma protein. Tumor P3K is a relative exception for plasmacytomas in possessing sufficient membrane-bound Ig to be detectable by direct immunofluorescence—light chains only detectable.
NT: not tested.

of the labeled isolated immunoglobulin, and we have found it extremely advantageous to use the γ-emitting isotope ^{75}Se as ^{75}Se methionine (GUTMAN et al., manuscript in preparation). Our results with a series of B-cell lymphomas are summarized in Table 1. The following brief description of these tumors and other known surface markers indicates some of the data suggestive of the concept of homogeneity of murine lymphomas and their arrest in differentiation. Complete details on many of these aspects are currently being prepared for publication.

ABE-8

This tumor was induced by Abelson virus [1, 29] and has been shown to belong to the B-cell series by virtue of expression of the Ly4.1 marker [15] and the absence of T-cell markers; it is nonphagocytic, requires 2-mercaptoethanol for culture, and has weak expression of membrane immunoglobulin. In its normal cultured state, the membrane Ig is barely detectable by indirect immunofluorescence; however, after culture for several days in theophylline, membrane Ig is quite readily demonstrable, possibly indicating that this tumor may represent an arrest in differentiation early in the B-cell series and that further differentiation in this line might be induced as a result of changes in intracellular cyclic nucleotide concentrations. Similar results have been reported by WEIMANN [37], and this concept of potential removal of the block of differentiation arrest requires considerable further experimentation, both in terms of basic concepts of differentiation arrest and possibly as a potential aid to lymphoma therapy.

WEHI-231, 259, and -279

These three tumors all represent tumors possessing extremely high densities of cell surface immunoglobulin of IgM type. As shown in Figure 2, the immunoglobulin can be labeled by cell surface iodination, isolated on anti-immunoglobulin columns, and quantitated by competitive radioimmunoassay. Preliminary results with these tumors indicate levels of cell surface immunoglobulin well in excess of the normal *average* values for B-cell immunoglobulin. The results thus suggest that these tumors are homogeneous, representing the high-density membrane immunoglobulin-bearing B-cell subpopulation. Studies on biosynthesis of immunoglobulins by these tumors, however, revealed no detectable secretion of immunoglobulin and extremely low levels of intracellular biosynthesis. The results thus suggest that these tumors have a relatively low biosynthetic capacity and that the immunoglobulin produced is accumulated and retained at the cell surface. Heterogeneity has, however, been observed between these tumors, in that tumor WEHI-231 appears not to express any I-region gene products, whereas tumor WEHI-279 shows some expression of an as yet uncharacterized I-subregion determinant.

WEHI-301, -267, and 2PK3

These three tumors might be proposed to represent the next stage in B-cell differentiation in that these tumors all bear readily detectable cell surface immunolglobulin and yet show moderate to good secretory activity.

The three tumors differ in the type of immunoglobulin present at the cell surface, with tumor WEHI-301 bearing both IgM and IgG_2, tumor WEHI-267 possessing cell surface IgA, and tumor 2PK3 having cell surface IgG_2. In all cases, biosynthetic studies with labeled amino acids have shown that each tumor synthesizes only one immunoglobulin class: IgM, IgA, and IgG2, respectively. Thus tumors WEHI-267 and 2PK3 would appear to represent a more mature B-cell population, possibly of immature plasma cell nature, which has reached the stage of differentiation where cell surface immunoglobulin is still readily detectable but secretion of this same ïmmunoglobulin is proceeding. It is of interest to note that tumor 2PK3 also shows strong expression of I-region gene products.

The situation with tumor WEHI-301 is more unusual in that two immunoglobulin classes are present at the cell surface although biosynthetic studies show the cell to be capable of synthesizing only IgM. Pretreatment of these tumor cells with nonfluorescent anti-μ-chain antiserum totally blocks the subsequent binding of either fluorescent conjugated anti-μ or anti-γ_2, indicating close spatial relationships between these two immunoglobulins. In contrast, pretreatment of the cells with anti-γ_{2b} antiserum (but not with anti-γ_2a antiserum) totally blocks the binding of fluorescent anti-γ_2 antibodies but does not show appreciable blocking of the binding of fluorescent anti-μ.These results might suggest that the cell bears a considerably greater excess of IgM than IgG_2 (the IgG_2 being restricted to the IgG_{2b} subclass). We would thus tentatively suggest that this tumor represents a murine analogue of a chronic lymphocytic leukemia tumor previously described in man, which bears surface IgM and IgG, with the IgM being of intrinsic origin and possessing rheumatoid factor reactivity [25]. Further studies on this tumor may provide a useful model for studying the biologic implications of such a situation.

These studies, with attempts to quantitate immunoglobulin production by a series of B-cell lymphomas both at the cell surface and biosynthetic levels, clearly indicate that different B-cell lymphomas are in themselves quite homogeneous in terms of cell surface immunoglobulin and biosynthetic capacity but can differ from one to another quite markedly in these respects. These data are thus compatible with the concept that each tumor represents an arrest in B-cell differentiation at different stages of immunoglobulin production. This conclusion is further borne out by preliminary studies with other cell surface markers, including Fc-receptor expression, expression of the B-cell alloantigens Ly4 and Ly7, and expression of I-region markers. The tumors have been found to differ in the expression of these different markers, again indicating a restriction or homogeneity of the tumor cell lines. Further studies are in progress to more clearly characterize the expression of a range of surface markers on these tumors. The preliminary information available is summarized in Table 2, which tentatively lists these tumors in order of differentiation lineage and indicates the available information on surface marker expression.

Plasmacytomas

In previous reports [23, 2b, 3b,], the induction and possible pathogenesis of murine plasma cell tumors has been considered in detail. Preliminary studies on surface marker characterization also indicate that this terminal stage of B-cell differentiation is associated with distinct changes in cell surface marker phenotypes. Thus, as indicated in Table 2, immunoglobulin secretory activity is quite marked although very few plasma cell tumors bear readily detectable membrane immunoglobulin. Fc-receptor expression is also usually absent [4], a marker which is expressed earlier in B-cell differentiation. Similarly, it is our experience that plasma cell tumors do not show readily detectable I-region determinants, whereas intense expression is apparent on tumors of a slightly earlier differentiation stage (e.g., 2PK3). The Ly4 and Ly7 markers [15] are not expressed on all plasma cell tumors (if on any), whereas the alloantigen Pca-1 [30], which was not present on some of the B-cell lymphomas, is expressed.

Table 2. Provisional scheme of differentiation arrest for murine B-cell lymphomas in relation to current marker assessment

Normal sequence:	Stem cell	Pro-B	Pre-B		B^1	B^2	Activated B cell		Immature plasma cell	Plasma cell
Tumor:			ABE-8	WEHI-231	WEHI-279		WEHI-301	2PK3 WEHI-267	P3K	MPC-11
Marker[a]										
I-region			−	±	+		++	+++	±	−
MIg			±	+++	+++		++	++	±	−
Ig.secr.			−	−	−		+	++	+++	+++
Ly4			+	+	+			+		−
Ly7			−	+	+			+		−
Pca-1			−	−	−					++
FcR			±	+	+			+	±	−

[a] This scheme provisionally lists the series of B-cell tumors in order of differentiation arrest as based on the current marker analysis. The markers studied were: I-region: polyvalent antiserum for I-region—ABJEC; MIg: membrane immunoglobulin assessed as described in the text; Ig. secr.: ability to secrete immunoglobulin as shown by biosynthetic studies; Ly4 and Ly7: B-cell surface alloantigens as described by McKenzie et al. [15]; Pca-1: plasma cell alloantigen [30]; FcR: Fc-receptor expression as tested by Warner et al. [35].

Conclusions

Further studies with these tumors are in progress to determine whether this concept of arrest and differentiation is applicable to this series of tumors and whether each tumor does indeed represent the equivalent of a normal B-cell subpopulation. Studies of this nature may provide a suitable working model for providing a rational basis for the characterization of human B-cell neoplasia according to the stages in B-cell differentiation. A considerably greater range of cell surface markers has yet to be explored with these tumors, particularly various heteroantisera prepared against the tumors and absorbed in various ways in attempts to produce heteroantisera specific for different differentiation antigens that might appear at particular stages. These types of antisera would clearly be more relevant to the human situation, and this may again be an example of where studies with a murine model provide considerable infomation relevant to further application in the human situation.

References

1. ABELSON, H. R., RABSTEIN, L. S.: Lymphosarcoma: virus induced thymic independent disease in mice. Cancer Res. *30*, 2213–2219 (1970)
2. ANDERSON, C. L., GREY, H. M.: Receptors for aggregated IgG on mouse lymphocytes: Their presence on thymocytes, thymus derived and bone marrow derived lymphocytes. J. Exp. Med. *139*, 1175–1188 (1974)
3. BASTEN, A., MILLER, J. F. A. P., WARNER, N. L., ABRAHAM, R., CHIA, E., GAMBLE, J.: A subpopulation of T cells bearing Fc receptors. J. Immunol. 1159–1165 (1975)
4. BASTEN, A., WARNER, N. L., MANDEL, T.: A receptor for antibody on B lymphocytes II. Immunochemical and electromicroscopy characteristics. J. Exp. Med. *135*, 627–642 (1972)
5. BOYLSTON, A. W., MOWBRAY, J. F.: Surface immunoglobulin of a mouse T cell lymphoma. Immunology *27*, 855–861 (1974)
6. BRAND, A., GILMOUR, D. G., GOLDSTEIN, G.: Lymphocyte differentiating hormone of bursa of Fabricius. Science *193*, 319–321 (1976)
7. COOPER, M. D., KEARNEY, J. F., LYDYARD, P. M., GROSSI, E. C., LAWTON, R. A.: Studies of generation of B cell diversity in mouse, man and chicken. Cold Spring Harbor Symp. Quant. Biol. *41*, 139–146 (1976)
8. FLAHERTY, L., STANTON, R., BOYSE, E. A.: Contamination of Ia antiserum A.TL anti A.TH with antibodies related to the Tla region. Immunogenetics *4*, 101–103 (1977)
9. GODING, J. W., WARR, G. W., WARNER, N. L.: Genetic polymorphism of IgD-like cell surface immunoglobulin in the mouse. Proc. Natl. Acad. Sci. USA *73*, 1305–1309 (1976)
10. HARRIS, A. W., BANKHURST, A. D., MASON, S., WARNER, N. L.: Differentiated functions expressed by cultured mouse lymphoma cells II. θ antigen, surface immunoglobulin, and a receptor for antibody on cells of a thymona cell line. J. Immunol. *110*, 431–438 (1973)
11. HAUSTEIN, D., MARCHALONIS, J. J., HARRIS, A. W.: Immunoglobulin of T lymphoma cells. Biosynthesis, surface representation and partial characterization. Biochemistry *14*, 1826–1834 (1975)
12. HERZENBERG, L. A., HERZENBERG, L. A., BLACK, J. J., LOKEN, M. R., OKUMURA, K., VAN DER LOO, W., OSBOURNE, B. A., HEWGILL, D., GODING, J. W., GUTMAN, G., WARNER, N. L.: Surface markers and functional relationships of cells involved in murine B-lymphocyte differentiation. Cold Spring Harbor Symp. Quant. Biol. *41*, 33–46 (1976)
13. KATZ, D., BENACERRAF, B.: The regulatory influence of activated T cells on B cell responses to antigen. Adv. Immunol. *15*, 2–94 (1972)
14. MARCHALONIS, J. J., WARR, G. W., BUCANA, C. D., HOYER, L. C., SZENBERG, A., WARNER, J. L.: Demonstration and partial characterization of murine B and T cell surface immunoglobulin using avian antibodies. ICN-UCLA symposium, Regulation of the immune system, E. SERCARZ, L. A. HERZENBERG, AND F. FOX, eds. Academic Press, 1977
15. MCKENZIE, I. F. C., GARDINER, J., CHERRY, M., SNELL, G. D.: Lymphocyte antigens: Ly-4, Ly-6 and Ly-7. Transplant. Proc. *9*, 667–670 (1970)
16. MELCHERS, F., BOEHMER, H. VON, PHILLIPS, R. A.: B lymphocyte subpopulations in the mouse. Organ distribution and ontogeny of immunoglobulin synthesizing and of mitogen sensitive cells. Transplant. Rev. *25*, 26–58 (1975)
17. MITCHELL, G. F.: T cell modification of B cell responses to antigen in mice. Contemp. Top. Immunobiol. *3*, 97–116 (1974)
18. MORETTA, L., FERRARINI, M., MINGARI, M. C., MORETTA, A., WEBB, S.: Subpopulations of human T cells identified by receptors for immunoglobulins and mitogen responsiveness. J. Immunol. *117*, 2171–2174 (1976)
19. MOSELY, J. M., MARCHALONIS, J. J., HARRIS, A. W., PYE, J.: Molecular properties of T lymphoma immunoglobulins. J. Immunogenet. in press (1977)
20. MURPHY, D. B., OKUMURA, K., HERZENBERG, L. A., HERZENBERG, L. A., MCDEVITT, H. O.: Selective expression of separate I region loci in functionally different lymphocyte subpopulations. Cold Spring Harbor Symp. Quant. Biol. *41*, 497–504 (1976)

21. PARKHOUSE, R. M. E., ABNEY, E. R., BOURGOIS, A., WILLCOX, H. N. A.: Functional and structural characterization of immunoglobulin on murine B lymphocytes. Cold Spring Harbor Symp. Quant. Biol. *41*, 193–200 (1976)
22. PERNIS, B., FORNI, L., LUSSATI, A. L.: Synthesis of multiple immunoglobulin classes by single lymphocytes. Cold Spring Harbor Symp. Quant. Biol. *41*, 175–184 (1976)
23. POTTER, M.: Immunoglobulin producing tumors and myeloma proteins of mice. Physiol. Rev. *52*, 631–719 (1972)
24. POTTER, M., WARNER, N. L., MELCHERS, F.: Functional properties of tumors of T and B lymphocytes. Natl. Cancer Inst. Workshop (1977)
25. PREUD'HOMME, J. L., SELIGMANN, M.: Anti-human immunoglobulin G activity of membrane-bound monoclonal immunoglobulin M in lymphoproliferative disorders. Proc. Natl. Acad. Sci. USA *69*, 2132–2135 (1972)
26. ROLLINGHOFF, M., ROUSE, B. T., WARNER, N. L.: Tumor immunity to murine plasma cell tumors I. Tumor associated transplantation antigens of NZB and BALB/c plasma cell tumors. J. Natl. Cancer Inst. *50*, 159–172 (1973)
27. RYSER, J. E., VASSALI, P.: Mouse bone marrow lymphocytes and their differentiation. J. Immunol. *113*, 159–172 (1973)
28. SHORTMAN, K., FIDLER, J. M., SCHLEGEL, R. A., NOSSAL, G. J. V., HOWARD, M., LIPP, J., BOEHMER, H. VON: Subpopulations of B lymphocytes: physical separation of functionally distinct stages of B cell differentiation. Contemp. Top. Immunobiol. *5*, 1–45 (1976)
29. SKLAR, M. D., WHITE, B. J., ROWE, W. P.: Initiation of oncogenic transformation of mouse lymphocytes in vitro by Abelson leukemia virus. Proc. Natl. Acad. Sci. USA *71*, 4077–4081 (1974)
30. TAKAHASHI, R., OLD, L. J., BOYSE, E. A.: Surface alloantigens of plasma cells. J. Exp. Med. *131*, 1325–1341 (1970)
31. TODA, R., TANIGUCHI, M., DAVID, C. S.: Suppressive and enhancing T-cell factors as I-region gene products: properties and the subregion assignment. Cold Spring Harbor Symp. Quant. Biol. *41*, 119–128 (1976)
32. WARNER, N. L.: Autoimmunity and the pathogenesis of plasma cell tumor induction in NZB inbred and hybrid mice. J. Immunogenet. *2*, 1–20 (1975)
33. WARNER, N. L., GODING, J. W.: I region transplantation antigens on T lymphomas of congenic resistant strain origin. In: Membrane Receptors of Lymphocytes. SELIGMANN, M., PREUD'HOMME, J. L., KOURILSKY, F. M. (eds.) North Holland Pub. 1975, pp. 287–292.
34. WARNER, N. L., GODING, J. W., GUTMAN, G. A., WARR, G. W., HERZENBERG, L. A., OSBORNE, B. A., VAN DER LOO, W., BLACK, S. J., LOKEN, M. R.: Allotypes of mouse IgM immunoglobulin. Nature *265*, 447–449 (1977)
35. WARNER, N. L., HARRIS, A. W., GUTMAN, G.: Membrane immunoglobulin and Fc receptors of murine T and B cell lymphomas. In: Membrane Receptors of Lymphomas, SELIGMANN, M., PREUD'HOMME, J. L., KOURILSKY, F. M. (eds.) North Holland Pub. 1975, pp. 203–216
36. WARNER, N. L., POTTER, M., METCALF, D. (eds.): Multiple myeloma and related immunoglobulin producing neoplasms. U.I.C.C. Technical report series, 1974, Vol. 13
37. WEIMANN, B. J. Induction of immunoglobulin synthesis in Abelson murine leukemia virus transformed mouse lymphoma cells in culture. Cold Spring Harbor Symp. Quant. Biol. *41*, 163–164 (1974)
38. VITETTA, E. S., CAMBIER, J., FORMAN, J., KETTMAN, J. R., YUAN, D., UHR, J. W.: Immunoglobulin receptors on murine B lymphocytes. Cold Spring Harbor Symp. Quant. Biol. *41*, 185–192 (1976)
39. YOSHIDA, T. O., ANDERSON, B.: Evidence for a receptor recognizing antigen complexed immunoglobulin on the surface of activated mouse thymus lymphocytes. Scand. J. Immunol. *1*, 401–408 (1972)

From Experimental Animal Models to Human Lymphoid Tissue Neoplasia: Search for a Viral Etiology

Henry S. Kaplan

Neoplasms of lymphoid and hematopoietic tissue origin in experimental and domestic animals [28] provide an important resource for investigators interested in the etiology, pathogenesis, biology, and immunology of the corresponding types of neoplasms in man. The most extensive studies have been performed on various strains of laboratory mice, and the types of lymphoid and hematopoietic neoplasms available for study in this species are considerably more diversified than those in other mammals. Mice readily develop lymphoblastic lymphomas, usually of thymic origin, either spontaneously or in response to exposure to ionizing radiation, various chemical agents, or the induction of autoimmune reactions. Such thymic lymphomas are composed of cells with T-lymphocyte markers and are morphologically indistinguishable from the corresponding tumors in man. Moreover, they resemble the human disease in their pattern of dissemination to other lymph nodes, to the viscera, to bone marrow, and to the central nervous system. Somewhat later in life, and in response to other types of agents, certain strains of mice develop B-cell lymphoblastic lymphomas, which are nonthymic in origin, and may arise in peripheral lymph nodes and other lymphoid tissues. Certain strains of mice also develop myeloid leukemias of bone marrow and/or spleen origin, as well as erythroblastic leukemias arising principally in the spleen. The spectrum of murine neoplasms also includes plasmacytomas, undifferentiated ("stem cell") lymphomas and leukemias, and pleomorphic tumors with morphologic features resembling those of human histiocytic lymphomas and, occasionally, of Hodgkin's disease [11, 12]. Rats also develop thymic T-cell lymphoblastic lymphomas, myeloid leukemias, and less frequently, B-cell lymphomas. Lymphoblastic lymphomas and lymphatic leukemias are also known to occur, or may be induced by appropriate treatment, in several other mammalian species, including cats, hamsters, guinea pigs, cattle, and subhuman primates.

Many important clues to the etiology and pathogenesis of human lymphomas and leukemias have emerged from experimental studies on these mammalian species. For example, it is known that ionizing radiation and certain chemicals are leukemogenic in both mice and men. There is today a strong renewal of interest in the somatic mutation hypothesis of carcinogenesis and an increased awareness of the important role that environmental chemical carcinogens almost certainly play in the etiology of human cancer. In this context, it is instructive to recall that somatic mutation was invoked some 30 years ago as the mechanism of action of ionizing radiation and chemical leukemogens in the induction of lymphomas and leukemias in mice. A series of careful dose-response and partial body irradiation studies, which are detailed elsewhere [27], demonstrated that the mechanism of induction of thymic lymphomas by whole body x-irradiation was completely indirect and that tumors of this type could develop in nonirradiated thymic grafts implanted into thymectomized, irradiated hosts [30, 32].

Meanwhile, the pioneering studies of Gross [18] had led to the discovery of the first murine leukemogenic virus in the high-susceptibility AKR strain. Accordingly, a search was undertaken for the presence of similar leukemogenic viruses in thymic lymphomas induced in low leukemia strains by x-irradiation, leading to the successful detection and isolation of the radiation leukemia virus [RadLV; 27, 38]. Viral agents similar to RadLV have also been isolated from lymphomas induced by several of the chemical leukemogenic agents [27]. Other murine leukemogenic viruses have been isolated from a variety of transplantable tumors of epithelial and connective tissue origin [27, 28]. Finally, C-type RNA viruses have been shown to be the etiologic agents of lymphomas and leukemias of higher mammalian species, including cats [24, 34], hamsters, guinea pigs, rats, cattle [14], and subhuman primates [33]. Collectively, these studies indicate that viruses are the universal etiologic agents of this group of neoplasms in all of the mammalian species studied to date and that the mechanism of action of ionizing radiation and the chemical leukemogens involves the activation of latent leukemogenic viruses rather than somatic mutation.

It has been shown that certain of the murine leukemogenic viruses, such as the Gross AKR virus and RadLV, are naturally occurring, vertically transmitted viruses, the DNA proviral form of which is integrated into the genome of the host and passed from generation to generation through the fetus [5, 19]. Mice also harbor other classes of endogenous C-type RNA viruses, some of which are known to induce sarcomas and others of which have no known oncogenic activity. Endogenous viral genomes have also been demonstrated in the other mammalian species studied, but in these instances the endogenous viruses have not been shown to have leukemogenic or other oncogenic potential. Instead, in cats and perhaps also in cattle and subhuman primates, the viruses responsible for lymphoma and leukemia induction appear to be horizontally transmitted [3, 25, 35]. Such viruses are perhaps generated as recombinants of endogenous viral genomes and host gene sequences [21, 23]. If human lymphomas and leukemias are also due to C-type RNA viruses, epidemiologic evidence for their existence would be much easier to obtain if they were transmitted horizontally, as in the cat, than if they were transmitted vertically, and perhaps activated from a latent state by exogenous leukemogenic agents, as in the low leukemia strains of mice. The fact that epidemiologic studies have revealed little or no convincing evidence suggestive of horizontal transmission may lend weight to the latter alternative.

The site(s) of integration, inducibility, and capacity for replication of endogenous viruses of different subclasses are known to be under genetic control in mice of different strains [43, 50]. Thus, the AKR Gross virus is spontaneously expressed at about the time of birth and spreads rapidly thereafter to many tissues throughout the body in the high leukemia AKR strain [22, 51], whereas spontaneous expression occurs very late in life in most of the low leukemia strains, such as C57BL and BALB/c, but may be induced in young animals of these strains by exposure to whole body irradiation, urethane, nitroquinoline oxides, and other agents [28]. Finally, there are certain low leukemia mouse strains, such as NIH/Swiss and C57L, in which endogenous virus expression does not occur at all, except for a curious class of C-type viruses which grow only in the cells of nonmurine species and are thus termed xenotropic [36]. The molecular mechanisms by which host cellular genes control murine C-type virus expression and replication have been partially elucidated [7, 26, 54].

Dramatic advances in our understanding of the molecular biology of the C-type RNA viruses have occurred during the past few years, beginning with the discovery by TEMIN and MIZUTANI [57] and BALTIMORE [1] of the presence within such virions of a unique enzyme, RNA-dependent DNA polymerase ("reverse transcriptase"), which, after viral penetration into the cell, synthesizes a complementary strand of DNA (cDNA) on the RNA template provided by the viral genome. A second DNA strand, complementary to the first, is then synthesized, and the double-stranded cDNA provirus is integrated by a recombinational process into the DNA of the host cell, where it may reside indefinitely without again expressing evidence of the presence of the viral genome. Alternatively, the virus may again emerge in a sequence of steps involving the synthesis of viral RNA, the synthesis of viral enzymes and structural proteins, and finally, the assembly and budding of complete virions from the cell membrane [56]. However, viral expression need not proceed through all of these steps to the replication of complete virions detectable in the extracellular fluids. Instances are now known in which expression proceeds only through the transcription step, leading to the presence of viral RNA but not of virus-specific antigens or of complete virions; in other instances, virus-specific RNA and some viral proteins are detectable, but complete virions are not produced.

A very instructive example is provided by recent studies of the expression of the radiation leukemia virus (RadLV) in thymic lymphomas induced by ionizing radiation in C57BL/Ka mice [42]. In this strain, several different classes of endogenous C-type RNA viruses are known to exist, but only one, RadLV, possesses the capacity to replicate in lymphoid cells of the thymus [9, 10], as well as their precursors in bone marrow, spleen, and fetal liver [40], and is able to induce thymic lymphoblastic lymphomas [8, 20, 39]. Although RadLV is consistently extractable from such radiation-induced thymic lymphomas, either in the autochthonous tumor or after serial in vivo or in vitro passage, viral antigens are seldom detectable in the early radiation-induced thymomas [42]. Moreover, only 1 of 16 cell lines established in vitro from such radiogenic thymomas spontaneously expressed virus during the first passage. Others required several subpassages, and some lines have remained virus-free after serial subpassage for many months. In these nonproducer cell lines, one might have been tempted to believe that the virus had played no significant role in the genesis of the neoplasm. Yet, superinfection of such nonproducer cells in vitro with a nonleukemogenic endogenous B-tropic virus promptly "rescues" RadLV, which is actively thymotropic and leukemogenic [37]. Moreover, the fact that the radiogenic tumors can be prevented by antiviral immunizing procedures, such as the inoculation of syngeneic cells infected with a nonleukemogenic endogenous virus [41] or treatment with passive antibody to RadLV or related viruses [47], strongly indicates that RadLV is the actual cause of the thymic lymphomas arising in these irradiated mice. Thus, the induction of a lymphoma by this virus occurs under circumstances in which complete viral expression is not required either for the initiation or the maintenance of the transformed phenotype.

From this it follows that, if we are to be successful in the search for possible human lymphoma- and leukemia-inducing viruses, we must search not only for complere virions in the extracellular culture fluids of cell lines established from such tumors but also use the techniques of modern molecular biology to search for the "fingerprints" of such C-type RNA viruses inside the tumor cells themselves. These fingerprints may involve the detection of incompletely matured particles with a density of approximately 1.16 g/ml which contain 70S RNA and reverse transcriptase or may require the detection by molecular hybridization techniques of virus-specific RNA in the absence of mature or immature virus particles.

Different classes of C-type RNA viruses have the capacity to induce lymphomas and leukemias of quite different types. Thus, whereas the Gross AKR, RadLV, and Moloney viruses induce T-cell thymic lymphoblastic lymphomas, the Abelson murine leukemia virus induces lymphoblastic lymphomas which are predominantly of B-cell origin [48], and the Friend and Rauscher viruses primarily induce splenic erythroblastic leukemias [15, 49], although they also contain a viral component with thymic lymphoma-inducing potential [49, 52]. If viruses are also involved in the induction of lymphomas and leukemias in man, it would clearly be a mistake to assume that all types of neoplasms arising from the lymphoid and hematopoietic tissues will be induced by a single class of virus. Instead, it is likely that such tumors will be caused by a family of human lymphoma-leukemia viruses. Nonetheless, if they resemble the murine viruses in this respect, such human viruses will synthesize certain virion proteins which share antigenic determinants and thus cross-react immunologically [53], even though they may differ in important ways with respect to their genetic sequences and other virion proteins.

It is also important to recognize that specificity for its oncogenic action is vested not only in the virus but also in the target cell. Thus, RadLV replicates well in and is capable of transforming T-lymphocytes of the thymus, as well as their precursors in bone marrow, spleen, and fetal liver, but replicates poorly, if at all, in syngeneic fibroblasts [8, 40]. Accordingly, if candidate human lymphoma-inducing viruses are isolated, it will be important to test their oncogenic potential in target cells of appropriate cell types. In light of our recent knowledge of differentiation-specific restriction mechanisms [8], the testing of candidate tumor viruses on cell types of inappropriate states of differentiation is no longer a biologically sound approach. It is thus clear that investigations aimed at the detection of possible human lymphoma-

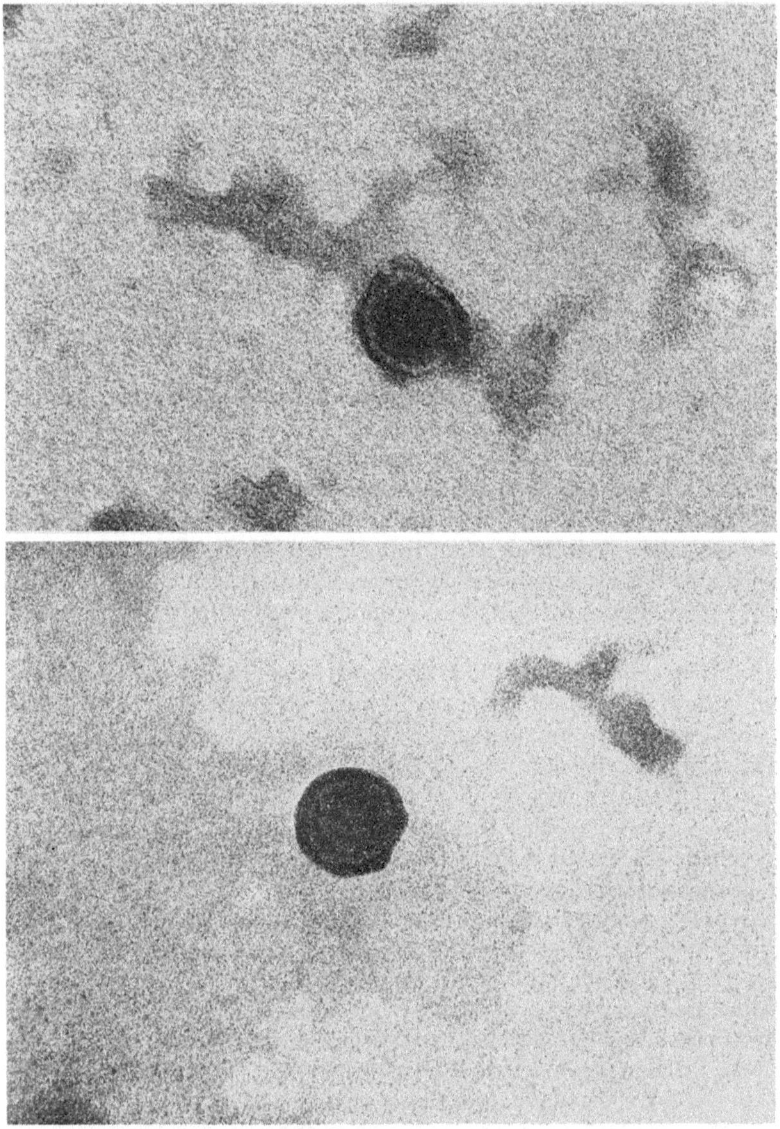

Fig. 1. The size and morphology of the C-type virus isolated from the culture fluids of the SU-DHL-1 human histiocytic lymphoma cell line (upper panel) closely resemble those of a typical murine lymphomagenic virus (RadLV of strain C57BL/Ka mice; lower panel) in electron micrographs made at the same magnification by Dr. Jack Griffith, Department of Biochemisty, Stanford University

leukemia viruses will involve a series of steps, beginning with the attempted establishment in culture of cell lines derived from the various types of human lymphomas. In those situations in which cell lines cannot be successfully established in culture, attempts to isolate virus from fresh peripheral blood, biopsy, or other tissue samples can also be undertaken. In instances in which cell lines are successfully established, proof of the neoplastic character of the cultured cells is important and usually requires the demonstration of aneuploidy and/or of heterotransplantability [29]. Next, a search for viruses in the extracellular culture fluids is made, using assays for reverse transcriptase or the electron microscopic detection of virus particles. Where no such particles are detected in the extracellular fluid, attempts may be made to detect intracytoplasmic enzymic, antigenic, and/or genetic viral information by the appropriate biochemical and immunologic procedures. Viral isolates obtained through such efforts must then be characterized to exclude the possibility that they represent contaminants of murine, feline, or simian origin, again using reference antisera prepared against virion structural proteins or reverse transcriptases of the corresponding C-type RNA viruses. Candidate viral isolates are next tested for their oncogenic potential by infecting cultures of normal human target cells homocytotypic, wherever possible, to the tumor cell of origin. Alterations in culture morphology, growth behavior, chromosome complement, and the acquisition of heterotransplantability are among the criteria that may be used to indicate transformation and the acquisition of neoplastic characteristics by the infected target cells [29]. A candidate virus that has passed all of these tests can be used for the preparation of specific antibodies with which seroepidemiologic studies can be undertaken in populations of normal individuals and patients having the same and other types of lymphomas, with the expectation that a virus having an etiologic role in the genesis of a particular type of lymphoma will reveal specific serologic reactivity in essentially all patients with that type of lymphoma and in few or no normal individuals or those with other types of neoplasms.

C-type viruses have been detected in culture fluids after short-term culture of hematopoietic cells from patients with leukemias [16, 44, 55] and of diploid human embryonic cell strains [46]. The viral isolates obtained in these studies have been shown to contain RNA genomes with extensive sequence homologies to the genomes of simian sarcoma virus as well as an endogenous virus of baboons [4, 45]. Moreover, the structural proteins and reverse transcriptases of these isolates are immunologically related to the corresponding proteins of simian sarcoma virus and the baboon endogenous virus [4, 45]. Incomplete C-type viruses have also been detected intracellularly in human neoplasms. Intracytoplasmic particles with a density characteristic of C-type viruses and reverse transcriptase activity have been reported in leukemic cells [2, 16, 17], as well as in the spleens of patients with leukemias and Hodgkin's disease [6, 58]. However, a serious obstacle to the further characterization of such C-type viruses has been the need to rely upon the inconsistent quality and sporadic availability of primary human tissue specimens.

Our studies in the Cancer Biology Research Laboratory at Stanford began with an attempt to

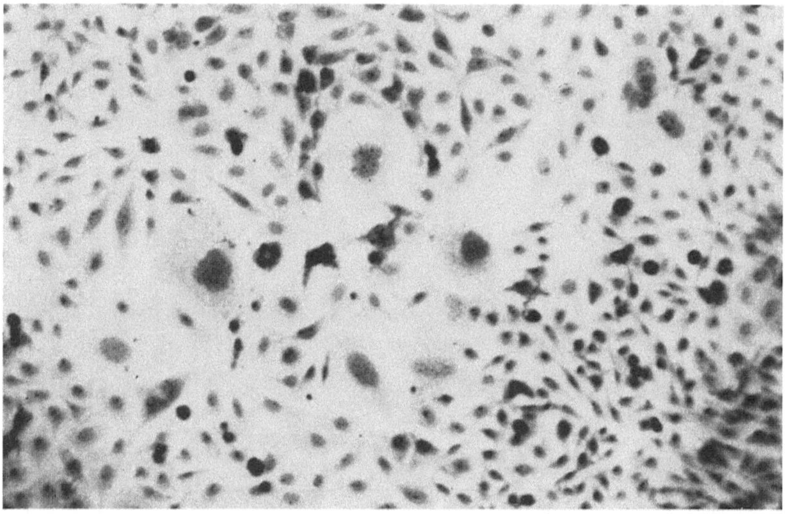

Fig. 2. Typical multinucleate giant cell syncytia induced in rat XC cells by cocultivation with SU-DHL-1 cells

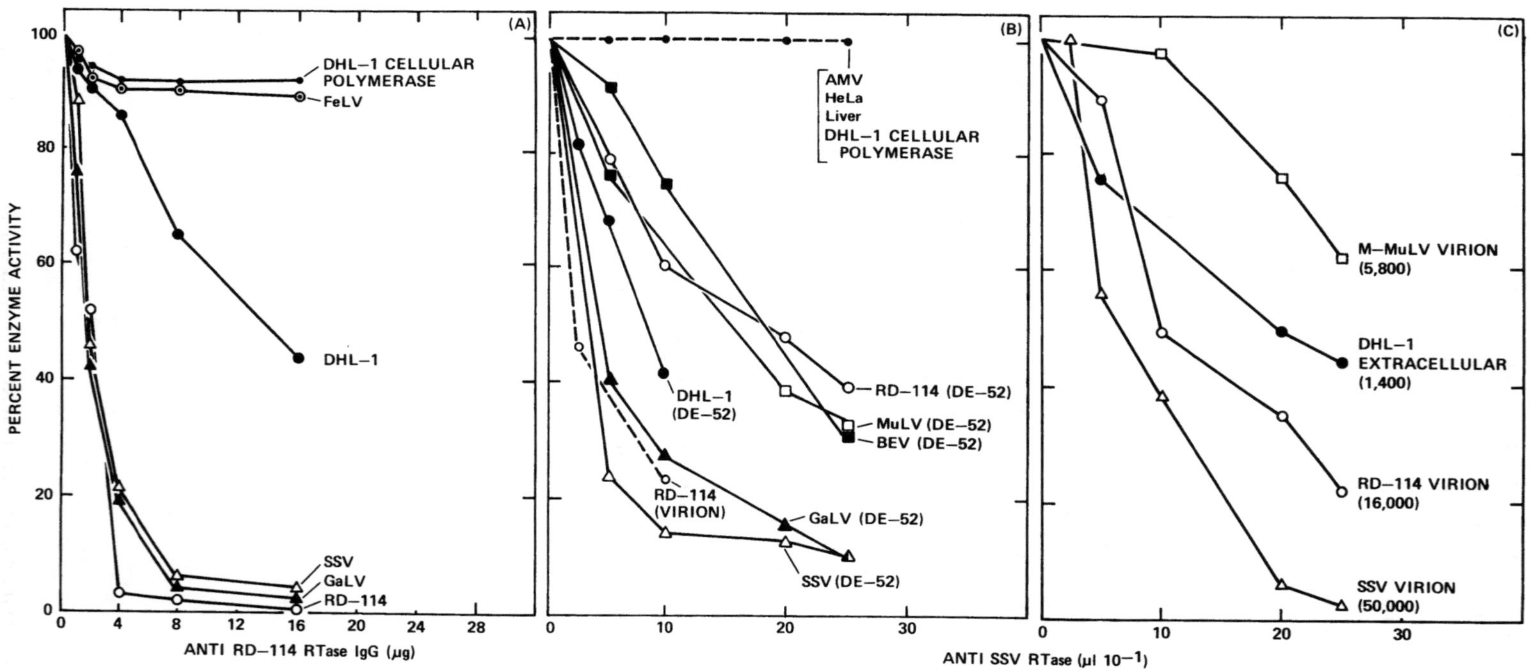

Fig. 3. Partial inhibition of the reverse transcriptase, partially purified on DE-52, from cytoplasmic particles (panels A and B) and from extracellular culture fluids (panel C) of SU-DHL-1 cell cultures by antibodies to the reverse transcriptases of RD-114, an endogenous feline C-type RNA virus (panel A) and simian sarcoma virus (SSV; panels B and C). The reaction conditions have been described elsewhere [31]. In similar experiments with antibody to murine leukemia virus (MuLV) reverse transcriptase, no inhibition of the activity of the SU-DHL-1 viral enzyme was observed. Note that the activities of cellular DNA polymerases (human liver β, HeLa cell γ, and SU-DHL-1 cell) were not affected by antibodies to SSV or RD-114 reverse transcriptases. GaLV: gibbon ape leukemia virus; AMV: avian myeloblastosis virus; BaEV: baboon endogenous virus; FeLV, feline leukemia virus

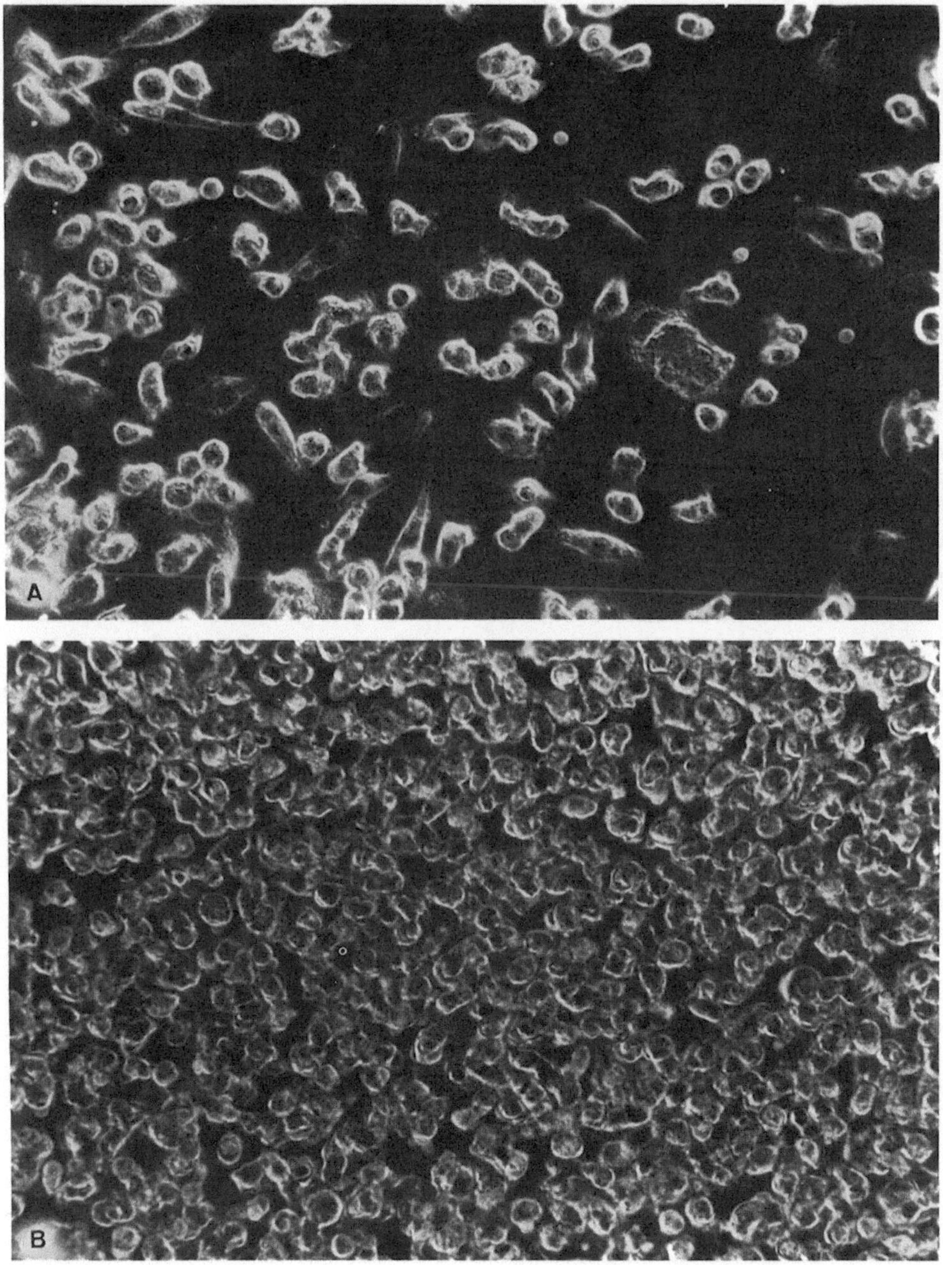

Fig. 4. (A) Control culture of adherent cells from a normal young adult human peripheral blood buffy coat preparation after 3 weeks; (B) Culture of adherent cells from the same buffy coat preparation 3 weeks after infection with filtered virus harvested from the supernatant fluids of SU-DHL-1 cell cultures

establish one or more types of human malignant lymphomas in continuous culture. Our first successful cell lines were obtained from patients with diffuse histiocytic lymphomas [13]. From the first of these lines, designated SU-DHL-1, a C-type RNA virus has now been isolated [31]. The virus has an equilibrium density of approximately 1.15 g/ml in sucrose gradients and has been shown to contain reverse transcriptase activity and 70S RNA. In negatively stained

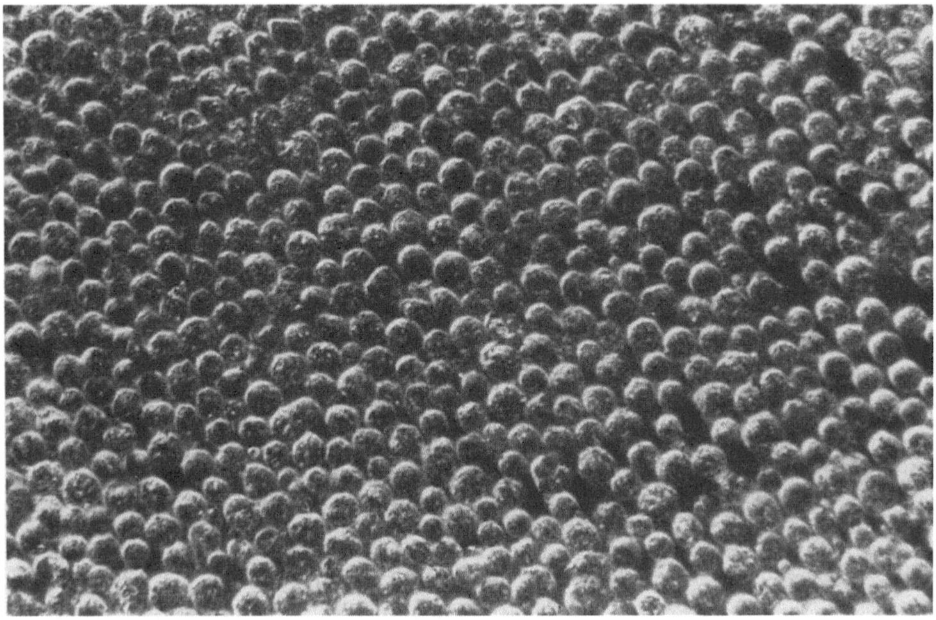

Fig. 5. Culture of adherent cells from a normal young adult rhesus monkey peripheral blood buffy coat preparation 5 weeks after infection with filtered virus harvested from the supernatant fluids of SU-DHL-1 cell cultures. The control cultures which received no virus (not shown) contained only a very small number of sparsely distributed macrophages at 5 weeks

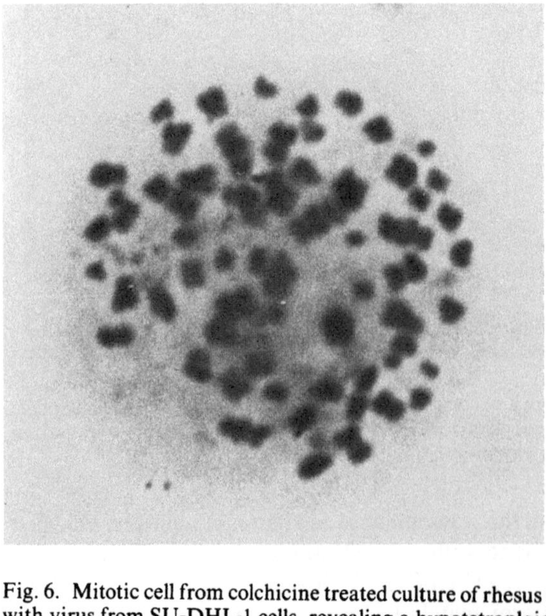

Fig. 6. Mitotic cell from colchicine treated culture of rhesus monkey buffy coat cells 3 weeks after infection with virus from SU-DHL-1 cells, revealing a hypotetraploid chromosome complement (approximately 75 chromosomes). The normal diploid number for rhesus is 42

electron micrographs, it closely resembles other mammalian C-type RNA viruses in size and morphology (Fig. 1). The virus exhibits the capacity to induce syncytia in rat XC cells (Fig. 2), a biologic attribute characteristic of murine, feline, and subhuman primate C-type RNA viruses. Studies of the inhibition of its reverse transcriptase activity by antibodies to the reverse transcriptases of other C-type RNA viruses suggest some degree of relatedness to viruses of subhuman primate origin (Fig. 3).

The virus failed to propagate, in the presence or absence of chemical-inducing agents, on a spectrum of fibroblastic and other nonlymphoid indicator cell lines. However, when filtered virus preparations were added to fresh human buffy coat mononuclear (or normal human spleen) cell cultures, or to the adherent cell subpopulation from such cultures, composed almost entirely initially of monocytes (histiocytes), and later of macrophages, significant alterations in culture morphology and growth behavior of the infected normal human cells have been consistently observed (Fig. 4). Similar alterations in growth behavior of buffy coat cultures from two of three rhesus monkeys were also noted (Fig. 5). After cultivation for 1–4 weeks, cells bearing aneuploid chromosome complements were observed in some of the human and rhesus cultures (Fig. 6). Heterotransplantation studies in nude mice will be undertaken if the confirmatory series of experiments currently in progress again reveal morphologic and growth behavioral changes indicative of the in vitro transformation of these normal monocytic and histiocytic cells.

Concomitantly, biochemical studies are underway to synthesize cDNA probes for molecular hybridization and for the possible detection of proviral DNA sequences in the SU-DHL-1 histiocytic lymphoma cell line from which the virus was isolated. Virion proteins are also being purified, injected into rabbits, and the antibodies thus harvested, after appropriate absorption, will be used as reagents for the detection of similar virion antigens in the cytoplasm of other histiocytic lymphoma cell lines, in biopsy specimens from patients with such lymphomas, and in comparison studies with normal lymphoid tissues and biopsy tissues from patients with other types of lymphomas.

Although the observations to date are of obvious interest, it is important to emphasize caution in the interpretation of these results. The in vitro studies now in progress should determine whether the virus does indeed have lymphoma-inducing potential for normal human cells of corresponding cell type. Demonstration that the virus is human in origin will require careful biochemical and seroepidemiologic studies and will clearly be the most difficult criterion to establish convincingly. Nonetheless, if this or subsequent isolates should indeed prove to be human lymphoma-inducing viruses, we will be deeply indebted to research on experimental animal models of lymphoid neoplasia, not only for an essential body of factual information but also for the conceptual framework which has guided these human studies to the threshold of important new advances.

Acknowledgements

These studies were supported by research contract NO1-CP-43228 from the National Cancer Institute, National Institutes of Health, Department of Health, Education and Welfare, and by gifts to the Joseph Edward Luetje Memorial Fund for lymphoma research.

References

1. BALTIMORE, D. RNA-dependent DNA polymerase in virions of RNA tumor viruses. Nature 226:1209–1211, 1970.
2. BAXT, W., HEHLMANN, R., and SPIEGELMAN, S. Human leukaemic cells contain reverse transcriptase associated with a high molecular weight virus-related RNA. Nature New Biology 240(98):72–75, 1972.

3. CALLAHAN, R., LIEBER, M. M., TODARO, G. J., GRAVES, D. C., and FERRER, J. F. Bovine leukemia virus genes in the DNA of leukemic cattle. Science 192:1005–1007, 1976.
4. CHAN, E., PETERS, W. P., SWEET, R. W., OHNO, T., KUFE, D. W., SPIEGELMAN, S., GALLO, R. C., and GALLAGHER, R. E. Characterization of a virus (HL23V) isolated from cultured acute myelogenous leukaemic cells. Nature 260:266–268, 1976.
5. CHATTOPADHYAY, S. K., ROWE, W. P., TEICH, N. M., and LOWY, D. R. Definitive evidence that the murine C-type virus inducing locus AKv-1 is viral genetic material. Proc. Nat. Acad. Sci, USA 72:906–910, 1975.
6. CHEZZI, C., DETTORI, G., MANZARI, V., AGLIANO, A. M., and SANNA, A. Simultaneous detection of reverse transcriptase and high molecular weight RNA in tissue of patients with Hodgkin's disease and patients with leukemia. Proc. Nat. Acad. Sci. USA 73:4649–4652, 1976.
7. DECLÈVE, A. and KAPLAN, H. S. Genetic control of naturally occurring murine ecotropic C-type virus replication in vitro and in vivo: A concise review. In: Radiation-induced Leukemogenesis and Related Viruses, J. F. Duplan, ed., Amsterdam, North-Holland Publishing Co., 1977, pp. 197–212.
8. DECLÈVE, A., LIEBERMAN, M., IHLE, J. N., and KAPLAN, H. S. Biological and serological characterization of radiation leukemia virus. Proc. Nat. Acad. Sci. USA 73:4675–4679, 1976.
9. DECLÈVE, A., SATO, C., LIEBERMAN, M., and KAPLAN, H. S. Selective thymic localization of murine leukemia virus-related antigens in C57BL/Ka mice after inoculation with radiation leukemia virus. Proc. Nat. Acad. Sci. USA 71:3124–3128, 1974.
10. DECLÈVE, A., TRAVIS, M., WEISSMAN, I. L., LIEBERMAN, M., and KAPLAN, H. S. Focal infection and transformation in situ of thymus cell subclasses by a thymotropic murine leukemia virus. Cancer Res. 35: 3585–3595, 1975.
11. DUNN, T. B. Normal and pathologic anatomy of the reticular tissue in laboratory mice, with a classification and discussion of neoplasms. J. Nat. Cancer Inst. 14:1281–1433, 1954.
12. DUNN, T. B. and DERINGER, M. K. Reticulum cell neoplasm, type B, or the "Hodgkin's-like lesion" of the mouse. J. Nat. Cancer. Inst. 40:771–821, 1968.
13. EPSTEIN, A. L. and KAPLAN, H. S. Biology of the human malignant lymphomas. I. Establishment in continuous cell culture and heterotransplantation of diffuse histiocytic lymphomas. Cancer 34:1851–1872, 1974.
14. FERRER, J. F., STOCK, N. D., and LIN, P. Detection of replicating C-type viruses in continuous cell cultures established from cows with leukemia: effect of the culture medium. J. Nat. Cancer Inst. 47:613–621, 1971.
15. FRIEND, C. Cell-free transmission in adult Swiss mice of a disease having the character of a leukemia. J. Exp. Med. 105:307–318, 1957.
16. GALLAGHER, R. E. and GALLO, R. C. Type C RNA tumor virus isolated from cultured human acute myelogenous leukemia cells. Science 187:350–353, 1975.
17. GALLO, R. C., MILLER, N. R., SAXINGER, W. C., and GILLESPIE, D. Primate RNA tumor virus-like DNA synthesized endogenously by RNA-dependent DNA polymerase in virus-like particles from fresh human acute leukemic blood cells. Proc. Nat. Acad. Sci. USA 70(11):3219–3224, 1972.
18. GROSS, L. "Spontaneous" leukemia developing in C3H mice following inoculation, in infancy, with AK-leukemic extracts, or AK-embryos. Proc. Soc. Exp. Biol. Med. 76:27–32, 1951.
19. GROSS, L. Pathologic properties, and "vertical" transmission of the mouse leukemia agent. Proc. Soc. Exp. Biol. Med. 78:342–348, 1951.
20. HARAN-GHERA, N., LIEBERMAN, M., and KAPLAN, H. S. Direct action of a leukemogenic virus on the thymus. Cancer Res. 26:438–441, 1966.
21. HARTLEY, J. W., WOLFORD, N. K., OLD, L. J., and ROWE, W. P. A new class of murine leukemia virus associated with development of spontaneous lymphomas. Proc. Nat. Acad. Sci. USA 74:789–792, 1977.
22. HILGERS, J., DECLÈVE, A., GALESLOOT, J., and KAPLAN, H. S. Murine leukemia virus group-specific antigen expression in AKR mice. Cancer Res. 34:2553–2561, 1974.
23. HOPKINS, N., SCHINDLER, J., and GOTTLIEB, P. D. Evidence for recombination between N- and B-tropic murine leukemia viruses. J. Virol. 21:1074–1078, 1977.
24. JARRETT, W. F. H., CRAWFORD, E. M., MARTIN, W. B., and DAVIE, F. Leukemia in the cat. A virus-like particle associated with leukaemia (lymphosarcoma). Nature 202:567–569, 1964.
25. JARRETT, W., JARRETT, O., MACKEY, L., LAIRD, H., HARDY, W., JR., and ESSEX, M. Horizontal transmission of leukemia virus and leukemia in the cat. J. Nat. Cancer Inst. 51:833–841, 1973.
26. JOLICOEUR, P. and BALTIMORE, D. Effect of Fv-1 gene product on proviral DNA formation and integration in cells infected with murine leukemia viruses. Proc. Nat. Acad. Sci. USA 73:2236–2240, 1976.
27. KAPLAN, H. S. On the natural history of the murine leukemias: Presidential address. Cancer Res. 27:1325–1340, 1967.
28. KAPLAN, H. S. Leukemia and lymphoma in experimental and domestic animals. Ser. Haematol. 7:94–163, 1974.

29. KAPLAN, H. S. Biological approaches to human cancer virus detection. Prog. Exp. Tumor Res. 21:2–18 (1977).
30. KAPLAN, H. S. and BROWN, M. B. Development of lymphoid tumors in nonirradiated thymic grafts in thymectomized irradiated mice. Science 119:439–446, 1954.
31. KAPLAN, H. S., GOODENOW, R. S., EPSTEIN, A. L., GARTNER, S., DECLÈVE, A., and ROSENTHAL, P. N. Isolation of a C-type RNA virus from an established human histiocytic lymphoma cell line. Proc. Nat. Acad. Sci. USA, 1977, in press.
32. KAPLAN, H. S., HIRSCH, B. B., and BROWN, M. B. Indirect induction of lymphomas in irradiated mice. IV. Genetic evidence of the origin of the tumor cells from the thymic grafts. Cancer Res. 16:434–436, 1956.
33. KAWAKAMI, T. G. and SUN, L. Type-C virus induced leukemia in gibbon. Cold Spring Harbor RNA Tumor Virus Meeting, Cold Spring Harbor Laboratory, N.Y., 1977, p. 114 (abstract).
34. KAWAKAMI, T. G., THEILEN, G. H., DUNGWORTH, D. L., MUNN, R. J., and BEALL, S. G. "C"-type viral particles in plasma of cats with feline leukemia. Science 158:1049–1050, 1067.
35. KETTMANN, R., PORTETELLE, D., MAMMERICKX, M., CLEUTER, Y., DEKEGEL, D., GALOUX, M., GHYSDAEL, J., BURNY, A., and CHANTRENNE, H. Bovine leukemia virus: an exogenous RNA oncogenic virus. Proc. Nat. Acad. Sci. USA 73:1014–1018, 1076.
36. LEVY, J. A. Xenotropic viruses: murine leukemia viruses associated with NIH Swiss, NZB, and other mouse strains. Science 192:1151–1153, 1973.
37. LIEBERMAN, M., DECLÈVE, A., and KAPLAN, H. S. Rescue of RadLV from cultured, non-producer lymphoma cells of strain C57BL/Ka mice. Cold Spring Harbor RNA Tumor Virus Meeting, Cold Spring Harbor Laboratory, N.Y., 1977, p. 43 (abstract).
38. LIEBERMAN, M. and KAPLAN, H. S. Leukemogenic activity of filtrates from radiation-induced lymphoid tumors of mice. Science 130:387–388, 1959.
39. LIEBERMAN, M. and KAPLAN, H. S. Lymphoid tumor induction by mouse thymocytes infected in vitro with radiation leukemia virus. Nat. Cancer Inst. Monogr. 22:549–564, 1966.
40. LIEBERMAN, M. and KAPLAN, H. S. The role of lymphoid and haematopoietic target cells in viral lymphomagenesis of C57BL/Ka mice. I. Susceptibility to viral replication. Blood Cells 2:291–299, 1976.
41. LIEBERMAN, M. and KAPLAN, H. S. Vaccination against x-ray or radiation leukemia virus-induced thymic lymphoma development by inoculation of mice with syngeneic fibroblastic cells infected with an endogenous B-tropic nonleukemogenic virus. In: "Radiation-Induced Leukemogenesis and Related Viruses, ed., J. F. Duplan, North-Holland Pub., Amsterdam, 1977, pp. 127–132.
42. LIEBERMAN, M., KAPLAN, H. S., and DECLÈVE, A. Anomalous viral expression in radiogenic lymphomas of C57BL/Ka mice. In: The Biology of Radiation Carcinogenesis, eds., J. M. Yuhas, R. M. Tennant, and J. D. Regan, Raven Press Books, Ltd., New York, 1977, pp. 237–244.
43. LILLY, F. and PINCUS, T. Genetic control of murine viral leukemogenesis. In: "Advances in Cancer Research", eds., Klein, G. and Weinhouse, S., New York. Academic Press, Vol. 17, 1973, pp. 231–277.
44. NOOTER, K., AARSSEN, A. M., BENTVELZEN, P., DE GROOT, F. G., and VAN PELT, F. G. Isolation of infectious C-type oncornavirus from human leukaemic bone marrow cells. Nature 256:595–597, 1975.
45. OKABE, H., GILDEN, R. V., HATANAKA, M., STEPHENSON, J. R., GALLAGHER, R. E., GALLO, R. C., TRONICK, S. R., and AARONSON, S. A. Immunological and biochemical characterisation of type C viruses isolated from cultured human AML cells. Nature 260:264–266, 1976.
46. PANEM, S., PROCHOWNIK, E. V., REALE, F. R., and KIRSTEN, W. H. Isolation of type C virions from a normal human fibroblast strain. Science 189:297–298, 1975.
47. PETERS, R. L., SASS, B., STEPHENSON, J. R., AL-GHAZZOULI, I. K., HINO, S., DONAHOE, R. M., KENDE, M., AARONSON, S. A., and KELLOFF, G. J. Immunoprevention of x-ray-induced leukemias in the C57BL mouse. Proc. Nat. Acad. Sci. USA 74:1697–1701, 1977.
48. RASCHKE, W. C., RALPH, P., WATSON, J., SKLAR, M., and COON, H. Oncogenic transformation of murine lymphoid cells by in vitro infection with Abelson leukemia virus. J. Nat. Cancer Inst. 54:1249–1253, 1975.
49. RAUSCHER, F. J. A virus-induced disease of mice characterized by erythrocytopoiesis and lymphoid leukemia. J. Nat. Cancer Inst. 29:515–543, 1962.
50. ROWE, W. P. Genetic factors in the natural history of murine leukemia virus infection: G. H. A. Clowes memorial lecture. Cancer Res. 33:3061–3068, 1973.
51. ROWE, W. P. and PINCUS, T. Quantitative studies of naturally occurring murine leukemia virus infection of AKR mice. J. Exp. Med. 135:429–436, 1972.
52. STEEVES, R. A., ECKNER, R. J., BENNETT, M., MIRAND, E. A., and TRUDEL, P. J. Isolation and characterization of a lymphatic leukemia virus in the Friend virus complex. J. Nat. Cancer Inst. 46:1209–1217, 1971.
53. STRAND, M. and AUGUST, J. T. Structural proteins of oncogenic ribonucleic acid viruses. J. Biol. Chem. 248:5627–5633, 1973.

54. SVEDA, M. M. and SOEIRO, R. Host restriction of Friend leukemia virus: synthesis and integration of the provirus. Proc. Nat. Acad. Sci. USA 73:2356–2360, 1976.
55. TEICH, N. M., WEISS, R. A., SALAHUDDIN, S. Z., GALLAGHER, R. E., GILLESPIE, D. H., and GALLO, R. C. Infective transmission and characterisation of a C-type virus released by cultured human myeloid leukaemia cells. Nature 256:551–555, 1975.
56. TEMIN, H. M and BALTIMORE, D. RNA-directed DNA synthesis and RNA tumor viruses. Adv. Virus Res. 17:129–186, 1972.
57. TEMIN, H. M. and MIZUTANI, S. RNA-dependent DNA polymerase in virions of Rous sarcoma virus. Nature 226:1211–1213, 1970.
58. WITKIN, S. S., OHNO, T., and SPIEGELMAN, S. Purification of RNA-instructed DNA polymerase from human leukemic spleens. Proc. Nat. Acad. Sci. USA 72:4133–4136, 1975.

Recent Results in Cancer Research

Sponsored by the Swiss League against Cancer. Editor in Chief: P. Rentchnick, Genève

For information about Vols. 1—9, please contact your bookseller or Springer-Verlag.

10 Nelson, R. S.: Radioactive Phosphorus in the Diagnosis of Gastrointestinal Cancer.

11 Freeman, R. G. and J. M. Knox: Treatment of Skin Cancer.

12 Lynch, H. T.: Hereditary Factors in Carcinoma.

13 Tumours in Children, 2nd Edition. Edited by H. B. Marsden and J. K. Steward.

14 Odartchenko, N.: Production Cellulaire Erythropoïétique.

15 Sokoloff, B.: Carcinoid and Serotonin.

16 Jacobs, M. L.: Malignant Lymphomas and Their Management.

17 Normal and Malignant Cell Growth. Edited by R. J. M. Fry, M. L. Griem, and W. H. Kirsten (Symposium).

18 Anglesio, E.: The Treatment of Hodgkin's Disease.

19 Bannasch, P.: The Cytoplasm of Hepatocytes during Carcinogenesis. Electron- and Lightmicroscopical Investigations of the Nitrosomorpholine-intoxicated Rat Liver.

20 Rubidomycin. A new Agent against Cancer. Edited by J. Bernard, R. Paul, M. Boiron, C. Jacquillat, and R. Maral.

21 Scientific Basis of Cancer Chemotherapy. Edited by G. Mathé (Symposium).

22 Koldovský, P.: Tumor Specific Transplantation Antigen.

23 Fuchs, W. A., J. W. Davidson, and H. W. Fischer: Lymphography in Cancer. With contributions by G. Jantet and H. Rösler.

24 Hayward, J.: Hormones und Human Breast Cancer. An Account of 15 Years Study.

25 Roy-Burman, P.: Analogues of Nucleic Acid Components. Mechanisms of Action.

26 Tumors of the Liver. Edited by G. T. Pack and A. H. Islami.

27 Szymendera, J.: Bone Mineral Metabolism in Cancer.

28 Meek, E. S.: Antitumour and Antiviral Substances of Natural Origin.

29 Aseptic Environments and Cancer Treatment. Edited by G. Mathé (Symposium).

30 Advances in the Treatment of Acute (Blastic) Leukemias. Edited by G. Mathé (Symposium).

31 Denoix, P.: Treatment of Malignant Breast Tumors. Indications and Results.

32 Nelson, R. S.: Endoscopy in Gastric Cancer.

33 Experimental and Clinical Effects of L-Asparaginase. Edited by E. Grundmann and H. F. Oettgen (Symposium).

34 Chemistry and Biological Actions of 4-Nitroquinolin 1-Oxide. Edited by H. Endo, T. Ono, and T. Sugimura.

35 Penn, I.: Malignant Tumors in Organ Transplant Recipients.

36 Current Concepts in the Management of Lymphoma and Leukemia. Edited by J. E. Ultmann, M. L. Griem, W. H. Kirsten, and R. W. Wissler (Symposium).

37 Chiappa, S., R. Musumeci, and C. Uslenghi: Endolymphatic Radiotherapy in Malignant Lymphomas. With contributions by G. Bonadonna, B. Damascelli, G. Fava, F. Pizzetti, U. Veronesi.

38 Koller, P. C.: The Role of Chromosomes in Cancer Biology.

39 Current Problems in the Epidemiology of Cancer and Lymphomas. Edited by E. Grundmann and H. Tulinius (Symposium).

40 Langley, F. A. and A. C. Crompton: Epithelial Abnormalities of the Cervix Uteri.

41 Tumours in a Tropical Country. A Survey of Uganda (1964—1968). Edited by A. C. Templeton.

42 Breast Cancer: A Challenging Problem. Edited by M. L. Griem, E. V. Jensen, J. E. Ultmann, and R. W. Wissler (Symposium).

43 Nomenclature, Methodology and Results of Clinical Trials in Acute Leukemias. Edited by G. Mathé, P. Pouillart, L. Schwarzenberg (Symposium).

44 Special Topics in Carcinogenesis. Edited by E. Grundmann (Symposium).

45 Koldovský, P.: Carcinoembryonic Antigens.

46 Diagnosis and Therapy of Malignant Lymphoma. Edited by K. Musshoff (Symposium).

47 Investigation and Stimulation of Immunity in Cancer Patients. Edited by G. Mathé and R. Weiner (Symposium).

48 Platinum Coordination Complexes in Cancer Chemotherapy. Edited by T. A. Connors and J. J. Roberts (Symposium).

49 Complications of Cancer Chemotherapy. Edited by G. Mathé and R. K. Oldham (Symposium).

50 Cancer Registry. Edited by E. Grundmann and E. Pedersen (Symposium).

51 Gliomas. Current Concepts in Biology, Diagnosis and Therapy. Edited by J. Hekmatpanah (Symposium).

52 The Ambivalence of Cytostatic Therapy. Edited by E. Grundmann and R. Gross (Symposium).

53 A. Clarysse, Y. Kenis, and G. Mathé: Cancer Chemotherapy.

54 Malignant Bone Tumors. Edited by E. Grundmann.

55 Mathé, G.: Cancer Active Immunotherapy, Immunoprophylaxis, and Immunorestoration.

56 Lymphocytes, Macrophages, and Cancer. Edited by G. Mathé, I. Florentin, and M.-C. Simmler (Symposium).

57 Breast Cancer: A Multidisciplinary Approach. Edited by G. St. Arneault, P. Band, and L. Israël (Symposium).

58 B. S. Schoenberg: Multiple Primary Malignant Neoplasms.

59 Selective Heat Sensitivity of Cancer Cells. Edited by A. Rossi-Fanelli, R. Cavaliere, B. Mondovi, and G. Moricca.

60 Tumors of the Male Genital System. Edited by E. Grundmann and W. Vahlensieck (Symposium).

61 D. Metcalf: Hemopoietic Colonies.

62 Tactics and Strategy in Cancer Treatment. Edited by G. Mathé (Symposium).

63 Antitumor Antibiotics. Edited by S. K. Carter, H. Umezawa, J. Douros, and Y. Sakurai (Symposium).

64 Lymphoid Neoplasias I: Classification, Categorization, Natural History.

65 Lymphoid Neoplasias II: Clinical and Therapeutic Aspects.
Lymphoid Neoplasias I & II. Proceedings of the 1977 CNRS-EORTC International Colloquium. Editors: G. Mathé, M. Seligmann, M. Tubiana. Devided into two volumes.

MIX
Papier aus verantwortungsvollen Quellen
Paper from responsible sources
FSC® C105338

If you have any concerns about our products,
you can contact us on
ProductSafety@springernature.com

In case Publisher is established outside the EU,
the EU authorized representative is:
Springer Nature Customer Service Center GmbH
Europaplatz 3, 69115 Heidelberg, Germany

Printed by Libri Plureos GmbH
in Hamburg, Germany